ELEVENTH EDITION

McKenzie's An Introduction to
Community & Public Health

Denise M. Seabert, PhD, MCHES
Professor Emeritus
Ball State University, Muncie, IN

James F. McKenzie, PhD, MPH, RMCHES, FAAHE
Professor Emeritus
Ball State University, Muncie, IN

Robert R. Pinger, PhD
Professor Emeritus
Ball State University, Muncie, IN

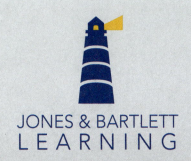

JONES & BARTLETT
LEARNING

World Headquarters
Jones & Bartlett Learning
25 Mall Road
Burlington, MA 01803
978-443-5000
info@jblearning.com
www.jblearning.com

Jones & Bartlett Learning books and products are available through most bookstores and online booksellers. To contact Jones & Bartlett Learning directly, call 800-832-0034, fax 978-443-8000, or visit our website, www.jblearning.com.

Substantial discounts on bulk quantities of Jones & Bartlett Learning publications are available to corporations, professional associations, and other qualified organizations. For details and specific discount information, contact the special sales department at Jones & Bartlett Learning via the above contact information or send an email to specialsales@jblearning.com.

30390-2

Production Credits

Senior Director, Content Production and Delivery: Christine Emerton
Director, Product Management: Melissa Kleeman Moy
Acquisition Editor: Sophie Teague
Content Manager: Bill Lawrensen
Content Manager: Jessica Covert
Content Coordinator: Samantha Gillespie
Manager, Intellectual Properties: Kristen Rogers
Content Production Manager: Erin Bosco
Intellectual Property Specialist: Carolyn Downer
Senior Product Marketing Manager: Susanne Walker

Procurement Manager: Wendy Kilborn
Composition: Exela Technologies
Project Management: Exela Technologies
Cover/Text Design: MPS
Intellectual Property Specialist: Faith Brosnan
Intellectual Property Specialist: Lisa Passmore
Cover Image (Title Page, Part Opener, Chapter Opener):
 © Art-Y/Getty Images
Printing and Binding: Lakeside Book Company

Library of Congress Cataloging-in-Publication Data
Library of Congress Cataloging-in-Publication Data unavailable at time of printing.

LCCN: 2024054308

6048

Printed in the United States of America
28 27 26 25   10 9 8 7 6 5 4 3 2 1

BRIEF CONTENTS

CONTENTS

How to Use This Book

Chapter Objectives

The chapter objectives identify the knowledge and competencies that students need to master as they read and study the chapter material, answer the end-of-chapter review questions, and complete the activities. To use the objectives effectively, students should review them before and after reading the chapters. This will help students focus on the major knowledge points in each chapter and facilitate answering the questions and completing the activities at the end of each chapter.

Chapter Objectives

After studying this chapter, you will be able to:

1. Define the terms *health, community, community health, population health, public health, public health system, global health,* and *social determinants of health.*
2. Briefly describe the social determinants of health.
3. Explain the difference between personal and community health activities.
4. List and discuss the factors that influence a community's health.
5. Briefly relate the history of community and public health, including the recent U.S. history of community and public health in the twentieth and early twenty-first centuries.
6. Provide a brief overview of the current health status of Americans.
7. Describe the purpose of the *Healthy People 2030* goals and objectives as they apply to the planning process of the health of Americans.
8. Summarize the major community and public health problems facing the United States and the world today.

Scenarios

Short scenarios are presented at the beginning of each chapter. The purpose of these scenarios is to bridge the gap between your students' personal experiences and ideas discussed within the chapter. The chapter content will enable your students to propose solutions to the community or public health problem posed in the scenario.

Scenario

Amy and Eric are a young working couple who are easing into a comfortable lifestyle. They have good-paying jobs, drive nice cars, have two healthy preschool children, and, after living in an apartment for several years, are now buying a home in a good neighborhood. When Amy picked her children up from daycare earlier in the day, she was told that another parent had reported that his child was diagnosed with RSV (respiratory syncytial virus). This news frightened Amy and made her begin to question the quality of the daycare center. Amy told Eric of this situation when he got home. As the couple discussed whether or not they should take their children to daycare as usual the following day, they discovered that they had many unanswered questions. How serious is RSV? What is the likelihood that their children will be at serious risk for getting the disease? What steps are being taken to control the outbreak? Is any state or local agency responsible for standardizing health practices at private daycare centers in the community? Does the city, county, or state carry out any type of inspection when they license these facilities? And, if the children do not attend daycare, which parent will stay home with them?

Introduction

Each chapter begins with a brief introduction that informs the reader of the topics to be presented and explains how these topics relate to others in the book.

Introduction

Since 1900, tremendous progress had been made in the health and life expectancy of people who live in the United States (see **Box 1.1**) and elsewhere in the world. Infant mortality has dropped, many infectious diseases have been brought under control, and better family planning has become available. However, much still needs to be done to improve health, especially when it comes to health disparities found among certain ethnic and racial groups. Individual health behaviors, such as the use of tobacco, poor diet, and physical inactivity, have given rise to an unacceptable number of cases of illness and death from noninfectious diseases, such as cancer, diabetes, and heart disease. Continued use of an outdated infrastructure, such as the old water pipes in Flint, Michigan, has exposed many people to unnecessary health risks. New, emerging infectious diseases (i.e., COVID-19), and diseases caused by "superbugs" (i.e., drug-resistant pathogens), have stretched resources available to control them. In addition, events stemming from natural disasters such as floods, tornadoes, and hurricanes; human-made disasters, such as the Gulf oil spill; and terrorism, such as the 2018 attack on a Pittsburgh synagogue have

Marginal Definitions

Understanding the key terms helps drive stronger comprehension of the core knowledge and competencies contained within the chapter. These terms are presented in **boldface** type in the text and defined in the margin. Before reading each chapter, we suggest that students review the chapter's key terms in preparation for encountering them in the text. The boldfaced terms also appear in the glossary at the end of the book.

Health is a dynamic state or condition of the human organism that is multidimensional in nature, a resource for living, and results from a person's interactions with and adaptations to their environment; therefore, it can exist in varying degrees and is specific to each individual and their situation

Chapter Summary

At the end of each chapter are several bulleted points that review the major concepts contained in each chapter. These provide a great way to review knowledge and comprehension of the material.

Chapter Summary

- A number of key terms are associated with the study of community and public health, including *health, community, community health, population health, public health, public health system, global health,* and *social determinants of health.*
- The four factors that affect the health of a community are physical (e.g., community size), social and cultural (e.g., religion), community organization, and individual behaviors (e.g., exercise and diet).
- It is important to be familiar with and understand the history of community health to be able to deal with the present and future community and public health issues.
- The earliest community and public health practices went unrecorded; however, archeological findings of ancient societies (before 500 BCE) show evidence of concern for community and public health. There is evidence during the time of the classical cultures (500 BCE–500 CE) that people were interested in physical strength, medicine, and sanitation.
- The belief of many living during the Middle Ages (500–1500 CE) was that health and disease were associated with spirituality. Many epidemics were seen during this period.
- During the Renaissance period (1500–1700 CE), there was a growing belief that disease was caused by the environment, not spiritual factors.
- The eighteenth century was characterized by industrial growth. Science was being used more in medicine, and
- it was during this century that the first vaccine was discovered.
- The nineteenth century ushered in the modern era of public health. Germ theory was introduced during this time, and the last quarter of the century is known as the bacteriological period of public health.
- The twentieth century can be divided into several periods. The health resources development period (1900–1960) was a time when many public and private resources were used to improve health. The period of social engineering (1960–1973) saw the U.S. government's involvement in health insurance through Medicare and Medicaid. The health promotion period began in 1974 and continues today.
- *Healthy People 2030* and the National Prevention Strategy are important components of the community and public health agenda in the United States.
- Great concern continues to exist in the United States regarding health care, the environment, diseases caused by an impoverished lifestyle, the spread of communicable diseases, the harm caused by alcohol and other substance use, and terrorism.
- Although the health of the world population is improving, communicable diseases, poor sanitation and unsafe drinking water, hunger, and migration are burdens for many and impact the people who live in poverty much more than those who do not.

Scenario: Analysis and Response

Following the chapter summary, students are provided with an opportunity to respond to the scenario presented earlier in the chapter. The content presented in the chapter will help students to formulate their responses or solutions.

Scenario: Analysis and Response

The Internet offers many sources of information that could help Amy and Eric with the decisions that they will have to make about the continued use of the daycare center for their children. Use a search engine (e.g., Google, Bing) and enter (a) RSV and (b) RSV and daycare centers. Print out the information that you find and use it in answering the following questions.

1. Based on the information you found on the Internet, if you were Amy or Eric, would you take your children to the daycare center the next day? Why or why not?

Review Questions

Review questions at the end of each chapter provide students with feedback regarding their mastery of the chapter's content. The questions reinforce the chapter objectives and key terms.

Activities

The activities at the end of each chapter provide an opportunity for students to apply new knowledge in a meaningful way. The activities, which are presented in a variety of formats, should appeal to the varying learning styles of students.

Learning and Teaching Tools

Instructor Resources

Qualified Instructors will receive a full suite of Instructor resources, including the following:

- Instructor Manual
- Slides in PowerPoint Format
- Test bank
- Web Links – Provides links to websites and articles related to content in the chapter
- Image Bank – Provides figures from the text in slide format

Student Resources

With the Navigate Advantage, students can reinforce comprehension of the course material.

- The Navigate eBook includes:
  - Chapter Review Slides
  - Flashcards
  - Image Bank

We Value Your Feedback

Do you love this text? Spot an error you'd like to report? Follow this QR code to give us your observations and suggestions for improvement.

ACKNOWLEDGMENTS

A project of this nature could not be completed without the assistance, expertise, and support of many individuals.

Special Thank You

A special thank you goes to James F. McKenzie, PhD, professor emeritus, and Robert R. Pinger, PhD, professor emeritus, Department of Nutrition and Health Science, Ball State University, for envisioning this valuable resource and making it available to teachers and learners for more than three decades—and for entrusting to me the future of this text. I am grateful for their vision, support, and mentorship.

Thank you to my boys for their love, support, and patience. In addition, gratitude goes to Clark Bailey for his editing and research skills as well as his contributions to revising the ancillaries.

Contributors

I would like to express my deepest gratitude to the following individuals, who have brought their expertise to the writing team:

Chapter 3 Epidemiology: The Study of Disease, Injury, and Death in the Community

Salma Haidar, MPH, PhD
Professor and Director of Division of Public Health
School of Health Sciences
Central Michigan University

Sameer Shepich, MPH student
School of Health Sciences
Central Michigan University

Chapter 4 Communicable and Noncommunicable Diseases: Prevention and Control of Diseases and Health Conditions

Kristina Jackson Behan, PhD, MLS (ASCP)
Professor Emeritus
Department of Medical Laboratory Sciences
University of West Florida

Chapter 5 Community Organizing/Building and Heath Promotion

Chapter 12 Alcohol, Tobacco, and Other Drugs: A Community Concern

Patricia Barrington, EdD, MCHES®
Department of Movement Sciences and Health
University of West Florida

Chapter 9 Older Adults

Amy Dunckel, MPT, DPT, GCS
Adjunct Faculty
Department of Health Sciences and Administration
University of West Florida

Chapter 10 Populations with Health Disparities in Community and Public Health

Ainna Flaminia, MPH, RN
Training and Prevention Specialist, Chicago Public Schools
Communications Director, Asian and Pacific Islander Caucus for Public Health, American Public Health Association

Chapter 11 Community Mental Health

Stephanie C. Bell, PhD, LPC, NCC, ACC
Associate Professor, School of Counseling
Marymount University

Mirian A. Campos, EdD, LPC
Assistant Professor, School of Counseling
Marymount University

Chapter 13 Healthcare Delivery in the United States

Tanisha Garcia, PhD, MHA
Associate Professor
Department of Public Health
California State University, Fresno

Chapter 14 Community and Public Health and the Environment

Jamie H. Wright, MHS, MS, CHMM
Emergency Management Hazards Analyst
Consolidated Nuclear Security, LLC

Chapter 15 Injuries as a Community and Public Health Problem

Katherine Greene, MPH
Adjunct Instructor
Department of Health Sciences and Administration
University of West Florida

Their expertise is both welcomed and appreciated.

Reviewers

We would like to express our appreciation to those professionals who took the time and effort to review and provide feedback on previous editions. Reviewers of the *Eleventh* and previous editions include:

- Teresa Drake, PhD, RD, CHES, Bradley University
- Marianne Jankowski, DHSC, MBA, MSPH, RRT

- Brent M. Peterson, PhD, MS, MPH
- Chad Rittle, DNP MPH, RN, FAAOHN
- Hans Schmalzried, PhD, Bowling Green State University
- Eric Sweeney, MEd, PhD, Baldwin Wallace University

Jones & Bartlett Learning Team

We would like to thank all of the employees of Jones & Bartlett Learning. Their hard work, support, guidance, and confidence in us have been most helpful in creating this and all previous editions of this text. Specifically, we would like to thank: Whitney Fekete, Product Manager; Jessica Covert, Content Manager; Erin Bosco, Content Production Manager; Lisa Passmore, Intellectual Property Specialist; Faith Brosnan, Intellectual Property Specialist; and Susanne Walker, Senior Product Marketing Manager.

Foundations of Community and Public Health

CHAPTER 1

Community and Public Health: Yesterday, Today, and Tomorrow

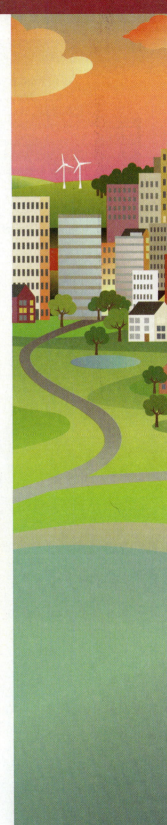

Chapter Objectives

After studying this chapter, you will be able to:

1. Define the terms *health, community, community health, population health, public health, public health system, global health,* and *social determinants of health.*
2. Briefly describe the social determinants of health.
3. Explain the difference between personal and community health activities.
4. List and discuss the factors that influence a community's health.
5. Briefly relate the history of community and public health, including the recent U.S. history of community and public health in the twentieth and early twenty-first centuries.
6. Provide a brief overview of the current health status of Americans.
7. Describe the purpose of the *Healthy People 2030* goals and objectives as they apply to the planning process of the health of Americans.
8. Summarize the major community and public health problems facing the United States and the world today.

Scenario

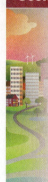

Amy and Eric are a young working couple who are easing into a comfortable lifestyle. They have good-paying jobs, drive nice cars, have two healthy preschool children, and, after living in an apartment for several years, are now buying a home in a good neighborhood. When Amy picked her children up from daycare earlier in the day, she was told that another parent had reported that his child was diagnosed with RSV (respiratory syncytial virus). This news frightened Amy and made her begin to question the quality of the daycare center. Amy told Eric of this situation when he got home. As the couple discussed whether or not they should take their children to daycare as usual the following day, they discovered that they had many unanswered questions. How serious is RSV? What is the likelihood that their children will be at serious risk for getting the disease? What steps are being taken to control the outbreak? Is any state or local agency responsible for standardizing health practices at private daycare centers in the community? Does the city, county, or state carry out any type of inspection when they license these facilities? And, if the children do not attend daycare, which parent will stay home with them?

Introduction

Since 1900, tremendous progress had been made in the health and life expectancy of people who live in the United States (see **Box 1.1**) and elsewhere in the world. Infant mortality has dropped, many infectious diseases have been brought under control, and better family planning has become available. However, much still needs to be done to improve health, especially when it comes to health disparities found among certain ethnic and racial groups. Individual health behaviors, such as the use of tobacco, poor diet, and physical inactivity, have given rise to an unacceptable number of cases of illness and death from noninfectious diseases, such as cancer, diabetes, and heart disease. Continued use of an outdated infrastructure, such as the old water pipes in Flint, Michigan, has exposed many people to unnecessary health risks. New, emerging infectious diseases (i.e., COVID-19) and diseases caused by "superbugs" (i.e., drug-resistant pathogens), have stretched resources available to control them. In addition, events stemming from natural disasters such as floods, tornadoes, and hurricanes; human-made disasters, such as the Gulf oil spill; and terrorism, such as the 2018 attack on a Pittsburgh synagogue have caused us to refocus our priorities. These events have severely disrupted Americans' sense of security and sense of safety in the environment.[1] In addition, many of these events revealed the vulnerability of the United States and the world in their ability to respond to such circumstances and highlighted the need for improvement in emergency response preparedness and the infrastructure of the public health system.

Despite all that has happened in recent years in the United States and around the world, the achievement of good health remains a worldwide goal of the twenty-first century. Governments, private organizations, and individuals throughout the world are working to improve health. Although individual actions to improve one's own personal health certainly contribute to the overall health of the community, organized community actions are often necessary when health problems exceed the resources of any one individual. When such actions are not taken, the health of the entire community is at risk.

This chapter introduces the concepts and principles of community and public health, explains how community and public health differ from personal health, and provides a brief history of community and public health. Some of the key health problems facing Americans are also described, and an outlook for the twenty-first century is provided.

Definitions

The word *health* means different things to different people. Similarly, there are other words that can be defined in various ways. Some basic terms we will use in this book are defined in the following paragraphs.

BOX 1.1   Ten Great Public Health Achievements—United States, 1900–1999 and 2001–2010

As the twentieth century came to a close, the overall health status and life expectancy in the United States were at all-time highs. Between 1900 and 2000, life expectancy at birth of U.S. residents increased by 62% from 47.3 years to 76.8 years[2]; 25 of these years have been attributed to advances in public health.[3] Currently, U.S. life expectancy is 77.5 years.[3] Many public health achievements can be linked to this gain in life expectancy. The Centers for Disease Control and Prevention (CDC), the U.S. government agency charged with protecting the public health of the nation, singled out "ten great public health achievements" in the United States between 1900 and 1999. Here is the list[4]:

1. Vaccination
2. Motor vehicle safety
3. Safer workplaces
4. Control of infectious diseases
5. Decline of deaths from coronary heart disease and stroke
6. Safer and healthier foods
7. Healthier mothers and babies
8. Family planning
9. Fluoridation of drinking water
10. Recognition of tobacco use as a health hazard

At the conclusion of 2010, public health scientists at the CDC were asked to nominate noteworthy public health achievements that occurred in the United States from 2001 to 2010. Below, in no specific order, are the ones selected from the nominations.[5]

- *Vaccine-preventable deaths*. Over the 10-year period, there was a substantial decline in cases, hospitalizations, deaths, and healthcare costs associated with vaccine-preventable diseases.
- *Prevention and control of infectious diseases*. Improvements in public health infrastructure, along with innovative and targeted prevention efforts, yielded significant progress in controlling infectious diseases (e.g., tuberculosis cases).

- *Tobacco control*. Tobacco still remains the single largest preventable cause of death and disease in the United States; adult smoking prevalence dropped to 11.5% in 2021[6] and 28 states have comprehensive smoke-free laws.[7]
- *Maternal and infant health*. During the 10-year period, there were significant reductions in the number of infants born with neural tube defects and an expansion of screening of newborns for metabolic and other heritable disorders.
- *Motor vehicle safety*. There were significant reductions in motor vehicle deaths and injuries, as well as pedestrian and bicyclist deaths. These reductions are attributed to safer vehicles, roads, and safer road use.
- *Cardiovascular disease prevention*. Death rates for both stroke and coronary heart disease continue to trend down. Most can be attributed to reduction in the prevalence of risk factors and improved treatments, medications, and quality of care.
- *Occupational safety*. Much progress was made in improving working conditions and reducing the risk for workplace-associated injuries over the 10-year period.
- *Cancer prevention*. A number of death rates due to various cancers dropped during the 10 years and much of the progress can be attributed to the implementation of the evidence-based screening recommendations.
- *Childhood lead poisoning prevention*. There was a steep decline in the percentage of children ages 1 to 5 years with blood levels ≥10 mcg/dL. Much of the progress can be traced to the 23 states in 2010 that had comprehensive lead poisoning prevention laws. As of 2021, experts use a reference level of 3.5 mcg/dL to identify children with high blood lead levels.[8]
- *Public health preparedness and response*. Following the terrorists' attacks of 2001 on the United States, great effort was put into both expanding and improving the capacity of the public health system to respond to public health threats.

Data from Centers for Disease Control and Prevention. (1999). "Ten Great Public Health Achievements—United States, 1900–1999." *Morbidity and Mortality Weekly Report*, 48(12): 241–243; and U.S. Department of Health and Human Services, Centers for Disease Control and Prevention (2011). "Ten Great Public Health Achievements – United States, 2001–2010." *Morbidity and Mortality Weekly Report*, 60(19): 619–623.

Health

The word *health* is derived from *hal*, which means "hale, sound, whole." When it comes to the health of people, the word health has been defined in a number of different ways—often in its social context, as when a parent describes the health of a child or when an avid fan defines the health of a professional athlete. The most widely quoted definition of health was the one created by the World Health Organization (WHO) in 1946, which states "health is a state of complete physical, mental, and social well-being and not merely the absence of disease and infirmity."[9] Furthermore, the WHO has indicated that health is a resource for living each day better, not the reason for living and includes social and personal resources, as well as physical capabilities.[10] Others have stated that health cannot be defined as a state because it is ever changing. Therefore, we have chosen to define **health** as a dynamic state or condition of the

Health is a dynamic state or condition of the human organism that is multidimensional in nature, a resource for living, and results from a person's interactions with and adaptations to their environment; therefore, it can exist in varying degrees and is specific to each individual and their situation

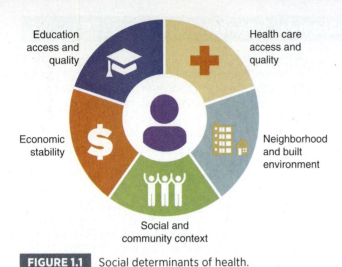

FIGURE 1.1 Social determinants of health.

Reproduced from Healthy People 2030, U.S. Department of Health and Human Services, Office of Disease Prevention and Health Promotion. Retrieved July 12, 2024, from https://health.gov/healthypeople/objectives-and-data/social-determinants-health

human organism that is multidimensional (i.e., physical, emotional, social, intellectual, spiritual, and occupational) in nature, a resource for living, and results from a person's interactions with and adaptations to their environment. Therefore, health can exist in varying degrees and is specific to each individual and their situation. A person can have a disease or injury and still be healthy. For example, a person with Type I Diabetes can manage their disease, feel well, and be in good health.

A person's health status is dynamic in part because of the many factors that determine one's health. The factors we study in public and community health are referred to as the **social determinants of health**. "Social determinants of health (SDOH) are the nonmedical factors that influence health outcomes. They are the conditions in which people are born, grow, work, live, and age, and the wider set of forces and systems shaping the conditions of daily life."[11] SDOH can be grouped into five domains: education access and quality, health care access and quality, neighborhood and built environment, social and community context, and economic stability.[11] Thus, the health fate of each of us is determined by the interconnectedness of these domains (see **Figure 1.1**). For example, unemployment could cause food and housing insecurity, and from there, individuals could experience additional impacts on their health. Furthermore, our social circumstances often impact the health care we receive. By addressing differences in the SDOH, we are working to ensure that every person has the opportunity to attain their highest level of health.[11]

Community

Traditionally, a community has been thought of as a geographic area with specific boundaries—for example, a neighborhood, city, county, or state. However, in the context of community and public health, a **community** is "a collective body of individuals identified by common characteristics such as geography, interests, experiences, concerns, values, race, ethnicity, or culture."[12] Communities are characterized by the following elements: (1) membership—a sense of identity and belonging; (2) common symbol systems—similar language, rituals, and ceremonies; (3) shared values and norms; (4) mutual influence—community members have influence and are influenced by each other; (5) shared needs and commitment to meeting them; and (6) shared emotional connection—members share common history, experiences, and mutual support.[13] Examples of communities include the people of the city of Columbus (location), the Asian community of San Francisco (race), the Hispanic community of Miami (ethnicity), seniors in the church (age), the business or the banking communities (occupation), the unhoused of Portland, OR (specific problem), those on welfare in Ohio (particular outcome), local union members (common bond), or those who are members of an electronic social network (cyber). A community may be as small as the group of people who live on a residence hall floor at a university or as large as all the individuals who make up a nation. A healthy community is one where people provide leadership in assessing their own resources and needs and continuously create and improve its physical and social environments, where public health and social infrastructure and policies support health, where essential public health services are available and accessible, and where people support one another in aspects of daily life to develop to their fullest potential.[14,15]

Public, Community, Population, and Global Health

Prior to defining the four terms *public health*, *community health*, *population health*, and *global health*, it is important to understand that the terms are often used interchangeably by both laypeople and professionals who work in the various health fields. When the terms are used

Social determinants of health are the nonmedical factors that influence health outcomes. They are the conditions in which people are born, grow, work, live, and age, and the wider set of forces and systems shaping the conditions of daily life

Community a collective body of individuals identified by common characteristics such as geography, interests, experiences, concerns, values, race, ethnicity, or culture

interchangeably, most people are referring to the collective health of those in society and the actions or activities taken to obtain and maintain that health. The definitions provided here for the four terms more precisely define the group of people in question and the origin of the actions or activities.

Of the four terms, public health is the most inclusive. The Institute of Medicine (IOM) defined **public health** in 1988 in its landmark report *The Future of Public Health* as "what we as a society do collectively to assure the conditions in which people can be healthy."[16] The **public health system**, which has been defined as "activities undertaken within the formal structure of government and the associated efforts of private and voluntary organizations and individuals,"[16] is the organizational mechanism for providing such conditions. Even with these formal definitions, some still see public health activities as only those efforts that originate in federal, state, and local governmental public health agencies such as the CDC and local (i.e., city and county) health departments.

Community health refers to the health status of a defined group of people and the actions and conditions to promote, protect, and preserve their health. For example, the health status of the people of Elizabethtown, PA, and the private and public actions taken to promote, protect, and preserve the health of these people would constitute community health.

The term *population health* is similar to community health. Although the term has been around for a number of years, it is appearing more commonly in the literature today. As such, it has been defined in several different ways. The most common definition used for **population health** is "the health outcomes of a group of individuals, including the distribution of such outcomes within the group."[17]

Another term that has been used increasingly in recent years is *global health*. **Global health** is "a term that describes a health problems, issues, and concerns that transcend national boundaries and places priority on improving health and achieving equity for all people worldwide through cooperative actions and solutions."[18] COVID-19 can be viewed as a global health issue. Much of the rise in concern about global health problems comes from the speed of international travel and how easy it is for people who may be infected with a disease to cross borders into another country.

Public health actions that society takes collectively to ensure that the conditions in which people can be healthy

Public health system the organizational mechanism of those activities undertaken within the formal structure of government and the associated efforts of private and voluntary organizations and individuals

Community health the health status of a defined group of people and the actions and conditions to promote, protect, and preserve their health

Population health "the health outcomes of a group of individuals, including the distribution of such outcomes within the group"[17]

Global health places priority on improving health and achieving health equity for all people worldwide and describes health problems, issues, and concerns that transcend national boundaries, may be influenced by circumstances or experiences in other countries, and are best addressed by cooperative actions and solutions

Personal Health Activities vs. Community and Public Health Activities

To further clarify the definitions presented in this chapter, it is important to distinguish between the terms *personal health activities* and *community and public health activities*.

Personal Health Activities

Personal health activities are individual actions and decision making that affect the health of an individual or their immediate family members or friends. These activities may be preventive or curative in nature but seldom directly affect the behavior of others. Choosing to eat wisely, to regularly wear a safety belt, and to visit the physician are all examples of personal health activities.

Community and Public Health Activities

Community and public health activities are activities that are aimed at protecting or improving the health of a population or community. Implementing childhood and adult vaccination programs, exploring the causes of injuries and how best to prevent them, and testing biological and environmental samples are examples of community health activities.

Factors That Affect the Health of a Community

Many factors affect the health of a community. As a result, the health status of each community is different. These factors may be physical, social, and/or cultural. They also include the ability of the community to organize and work together as a whole as well as the individual behaviors of those in the community (see **Figure 1.2**).

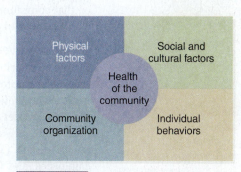

FIGURE 1.2 Factors that affect the health of the community.

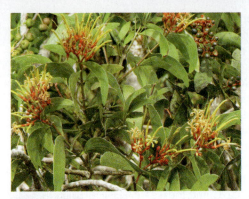

FIGURE 1.3   In tropical countries, parasitic and infectious diseases are leading community health problems.

© Guentermanaus/Shutterstock

Physical Factors

Physical factors include the influences of geography, the environment, community size, and industrial development.

Geography

A community's health problems can be directly influenced by its altitude, latitude, and climate. In tropical countries where warm, humid temperatures and rain prevail throughout the year, parasitic and infectious diseases are a leading community health problem (see **Figure 1.3**). In many tropical countries, survival from these diseases is made more difficult because poor soil conditions result in inadequate food production and malnutrition. In temperate climates with fewer parasitic and infectious diseases and a more than adequate food supply, obesity and heart disease are important community and public health problems.

Environment

The quality of our natural environment is directly related to the quality of our stewardship of it. Many experts believe that if we continue to allow uncontrolled population growth and continue to deplete nonrenewable natural resources, succeeding generations will inhabit communities that are less desirable than ours. Many feel that we must accept responsibility for this stewardship and drastically reduce the rate at which we foul the soil, water, and air.

When speaking about the environment, we must also consider the impact the built environment has on community and public health. The term **built environment** refers to "the design, construction, management, and land use of human-made surroundings as an interrelated whole, as well as their relationship to human activities over time."[19] It includes but is not limited to: transportation systems (e.g., mass transit); urban design features (e.g., bike paths, sidewalks, adequate lighting); parks and recreational facilities; land use (e.g., community gardens, location of schools, trail development); building with health-enhancing features (e.g., green roofs, stairs); road systems; and housing free from environmental hazards.[19-21] The built environment can be structured to give people more or fewer opportunities to behave in health-enhancing ways.

Community Size

The larger the community, the greater its range of health problems and the greater its number of health resources. For example, larger communities have more health professionals and better health facilities than smaller communities. These resources are often needed because communicable diseases can spread more quickly and environmental problems are often more severe in densely populated areas. For example, the amount of trash generated by the approximately 8.5 million people in New York City is many times greater than that generated by the entire state of Wyoming, with its population of 578,803.

It is important to note that a community's size can have both a positive and negative impact on that community's health. The ability of a community to effectively plan, organize, and use its resources can determine whether its size can be used to good advantage.

Industrial Development

Industrial development, like size, can have either positive or negative effects on the health status of a community. Industrial development provides a community with added resources for community health programs, but it may bring with it environmental pollution and occupational injuries and illnesses. Communities that experience rapid industrial development must eventually regulate (e.g., laws and ordinances) the way in which industries (1) obtain raw materials, (2) discharge by-products, (3) dispose of wastes, (4) treat and protect their employees, and (5) clean up environmental accidents. Unfortunately, many of these laws are usually passed only after these communities have suffered significant reductions in the quality of their life and health.

Built environment "the design, construction, management, and land use of human-made surroundings as an interrelated whole, as well as their relationship to human activities over time"[19]

Social and Cultural Factors

Social factors are those that arise from the interaction of individuals or groups within the community. For example, people who live in urban communities, where life is fast paced, experience higher rates of stress-related illnesses than those who live in rural communities, where life is more leisurely. On the other hand, those in rural areas may not have access to the same quality or selection of health care (i.e., hospitals or medical specialists) that is available to those who live in urban communities.

Cultural factors arise from guidelines (both explicit and implicit) that individuals "inherit" from being a part of a particular society. Some of the factors that contribute to culture are discussed in the following sections.

Beliefs, Traditions, and Prejudices

The beliefs, traditions, and prejudices of community members can affect the health of the community. The beliefs of those in a community about such specific health behaviors as exercise and smoking can influence policymakers on whether they will spend money on bike lanes on the roads and recreational bike trails and work toward smoke-free policies. The traditions of specific ethnic groups can influence the types of food, restaurants, retail outlets, and services available in a community. Prejudices of one specific ethnic or racial group against another can result in acts of violence and crime. Racial and ethnic disparities will continue to put certain groups, such as Blacks or certain religious groups, at greater risk.

Economy

Both national and local economies can affect the health of a community through reductions in health and social services. An economic downturn means lower tax revenues (fewer tax dollars) and fewer contributions to charitable groups. Such actions will result in fewer dollars being available for programs such as food and housing assistance, community health care, and other community services. This occurs because revenue shortfalls cause agencies to undergo budget cuts. With fewer dollars available, these agencies often alter their eligibility guidelines, thereby restricting aid to just individuals with the greatest need. In this situation, many people who had been eligible for assistance before the economic downturn become ineligible.

As their income drops, employers usually find it increasingly difficult to provide health benefits for their employees. Those who are unemployed and underemployed face poverty and deteriorating health. Thus, the cumulative effect of an economic downturn significantly affects the health of the community.

Politics

Politicians and government workers can improve or jeopardize the health of their community by the decisions (i.e., laws and ordinances) they make. In the most general terms, the argument is over greater or lesser governmental participation in health issues. For example, there has been a long-standing discussion in the United States regarding the extent to which the government should involve itself in health care. Historically, Democrats have been in favor of such action while Republicans have been against it. State and local politicians also influence the health of their communities each time they vote on health-related measures brought before them, such as increasing the minimum legal sales age for tobacco products to 21 years.

Religion

A number of religions have taken a position on health care and health behaviors. For example, some religious communities limit the type of medical treatment their members may receive. Some do not permit immunizations; others do not permit their members to be treated by physicians. Others prohibit certain foods. For example, kosher dietary regulations permit Jews to eat only the meat of animals that chew cud and have cloven hooves and the flesh of fish that have both fins and scales. Still others, like the Native American Church of the Morning Star, use peyote, a hallucinogen, as a sacrament.

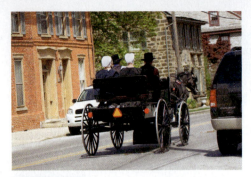

FIGURE 1.4 Religion can affect a community's health either positively or negatively.

© James F. McKenzie

Some religious communities actively address moral and ethical issues such as abortion, premarital intercourse, and homosexuality. Still other religions teach health-promoting codes of living to their members. For these reasons, religion can affect a community's health positively or negatively (see **Figure 1.4**).

Social Norms

The influence of social norms on community and public health can be positive or negative and can change over time. Cigarette smoking is a good example. During the 1940s, 1950s, and 1960s, it was socially acceptable to smoke in most settings. As a matter of fact, in 1965, 51.2% of American men and 33.7% of American women smoked. Thus, in 1965, it was socially acceptable to be a smoker, especially if you were male. Now, in the third decade of the twenty-first century, those percentages have dropped to 13.1% of males and 10.1% of females[6] and in most public places, it has become socially unacceptable to smoke. The lawsuits against tobacco companies by both the state attorneys general and private citizens provide further evidence that smoking has fallen from social acceptability. Because of this change in the social norm, there is less secondhand smoke in public places, and in turn, the health of the community has improved.

Unlike smoking, alcohol consumption represents a continuing negative social norm in America, especially on college campuses. The normal expectation seems to be that drinking is fun (and almost everyone wants to have fun). Despite the fact that most college students are too young to drink legally, approximately 65.9% of college students drink.[22] In past surveys, when college students were asked what percentage of other college students consumed alcohol, they regularly reported more than 90%,[23] suggesting that the American alcoholic-beverage industry has influenced our social norms.

Socioeconomic Status

Differences in socioeconomic status (SES), whether "defined by education, employment, or income, both individual- and community-level socioeconomic status have independent effects on health."[24] There is a strong correlation between SES and health status—individuals in lower SES groups, regardless of other characteristics, have poorer health status. This correlation applies both across racial groups and within racial groups.[25]

Community Organizing

The way in which a community organizes its resources directly influences its ability to intervene and solve problems, including health problems. **Community organizing** is "the process by which community groups are helped to identify common problems or change targets, mobilize resources, and develop and implement strategies for reaching their collective goals."[26] It is not a science but an art of building a consensus within a democratic process.[27] If a community can organize its resources effectively into a unified force, it "is likely to produce benefits in the form of increased effectiveness and productivity by reducing duplication of efforts and avoiding the imposition of solutions that are not congruent with the local culture and needs."[15] For example, many communities in the United States have faced community-wide drug problems. Some have been able to organize their resources to reduce or resolve these problems, whereas others have not.

Individual Behavior

The behavior of the individual community members contributes to the health of the entire community. It takes the concerted effort of many, if not most, of the individuals in a community to make a program work. For example, if each individual consciously engages in recycling practices, community recycling will be successful. Likewise, the more individuals who become immunized against a specific communicable disease, the slower the disease will spread and the fewer people will be exposed. This concept is known as **herd immunity**.

Community organizing the process by which community groups are helped to identify common problems or change targets, mobilize resources, and develop and implement strategies for reaching their collective goals

Herd immunity the resistance of a population to the spread of an infectious agent based on the immunity of a high proportion of individuals

A History of Community and Public Health

The history of community and public health is almost as long as the history of civilization. This summary provides an account of some of the historic accomplishments and failures in community and public health. We hope that knowledge of the past will enable us to better prepare for future challenges to our community's health.

Earliest Civilizations

In all likelihood, the earliest community health practices went unrecorded. Perhaps these practices involved taboos against defecation within the tribal communal area or near the source of drinking water. Perhaps they involved rites associated with burial of the dead. Certainly, the use of herbs for the prevention and curing of diseases, and communal assistance with childbirth are practices that predate archeological records.

Excavations at sites of some of the earliest known civilizations, dating from about 2000 BCE, have uncovered archeological evidence of community health activities (see **Figure 1.5**). A combination of additional archeological findings and written history provides much more evidence of community and public health activities throughout the seventeenth century. **Box 1.2** provides a timeline and some of the highlights of that history for the Ancient Societies (before 500 BCE), the Classical Cultures (500 BCE–500 CE), the Middle Ages (500–1500 CE), and the period of Renaissance and Exploration (1500–1700 CE).

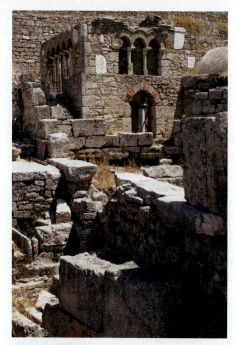

FIGURE 1.5 Archeological findings reveal community and public health practices of the past.

© Styve Reineck/Shutterstock

The Eighteenth Century

The eighteenth century was characterized by industrial growth. Despite the beginnings of recognition of the nature of disease, living conditions were hardly conducive to good health. Cities were overcrowded, and water supplies were inadequate and often unsanitary. Streets were usually unpaved, filthy, and heaped with trash and garbage. Many homes had unsanitary dirt floors.

Workplaces were unsafe and unhealthy. A substantial portion of the workforce was made up of people living in poverty, which included children, who were forced to work long hours as indentured servants. Many of these jobs were unsafe or involved working in unhealthy environments, such as textile factories and coal mines (see **Box 1.3**).

The Nineteenth Century

Epidemics continued to be a problem in the nineteenth century, with outbreaks in major cities in both Europe and America. In 1854, another cholera epidemic struck London. Dr. John Snow studied the epidemic and hypothesized that the disease was caused by the drinking water from the Broad Street pump. He obtained permission to remove the pump handle, and the epidemic was abated (see **Figure 1.6**). Snow's action was remarkable because it predated the discovery that micro-organisms can cause disease. The predominant theory of contagious disease at the time was the "miasmas theory," which postulated that vapors, or miasmas, were the source of many diseases. The miasmas theory remained popular throughout much of the nineteenth century.

In the United States in 1850, Lemuel Shattuck drew up a health report for the Commonwealth of Massachusetts that outlined the public health needs for the state. It included recommendations for the establishment of boards of health, the collection of vital statistics, the implementation of sanitary measures, and research on diseases. Shattuck also recommended

BOX 1.2   Timeline and Highlights of Community and Public Health Prior to 1700 CE

A. Early Civilizations
1. Ancient Societies (before 500 BCE)
   a. Prior to 2000 BCE: Archeological findings provide evidence of sewage disposal and written medical prescriptions.
   b. Circa 1900 BCE: Perhaps the earliest written record of public health was the Code of Hammurabi; it included laws for physicians and health practices.[26,28]
   c. Circa 1500 BCE: Bible's Book of Leviticus written; includes guidelines for personal cleanliness and sanitation.[26,28]
2. Classical Cultures (500 BCE–500 CE)
   a. Fifth and sixth centuries BCE: Evidence that Greek men participated in games of strength and skill and swam in public facilities.[27,29]
   b. Greeks were involved in practice of community sanitation; involved in obtaining water from sources far away and not just local wells.[28,30]
   c. Romans were community-minded; improved on community sanitation of Greeks; built aqueducts to transport water from miles away; built sewer systems; created regulation for building construction, refuse removal, and street cleaning and repair[27,29]; created hospitals as infirmaries for slaves.[29,31]
   d. Christians created hospitals as benevolent charitable organizations.[29,31]
   e. 476 CE: Roman Empire fell, and most public health activities ceased.

B. Middle Ages (500–1500 CE)
1. 500–1000 CE (Dark Ages): Growing revulsion for Roman materialism and a growth of spirituality; health problems were considered to have both spiritual causes and spiritual solutions,[29,31] a time referred to as the **spiritual era of public health**.
2. Failure to consider the role of the physical and biological environment in the causation of communicable diseases resulted in many unrelenting epidemics in which millions suffered and died.
   a. Deadliest epidemics were from plague ("Black Death"); occurred in 543 CE and 1348 CE (this one killed 25 million; half of the population of London lost and in some parts of France, only one in 10 survived).[26,28]
   b. 1200 CE: More than 19,000 leper houses.
   c. Other epidemics of the period: Smallpox, diphtheria, measles, influenza, tuberculosis, anthrax, and trachoma.
   d. 1492 CE: Syphilis epidemic was the last epidemic of the period.

C. Renaissance and Exploration (1500–1700 CE)
1. Rebirth of thinking about the nature of the world and humankind.
2. Belief that disease was caused by environmental, not spiritual, factors; for example, the term malaria, meaning bad air, is a direct reference to humid or swampy air.
3. Observation of ill led to more accurate descriptions of symptoms and outcomes of diseases; observations led to first recognition of whooping cough, typhus, scarlet fever, and malaria as distinct and separate diseases.[28,30]
4. 1662: John Graunt published the *Observations on the Bills of Mortality*, which was the beginning of vital statistics.
5. Epidemics (e.g., smallpox, malaria, and plague) still rampant; plague epidemic killed 68,596 (15% of the population) in London in 1665.
6. Explorers, conquerors, and merchants and their crews spread disease to colonists and indigenous people throughout the New World.

health education and controlling exposure to alcohol, smoke, adulterated food, and nostrums (quack medicines).[28] Although some of his recommendations took years to implement (the Massachusetts Board of Health was not founded until 1869), the significance of Shattuck's report is such that 1850 is a key date in American public health; it marks the beginning of the **modern era of public health**.

Real progress in the understanding of the causes of many communicable diseases occurred during the last third of the nineteenth century. One of the obstacles to progress

BOX 1.3   Timeline and Highlights of Community and Public Health from 1700 to 1848

A. Eighteenth Century (1700s)
1. 1790: First U.S. census.
2. 1793: Yellow fever epidemic in Philadelphia.[32]
3. 1796: Dr. Edward Jenner successfully demonstrated smallpox vaccination.
4. 1798: Marine Hospital Service (forerunner to U.S. Public Health Service) was formed.
5. By 1799: Several of America's largest cities, including Boston, Philadelphia, New York, and Baltimore, had municipal boards of health.

B. First Half of the Nineteenth Century (1800–1848)
1. U.S. government's approach to health was *laissez faire* (i.e., noninterference).
2. 1813: First visiting nurse in United States.

was the theory of spontaneous generation, the idea that living organisms could arise from inorganic or nonliving matter. Akin to this idea was the thought that one type of contagious microbe could change into another type of organism.

In 1862, Louis Pasteur of France proposed his germ theory of disease. Throughout the 1860s and 1870s, he and others carried out experiments and made observations that supported this theory and disproved spontaneous generation. Pasteur is generally given credit for providing the death blow to the theory of spontaneous generation.

It was the German scientist Robert Koch who developed the criteria and procedures necessary to establish that a particular microbe, and no other, causes a particular disease. His first demonstration, with the anthrax bacillus, was in 1876. Between 1877 and the end of the century, the identity of numerous bacterial disease agents was established, including those that caused gonorrhea, typhoid fever, leprosy, tuberculosis, cholera, diphtheria, tetanus, pneumonia, plague, and dysentery. This period (1875–1900) has come to be known as the **bacteriological period of public health**.

Although most scientific discoveries in the late nineteenth century were made in Europe, significant public health achievements were occurring in America as well. The first law prohibiting the adulteration of milk was passed in 1856, the first sanitary survey was carried out in New York City in 1864, and the American Public Health Association was founded in 1872. The Marine Hospital Service gained new powers of inspection and investigation under the Port Quarantine Act of 1878.[28] In 1890, the pasteurization of milk was introduced, and in 1891, meat inspection began. It was also during this time that nurses were first hired by industries (in 1895) and schools (in 1899). Also in 1895, septic tanks were introduced for sewage treatment. In 1900, Major Walter Reed of the U.S. Army announced that mosquitoes transmitted yellow fever (see **Box 1.4**).

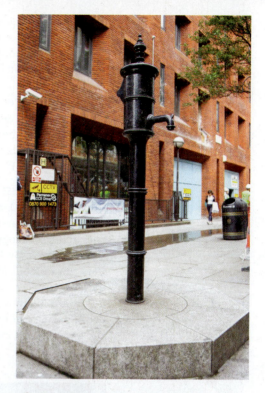

FIGURE 1.6   In London, England, in 1854, John Snow helped interrupt a cholera epidemic by having the handle removed from this pump, located on Broad Street.

© Nathaniel Noir/Alamy Stock Photo

The Twentieth Century

As the twentieth century began, life expectancy was still less than 50 years.[2] The leading causes of death were communicable diseases—influenza, pneumonia, tuberculosis, and infections of the gastrointestinal tract. Other communicable diseases, such as typhoid fever, malaria, and diphtheria, also killed many people.

There were other health problems as well. Thousands of children were afflicted with conditions characterized by noninfectious diarrhea or by bone deformity. Although the symptoms of pellagra and rickets were known and described, the causes of these ailments remained a mystery at the turn of the century. Discovery that these conditions resulted from vitamin deficiencies was slow because some scientists were searching for bacterial causes.

Spiritual era of public health a time during the Middle Ages when the causation of communicable disease was linked to spiritual forces

Modern era of public health the era of public health that began in 1850 and continues today

Bacteriological period of public health the period from 1875–1900, during which the causes of many bacterial diseases were discovered

---

BOX 1.4   Timeline and Highlights of Community and Public Health for the Second Half of Nineteenth Century (1848–1900)

1. 1849, 1854: London cholera epidemics.
2. 1850: Modern era of public health begins.
3. 1850: Shattuck's report was published.
4. 1854: Snow had pump handle removed from Broad Street pump.
5. 1863: Pasteur proposed germ theory.
6. 1872: American Public Health Association founded.
7. 1875–1900: Bacteriological period of public health.
8. 1876: Koch established relationship between a particular microbe and a particular disease.
9. 1900: Reed announced that yellow fever was transmitted by mosquitos.

Vitamin deficiency diseases and one of their contributing conditions, poor dental health, were extremely common in the slum districts of both European and American cities. The unavailability of adequate prenatal and postnatal care meant that deaths associated with pregnancy and childbirth were also high.

Health Resources Development Period (1900–1960)

Much growth and development took place during the 60-year period from 1900 to 1960. Because of the growth of healthcare facilities and providers, this period of time is referred to as the **health resources development period**. This period can be further divided into the reform phase (1900–1920), the 1920s, the Great Depression and World War II, and the postwar years.

The Reform Phase (1900–1920)

During the first 20 years of the twentieth century (i.e., the **reform phase of public health**), there was a growing concern about the many social problems in America. The remarkable discoveries in microbiology made in previous years had not dramatically improved the health of the average citizen. By 1910, the urban population had grown to 45% of the total population (up from 19% in 1860). Much of the growth was the result of immigrants who came to America for the jobs created by new industries (see **Figure 1.7**). Northern cities were also swelling from the northward migration of Blacks from the southern states. Many of these workers had to accept poorly paying jobs involving hard labor. There was also a deepening chasm between the upper and lower classes, and social critics began to clamor for reform.

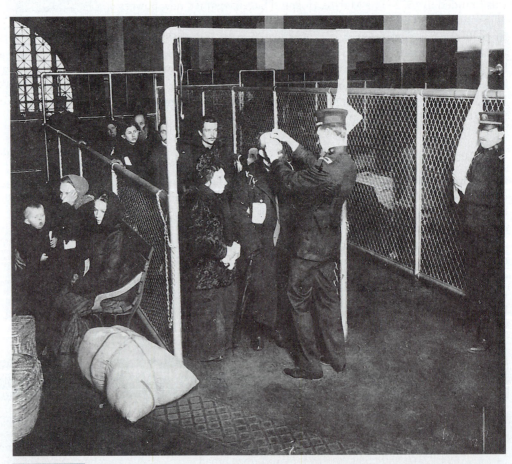

FIGURE 1.7   Ellis Island immigration between 1860 and 1910 resulted in dramatic increases in urban population in America.

Courtesy of Library of Congress, Prints & Photographs Division, [reproduction number LC-USZ62-7386].

In 1906, the plight of the immigrants working in the meat packing industry was graphically depicted by Upton Sinclair in his book *The Jungle*. Sinclair's goal was to draw attention to unsafe working conditions. What he achieved was greater governmental regulation of the food industry through the passage of the Pure Food and Drugs Act of 1906.

The reform movement was broad, involving both social and moral as well as health issues. In 1909, it was noted that "[i]ll health is perhaps the most constant of the attendants of poverty."[33] The reform movement finally took hold when it became evident to the majority that neither the discoveries of the causes of many communicable diseases nor the continuing advancement of industrial production could overcome continuing disease and poverty. Even by 1917, the United States ranked 14th of 16 "progressive" nations in maternal death rate.[33]

Although the relationship between occupation and disease had been pointed out 200 years earlier in Europe, occupational health in America in 1900 was an unknown quantity. However, in 1910, the first International Congress on Occupational Diseases was held in Chicago.[34] That same year, the state of New York passed a tentative Workman's Compensation Act, and over the next 10 years, most other states passed similar laws. Also in 1910, the U.S. Bureau of Mines was created and the first clinic for occupational diseases was established in New York at Cornell Medical College.[33] By 1910, the movement for healthier conditions in the workplace was well established.

This period also saw the birth of the first national-level volunteer health agencies. The first of these agencies was the National Association for the Study and Prevention of Tuberculosis (TB), which was formed in 1902. It arose from the first local voluntary health agency, the Pennsylvania Society for the Prevention of Tuberculosis, organized in 1892.[35] The American Cancer Society was founded in 1913. That same year, the Rockefeller Foundation was established in New York. This philanthropic foundation has funded a great many public health projects, including work on hookworm and pellagra and the development of a vaccine against yellow fever.

Another movement that began about this time was that of public health nursing. The first school nursing program was begun in New York City in 1902. In 1918, the first school of public health was established at Johns Hopkins University in Baltimore. This was followed by establishment of the Harvard School of Public Health in 1923. Also occurring in 1918 was the birth of school health instruction as we know it today.

These advances were matched with similar advances by governmental bodies. The Marine Hospital Service was renamed the Public Health and Marine Hospital Service in 1902 in keeping with its growing responsibilities. In 1912, it became the U.S. Public Health Service.[28]

By 1900, 38 states had state health departments. The rest followed during the first decades of the twentieth century. The first two local (county) health departments were established in 1911, one in Guilford County, North Carolina, and the other in Yakima County, Washington.

The 1920s

In comparison with the preceding period, the 1920s represented a decade of slow growth in public health, except for a few health projects funded by the Rockefeller and Millbank Foundations. Prohibition resulted in a decline in the number of alcoholics and alcohol-related deaths. Although the number of county health departments had risen to 467 by 1929, 77% of the rural population still lived in areas with no health services.[35] However, it was during this period in 1922 that the first professional preparation program for health education specialists was begun at Columbia University by Thomas D. Wood, MD, whom many consider the father of health education. The life expectancy in 1930 had risen to 59.7 years.

The Great Depression and World War II

Until the Great Depression (1929–1935), individuals and families in need of social and medical services were dependent on friends and relatives, private charities, voluntary agencies, community chests, and churches. By 1933, after 3 years of economic depression, it became evident that private resources could never meet the needs of all the people who needed assistance. The drop in tax revenues during the Depression also reduced health department budgets and caused a virtual halt in the formation of new local health departments.[35]

Beginning in 1933, President Franklin D. Roosevelt created numerous agencies and programs for public works as part of his New Deal. Much of the money was used for public health, including the control of malaria, the building of hospitals and laboratories, and the construction of municipal water and sewer systems.

The Social Security Act of 1935 marked the beginning of the government's major involvement in social issues, including health. This legislation provided substantial support for state health departments and their programs, such as maternal and child health, and sanitary facilities. As progress against communicable diseases became visible, some turned their attention toward other health problems, such as cancer. The National Cancer Institute was formed in 1937.

America's involvement in World War II resulted in severe restrictions on resources available for public health programs. Immediately following the conclusion of the war, however, many of the medical discoveries made during wartime made their way into civilian practice. Two examples are the antibiotic penicillin, used for treating pneumonia, rheumatic fever, syphilis, and strep throat; and the insecticide DDT, used for killing insects that transmit diseases.

During World War II, the Communicable Disease Center was established in Atlanta, Georgia. Now called the Centers for Disease Control and Prevention (CDC), it has become the premier epidemiologic center of the world.

The Postwar Years

Following the end of World War II, there was still concern about medical care and the adequacy of the facilities in which that care could be administered. In 1946, the U.S. Congress passed the National Hospital Survey and Construction Act (the Hill-Burton Act). The goal of the legislation was to improve the distribution of medical care and to enhance the quality of hospitals. From 1946 through the 1960s, hospital construction occurred at a rapid rate with relatively little thought given to planning. Likewise, attempts to set national health priorities or to establish a national health agenda were virtually nonexistent.

The two major health events in the 1950s were the development of a vaccine to prevent polio and President Eisenhower's heart attack. The latter event helped America to focus on its number one killer, heart disease. When the president's physician suggested exercise, some Americans heeded his advice and began to exercise on a regular basis.

Period of Social Engineering (1960–1973)

The 1960s marked the beginning of a period when the federal government once again became active in health matters. The primary reason for this involvement was the growing realization that many Americans were still not reaping any of the benefits of 60 years of medical advances. These Americans, most of whom were older adults or living in poverty, either lived in underserved areas or simply could not afford to purchase medical services.

In 1965, Congress passed the Medicare and Medicaid bills (amendments to the Social Security Act of 1935). **Medicare** assists in the payment of medical bills for older adults and certain people with disabilities, and **Medicaid** assists in the payment of medical bills for low-income people. These pieces of legislation helped provide medical care for millions who would not otherwise have received it; this legislation also improved standards in healthcare facilities. Unfortunately, this influx of federal dollars accelerated the rate of increase in the cost of health care for everyone. As a result, the 1970s, 1980s, and 1990s saw repeated attempts and failures to bring the growing costs of health care under control (see **Box 1.5**).

Period of Health Promotion (1974–Present)

By the mid-1970s, it had become apparent that the greatest potential for saving lives and reducing healthcare costs in America was to be achieved through means other than health care.

Most scholars, policymakers, and practitioners in health promotion would pick 1974 as the turning point that marks the beginning of health promotion as a significant component of national health policy in the twentieth century. That year, Canada published its landmark policy statement, *A New Perspective on the Health of Canadians*.[36] In 1976, the United States Congress passed PL 94-317, the Health Information and

Medicare government health insurance for older adults and those with certain disabilities

Medicaid government health insurance for low-income people

BOX 1.5   Timeline and Highlights of Community and Public Health for the Health Resources Development Period (1900–1960)

A. The Reform Phase (1900–1920)
1. 1902: First national-level voluntary health agency created.
2. 1906: Sinclair's *The Jungle* published.
3. 1910: First International Congress on Diseases of Occupation.
4. 1910: 45% of U.S. population was in the cities.
5. 1911: First local health department established.
6. 1913: American Cancer Society founded.
7. 1917: United States ranked 14th of 16 in maternal death rate.
8. 1918: Birth of school health instruction.
9. 1918: First school of public health established in United States.

B. 1920s
1. 1922: Wood created first professional preparation program for health education specialists.

2. 1930: Life expectancy in the United States was 59.7 years.

C. The Great Depression and World War II
1. 1933: New Deal; included unsuccessful attempt at national healthcare program.
2. 1935: Social Security Act passed.
3. 1937: National Cancer Institute formed.

D. Postwar Years
1. 1946: National Hospital Survey and Construction (Hill-Burton) Act passed.
2. 1952: Development of polio vaccine.
3. 1955: Eisenhower's heart attack.

E. Period of Social Engineering (1960–1973)
1. 1965: Medicare and Medicaid bills passed.

Health Promotion Act, which created the Office of Health Information and Health Promotion, later renamed the Office of Disease Prevention and Health Promotion.[37]

In the late 1970s, the CDC conducted a study that examined premature deaths (defined then as deaths prior to age 65, but now as deaths prior to age 75) in the United States in 1977. That study revealed that approximately 48% of all premature deaths could be traced to one's lifestyle or health behavior—choices that people make. Lifestyles characterized by a lack of exercise, unhealthy diets, smoking, uncontrolled hypertension, and the inability to control stress were found to be contributing factors to premature mortality.[38] This led the way for the U.S. government's publication *Healthy People: The Surgeon General's Report on Health Promotion and Disease Prevention.*[39] This report was one of the first formal reports to discuss the relationship between personal behavior and health status. Additionally, it documented a "personal responsibility" model that provided Americans with specific guidance for reducing health risks and increasing good health.[40]

Healthy People was followed by the release of the first set of health goals and objectives for the nation, called *Promoting Health/Preventing Disease: Objectives for the Nation.*[41] **Healthy People 2030** is the fifth edition of these goals and objectives. Since their inception, these *Healthy People* documents have defined the nation's health agenda and guided its health policy since their inception (see **Box 1.6**).

Healthy People 2030 the fifth set of health goals and objectives for the United States that defines the nation's health agenda and guides its health policy

---

BOX 1.6   Timeline and Highlights of Community and Public Health for the Period of Health Promotion (1974–Present)

A. Late Twentieth Century
1. 1974: Nixon's unsuccessful attempt at national health-care program.
2. 1974: *A New Perspective on the Health of Canadians* published.
3. 1976: Health Information and Health Promotion Act passed.
4. 1979: *Healthy People* published.
5. 1980: *Promoting Health/Preventing Disease: Objectives of the Nation* published.

6. 1990: *Healthy People 2000* published.
7. 1997: Clinton's unsuccessful attempt at a national healthcare program.

B. Early Twenty-First Century
1. 2000: *Healthy People 2010* published.
2. 2010: Affordable Care Act becomes law.
3. 2010: *Healthy People 2020* published.
4. 2020: *Healthy People 2030* published.

All five editions of the *Healthy People* documents include several overarching goals and many supporting objectives for the nation's health. The goals provide a general focus and direction, whereas the objectives are used to measure progress within a specified period of time. Formal reviews (i.e., measured progress) of these objectives are conducted both at midcourse (i.e., halfway through the 10-year period) and again at the end of 10 years. The midcourse review provides an opportunity to update the document based on the events of the first half of the decade for which the objectives were written.

Healthy People 2030 was released in August of 2020, and it includes a vision statement, a mission statement, foundational principles, five overarching goals (see **Table 1.1**), a plan of action, and 359 core science-based objectives spread over 62 different topic areas (see **Table 1.2**).[42] On the Healthy People.gov website, each topic has its own webpage. At a minimum, each page

---

TABLE 1.1 *Healthy People 2030* **Vision, Mission, Foundational Principles, Overarching Goals, and Plan of Action**

Vision

A society in which all people can achieve their full potential for health and well-being across the lifespan.

Mission

To promote, strengthen, and evaluate the nation's efforts to improve the health and well-being of all people.

Foundational Principles

The following foundational principles guide decisions about *Healthy People 2030*:
- The health and well-being of all people and communities is essential to a thriving, equitable society.
- Promoting health and well-being and preventing disease are linked efforts that encompass physical, mental, and social health dimensions.
- Investing to achieve the full potential for health and well-being for all provides valuable benefits to society.
- Achieving health and well-being requires eliminating health disparities, achieving health equity, and attaining health literacy.
- Healthy physical, social, and economic environments strengthen the potential to achieve health and well-being.
- Promoting and achieving health and well-being nationwide is a shared responsibility that is distributed across the nation, state, tribal, and community levels, including the public, private, and not-for-profit sectors.
- Working to attain the full potential for health and well-being of the population is a component of decision-making and policy formulation across all sectors.

Overarching Goals

- Attain healthy, thriving lives and well-being free of preventable disease, disability, injury, and premature death.
- Eliminate health disparities, achieve health equity, and attain health literacy to improve the health and well-being of all.
- Create social, physical, and economic environments that promote attaining the full potential for health and well-being for all.
- Promote healthy development, healthy behaviors, and well-being across the life stages.
- Engage leadership, key constituents, and the public across multiple sectors to take action and design policies that improve the health and well-being of all.

Plan of Action

- Set national goals and measurable objectives to guide evidence-based policies, programs, and other actions to improve health and well-being.
- Provide accurate, timely, and accessible data that can drive targeted actions to address regions and populations that have poor health or are at high risk for poor health.
- Foster impact through public and private efforts to improve health and well-being for people of all ages and the communities in which they live.
- Provide tools for the public, programs, policymakers, and others to evaluate progress toward improving health and well-being.
- Share and support the implementation of evidence-based programs and policies that are replicable, scalable, and sustainable.
- Report biennially on progress throughout the decade from 2020 to 2030.
- Stimulate research and innovation toward meeting *Healthy People 2030* goals and highlight critical research, data, and evaluation needs.
- Facilitate the development and availability of affordable means of health promotion, disease prevention, and treatment.

Reproduced from U.S. Department of Health and Human Services. (2024). *About: Healthy People 2030 Framework*. Available at https://health.gov/healthypeople/about/healthy-people-2030-framework

TABLE 1.2 *Healthy People 2030* Topic Areas

Health Conditions

Addiction	Heart Disease and Stroke
Arthritis	Infectious Disease
Blood Disorders	Mental Health and Mental Disorders
Cancer	Oral Conditions
Chronic Kidney Disease	Osteoporosis
Chronic Pain	Overweight and Obesity
Dementia	Pregnancy and Childbirth
Diabetes	Respiratory Disease
Foodborne Illness	Sensory or Communication Disorders
Healthcare-Associated Infections	Sexually Transmitted Diseases

Health Behaviors

Child and Adolescent Development	Physical Activity
Drug and Alcohol Use	Preventive Care
Emergency Preparedness	Safe Food Handling
Family Planning	Sleep
Health Communication	Tobacco Use
Injury Prevention	Vaccination
Nutrition and Healthy Eating	Violence Prevention

Populations

Adolescents	Older Adults
Children	Parents or Caregivers
Infants	People with Disabilities
LGBT	Women
Men	Workforce

Settings and Systems

Community	Hospital and Emergency Services
Environmental Health	Housing and Homes
Global Health	Public Health Infrastructure
Health Care	Schools
Health Insurance	Transportation
Health IT	Workplace
Health Policy	

Social Determinants of Health

Economic Stability	Neighborhood and Built Environment
Education Access and Quality	Social and Community Context
Health Care Access and Quality	

Reproduced from U.S. Department of Health and Human Services. (2024). *Healthy People 2030: Objectives and Data*. Available at https://health.gov/healthypeople/objectives-and-data

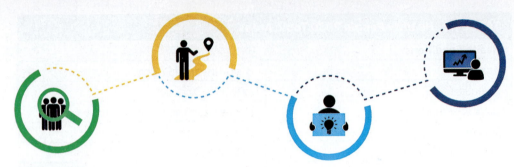

FIGURE 1.8   Practical steps to follow to achieve *Healthy People* goals.

Reproduced from U.S. Department of Health and Human Services. (2024). *Healthy People 2030: Tools for Action.* Available at https://health
.gov/healthypeople/tools-action

contains a concise goal statement, a brief overview of the topic that provides the background and context for the topic, a statement about the importance of the topic backed up by appropriate evidence, and references.

The developers of *Healthy People 2030* have developed Tools for Action to support communities, states, and organizations to use the *Healthy People* objectives to priorities (see **Figure 1.8**). *Healthy People 2030* users are encouraged to follow four steps: (1) Identify needs and priority populations in order to make the case for a program, secure resources, and build partnerships; (2) Set local targets that contribute to national success; (3) Find inspiration and practical tools by reviewing successful programs, policies, and interventions; and (4) Monitor national progress and use local data to inform policy and planning.[42]

In addition to the *Healthy People* initiative, the United States developed the National Prevention Strategy (Strategy), which was released in 2011. The Affordable Care Act (ACA) "created the National Prevention Council (NPC) and called for the development of the Strategy to realize the benefits of prevention for the health of all Americans. The Strategy is critical to the prevention focus of the ACA and builds on the law's efforts to lower healthcare costs, improve the quality of care, and provide coverage options for the uninsured."[43]

The NPC provided leadership for the Strategy under the guidance of representatives from 20 federal departments, agencies, and offices and the U.S. Surgeon General. Although the NPC "provides coordination and leadership at the federal level and identifies ways that agencies can work individually, as well as together, to improve our nation's health,"[43] public and private partners provided much input in creating the Strategy. Such input was provided by the Advisory Group on Prevention, Health Promotion, and Integrative and Public Health, referred to as the Prevention Advisory Group. This group was also created by the ACA and comprised 21 nonfederal members appointed by the president.[43]

The goal of the Strategy was to "increase the number of Americans who are healthy at every stage of life."[43] At the foundation of the Strategy are four strategic directions that include Healthy and Safe Community Environments, Clinical and Community Preventive Services, Empowered People, and Elimination of Health Disparities (see **Figure 1.9**). "Each Strategy direction can stand alone and can guide actions that will demonstrably improve health. Together, the strategic directions create the web needed to fully support Americans in leading longer and healthier lives."[43] The Strategy included seven targeted priorities (Tobacco-Free Living, Preventing Drug Abuse and Excessive Alcohol Use, Healthy Eating, Active Living, Injury and Violence Free Living, Reproductive and Sexual Health, and Mental and Emotional Well-Being). The priorities were "designed to improve health and wellness for the entire U.S. population, including those groups disproportionately affected by disease and injury."[43] Preference was given to efforts that would "have the greatest impact on the largest number of people and can be sustained over time."[43]

The Strategy includes: key facts and documents; a list of recommended policies, programs, and system approaches to address each of the strategic directions and priorities; and actions for both the federal government and for the partners. The actions for the partners are

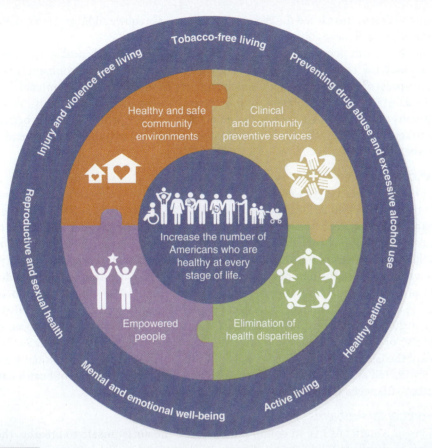

FIGURE 1.9 National Prevention Strategy.

Reproduced from National Prevention Council, U.S. Department of Health and Human Services, Office of the Surgeon General. (2011). *National Prevention Strategy*. Available at https://www.hhs.gov/sites/default/files/disease-prevention-wellness-report.pdf

specific to type of partners, which include: (1) state, tribal, local, and territorial governments; (2) employers; (3) healthcare organizations, insurers, and clinicians; (4) educational organizations; (5) community groups; and (6) faith-based organizations. In addition, within each of the strategic directions and priorities are key indicators that will be used to measure progress toward the overarching goal based on 10-year targets. In addition to measuring progress in prevention, the indicators "will be used to plan and implement future prevention efforts. Key indicators will be reported for the overall population and by subgroups, as data become available. Indicators and 10-year targets are drawn from existing measurement efforts, especially *Healthy People 2020*. As data sources and metrics are developed or enhanced, the key indicators and targets of the National Prevention Strategy will be updated."[43]

The Twenty-First Century

Now, in the third decade of the twenty-first century, the need to improve community and public health continues. In the sections that follow, we have outlined some of the major problems still facing the United States and the world.

U.S. Community and Public Health in the Twenty-First Century

With one-quarter of the twenty-first century behind us, it is widely agreed that although decisions about health are an individual's responsibility to a significant degree, society has an obligation to provide an environment in which the achievement of good health is possible and encouraged. Furthermore, many recognize that certain segments of our population whose disease and death rates exceed the general population may require additional resources, including education, to achieve good health.

The American people face a number of serious public health problems. These problems include the continuing rise in healthcare costs, growing environmental concerns, the ever-present lifestyle diseases, emerging and re-emerging communicable diseases, serious substance abuse problems, and disasters, both natural and human-made. In the paragraphs that follow, we have elaborated on each of these problems briefly because they seem to represent a significant portion of the community and public health agenda for the years ahead.

Healthcare Delivery

In 2010, significant changes were made to the U.S. healthcare system with the passage of the Patient Protection and Affordable Care Act (PPACA; Public Law 111-148) and the Health Care and Education Reconciliation Act of 2010 (HCERA; Public Law 111-152). These two acts were consolidated shortly thereafter with other approved legislation and are now referred to as the *Affordable Care Act* (ACA). Although the law has many components, the primary focus was to increase the number of Americans with health insurance. The ACA does this, but by providing health insurance to millions of Americans who did not have it before, the costs will also go up, which will continue to make U.S. health care the most expensive in the world. In 2021, national health expenditures grew by 2.7%, reaching $4.3 trillion, accounting for 18.3%[44] of the gross domestic product (GDP), and are expected to reach $5.96 trillion (19.4% of the GDP) by 2027.[45] The United States spends more per person annually on health care (estimated at $12,914 in 2021)[44] than any other nation. The cost of health care is an issue that still needs to be addressed.

Environmental Problems

Millions of Americans live in communities where the air is unsafe to breathe, the water is unsafe to drink, or solid waste is disposed of improperly. With a few minor exceptions, the rate at which we pollute our environment continues to increase. Many Americans still believe that our natural resources are unlimited and that their individual contributions to the overall pollution are insignificant. We must improve on our efforts in resource preservation and energy conservation if our children are to enjoy an environment as clean as ours. These environmental problems are compounded by the fact that the world population continues to grow; it is now more than 8 billion people and expected to grow to 14 billion over the next 14 years.[46]

Lifestyle Diseases

Over the past nearly 40 years, the leading causes of death in the United States had been related to chronic illnesses and unintentional injuries. But the COVID-19 pandemic caused a significant number of deaths, bringing communicable disease back into the top leading causes of death and had an indirect effect on the other leading causes of death.[47] Although it is true that everyone has to die from some cause, at some time, too many Americans die prematurely. Two-thirds of all deaths among Americans each year are from one or more of these five chronic diseases: heart disease, cancer, stroke, chronic lower respiratory disease, and diabetes.[48] In addition, 90% of all healthcare spending in the United States is for people with chronic and mental health conditions.[49] Chronic diseases are not only the most common, deadly, and costly conditions, but they are also the most preventable of all health problems in the United States.[50] They are the most preventable because four modifiable risk behaviors—physical inactivity, poor nutrition, tobacco use, and excessive alcohol use—are responsible for much of the illness, suffering, and early death related to chronic diseases.[50] In fact, one study found that mortality decreases progressively as the number of health behaviors increases. Specifically, study participants who were nonsmokers, were physically active, and consumed a healthy diet had a risk for mortality from all causes that was 82% lower than study participants not engaging in these three preventative behaviors[49] (see **Table 1.3**).

TABLE 1.3 Comparison of the Most Common Causes of Death and Actual Causes of Death

Most Common Causes of Death, United States, 2011	Actual Causes of Death, United States, 2000
1. Heart disease	1. Tobacco
2. Cancer	2. Poor diet and physical inactivity
3. COVID-19	3. Alcohol consumption
4. Unintentional injuries	4. Microbial agents
5. Stroke	5. Toxic agents
6. Chronic lower respiratory disease	6. Motor vehicles
7. Alzheimer's disease	7. Firearms
8. Diabetes	8. Sexual behavior
9. Liver disease	9. Illicit drug use
10. Nephritis	

Data from: Centers for Disease Control and Prevention. *Exploring leading causes of death.* 2023. Available at https://www.cdc.gov/injury/wisqars/leadingcauses.html; Mokdad AH, Marks JS, Stroup DF, Gerberding JL. Actual causes of death in the United States, 2000. *JAMAssociation.* 2000;*291*(10):1238–1245; Mokdad AH, Marks JS, Stroup DF, Gerberding JL. Correction: actual causes of death in the United States, 2000. *JAMA.* 2005;*293*(3):293–294.

Communicable Diseases

With the COVID-19 pandemic hitting the United States in 2020, everything written about the impact of communicable diseases on the health of Americans has significantly changed (see **Figure 1.10**). Prior to the COVID-19 pandemic, there was concern about the impact on the lives of Americans, but the concern about an early death because of a communicable disease was not a regular thought. In general, communicable diseases cause concern because they are the primary reason for days missed at school or at work. The success in reducing the life-threatening nature of these diseases has made many Americans complacent about obtaining vaccinations or taking other precautions against contracting these diseases. With the exception of smallpox, none of the communicable diseases have been eradicated, although several should have been, such as measles.

Second, as new communicable diseases emerge, old ones, such as tuberculosis re-emerge, sometimes in drug-resistant forms (i.e., caused by superbugs), demonstrating that communicable diseases still represent a serious community health problem in America. Legionnaires' disease, Lyme disease, acquired immunodeficiency syndrome (AIDS), severe acute respiratory syndrome (SARS), Zika virus, and COVID-19 are diseases that were unknown only 60 years ago. The first cases of AIDS were reported in June of 1981.[52] By August of 1989, 100,000 cases had been reported,[53] and it took only an additional 2 years to report the second 100,000 cases.[54] At the end of 2021, an estimated 1.2 million people in the United States had HIV.[55] The total number of cases continues to grow with more than 35,000 new HIV cases being diagnosed each year.[55] In addition, diseases that were once only found in animals are crossing over to human populations and causing much concern and action. Included in this group of diseases are avian flu, *Escherichia coli* O157:H7, hantavirus, mad cow disease, and SARS.

Third, and maybe the most disturbing, is the use of communicable diseases for bioterrorism. **Bioterrorism** is "the deliberate use of viruses, bacteria, or toxins or other agents to cause illness or death in people, animals, or plants."[56] Concern in the United States over bioterrorism was heightened after September 11, 2001 (9/11), and the subsequent intentional distribution of *Bacillus anthracis* spores through the U.S. postal system (the anthrax mailings).

Bioterrorism the deliberate use of viruses, bacteria, or toxins or other agents to cause illness or death in people, animals, or plants

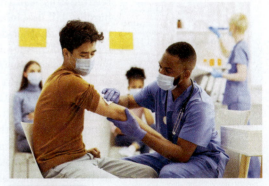

FIGURE 1.10   The COVID-19 pandemic reshaped how the U.S. approaches communicable disease prevention.

© Prostock-studio/Shutterstock

Since then, a heightened awareness of potential threats posed by chemical and biological weapons and low-grade nuclear materials has prompted public officials nationwide to review and revamp the [public health] system. Large-scale bioterrorism has not yet occurred, but global unrest amid the rise of extremism makes it a real possibility in the future.

Alcohol and Other Substance Use

Substance use disorder and addiction due to the use of tobacco, alcohol, and illegal drugs have a number of negative effects on individuals and society, including but not limited to failure in school, child abuse, disintegration of the family, domestic violence, loss of employment, violent crimes, and even death. Estimates of the total overall costs of substance abuse in the United States, including lost productivity and health- and crime-related costs, exceed $740 billion annually.[57] Federal, state, and local governments as well as private agencies attempt to address the supply and demand problems associated with the abuse of alcohol and other drugs, but a significant challenge remains for America. A recent example of this challenge has been the response to opioid pain reliever overdose. In 2022, more than 80,000 overdose deaths from opioids (primarily fentanyl) were reported, a rate that quadrupled since 2010. Due to the addictive nature of opioids, opioid users are seeking nonprescription pain relief from withdrawal symptoms caused by addiction to doctor-prescribed opioids.[58] In response to the increase in major overdose deaths, two major steps have been taken. The first was the approval of intranasal naloxone—a nasal spray formulation of the medication designed to rapidly reverse opioid overdose, by the U.S. Food and Drug Administration (FDA). This provides family members, caregivers, and first responders with an alternative to injectable naloxone for use during a suspected opioid overdose. This was originally available only with a prescription, but in 2023, the FDA approved naloxone hydrochloride nasal spray for over-the-counter, nonprescription use, the first product approved for use without a prescription.[59] Access to naloxone has resulted in many public health campaigns to educate individuals on the importance of naloxone in saving lives and how to effectively use it in an emergency situation. The second was the development by the CDC of guidelines for prescribing opioids for chronic pain that provided recommendations for the prescribing of opioid pain medication for patients ages 18 years and older in primary-care settings.[60] Making naloxone so easily accessible is an example of using harm reduction to reduce certain health and safety issues associated with drug use. Federal public health efforts, including research supported by NIDA, are helping explore new and emerging approaches to keeping individuals and communities safe, particularly in resource-challenges.[61]

Health Disparities

It has long been recognized that some individuals lead longer and healthier lives than others, and that these differences are often closely associated with social characteristics such as race, ethnicity, gender, geographic location, and income.[62] These gaps between groups have been referred to as health disparities. More formally, **health disparities** have been defined as "a higher burden of illness, injury, disability, and/or mortality that is experienced by one group of people relative to another due to current or historic disadvantage, oppression, or racism, which is manifested through inequitable social, economic, and environmental systems."[63] Health disparities are a problem in the United States in that the health status of many minority groups, on many different measures, is not as good as that of the white population. Efforts have been put forth to eliminate the disparities, as evidenced by one of the *Healthy People 2030* overarching goals to "eliminate health disparities, achieve health equity, and attain health literacy to improve the health and well-being for all."[42]

The COVID-19 pandemic heightened the focus on health disparities in the U.S. COVID-19 cases, hospitalizations, and deaths were significantly higher for Native Americans, Alaska natives, Hispanics, and Black people compared with White people.[64] As has been discussed throughout this text, most deaths have underlying causes and COVID-19 is no different. Sociodemographic and health characteristics, race/ethnicity, sex, and gender are some of the underlying causes of death attributed to COVID-19. Specifically, COVID-19 mortality was five times higher for adults in low socioeconomic positions than those in high socioeconomic

Health disparities is the higher burden of illness, injury, disability, and/or mortality that is experienced by one group of people relative to another due to current or historic disadvantage, oppression, or racism, which is manifested through inequitable social, economic, and environmental systems

positions. The combination of low socioeconomic status, Hispanic ethnicity, and male gendered carried a COVID-19 mortality risk that was 27 times higher.[64] White, high socioeconomic standing women had the lowest mortality risk. The point of sharing these data is to demonstrate how the COVID-19 pandemic emphasized how deep the disparities are in the United States. Many experts think these differences have been caused by two health inequities: (1) lack of access to health care, and (2) when health care is received, the quality has not been as good for those in racial and ethnic minority groups. Whatever the reason, health disparities continue to be a problem, and much more needs to be done.

Disasters

Disasters can be classified into two primary categories—natural and human-caused, including technological disasters. Whereas natural disasters are the result of the combination of the forces of nature (e.g., hurricane, flood, blizzard, tornado, earthquake, landslide), human-caused disasters result from either unintentional (e.g., spill of a toxic substance into the environment) or intentional (e.g., bioterrorism) human activities, often associated with the use or misuse of technology. Both types of disasters have the potential to cause injury, death, disease, and damage to property on a large scale.[65] In recent years, the United States has felt the large-scale impact of both types of disasters via wildfires, the BP Gulf oil spill, Hurricane Harvey and Major Hurricane Ida, severe flooding, and mass shootings. These events showed us that the preparation for such disasters was not adequate and that each type of disaster required different resources and responses.

Although the causes of the two categories of disasters are different, preparedness for them has many common elements. Due to this overlap in challenges between natural and human disasters, by preparing for natural disasters, a general, basic disaster response system is established. Beyond general disaster response preparedness, specific steps must be taken to deal with the peculiarity of the human-caused disasters. An example of this would be the need for decontamination following exposure to a biological agent.

Despite the devastating consequences of natural disasters, such as hurricanes, flooding, or the wildfires that consume many thousands of acres of woodlands each year, the intentional human-caused disasters—specifically, terrorism—have occupied much of our attention in recent years (see **Figure 1.11**).

Mention was made earlier of the use of a communicable disease as part of terrorism. In fact, a number of agents could be used for terrorism. Since the anthrax mailings, community and public health professionals have focused on the possibility that future terrorism could include chemical, biological, radiological, and/or nuclear (CBRN) agents, resulting in mass numbers of casualties. Such concern led to an evaluation of community and public health emergency preparedness and response. "Determining the level of state and local health departments' emergency preparedness and response capacities is crucial because public health officials are among those, along with firefighters, emergency medical personnel, and local law enforcement personnel, who serve on "rapid response" teams when large-scale emergency situations arise."[15] Results of that evaluation showed that the public health infrastructure was not where it should be to handle large-scale emergencies, as well as a number of more common public health concerns. These public health infrastructure and strategic shortcomings were highlighted during the COVID-19 pandemic. While the pandemic was hard to predict and extremely challenging to manage, many national and local public health flaws were exposed.

Based on the results of several different evaluations that exposed many weaknesses in emergency preparedness in general and in the public health infrastructure more specifically, investment in public health preparedness has increased since 9/11. Those federal departments that have been responsible for

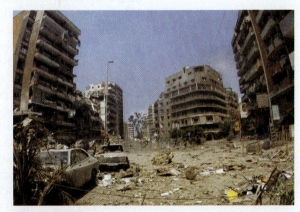

FIGURE 1.11   Terrorism has become a concern throughout the world.

© Sadik Gulec/Shutterstock

Public health preparedness the capability of the public health and healthcare systems, community, and individuals to prevent, protect against, quickly respond to, and recover from health emergencies, particularly those in which scale, timing, or unpredictability threatens to overwhelm routine capabilities

most of the effort have been the U.S. Departments of Homeland Security (DHS) and Health and Human Services (HHS). The DHS has the responsibility of protecting America, whereas the HHS has taken the leadership for public health and medical preparedness. **Public health preparedness** has been defined as "the capability of the public health and health care systems, communities, and individuals, to prevent, protect against, quickly respond to, and recover from health emergencies, particularly those in which scale, timing, or unpredictability threatens to overwhelm routine capabilities."[66] Information about emergency preparedness and response can be found on the websites of all HHS agencies; however, those that have been most visible have been the CDC, the Health Resources and Services Administration (HRSA), and the Agency for Healthcare Research and Quality (AHRQ).

After 9/11, the federal government, through a variety of funding sources and programs, has worked to strengthen homeland security, emergency preparedness, and response at all levels. The funding was used to create or enhance the various components needed in disaster situations (i.e., communication, coordination, and the workforce). The funding also had to be used to bring much of the public health system up to date (e.g., laboratories, personnel, and surveillance) after many years of neglect. Several years leading up to the COVID-19 pandemic, there had been a decrease in public health preparedness funding, which had begun to erode a decade's worth of progress.[63] Since the outbreak of the COVID-19 pandemic, public health preparedness funding has rebounded on the state and local level.

Although the United States is better prepared than prior to 9/11, much still needs to be done. In March of 2024, the Trust for America's Health (TFAH), a nonprofit, nonpartisan organization, released their report on the state of public health preparedness in the United States.[67] Central to the report is a scorecard that rates all 50 states and the District of Columbia based on nine priority indicators to assess health emergency preparedness capabilities. States are making progress in public health funding, laboratory surge capacity, and participation in health worker licensing compacts; however, we have stalled or lost ground in areas such as flu vaccination, hospital patient safety, and access to paid time off.[67]

Data from the report showed that 13 states cut public health funding during the 2023 fiscal year. Flu vaccination coverage was 49% during the 2022–2023 season,[67] far below the 70% coverage goal of *Healthy People 2030*.[42] In addition, with only 55% of employed state residents, on average, having access to paid time off, there is a risk of spreading infectious disease in the work setting.[65] Obviously, there is still much work to be done and, unfortunately, the status of most of these problems has not significantly improved in the past 8 years.

World Community and Public Health in the Twenty-First Century

Like the United States, much progress has been made in the health of people throughout the world in recent years. Yet, in just 2 years, the COVID-19 pandemic reversed over a decade of gains in life expectancy. Between 2019 and 2021, the global life expectancy dropped by 1.7 years to 71.9 years in 2021, back to the same level of 2012.[68] Over the past decade, like has been observed in the United States, deaths from noncommunicable diseases have risen steadily (79.1% of deaths in 2019), while communicable disease deaths have continued to drop. However, with the emergence of COVID-19, the percentage of deaths from communicable diseases surged from 18.2% in 2019 to 28.1% of all deaths in 2021—a return to 2005 levels.[68] Progress on global health-related goals has been greatly challenged by COVID-19. Goals related to universal health coverage, health emergency preparedness, and healthier population targets are off track for 2025. Furthermore, the world continues to struggle with the double burden of malnutrition and overweight/obesity, demonstrating the need to respond to changing demographics and persisting inequities around the world with individuals in high-income countries having a much better chance of living longer than people in low-income countries.[68] And, as in the United States, a number of public health achievements took place in the early part of the twenty-first century (see **Box 1.7**). However, all people of the world do not share in this increased life expectancy and better health.

In the following sections, we have identified some of the community and public health issues that the people of the world will be facing in years ahead.

BOX 1.7   Ten Great Public Health Achievements—Worldwide 2001–2010

At the conclusion of 2010, experts in global public health were asked to nominate noteworthy public health achievements that occurred outside of the United States during 2001–2010. From their responses, 10 were selected. Below, in no specific order, are the ones selected from the nominations.[69]

- *Reductions in child mortality.* Currently, an estimated 4.9 million children die each year before reaching their fifth birthday, which is a 51% decline in the global under-5 mortality rate since 2000. Significant disparities exist. For example, the African Region accounted for over half of the total under-5 deaths in 2022, while only accounting for 30% of the global live births.[68]

- *Vaccine-preventable deaths.* Vaccines are now available to prevent more than 20 life-threatening diseases and preventing 3.5 to 5 million deaths every year from diseases like COVID-19, diphtheria, tetanus, pertussis, influenza, and measles.[70]

- *Access to safe water and sanitation.* In 2022, 73% (6 billion people) of the global population had access to safe drinking water, yet there continues to be a significant health burden due to lack of access to safe drinking water.[69] Annually, an estimated 1.4 million deaths, 395,000 of these among children under 5 years of age, could be prevented annually through safe water, sanitation, and hygiene (WASH).[71]

- *Malaria prevention and control.* Malaria is a leading cause of death from infectious disease worldwide. Increased coverage with insecticide-treated bed nets, indoor residual spraying, rapid diagnosis and prompt treatment with artemisinin combination therapy, and intermittent preventive treatment during pregnancy resulted in a 21% decrease in estimated global malaria deaths between 2000 and 2009. But in recent years, that progress has stalled. Thus, the WHO Global Malaria Programme has developed a new strategy for 2024–2030 that will focus on establishing standards, new tools, strategic communication, and leadership.[70] The first doses of a malaria vaccine were to be disseminated in early 2024. Twenty-nine countries account for approximately 95% of malaria cases globally reinforcing the disparities among countries and the importance of continuous government efforts to strategically address infectious diseases.[72]

- *Prevention and control of HIV/AIDS.* HIV remains a global public health challenge with 39.0 million people living with HIV at the end of 2022. Efforts to address HIV globally are inconsistent with some countries reporting increasing trends in new infections when previously on the decline.[73] A number of public health interventions, including provider-initiated HIV testing and counseling, prevention of mother-to-child HIV transmission, expanded availability and use of condoms and sterile injection equipment, improved blood safety, and antiretroviral therapy (ART) have helped to reduce the number of new infections.

- *Tuberculosis control.* Due in large part to the WHO's directly observed therapy(DOTS), short-course strategy for TB control; focusing on finding and successfully treating TB cases with standardized regimens and rigorous treatment; and program monitoring, during the decade case detection and treatment success rates each have risen nearly 20%, with incidence and prevalence declining in every region. An estimated 76 million lives have been saved since 2000 due to global efforts to combat TB. However, in 2022, tuberculosis was the second-leading cause of death from infectious diseases after COVID-19. Multidrug-resistant TB remains a public health crisis and security threat.[74]

- *Control of neglected tropical diseases.* Neglected tropical diseases affect approximately 1 billion people worldwide. Three of these diseases have been targeted for elimination or eradication: dracunculiasis (Guinea worm disease), onchocerciasis (river blindness) in the Americas, and lymphatic filariasis. Programs targeting dracunculiasis and onchocerciasis in the Americas are on the verge of success, and the lymphatic filariasis programs are making progress.

- *Tobacco control.* The global tobacco epidemic kills more than 8 million people each year with 7 million of the deaths a direct result of tobacco use with the other deaths the result of exposure to second-hand smoke.[75] However, during the decade, 168 countries adopted WHO's first global health treaty aimed at tobacco, 163 countries tracked tobacco use via surveys, and the total global population covered by smoke-free laws increased. Currently, 182 countries have joined this treaty.

- *Increased awareness and response for improving global road safety.* Approximately 1.19 million people die each year as a result of road traffic crashes, the leading cause of death for children and young adults aged 5 to 29 years.[76] This is a 5% decrease since 2010. With more than 90% of road traffic deaths occurring in low- and middle-income countries, road crashes remain a persistent global health crisis. A significant global effort has been made to create a plan to reduce the forecasted growth in road fatalities, but there is still progress to be made.

- *Improved preparedness and response to global health threats.* During the 10-year period of time, the public health community has improved preparedness for and detection of pandemic threats and is now responding more effectively than before. This is due in part to modernization of the international legal framework, better disease surveillance techniques, better public health networking, and better global disease detection systems.

Data from: U.S. Department of Health and Human Services, Centers for Disease Control and Prevention. (2011). Ten Great Public Health Achievements—Worldwide, 2001–2010. *Morbidity and Mortality Weekly Report, 60*(24), 814–818. Available at http://www.cdc.gov/mmwr/preview/mmwrhtml/mm6024a4.htm

Communicable Diseases

Even though information presented in Box 1.7 suggests that there have been a number of achievements with regard to communicable diseases throughout the world between 2001 and 2010, the burden of communicable diseases worldwide is still great. It is most vivid when looking at mortality. The leading causes of death in the world do not look much different from the leading causes of death in the United States. In fact, prior to the COVID-19 pandemic, heart disease and stroke were the number one and two killers worldwide. However, when the leading causes of death are broken down by the wealth of the countries, big differences appear. Six of the 10 leading causes of death are infectious diseases (e.g., lower respiratory infections, malaria, tuberculosis, diarrheal disease, COVD-19, and HIV/AIDS) in low-income countries, whereas eight to nine of the 10 leading causes are noncommunicable diseases in high-income countries.[69] Similar trends appear when life expectancy is compared with the wealth of the countries. A boy born in 2021 in a high-income country can expect to live to approximately 75 years—more than 13 years longer than a boy born in a low-income country (62 years). For girls, the difference is slightly more; a gap of 14 years separates life expectancy in high-income (81.0 years) and low-income countries (67.0 years)."[69]

Poor Sanitation and Unsafe Drinking Water

Closely related to the problem of communicable diseases and related death are unsafe drinking water and poor sanitation. Worldwide, approximately 1 million people die each year from diarrhea as a result of unsafe drinking water, sanitation, and hand hygiene.[77] For those individuals who grew up in a high-income country, the thought of not having clean water and sanitary conditions is hard to understand. Yet, worldwide, one in four people do not have access to safely managed drinking water, with less than half of the population in sub-Saharan Africa with access to basic drinking water and nearly half (45%) of this population collecting water from sources not at home.[77] In addition, an estimated 1.7 billion people lack basic sanitation, which includes safe disposal of human waste and access to handwashing stations with soap and water at home.[78]Access to safe drinking water, adequate sanitation, and proper hygiene education are essential to reducing illness and death, which, in turn, leads to improved health, poverty reduction, and socioeconomic development. Access to safe drinking water, sanitation, and hygiene (WASH) are basic human rights. Public health efforts do make a difference as it is estimated that for every $1 invested in hand hygiene results in $15 return on investment.[78] There is much more work to be done.

Hunger

Hunger can be defined in several different ways, but the definition that applies here is a severe lack of food.[79] World hunger is not merely a problem of the amount of food but also the maldistribution of the available food. Too many people cannot afford to buy the available food, lack the land and resources to grow it themselves, or live in a climate that is not conducive to food production. The increase in conflict and violence in several parts of the world and climate-related events also contribute to food security and nutrition problems.[80] Despite a 27% reduction in hunger worldwide since 2000[81] and an 11% decline in malnourished children in developing countries since 1990,[82] an estimated one in 10 people were food insecure in 2022.[83] Efforts are being implemented globally to address inequalities in food systems as well as inequalities in food security and nutrition.[84]

Migration and Health

Recent political events in the Middle East, Sudan, Ukraine, and the Democratic Republic of Congo have ignited a dramatic increase in migration and the number of displaced people. In 2023, 117.3 million individuals worldwide who had been forcibly displaced because of persecution, conflict, human rights violations, and events seriously disturbing the public order. In other words, one in every 69 people in the world's population is now forcibly displaced, which is nearly double the number a decade ago.[85] Of this number, 31.64 million were refugees, 67.08 million were internally displaced persons (IDPs), 6.86 million were asylum seekers, and 5.97 million were Palestine refugees under the United Nations Relief and Works Agency (UNRWA) mandate.[86] Millions of people have lost everything.

The surge of refugees and migrants creates challenges that require adequate preparedness, rapid humanitarian responses, and increased technical assistance. Unexpected pressure on health systems, social services, and employment systems can result in economic crises and other resource challenges when host countries are not adequately prepared for the influx. Consider how difficult it is sometimes to get the appropriate health care in a resource-rich country like the United States, then consider how difficult it might be to receive appropriate health care in a new country where you are not familiar with the structure of the healthcare system, where you do not speak the language, where you lack transportation, and where you lack resources to pay for the services. What makes this situation even worse is that many of the refugees and migrants are in countries that lack enough resources for their own residents and are, therefore, overwhelmed by the influx of people.[86]

Chapter Summary

- A number of key terms are associated with the study of community and public health, including *health, community, community health, population health, public health, public health system, global health, and social determinants of health.*

- The four factors that affect the health of a community are physical (e.g., community size), social and cultural (e.g., religion), community organization, and individual behaviors (e.g., exercise and diet).

- It is important to be familiar with and understand the history of community health to be able to deal with the present and future community and public health issues.

- The earliest community and public health practices went unrecorded; however, archeological findings of ancient societies (before 500 BCE) show evidence of concern for community and public health. There is evidence during the time of the classical cultures (500 BCE–500 CE) that people were interested in physical strength, medicine, and sanitation.

- The belief of many living during the Middle Ages (500–1500 CE) was that health and disease were associated with spirituality. Many epidemics were seen during this period.

- During the Renaissance period (1500–1700 CE), there was a growing belief that disease was caused by the environment, not spiritual factors.

- The eighteenth century was characterized by industrial growth. Science was being used more in medicine, and it was during this century that the first vaccine was discovered.

- The nineteenth century ushered in the modern era of public health. Germ theory was introduced during this time, and the last quarter of the century is known as the bacteriological period of public health.

- The twentieth century can be divided into several periods. The health resources development period (1900–1960) was a time when many public and private resources were used to improve health. The period of social engineering (1960–1973) saw the U.S. government's involvement in health insurance through Medicare and Medicaid. The health promotion period began in 1974 and continues today.

- *Healthy People 2030* and the National Prevention Strategy are important components of the community and public health agenda in the United States.

- Great concern continues to exist in the United States regarding health care, the environment, diseases caused by an impoverished lifestyle, the spread of communicable diseases, the harm caused by alcohol and other substance use, and terrorism.

- Although the health of the world population is improving, communicable diseases, poor sanitation and unsafe drinking water, hunger, and migration are burdens for many and impact the people who live in poverty much more than those who do not.

Scenario: Analysis and Response

The Internet offers many sources of information that could help Amy and Eric with the decisions that they will have to make about the continued use of the daycare center for their children. Use a search engine (e.g., Google, Bing) and enter (a) RSV and (b) RSV and daycare centers. Print out the information that you find and use it in answering the following questions.

1. Based on the information you found on the Internet, if you were Amy or Eric, would you take your children to the daycare center the next day? Why or why not?

2. Do you believe the RSV problem in daycare centers is a personal health concern or a community health concern? Why?

3. Which of the factors noted in this chapter that affect the health of a community play a part in the RSV problem that Amy and Eric faced?

4. Why does the RSV problem remind us of the health problems faced by people in this country prior to 1900?

5. Under which of the focus areas in the *Healthy People 2030* would RSV fall? Why?

Review Questions

1. How did the WHO define health in 1946? How has that definition been modified?

2. What is public health?

3. What are the differences among community health, population health, and global health?

4. What are the components of the social determinants of health and how do they impact the health of an individual?

5. What is the difference between personal health activities and community and public health activities?

6. Define the term *community*.

7. What are four major factors that affect the health of a community? Provide an example of each.

8. Identify some of the major events of community and public health in each of the following periods of time:

   Early civilizations (prior to 500 CE)

   Middle Ages (500–1500 CE)

   Renaissance and Exploration (1500–1700 CE)

   The eighteenth century

   The nineteenth century

9. Provide a brief explanation of the origins from which the following twentieth-century periods get their names:

   Health resources development period

   Period of social engineering

   Period of health promotion

10. What significance do the *Healthy People* documents have in community and public health development in recent years?

11. What significance do you think *Healthy People 2030* will have in the years ahead?

12. What is the National Prevention Strategy, and who is responsible for it?

13. What are the major community and public health problems facing the United States and the world in the twenty-first century?

Activities

1. Write your own definition for health.

2. Create a visual presentation using photos to explain how the social determinants of health could interact to reduce the risk of chronic disease in a community.

3. Create a public service announcement explaining why heart disease can be both a personal health problem and a community and public health problem.

4. Select a community and public health problem that exists in your hometown; then, using the factors that affect the health of a community noted in this chapter, analyze and discuss at least three factors that contribute to this problem.

5. Select one of the following individuals (all have been identified in this chapter). Using the Internet, find three reliable websites that provide information on the individual, and then write a two-page paper on the person's contribution to community and public health.

   Edward Jenner

   John Snow

   Lemuel Shattuck

   Louis Pasteur

   Robert Koch

   Walter Reed

6. Review the *Healthy People* website. Then, set up a time to talk with an administrator in your hometown health department. Find out which of the objectives the health department has been working on as priorities. Summarize in a paper what the objectives are, what the health department is doing about them, and what it hopes to accomplish by the year 2030.

7. Examine state and local COVID-19 data. Discuss the evidence you find to demonstrate the health disparities in your community? Based on what you have learned so far and your Internet search skills, recommend two strategies to help improve the situation experienced by those disparate groups. Explain your decision.

8. Share something learned from this chapter with a roommate, parent, friend, or colleague. Discuss how politics may have helped or hurt this situation. Submit a discussion board response or reflection response about the impact of politics on health.

References

1. Schneider, M. J. (2017). *Introduction to public health* (5th ed.). Jones & Bartlett Learning.

2. National Center for Health Statistics. (2016). *Health, United States, 2015: With special feature on racial and ethnic health disparities.* CDC, National Center for Health Statistics. Retrieved from http://www.cdc.gov/nchs/data/hus/hus15.pdf

3. Centers for Disease Control and Prevention, National Center for Health Statistics. (2024). *Life expectancy.* Retrieved from https://www.cdc.gov/nchs/fastats/life-expectancy.htm

4. Centers for Disease Control and Prevention. (1999). Ten great public health achievements—United States, 1900–1999. *Morbidity and Mortality Weekly Report, 48*(12), 241–243.

5. U.S. Department of Health and Human Services, Centers for Disease Control and Prevention. (2011). Ten great public health achievements—United States, 2001–2010. *Morbidity and Mortality Weekly Report, 60*(19), 619–623. Retrieved from https://www.cdc.gov/mmwr/preview/mmwrhtml/mm6019a5.htm?s_cid=mm6019a5_w

6. Centers for Disease Control and Prevention. (2023). *Cigarette smoking in the U.S.* Retrieved from https://www.cdc.gov/tobacco/data_statistics/fact_sheets/fast_facts/cigarette-smoking-in-the-us.html

7. Campaign for Tobacco-Free Kids. (2024). *U.S. state and local issues: Smoke-free laws.* Retrieved from https://www.tobaccofreekids.org/what-we-do/us/smoke-free-laws

8. Centers for Disease Control and Prevention. (2024). *Childhood lead poisoning prevention: About the data: Blood level surveillance.* Retrieved from https://www.cdc.gov/lead-prevention/php/data/blood-lead-surveillance.html

9. World Health Organization. (2024). *Frequently asked questions: What is the WHO definition of health?* Retrieved from https://www.who.int/about/frequently-asked-questions

10. World Health Organization. (2024). *Health promotion.* Retrieved from https://www.who.int/teams/health-promotion/enhanced-wellbeing/first-global-conference

11. Centers for Disease Control and Prevent. (CDC). (2024). *Social determinants of Health.* Retrieved from https://www.cdc.gov/about/priorities/why-is-addressing-sdoh-important.html

12. Joint Committee on Health Education and Promotion Terminology. (2012). Report of the 2011 Joint Committee on Health Education and Promotion Terminology. *American Journal of Health Education, 43*(2), 1–19.

13. Israel, B. A., Checkoway, B., Schulz, A., & Zimmerman, M. (1994). Health education and community empowerment: Conceptualizing and measuring perceptions of individual, organizational, and community control. *Health Education Quarterly, 21*(2), 149–170.

14. Carrillo, A., Nava, M., Rothschild, S. K., & Saw, A. (2017). What is a healthy community? *Working paper No. 7.* Center for Community Health Equity. Chicago, IL.

15. Institute of Medicine. (2003). *The future of the public's health in the 21st century.* National Academies Press.

16. Institute of Medicine. (1988). *The future of public health.* National Academies Press.

17. Kindig, D., & Stoddart, G. (2003). What is population health? *American Journal of Public Health, 93*(3), 380–383.

18. Institute of Medicine. (1997). *America's vital interest in global health: Protecting our people, enhancing our economy, and advancing our international interests.* National Academies Press. Retrieved from http://books.nap.edu/openbook.php?record_id=5717&page=R1

19. Coupland, K., Rikhy, S., Hill, K., & McNeil, D. (2011). *State of evidence: The built environment and health 2011–2015.* Public Health Innovation and Decision Support, Population, & Public Health, Alberta Health Services.

20. Davidson, A. (2015). *Social determinants of health: A comparative approach.* Oxford University Press.

21. Institute of Medicine. (2005). *Does the built environment influence physical activity? Examining the evidence.* National Academies Press.

22. American College Health Association. (2019). *American College Health Association—National College Health Assessment II (ACHA NCHA II) Spring 2019 Reference Group Executive Summary Spring 2023.* Retrieved from https://www.acha.org/documents/ncha/NCHA-III_SPRING_2023_REFERENCE_GROUP_EXECUTIVE_SUMMARY.pdf

23. American College Health Association. (2019). *American College Health Association—National College Health Assessment II (ACHA-NCHA II) Spring 2019: Reference Group Executive Summary.* Retrieved from https://www.acha.org/documents/ncha/NCHA-II_SPRING_2019_US_REFERENCE_GROUP_EXECUTIVE_SUMMARY.pdf

24. Shi, L., & Singh, D. A. (2017). *Essentials of the U.S. health care system* (4th ed.). Jones & Bartlett Learning.

25. Issel, L. M. (2014). *Health program planning and evaluation: A practical systematic approach for community health* (3rd ed.). Jones & Bartlett Learning.

26. Minkler, M., & Wallerstein, N. (2012). Improving health through community organization and community building: Perspectives from health education and social work. In M. Minkler (Ed.), *Community organizing and community building for health and welfare* (3rd ed.; pp. 37–58). Rutgers University Press.

27. Ross, M. G. (1967). *Community organization: Theory, principles, and practice.* Harper & Row.

28. Pickett, G., & Hanlon, J. J. (1990). *Public health: Administration and practice* (9th ed.). Times Mirror/Mosby.

29. Legon, R. P. (1986). Ancient Greece. In *World Book Encyclopedia.* World Book.

30. Rosen, G. (1958). *A history of public health.* MD Publications.

31. Burton, L. E., Smith, H. H., & Nichols, A. W. (1980). *Public health and community medicine* (3rd ed.). Williams & Wilkins.

32. Woodruff, A. W. (1977). Benjamin Rush, his work on yellow fever and his British connections. *American Journal of Tropical Medicine and Hygiene, 26*(5), 1055–1059.

33. Rosen, G. (1975). *Preventive medicine in the United States, 1900–1975.* Science History Publications.

34. Smillie, W. G. (1955). *Public health: Its promise for the future.* Macmillan.

35. Duffy, J. (1990). *The sanitarians: A history of American public health.* University of Illinois Press.

36. Lalonde, M. (1974). *A new perspective on the health of Canadians: A working document.* Minister of Health.

37. Green, L. W. (1999). Health education's contributions to the twentieth century: A glimpse through health promotion's rearview mirror. In J. E. Fielding, L. B. Lave, & B. Starfield (Eds.), *Annual review of public health* (pp. 67–88). Annual Reviews.

38. U.S. Department of Health and Human Services, Public Health Service. (1980). *Ten leading causes of death in the United States, 1977.* U.S. Government Printing Office.

39. U.S. Department of Health, Education, and Welfare. (1979). *Healthy People: The Surgeon General's report on health promotion and disease prevention* (DHEW pub. No. 79-55071). U.S. Government Printing Office.

40. McKenzie, J. F., Neiger, B. L., & Thackeray, R. (2017). *Planning, implementing, and evaluating health promotion programs: A primer* (7th ed.). Pearson.

41. U.S. Department of Health and Human Services. (1980). *Promoting health/preventing disease: Objectives for the nation.* U.S. Government Printing Office.

42. U.S. Department of Health and Human Services. (2024). *Healthy People 2030.* Retrieved from https://health.gov/healthypeople

43. U.S. Department of Health and Human Services, Office of the Surgeon General. (2011). *National Prevention Strategy.* Retrieved from https://www.hhs.gov/sites/default/files/disease-prevention -wellness-report.pdf

44. Centers for Medicare and Medicaid Services. (2024). *National health expenditure fact sheet.* Retrieved from https://www .cms.gov/data-research/statistics-trends-and-reports/national -health-expenditure-data/nhe-fact-sheet

45. Sisko, A. M., Keehan, S. P., Poisal, J. A., Cuckler, G. A., Smith, S. D., Madison, A. J., Rennie, K. E., & Hardesty, J. C. (2019). National health expenditure projections, 2018–27: Economic and demographic trends drive spending and enrollment. *Health Affairs, 38*(3). Retrieved from https://www.healthaffairs.org/doi/abs/10.1377 /hlthaff.2018.05499

46. U.S. Census Bureau. (2023). *U.S. and World Population Clock. Retrieved from* https://www.census.gov/popclock/

47. Shiels, M., Haque, A., Berrington de Gonzalez, A., & Freedman, N. D. (2022). Leading causes of death in the US during the COVID-19 pandemic, March 202 to October 2021. *JAMA Intern Med. 182*(8), 883–886.

48. Centers for Disease Control and Prevention. (2024). *Leading causes of death and injury.* Retrieved from https://www.cdc.gov/injury /wisqars/LeadingCauses.html

49. Centers for Disease Control and Prevention. (CDC). (2023). *Health and economic costs of chronic diseases.* Retrieved from https://www .cdc.gov/chronicdisease/about/costs/index.htm

50. Centers for Disease Control and Prevention. (CDC). (2024). *About chronic diseases.* Retrieved from https://www.cdc.gov /chronic-disease/about/

51. Ford, E., Bergmann, M., Boening, H., Li, Ch., Capewell, S. (2015). Healthy lifestyle behaviors and all-cause mortality among adults in the United States. *Prev Med, 2012 Jul: 55*(1), 23–27. Retrieved from https://www.ncbi.nlm.nih.gov/pmc/articles/PMC4688898/

52. Centers for Disease Control and Prevention. (1981). Pneumocystis pneumonia—Los Angeles. *Morbidity and Mortality Weekly Report, 30,* 250–252.

53. Centers for Disease Control and Prevention. (1989). First 100,000 cases of acquired immunodeficiency syndrome—United States. *Morbidity and Mortality Weekly Report, 38,* 561–563.

54. Centers for Disease Control and Prevention. (1992). The second 100,000 cases of acquired immunodeficiency syndrome—United States, June 1981–December 1991. *Morbidity and Mortality Weekly Report, 42*(2), 28–29.

55. Centers for Disease Control and Prevention. (2024). *HIV.* Retrieved from https://www.cdc.gov/hiv/index.html

56. Interpol. (2024). *Bioterrorism.* Retrieved from https://www.interpol .int/en/Crimes/Terrorism/Bioterrorism

57. National Institute on Drug Abuse. (2020). *Trends & statistics: Costs of substance abuse.* Retrieved from https://www.drugabuse.gov /related-topics /trends-statistics

58. National Institute on Drug Abuse. (2024). *Drug overdose death rates.* Retrieved from https://nida.nih.gov/research-topics/trends-statistics /overdose-death-rates

59. U.S. Food & Drug Administration. (2023). *FDA news release: FDA approves first over-the-counter naloxone nasal spray.* Retrieved from https://www.fda.gov/news-events/press-announcements /fda-approves-first-over-counter-naloxone-nasal-spray

60. Centers for Disease Control and Prevention. (2019). *CDC guideline for prescribing opioids for chronic pain.* Retrieved from https:// emergency.cdc.gov/coca/calls/opioidresources.asp

61. National Institute on Drug Abuse. (2024). *Harm reduction.* Retrieved from https://nida.nih.gov/research-topics/harm-reduction

62. Videto, D. M. & Dennis, D. L. (2021). Report of the 2020 joint committee on health education and promotion terminology. *The Health Educator, 53*(1):3–19.

63. King, N. B. (2014). Health inequalities and health inequities. In E. E. Morrison & B. Furlong (Eds.), *Health care ethics: Critical issues for the 21st century* (pp. 301–316). Jones & Bartlett Learning.

64. Mheidly, M., Fares, N. Y., Fares, M. Y., & Fares, J. (2023). Emerging health disparities during the COVID-19 pandemic. *Avicenna J Med 13*(1):60–64. doi: 10.1055/s-0042-1759842 Retrieved from https:// www.ncbi.nlm.nih.gov/pmc/articles/PMC10038746/

65. U.S. Department of Homeland Security. (2024). *Ready: Disasters and emergencies.* Retrieved from https://www.ready.gov/be-informed

66. Nelson, C., Lurie, N., Wasserman, J., & Zakowski, S. (2007). Conceptualizing and defining public health emergency preparedness. *American Journal of Public Health, 97* (Suppl 1), S9–S11. Retrieved from https://www.ncbi.nlm.nih.gov/pmc/articles/PMC1854988/

67. Trust for America's Health. (2024). *Ready or not? Protecting the public's health from disease, disasters, and bioterrorism.* Retrieved from https://www.tfah.org/wp-content/uploads/2024/03/2024-ReadyOrNot -FINAL

68. World Health Organization. (2024). *World health statistics 2024: Monitoring health for the SDGs, sustainable development goals. Geneva: World Health Organization.* Retrieved from https://www .who.int/data/gho/publications/world-health-statistics

69. U.S. Department of Health and Human Services, Centers for Disease Control and Prevention. (2011). Ten great public health achievements—worldwide, 2001–2010. *Morbidity and Mortality Weekly Report, 60*(24), 814–818. Retrieved from https://www.cdc .gov/mmwr/preview/mmwrhtml/mm6024a4.htm

70. World Health Organization. (2024). *Vaccines and immunizations.* Retrieved from https://www.who.int/health-topics/vaccines -and-immunization#tab=tab_1

71. World Health Organization. (2024). *Drinking water.* Retrieved from https://www.who.int/news-room/fact-sheets/detail/drinking-water

72. World Health Organization. (2023). *World malaria report 2023.* Geneva: World Health Organization.

73. World Health Organization. (2023). *HIV and AIDS.* Retrieved from https://www.who.int/news-room/fact-sheets/detail/hiv-aids

74. World Health Organization. (2023). *Tuberculosis.* Retrieved from https://www.who.int/news-room/fact-sheets/detail/tuberculosis

75. World Health Organization. (2023). *Tobacco.* Retrieved from https:// www.who.int/news-room/fact-sheets/detail/tobacco

76. World Health Organization. (2023). *Despite notable progress, road safety remains urgent global issue.* Retrieved from https://www.who .int/news/item/13-12-2023-despite-notable-progress-road-safety -remains-urgent-global-issue

77. World Health Organization. (2023). *Facts about water: Statistics of the water crisis.* Retrieved from https://thewaterproject.org /water-scarcity/water_stats

78. Centers for Disease Control and Prevention. (2024). *Global water, sanitation & hygiene (WASH): About global sanitation.* Retrieved from https://www.cdc.gov/global-water-sanitation-hygiene/about /about-global-sanitation.html

79. Hunger. (n.d.). *Merriam-Webster Dictionary.* Retrieved from http:// www.merriam-webster.com/dictionary/hunger

80. World Health Organization. (2023). *The state of food security and nutrition in the world 2023.* Retrieved from https:// www.who.int/publications/m/item/the-state-of-food-security -and-nutrition-in-the-world-2023

81. International Food Policy Research Institute. (2020). *2017 global hunger index: The inequalities of hunger.* Retrieved from https://www .ifpri.org /publication/2017-global-hunger-index-inequalities-hunger

82. World Health Organization. (2014). *Twelfth general programme of work: Not merely the absence of disease.* Retrieved from http://www .who.int/about /resources_planning/twelfth-gpw/en/

83. Ritchie, H., Rosado, P., & Roser, M. (2024). *Hunger and undernourishment.* Retrieved from https://ourworldindata.org/hunger -and-undernourishment

84. High Level Panel Experts (HLPE). (2023). *Reducing inequalities for food security and nutrition.* Rome, CFS HLPE-FSN. Retrieved from https://www.fao.org/cfs/cfs-hlpe/publications/hlpe-18

85. United Nations High Commission for Refugees (UNHCR). (2024). *Data and statistics: Global trends.* Retrieved from https://www.unhcr.org/us/global-trends

86. World Health Organization. (2022). *Refugee and migrant health.* Retrieved from https://www.who.int/news-room/fact-sheets/detail/refugee-and-migrant-health

CHAPTER 2

Organizations That Help Shape Community and Public Health

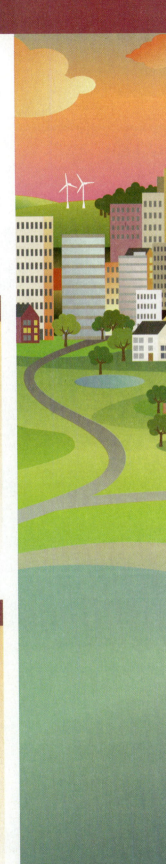

Chapter Objectives

After studying this chapter, you will be able to:

1. Summarize the need for organizing to improve community and public health.

2. Explain what a governmental health organization is and give an example of one at each of the following levels— international, national, state, and local.

3. Discuss the role the World Health Organization (WHO) plays in community and public health.

4. Briefly describe the structure and function of the U.S. Department of Health and Human Services (HHS).

5. State the three core functions of public health.

6. List the 10 essential public health services.

7. Describe the relationship between a state and local health department.

8. Explain what is meant by Whole School, Whole Community, Whole Child (WSCC).

9. Define the term *quasi-governmental* and explain why some health organizations are classified under this term.

10. List the four primary activities of most voluntary health organizations.

11. Explain the purpose of a professional health organization/association.

12. Demonstrate how philanthropic foundations contribute to community and public health.

Chapter Objectives   *(continued)*

13. Discuss the role that service, social, and religious organizations play in community and public health.

14. Identify the major reason why corporations are involved in community and public health, and describe some corporate activities that contribute to community and public health.

Scenario

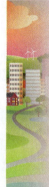

Mary is a hardworking senior at the local university. She is majoring in physical education and looking forward to teaching elementary physical education after graduation. Mary has always been involved in team sports and has been a lifeguard at the local swimming pool for the past 4 years. Mary has a fair complexion with honey-blonde hair and blue eyes. She has always tanned easily, so has not bothered very much with sunscreens. For the past few weeks, Mary has noticed a red, scaly, sharply outlined patch of skin on her forehead. She has put creams and ointments on it, but it will not go away and may be getting larger. Her roommate, Clare, suggests that she make an appointment with the campus health services office. Mary lets it go another week and then decides to see the doctor.

After looking at the patch of skin, the doctor refers Mary to a specialist, Dr. Rice, who is a dermatologist. The dermatologist suggests a biopsy be taken of the lesion to test for skin cancer. The specialist tells Mary that if it is cancer, it is probably still in its early stages and so the prognosis is good.

A potential diagnosis of cancer often raises a lot of questions and concerns. Are there any resources in the community to which Mary can turn for help?

Introduction

The history of community and public health dates to antiquity. For much of that history, community and public health issues were addressed only on an emergency basis. For example, if a community faced a drought or an epidemic, a town meeting would be called to deal with the problem. Only in the last 100 years or so have communities taken explicit actions to deal aggressively with health issues on a continual basis.

Today's communities differ from those of the past in several important ways. Although individuals are better educated, more mobile, and more independent than in the past, communities are less autonomous and are more dependent on state and federal funding for support. Contemporary communities are too large and complex to respond effectively to sudden health emergencies or to make long-term improvements in community and public health without community organization and careful planning. Better community organizing and careful long-term planning are essential to ensure that a community makes the best use of its resources for health, both in times of emergency and over the long run.

The ability of today's communities to respond effectively to their own problems is hindered by the following characteristics: (1) highly developed and centralized resources in our national institutions and organizations; (2) continuing concentration of wealth and population in the largest metropolitan areas; (3) rapid movement of information, resources, and people made possible by advanced communication and transportation technologies that eliminate the need for local offices where resources were once housed; (4) the globalization of health; (5) limited horizontal relationships between/among organizations; and (6) a system of **top-down funding** (an approach where money is transmitted from either the federal or state government to the local level) for many community programs.[1]

In this chapter, we discuss organizations that help to shape a community's ability to respond effectively to health-related issues by protecting and promoting the health of the community and its members. These community organizations can be classified as governmental, quasi-governmental, and nongovernmental—according to their sources of funding, responsibilities, and organizational structure.

Top-down funding a method of funding in which funds are transmitted from federal or state government to the local level

Governmental Health Agencies

Governmental health agencies are part of the governmental structure (federal, state, tribal and/or territorial, or local). They are funded primarily by tax dollars and managed by government officials. Each governmental health agency is designated as having authority over some geographic area. Such agencies exist at the four governmental levels—international, national, state, and local.

International Health Agencies

The most widely recognized international governmental health organization today is the **World Health Organization (WHO)** (see **Figure 2.1**). The WHO headquarters is in Geneva, Switzerland, and there are six regional offices around the world. The names, acronyms, and cities and countries of location for WHO regional offices are as follows: Africa (AFRO), Brazzaville, Congo; Americas (PAHO), Washington, D.C., United States; Eastern Mediterranean (EMRO), Cairo, Egypt; Europe (EURO), Copenhagen, Denmark; Southeast Asia (SEARO), New Delhi, India; and Western Pacific (WPRO), Manila, Philippines.[2]

Although the WHO is now the largest international health organization, it is not the oldest. Among the organizations (listed with their founding dates) that predate WHO are the following:

- International D'Hygiène Publique (1907); absorbed by the WHO
- Health Organization of the League of Nations (1919); dissolved when the WHO was created
- United Nations Relief and Rehabilitation Administration (1943); dissolved in 1946—its work is carried out today by the Office of the United Nations High Commissioner for Refugees (UNHCR) (1950)
- United Nations Children's Fund (UNICEF) (1946); formerly known as the United Nations International Children's Emergency Fund
- Pan American Health Organization (PAHO) (1902); still an independent organization but is integrated with WHO in a regional office

Because the WHO is the largest and most visible international health agency, it is discussed at greater length in the following sections.

History of the World Health Organization

Planning for the WHO began when a charter of the United Nations was adopted at an international meeting in 1945. Contained in the charter was an article calling for the establishment of a health agency with wide powers. In 1946, at the International Health Conference, representatives from all of the countries in the United Nations succeeded in creating and ratifying the constitution of the WHO. However, it was not until April 7, 1948, that the constitution went into force and the organization officially began its work. In recognition of this beginning, April 7 is commemorated each year as World Health Day with a theme reflecting a priority area of current concern to WHO.[2]

Organization of the World Health Organization

"WHO works worldwide to promote health, keep the world safe, and serve the vulnerable" with the goal of ensuring universal health coverage, protect people from health emergencies, and provide individuals with better health and well-being.[3] Membership in the WHO is open to any nation that has ratified the WHO constitution and receives a majority vote of the World Health Assembly. Currently, there are 194 member states. The

Governmental health agencies health agencies that are part of the governmental structure (federal, state, or local) and that are funded primarily by tax dollars

World Health Organization (WHO) the most widely recognized international governmental health organization

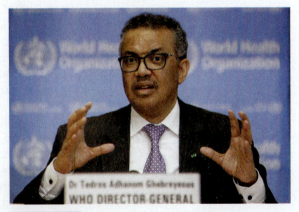

FIGURE 2.1   Ethiopia's Dr. Tedros Adhanom Ghebreyesus, Director–General of the World Health Organization, is serving his second term.

World Health Assembly comprises the delegates of the member nations. This assembly, which meets in general sessions annually and in special sessions when necessary, has the primary tasks of determining policies, appointing the director–general, supervising financial policies, and reviewing and approving the proposed program budget.[4]

The WHO is administered by a staff that includes an appointed director–general, a deputy director–general, seven assistant directors–general, and six regional directors. Great care is taken to ensure political balance in staffing WHO positions, particularly at the higher levels of administration. The WHO includes more than 8,000 people working in 150 country offices, six regional offices, as well as the headquarters in Geneva, Switzerland.[2]

Purpose and Work of the World Health Organization

The purpose of the WHO is "to help people achieve the highest possible level of health for all people." The WHO supports this through the following types of activities:

- Providing technical assistance to countries
- Setting international health standards
- Providing guidance on important health issues
- Coordinating and supporting international response to health emergencies, such as disease outbreaks
- Promoting and advocating for better global health

The WHO's overarching vision for the 2025–2028 period is to "promote, provide, and protect the health and well-being of all people, everywhere." The WHO has established six strategic priorities[5]:

1. Respond to climate change, an escalating health threat in the 21st century.
2. Address health determinants and the root causes of ill health in key policies across sectors.
3. Advance the primary health care approach and essential health system capacities for universal health coverage.
4. Improve health service coverage and financial protection to address inequity and gender inequalities.
5. Prevent, mitigate, and prepare for risks to health from all hazards.
6. Rapidly detect and sustain an effective response to all health emergencies, as outlined in its "general programme of work."

This document, which is a requirement of the WHO constitution, sets a high-level roadmap and agenda for global health, identifies priorities and strategic direction, as well as a framework for resource allocation and decision-making. The Fourteenth General Programme of Work,[5] covers the years 2025–2028.

The work of the WHO is financed by its member states with assessed and voluntary contributions. Each member state is assessed according to its ability to pay; the wealthiest countries contribute the most. Voluntary contributions also come from the member states and account for 80% of the budget financing.[6]

The WHO has sponsored and continues to sponsor many worthwhile programs. An especially noteworthy program was the work of the WHO in helping to eradicate smallpox. At one time, smallpox was the world's most feared disease, until it was eradicated by a collaborative global vaccination program led by the WHO.[2] The year 2019 marked the fortieth anniversary of smallpox eradication.[7] In 1967, smallpox was active in 31 countries. During that year, 10 to 15 million people contracted the disease, and of those, approximately 2 million died. Many millions of others were permanently disfigured or blinded. The last known natural case of smallpox was diagnosed on October 26, 1977, in Somalia.[2] In 1978, a laboratory accident in Birmingham, England, resulted in one death and a limited outbreak of the acute disease. In 1979, the World Health Assembly declared the global eradication of this disease. Using the smallpox mortality figures from 1967, it can be estimated that more than 60 million lives have been saved since the eradication.

More recently, the WHO has led the efforts to contain the outbreaks of the coronavirus (COVID-19). Within weeks of the outbreak, the WHO convened a global research and innovation forum to mobilize response to the outbreak. Major research funders and over 300 scientists and researchers gathered to examine all aspects of the outbreak, ways to control it, and urgent global research priorities.[8] At time of publication, the COVID-19 pandemic is in its fourth year and surveillance efforts have declined dramatically. WHO has updated its Strategic Preparedness and Response plan for 2023–2025 and is working to support countries as they transition their emergency response activities to longer-term sustained COVID-19 disease prevention, control, and management.[9]

In 2015, the countries in the United Nations adopted the 2030 Agenda for **Sustainable Development Goals (SDGs)**. These 17 goals were established to be interconnected and are concentrated toward ending poverty and inequality, addressing climate change, and ensuring that all people enjoy health, justice, and prosperity. Most of the Goals have some direct health targets and are associated with specific indicators in which progress can be measured.[10] The WHO publishes an annual compilation of health and health-related indicators associated with the SGDs and WHO's General Programme of Work.[11]

Table 2.1 provides a list of the 17 SDGs.

Sustainable Development Goals (SDGs) a shared set of goals adopted by the United Nations member states focused on ending poverty and inequality, protecting the planet, and ensuring health for all adopted by all

National Health Agencies

Each national government has a department or agency that has the primary responsibility for the protection of the health and welfare of its citizens. These national health agencies meet their responsibilities through the development of health policies, the enforcement of health regulations, the provision of health services and programs, the funding of research, and the support of their respective state and local health agencies.

TABLE 2.1 Seventeen Sustainable Development Goals	
Goal 1	End poverty in all its forms everywhere.
Goal 2	Zero hunger—end hunger, achieve food security, and improved nutrition and promote sustainable agriculture.
Goal 3	Ensure healthy lives and promote well-being for all at all ages.
Goal 4	Ensure inclusive and equitable quality education and promote lifelong learning opportunities for all.
Goal 5	Achieve gender equality and empower all women and girls.
Goal 6	Ensure availability and sustainable management of water and sanitation for all.
Goal 7	Ensure access to affordable, reliable, sustainable, and modern energy for all.
Goal 8	Promote sustained, inclusive, and sustainable economic growth, full and productive employment, and decent work for all.
Goal 9	Build resilient infrastructure, promote inclusive and sustainable industrialization, and foster innovation.
Goal 10	Reduce inequality within and among countries.
Goal 11	Make cities and human settlements inclusive, safe, resilient, and sustainable.
Goal 12	Ensure sustainable consumption and production patterns.
Goal 13	Take urgent action to combat climate change and its impacts.
Goal 14	Conserve and sustainably use the oceans, seas, and marine resources for sustainable development.
Goal 15	Protect, restore, and promote sustainable use of terrestrial ecosystems; sustainably manage forests; combat desertification; and halt and reverse land degradation and halt biodiversity loss.
Goal 16	Promote peaceful and inclusive societies for sustainable development, provide access to justice for all, and build effective, accountable, and inclusive institutions at all levels.
Goal 17	Strengthen the means of implementation and revitalize the Global Partnership for Sustainable Development.

Data from United Nations. (2024). *Sustainable Development Goals: The 17 Goals*. Available at https://sdgs.un.org/goals

In the United States, the primary national health agency is the Department of Health and Human Services (HHS). The mission of HHS is to enhance the health and well-being of all Americans. HHS does this by providing health and human services and advancing medicine, public health, and social services.[12] Many other federal agencies also contribute to the betterment of our nation's health. For example, the U.S. Department of Agriculture (USDA) inspects meat and dairy products and coordinates the Special Supplemental Nutrition Program for Women, Infants, and Children, better known as the WIC food assistance program; the Environmental Protection Agency (EPA) regulates hazardous wastes; the Department of Labor houses the Occupational Safety and Health Administration (OSHA), which is concerned with safety and health in the workplace; the Department of Commerce, which includes the Bureau of the Census, collects much of the national data that drive our nation's health programs; and the Department of Homeland Security (DHS) deals with all aspects of terrorism within the United States. A detailed description of the HHS follows.

Department of Health and Human Services

The HHS is headed by the Secretary of Health and Human Services, who is appointed by the president and is a member of the cabinet. The Department of Health and Human Services was formed in 1980 (during the administration of President Jimmy Carter), when the Department of Health, Education, and Welfare (HEW) was divided into two new departments—HHS and the Department of Education. HHS is the department most involved with the nation's human concerns. In one way or another it touches the lives of more Americans than any other federal agency. It is literally a department of people serving people, from newborn infants to persons requiring health services to our most older citizens, with an annual budget of $1.7 trillion.[13]

The 2024 fiscal year budget proposed $144.3 billion in discretionary budget authority and $1.7 trillion in mandatory HHS funding. The budget proposal addresses urgent challenges, including a growing behavioral health crisis, the need to prepare for future public health threats, and the large arrival of unaccompanied children and refugees. In an effort to secure a healthier, more vibrant future for all Americans, specific investments are being made to expand coverage and access to care; address the needs of those most at risk, including Indian Country, children, families, and older adults; growing the health workforce; and advancing science to improve health.[13]

Since its formation, HHS has undergone several reorganizations. Some of the more recent changes include the addition of the Advanced Research Projects Agency for Health and Office of the National Coordinator for Health Information Technology. Furthermore, the Administration for Strategic Preparedness and Response has changed from an Office of the Secretary to an official operating division. Currently, the HHS is organized into 12 operating divisions/agencies (see **Figure 2.2**) whose heads report directly to the Secretary. In addition, the HHS has 10 regional offices . These offices serve as representatives of the Secretary of HHS in direct, official dealings with state and local governmental organizations. Ten of the 13 operating divisions of HHS (AHRQ, ARPA-H, ASPR, ATSDR, CDC, FDA, HRSA, IHS, NIH, and SAMHSA—see their descriptions in the following sections), along with the Office of Global Affairs (OGA), constitute the Public Health Service (PHS). Another three operating divisions (CMS, ACF, and ACL, described later) comprise the human services operating divisions.

Administration for Children and Families (ACF)

The ACF is a division of HHS that promotes the economic and social well-being of families, children, individuals, and communities. One of the better-known programs originating from this division is Head Start, which serves more than 800,000 preschool children annually, promotes school readiness for children birth to age 5 in low-income families through services that support early learning and development.[14] Other programs focus on family assistance, refugee resettlement, and child support enforcement.

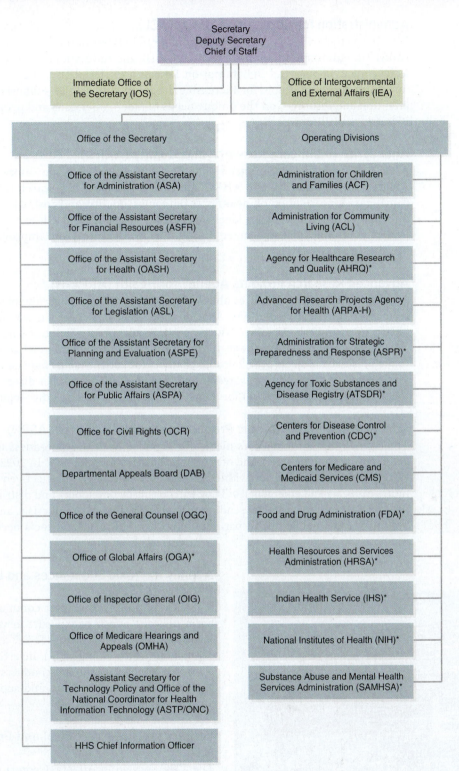

FIGURE 2.2   Organizational chart for the U.S. Department of Health and Human Services (HHS).

*Designates a component of the U.S. Public Health Service.

Reproduced from U.S. Department of Health and Human Services. (2024). *U.S. Department of Health and Human Services Organizational Chart.* Available at https://www.hhs.gov/about/agencies/orgchart/index.html. Accessed June 28, 2024.

Administration for Community Living (ACL)

The ACL is the division of the HHS that integrates efforts of the Administration on Aging (AoA), the Administration on Disabilities (AoD), and the National Institute on Disability, Independent Living, and Rehabilitation Research (NIDILRR).[15] The ACL serves as the federal agency responsible for increasing access to community supports while focusing attention and resources on the unique needs of older Americans and people with disabilities across the life span.[15]

Agency for Healthcare Research and Quality (AHRQ)

AHRQ is the lead federal agency charged with improving the safety and quality of America's healthcare system. AHRQ sponsors and conducts research that provides evidence-based information on healthcare outcomes; quality; and cost, use, and access. The information helps healthcare decision-makers—patients and clinicians, health system leaders, and policymakers—make more informed decisions and improve the quality of healthcare services.[16]

Advanced Research Projects Agency for Health (ARPA-H)

Created in 2022, ARPA-H was established to improve the U.S. government's ability to speed biomedical and health solutions. As a funding agency, ARPA-H invests in breakthrough technologies and solutions "with the potential to advance medicine and health that cannot readily be accomplished through traditional research or commercial activity."[17] Current funded research projects are exploring chatbots for patient-facing applications, treatments for neurodegenerative diseases, retraining immune cells to combat diseases, autonomous robotic surgery, restoring sight for people who are blind, among other topics.[18]

Administration for Strategic Preparedness and Response (ASPR)

This agency "leads the nation's medical and public health preparedness for, response to, and recovery from disasters and other public health emergencies."[19] In 2022, ASPR was elevated to an operating division within HHS to more efficiently and effectively respond during future disasters and emergencies. They will do this by developing and distributing response tools against multiple threats, sending response teams in times of crisis, and ensuring that health care and public health partners have the knowledge and tools needed to navigate whatever challenges are ahead.[19]

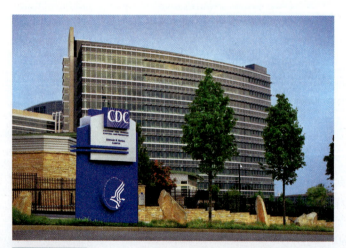

FIGURE 2.3   The Centers for Disease Control and Prevention in Atlanta, Georgia, is one of the major operating divisions of the Department of Health and Human Services.

Courtesy of James Gathany/CDC.

Agency for Toxic Substances and Disease Registry (ATSDR)

ATSDR's purpose is to protect communities from the harmful health effects of exposure to natural and man-made hazardous substances. ATSDR responds to environmental health emergencies, investigates emerging environmental health threats, conducts research on the health impacts of waste sites, and supports state and local health partners.[20]

Centers for Disease Control and Prevention (CDC)

The CDC, located in Atlanta, Georgia (see **Figure 2.3**), is the nation's leading health protection agency, dedicated to saving lives and protecting people from health threats. Once known solely for its work to control communicable diseases, the CDC now also maintains records, analyzes disease trends, and publishes epidemiologic reports on all types of diseases, including those that result from lifestyle, occupational, and environmental causes. Beyond its own specific responsibilities, the CDC also supports state and local health departments and cooperates with similar national health agencies from other WHO member nations.

The CDC prides itself on working 24/7 to protect America from health, safety, and security threats. They do this by:

- Detecting and responding to new and emerging health threats
- Tackling the biggest health problems causing death and disability for Americans
- Putting science and advanced technology into action to prevent disease
- Promoting healthy and safe behaviors, communities, and environment
- Developing leaders and training the public health workforce, including disease detectives
- Taking the health pulse of our nation[21]

To carry out its work, the CDC is organized into centers, institutes, and offices (CIOs). The CIOs allow the agency to be more responsive and effective when dealing with public health concerns. Each group implements the CDC's response in their areas of expertise, while also providing intra-agency support and resource sharing for cross-cutting issues and specific health threats.[22] **Figure 2.4** shows how the CIOs are organized in the CDC.

Like other public health agencies, the CDC's most important achievements are the outbreaks that do not happen, the communicable diseases that are stopped before spreading, and the lives saved from preventable chronic diseases and injuries. Learning from the commitment to equity and diversity during the COVID-19 pandemic, the CDC is dedicated to "use timely data and science to drive and communicate customer-centered, high-impact public health action."[21]

Food and Drug Administration (FDA)

The FDA touches the lives of virtually every American, every day. It is responsible for "protecting the public health by ensuring the safety, efficacy, and security of human and veterinary drugs, biological products, and medical devices; and by ensuring the safety of our nation's food supply, cosmetics, and products that emit radiation."[22]

Specifically, the FDA is responsible for advancing the public health by doing the following:

- Helping to speed innovations that make medical products safer, more effective, and more affordable
- Providing the public with the accurate, science-based information they need to use medical products and foods to maintain and improve their health
- Regulating the manufacturing, marketing, and distribution of tobacco products to protect the public and reduce tobacco use by minors
- Addressing the nation's counterterrorism capability and ensuring the security of the supply of foods and medical products[22]

Much of this work revolves around regulatory activities and the setting of health and safety standards as spelled out in the Federal Food, Drug, and Cosmetic Act and other related laws. However, because of the complex nature of its standards and the agency's limited resources, enforcement of many FDA regulations is left to other federal agencies and to state and local agencies. For example, the USDA is responsible for the inspection of many foods, such as meat and dairy products. Restaurants, supermarkets, and other food outlets are inspected by state and local public health agencies.

Centers for Medicare and Medicaid Services (CMS)

Established as the Health Care Financing Administration (HCFA) in 1977, the CMS is responsible for overseeing the Medicare program (health care for people 65 and older and people with disabilities), the federal portion of the Medicaid program (health care for low-income children and adults), and the related quality assurance activities. Both Medicare and Medicaid were created in 1965 to ensure that the special groups covered by these programs would not be deprived of health care because of cost. Currently, approximately one-third of Americans are covered by these programs.[23] In 1997, the State Children's Health Insurance

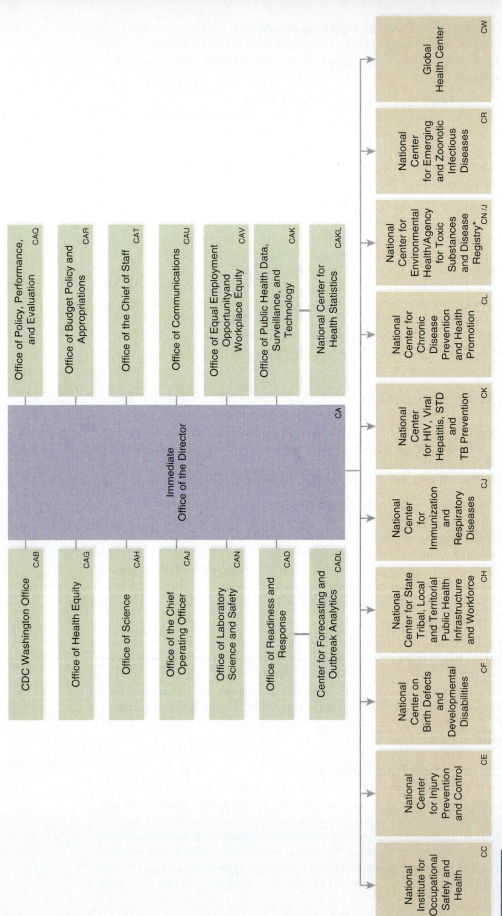

FIGURE 2.4   Organizational chart of the Centers for Disease Control and Prevention.

Program (SCHIP), now known as the Children's Health Insurance Program (CHIP), also became the responsibility of the CMS. Medicare, Medicaid, and CHIP are discussed in greater detail elsewhere in the text.

Health Resources and Services Administration (HRSA)

The HRSA is the principal primary healthcare service agency of the federal government that provides access to essential healthcare services for people who are geographically isolated and economically or medically vulnerable. The cited mission of HRSA is "to improve health outcomes and achieve health equity through access to quality services, a skilled health workforce, and innovative, high-value programs."[24] HRSA maintains the National Health Service Corps and helps build the healthcare workforce through training and education programs. HRSA is also responsible for overseeing the nation's organ, bone marrow, and cord blood donation system.[24]

Indian Health Service (IHS)

The IHS provides federal health services to American Indians and Alaska Natives. As the principal federal healthcare provider and health advocate for Indian people, IHS serves approximately 2.6 million American Indians and Alaska Natives who belong to 574 federally recognized tribes in 37 states. With the goal of raising their physical, mental, social, and spiritual health to the highest possible level, IHS works to ensure that comprehensive, culturally appropriate services are available and accessible.[25]

Although health services have been provided sporadically by the United States government since the early nineteenth century, it was not until 1989 that the IHS was elevated to an agency level; prior to that time, it was a division in HRSA.

National Institutes of Health (NIH)

Begun as a one-room Laboratory of Hygiene in 1887, the NIH today is one of the world's foremost medical research centers and the federal focal point for medical research in the United States.[27] The mission of the NIH "is to seek fundamental knowledge about the nature and behavior of living systems and the application of that knowledge to enhance health, lengthen life, and reduce the burdens of illness and disability."[26] Although a significant amount of research is carried out by NIH scientists at NIH laboratories in Bethesda and elsewhere, a much larger portion of this research is conducted by scientists at public and private universities and other research institutions. These scientists receive NIH funding for their research proposals through a competitive, peer-review grant application process. Through this process of proposal review by qualified scientists, NIH seeks to ensure that federal research funds are spent on the best-conceived research projects. **Table 2.2** presents a listing of all of the institutes and centers located in the NIH.

Substance Abuse and Mental Health Services Administration (SAMHSA)

The SAMHSA is the agency that leads public health efforts to advance the behavioral health of the nation and improve the lives of individuals living with mental health and substance use disorders. The SAMHSA directs its efforts on mental health promotion, prevention, and treatment with an emphasis on ensuring equity, trauma-informed approaches, recovery, and a commitment to data and evidence.[27] Within SAMHSA, there are four centers—the Center for Substance Abuse Treatment (CSAT), the Center for Substance Abuse Prevention (CSAP), the Center for Mental Health Services (CMHS), and the Center for Behavioral Health Statistics and Quality (CBHSQ).[27] Each of these centers has its own mission that contributes to the overall mission of SAMHSA.

State Health Agencies

All 50 states have their own state health departments (see **Figure 2.5**). Although the names of these departments may vary from state to state (e.g., Ohio Department of Health, Indiana State Department of Health), their purposes remain the same: to promote, protect, and maintain

TABLE 2.2 Units Within the National Institutes of Health (NIH)

National Cancer Institute (NCI)	National Institute of Environmental Health Sciences (NIEHS)
National Eye Institute (NEI)	National Institute of General Medical Sciences (NIGMS)
National Heart, Lung, and Blood Institute (NHLBI)	National Institute of Mental Health (NIMH)
National Human Genome Research Institute (NHGRI)	National Institute on Minority Health and Health Disparities (NIMHD)
National Institute on Aging (NIA)	National Institute of Neurological Disorders and Stroke (NINDS)
National Institute on Alcohol Abuse and Alcoholism (NIAAA)	National Institute of Nursing Research (NINR)
National Institute of Allergy and Infectious Diseases (NIAID)	National Library of Medicine (NLM)
National Institute of Arthritis and Musculoskeletal and Skin Diseases (NIAMS)	NIH Clinical Center (CC)
National Institute of Biomedical Imaging and Bioengineering (NIBIB)	Center for Information Technology (CIT)
Eunice Kennedy Shriver National Institute of Child Health and Human Development (NICHD)	National Center for Complementary and Integrative Health (NCCIH)
National Institute on Deafness and Other Communication Disorders (NIDCD)	Fogarty International Center (FIC)
National Institute of Dental and Craniofacial Research (NIDCR)	Center for Scientific Review (CSR)
National Institute of Diabetes and Digestive and Kidney Diseases (NIDDK)	National Center for Advancing Translational Sciences (NCATS)
National Institute on Drug Abuse (NIDA)	

Reproduced from National Institutes of Health. (2024). *List of Institutes and Centers*. Available at https://www.nih.gov/institutes-nih/list-institutes-centers

Core functions of public health assessment, policy development, and assurance

the health and welfare of their citizens. These purposes are represented in the **core functions of public health**, which include assessment of information on the health of the community, comprehensive public health policy development, and assurance that public health services are provided to the community.[28] These core functions have been defined further with the following 10 essential public health services.[29]

1. Assess and monitor population health status, factors that influence health, and community needs and assets.

2. Investigate, diagnose, and address health problems and hazards affecting the population.

3. Communicate effectively to inform and educate people about health, factors that influence it, and how to improve it.

4. Strengthen, support, and mobilize communities and partnerships to improve health.

5. Create, champion, and implement policies, plans, and laws that impact health.

6. Utilize legal and regulatory actions designed to improve and protect the public's health.

7. Assure an effective system that enables equitable access to the individual services and care needed to be healthy.

8. Build and support a diverse and skilled public health workforce.

9. Improve and innovate public health functions through ongoing evaluation, research, and continuous quality improvement.

10. Build and maintain strong organizational infrastructure for public health (see **Figure 2.6**).

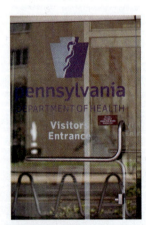

FIGURE 2.5 Each of the 50 states has its own health department.

© James F. McKenzie

The head of the state health department is usually a medical doctor, appointed by the governor, who may carry the title of director, commissioner, or secretary. However, because of the political nature of the appointment, this individual may or may not have extensive experience

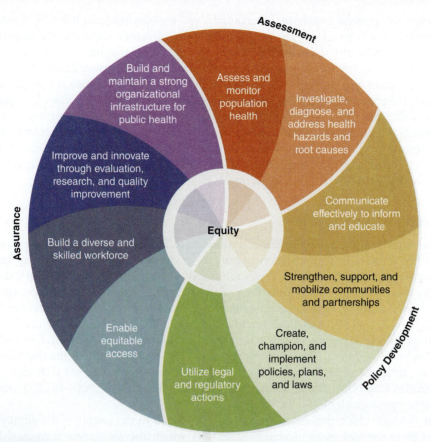

FIGURE 2.6   The 10 essential public health services.

Reproduced from Centers for Disease Control and Prevention. (2020). *The 10 Essential Public Health Services*. Available at https://www.cdc.gov/public-health-gateway/php/about/index.html

in community or public health. Unfortunately, political influence sometimes reaches below the level of commissioner to the assistant commissioners and division chiefs; it is the commissioner, assistant commissioners, and division chiefs who set policy and provide direction for the state health department. Middle- and lower-level employees are usually hired through a merit system and may or may not be able to influence health department policy. These employees, who carry out the routine work of the state health department, are usually professionally trained health specialists, such as microbiologists, engineers, sanitarians, epidemiologists, nurses, and health education specialists.

Most state health departments are organized into divisions or bureaus that provide certain standard services. Typical divisions include administration, communicable disease prevention and control, chronic disease prevention and control, vital and health statistics, environmental health, health education or promotion, health services, maternal and child health, mental health, occupational and industrial health, dental health, laboratory services, public health nursing, veterinary public health, and most recently, a division of Public Health Preparedness to deal with bioterrorism issues.

In promoting, protecting, and maintaining the health and welfare of their citizens, state health departments play many different roles. They can establish and promulgate health regulations that have the force and effect of law throughout the state. The state health departments also provide an essential link between federal and local (city and county) public health agencies. As such, they serve as conduits for federal funds aimed at local health problems. Federal funds come to the states as block grants. Funds earmarked for specific health projects are distributed to local health departments by their respective state health departments in accordance with previously agreed-upon priorities. State health departments may also link local needs with federal expertise. For example, epidemiologists from the CDC are some-times made available to investigate local disease outbreaks at the request of the state health department. State health departments usually must approve appointments of local health officers and can also remove any local health officers who neglect their duties.

The resources and expertise of the state health department are also at the disposal of local health departments. One area where the state health departments can be helpful is laboratory services; many modern diagnostic tests are simply too expensive for local health departments. Another area is environmental health. Water and air pollution problems usually extend beyond local authorities, and their detection and measurement often require equipment that is too expensive for local governments to afford. This equipment and expertise are often provided by the state health department.

Local Health Departments

Local-level governmental health organizations, referred to as local health departments (LHDs), are usually the responsibility of the city or county governments. In large metropolitan areas, community health needs are usually best served by a city health department. In smaller cities with populations of up to 50,000, people often come under the jurisdiction of a county health department. When most of the population is concentrated in a single city, an LHD may have jurisdiction over both city and county residents. In sparsely populated rural areas, it is common to find more than one county served by a single health department. There are approximately 2,510 agencies or units that meet the profile definition of an LHD. According to the 2022 Profile study, 62% of LHDs serve small communities (<50,000), 33% serve medium-size communities (50,000–499,999), and 6% serve large communities (500,000+).[30]

It is through LHDs that health services are provided to the people of the community. Many of these services are mandated by state laws, which also set standards for health and safety. Examples of mandated local health services include the inspection of restaurants, public buildings, and public transportation systems; the detection and reporting of certain diseases; and the collection of vital statistics, such as births and deaths. Other programs, such as car seat programs and immunization clinics may be locally planned and implemented. In this regard, local health jurisdictions are permitted (unless pre-emptive legislation is in place) to enact ordinances that are stricter than those of the state, but these jurisdictions cannot enact codes that fall below state standards. It is at this level of governmental health agencies that sanitarians implement the environmental health programs, nurses and physicians offer clinical services, and health education specialists present health education and promotion programs.

Organization of Local Health Departments

Each LHD is led by a health officer/administrator/commissioner (see **Figure 2.7**). In most states, there are laws that prescribe who can hold such a position. Those often noted are physicians, dentists, veterinarians, or individuals with a master's or doctoral degree in public

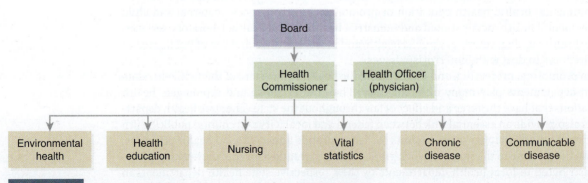

FIGURE 2.7   Organizational chart of a local public health department.

health. If the health officer is not a physician, a physician is usually hired on a consulting basis to advise as needed. Usually, this health officer is appointed by a board of health, the members of which are themselves appointed by officials in the city or county government or, in some situations, elected by the general public. The health officer and administrative assistants may recommend which programs will be offered by the LHDs. However, they may need final approval from a board of health. Although it is desirable that those serving on the local board of health have some knowledge of community health programs, most states have no such requirement. Often, politics plays a role in deciding the makeup of the local board of health.

The local health officer, like the state health commissioner, has far-reaching powers, including the power to arrest someone who refuses to undergo treatment for a communicable disease (tuberculosis, for example) and who thereby continues to spread disease in the community. The local health officer has the power to close a restaurant on the spot if it has serious health law violations or to impound a shipment of food if it is contaminated. Because many local health departments cannot afford to employ a full-time physician, the health officer may be hired on a part-time basis. In such cases, the day-to-day activities of the LHD are carried out by an administrator trained in public health. The administrator is also hired by the board of health based on qualifications and the recommendation of the health officer.

The greatest percentage of LHD revenues comes from local funds, followed by state and federal pass-through funds. A limited number of LHD services are provided on a fee-for-service basis. For example, there is usually a fee charged for birth and death certificates issued by the LHD. Also, in some communities, minimal fees are charged to offset the cost of providing immunizations, lab work, or inspections. Seldom do these fees cover the actual cost of the services provided. Therefore, income from service fees usually makes up a very small portion of any LHD budget. Additionally, it is not unusual to find that many LHDs use a **sliding scale** to determine the fee for a service.

Public Schools

Few people think of public schools as governmental health agencies. Consider, however, that schools are funded by tax dollars, are under the supervision of an elected school board, and include as a part of their mission the improvement of the health of those in the school community. Because school attendance is required throughout the United States, the potential for school health programs to make a significant contribution to community and public health is enormous, especially when it comes to promoting the health and safety of young people and helping them establish lifelong healthy behavior patterns.[31] In fact, it has been stated that schools "could do more perhaps than any other single agency in society to help young people, and the adults they will become, to live healthier, longer, more satisfying, and more productive lives."[32]

Current thinking is that schools, along with government agencies, community organizations, and other community members, can be a part of a collaborative and comprehensive approach to have a positive impact on the health outcomes of young people.[31] To create such a program, the CDC and the ASCD (previously known as the Association for Supervision and Curriculum Development) developed the Whole School, Whole Community, Whole Child (WSCC) model. The WSCC model is "student-centered and emphasizes the role of the community in supporting the school, the connections between health and academic achievement, and the importance of evidence-based school policies and practices."[31] The WSCC model includes 10 components: physical education and physical activity; nutrition environment and services; health education; social and emotional school climate; physical environment; health services; counseling, psychological, and social services; employee wellness; community involvement; and family engagement.[31] If communities are willing to work with the public health and education sectors, the contribution of WSCC model programs to community and public health could be almost unlimited.

Sliding scale a method used to determine the fee for services based on ability to pay

Quasi-Governmental Health Organizations

The **quasi-governmental health organizations**—organizations that have some official health responsibilities but operate, in part, like voluntary health organizations—make important contributions to community health. Although they derive some of their funding and legitimacy from governments and carry out tasks that may be normally thought of as government work, they operate independently of government supervision. In some cases, they also receive financial support from private sources. Examples of quasi-governmental agencies are the American Red Cross (ARC), the National Science Foundation, and the National Academy of Sciences.

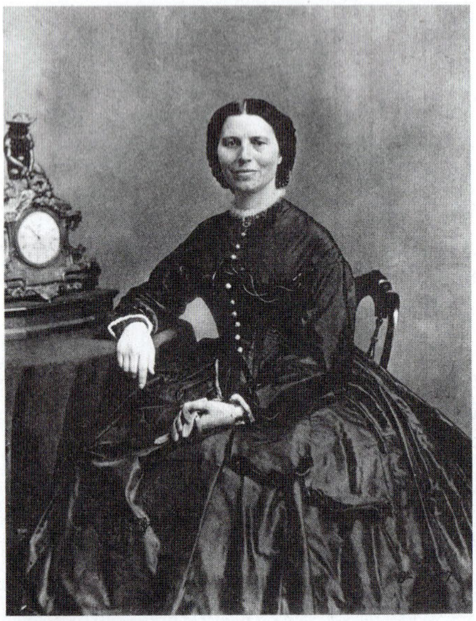

The American Red Cross (ARC)

The ARC, founded in 1881 by Clara Barton[34] (see **Figure 2.8**), is a prime example of an organization that has quasi-governmental status. Although it has certain "official" responsibilities placed on it by the federal government, it is funded by voluntary contributions. These official duties include: (1) providing relief to victims of natural disasters, such as floods, tornadoes, hurricanes, and fires and (2) serving as the liaison between members of the military, veterans and their families prepare for, cope with, and respond to, the challenges of military service. In this latter capacity, the ARC can assist active-duty members of the military in contacting their families in case of an emergency, or vice versa.

In addition to these official duties, the ARC also engages in many nongovernmental services. These include blood donor services and drives; training and certification services, such as water safety, first aid, CPR, and babysitting and child care; and international disaster services.

The ARC was granted a charter by Congress in 1900, and the ARC and the federal government have had a special relationship ever since. The President of the United States is the honorary chairperson of the ARC.[33] The U.S. Attorney General and Secretary of the Treasury are honorary counselor and treasurer, respectively.

The Red Cross began in 1863 by five Swiss men in Geneva, Switzerland, who were concerned with the treatment provided to the wounded during times of war.[34] The group, which was called the International Committee for the Relief to the Wounded, was led by Henry Dunant (1828–1910 CE). With the assistance of the Swiss government, the International Committee brought together delegates from 16 nations in 1864 to the Geneva Convention for the Amelioration of the Condition of the Wounded in Armies in the Field (known as the first Geneva Convention) to sign the Geneva Treaty.[34]

The efforts of Henry Dunant and the rest of the international committee led to the eventual establishment of the International Committee of the Red Cross (ICRC). The ICRC, which is still headquartered in Geneva and governed by the Swiss, continues to work during times of disaster and international conflict. It is the organization that visits prisoners of war to ensure they are being treated humanely.[34]

Today, the international movement of the Red Cross comprises the Geneva-based ICRC, the International Federation of Red Cross and Red Crescent Societies (the red crescent emblem is used in Moslem countries), and the over 190 National Red Cross and Red Crescent Societies.[34] There are a number of other countries that believe in the principles of the Red Cross Movement but have not officially joined because the emblems used by the movement are offensive. Thus, the ICRC created a third emblem that meets all the criteria for use as a protective device and at the same time, is free of any national, political, or religious connotations. The design is with a red frame in the shape of a square on the edge of a white background. The name chosen for this distinctive emblem was "red crystal," to signify purity[35] (see **Figure 2.9**).

FIGURE 2.8   The American Red Cross was founded by Clara Barton in 1881.

© National Library of Medicine

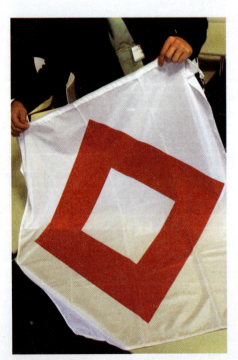

FIGURE 2.9   The red crystal: an additional emblem of the ICRC

© Laurent Gillieron/EPA/Shutterstock

Other Quasi-Governmental Organizations

Two other examples of quasi-governmental organizations in the United States are the National Science Foundation (NSF) and the National Academy of Sciences (NAS). The purpose of the NSF is the funding and promotion of scientific research and the development of individual scientists. NSF receives and disperses federal funds but operates independently of governmental supervision. Chartered by Congress in 1863, NAS acts as an advisor to the government on questions of science and technology. Included in its membership are some of America's most renowned scientists. Although neither of these agencies exists specifically to address health problems, both organizations fund projects, publish reports, and take public stands on health-related issues.

Voluntary health agencies
nonprofit organizations created by concerned citizens to deal with a health need not met by governmental health agencies

Nongovernmental Health Agencies

Nongovernmental health agencies are funded by private donations or, in some cases, by membership dues. There are thousands of these organizations, but they all have one thing in common: They arose because there was an unmet need. For the most part, the agencies operate free from governmental interference as long as they meet Internal Revenue Service guidelines with regard to their specific tax status. In the following sections, we discuss the different types of nongovernmental health agencies—voluntary, professional, philanthropic, service, social, religious, and corporate.

Voluntary Health Agencies

Voluntary health agencies are an American creation. Each of these agencies was created by one or more concerned citizens who thought that a specific health need was not being met by existing governmental agencies. In a sense, these new voluntary agencies arose by themselves, in much the same way as a "volunteer" tomato plant arises in a vegetable garden. New voluntary agencies continue to emerge each year. A discussion of the commonalities of voluntary health agencies follows.

Organization of Voluntary Health Agencies

Most voluntary agencies exist at three levels—national, state, and local. At the national level, policies that guide the agency are formulated. A significant portion of the money raised locally is forwarded to the national office, where it is allocated according to the agency's budget. Much of the money is designated for research. By funding research, the agencies hope to discover the cause of and cure for a particular disease or health problem. There have been some major successes. The March of Dimes, for example, helped to eliminate polio as a major disease problem in the United States through its funding of immunization research.

There is not always a consensus of opinion about budget decisions made at the national level; some believe that less should be spent for research and more for treating those who have the disease. Another common internal disagreement concerns how much of the funds raised at the local level should be sent to the national headquarters instead of being retained for local use. Those outside the agency sometimes complain that when an agency achieves success, as the March of Dimes did in its fight against polio, it should dissolve. This does not usually occur; instead, successful agencies often find a new health concern. The March of Dimes now fights birth defects, and when tuberculosis was under control, the Tuberculosis Society changed its name to the American Lung Association to fight all lung diseases.

The state-level offices of voluntary agencies are analogous to the state departments of health in the way that they link the national headquarters with local offices. The primary work at this level is to coordinate local efforts and to ensure that policies developed at the national headquarters are carried out. The state-level office may also provide training services for employees and volunteers of local-level offices and are usually available as consultants and problem solvers. In recent years, some voluntary agencies have been merging several state offices into one to help reduce overhead expenses.

The local-level office of each voluntary agency is usually managed by paid staff who has been hired either by the state-level office or by a local board of directors. Members of the local board of directors usually serve in that capacity on a voluntary basis. Working under the manager of each agency are local volunteers, who are the backbone of voluntary agencies. It has been said that the local level is where the "rubber meets the road." In other words, this is where most of the money is raised, most of the education takes place, and most of the service is rendered. Volunteers are of two types, professional and lay. Professional volunteers have had training in a medical profession, while lay volunteers have had no medical training. The paid employees help facilitate the work of the volunteers with expertise, training, and other resources.

Purpose of Voluntary Health Agencies

Voluntary agencies share four basic objectives: (1) to raise money to fund their programs, with the majority of the money going to fund research; (2) to provide education both to professionals and to the public; (3) to provide service to those individuals and families that have the disease or health problem; and (4) to advocate for beneficial policies, laws, and regulations that affect the work of the agency and in turn the people they are trying to help (see **Box 2.1**).

Fundraising is a primary activity of many voluntary agencies. Whereas in the past, this was accomplished primarily by door-to-door solicitations; today, mass-mailing, emailing, and telephone solicitation are more common. In addition, most agencies sponsor special events, such as golf outings, dances, or dinners. One type of special event that is very popular today is the "a-thon" (see **Figure 2.10**). The term *a-thon* is derived from the name of the ancient Greek city Marathon and usually signified some kind of "endurance" event. Examples include bike-a-thons, rock-a-thons, telethons, skate-a-thons, and dance-a-thons. These money-making

---

BOX 2.1   A Closer Look at One Voluntary Health Agency: The American Cancer Society

The American Cancer Society (ACS) was founded in 1913 by 10 physicians and five laypeople.[36] At that time, it was known as the American Society for the Control of Cancer. Today, with offices throughout the country and 1.3 million volunteers, ACS is the pre-eminent cancer fighting organization in the United States.[37]

The mission of the ACS is "to improve the lives of people with cancer and their families through advocacy, research, and patient support, to ensure everyone has an opportunity to prevent, detect, treat, and survive cancer."[37]

The American Cancer Society's educational programs are targeted at two different groups—the general public and the health professionals who treat cancer patients. The public education programs promote prevention by taking steps to reduce cancer risk, quitting smoking, getting recommended cancer screenings, and living healthier lifestyles. ACS provides resources, information, and support for individuals and loved ones. A few of their better-known programs include Stay Healthy and Reach to Recovery.[37]

The ACS's professional education program is aimed at the professionals who work with cancer patients. The objective of this program is to motivate physicians and other healthcare professionals to maintain and improve their knowledge of cancer prevention, detection, diagnosis, treatment, and palliative care. Such education is provided through professional publications, podcasts, online resources, conferences, and grants that fund specialized education experiences.

The ACS offers patient service and survivor programs that ease the impact of cancer on those affected. The mobile app ACS CARESTM provides curated content, programs, and services to fit an individual's specific cancer journey. The services offered include information and referral to appropriate professionals, transportation of patients to maintain their medical and continuing care programs, as well as social support for cancer patients.

The ACS is the largest source of private, not-for-profit cancer research funds in the United States, second only to the federal government in total dollars spent. Since 1946, when the ACS first started awarding grants, it has invested more than $5 billion in cancer research. The research program consists of three components: extramural grants, intramural epidemiology and surveillance research, and the intramural behavioral research center.[37] The most recent addition to the work of the ACS is in the area of advocacy through their Cancer Action Network (CAN). Specifically, the ACS CAN's work has resulted in increased funding for cancer research and prevention programs, stronger tobacco control policies nationwide, and improved access to a full range of cancer care for people diagnosed with cancer and their families.[37]

All ACS programs—education, service, research, and advocacy—are planned primarily by the society's volunteers. However, the society does employ staff members to carry out the day-to-day operations and to help advise and support the work of the volunteers. This arrangement of volunteers and staff working together has created a very strong voluntary health agency.

"a-thons" seem to be limited in scope only by the creativity of those planning them. In addition, some of these agencies have become United Way agencies and receive some funds derived from the annual United Way campaign, which conducts fundraising efforts at worksites.

Over the years, the number of voluntary agencies formed to help meet special health needs has increased. Because of the growth in the number of new agencies, several consumer "watchdog" groups have taken a closer look into the practices of these agencies. A major concern of these consumer groups has been the amount of money that the voluntary agencies spend on the cause (e.g., cancer, heart disease, AIDS) and how much they spend on fundraising and overhead (e.g., salaries, office furniture, leasing of office space). Well-run agencies will spend 15% to 20% of what they raise on fundraising and overhead. Some of the not-so-well-run agencies spend as much as 80% to 90% of money raised on fundraising and overhead. All consumers should ask agencies how they spend their money prior to contributing.

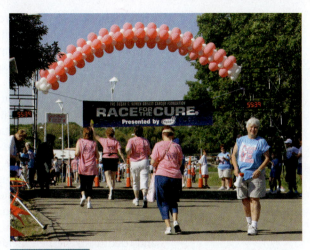

FIGURE 2.10 Most voluntary health agencies hold special events to raise money for their causes.
© Suzanne Tucker/Shutterstock

Professional Health Organizations/Associations

Professional health organizations and associations are composed of health professionals who have completed specialized education and training programs and have met the standards of registration, certification, and/or licensure for their respective fields. Their mission is to promote high standards of professional practice for their specific profession, thereby improving the health of society by improving the people in the profession. Professional organizations are funded primarily by membership dues. Examples of such organizations are the American Medical Association, the American Dental Association, the American Nursing Association, the American Public Health Association, and the Society for Public Health Education.

Although each professional organization is unique, most provide similar services to their members. These services include the certification of continuing education programs for professional renewal, the hosting of annual conventions where members share research results and interact with colleagues, and the publication of professional journals and other reports. Some examples of journals published by professional health associations are the *Journal of the American Medical Association* (*JAMA*), the *American Journal of Public Health*, and *Health Promotion Practice*.

Like voluntary health agencies, another important activity of some professional organizations is advocating for issues important to their membership. The American Medical Association, for example, has a powerful lobby nationally and in some state legislatures. Their purpose is to affect legislation in such a way as to benefit their membership and their profession. Many professional health organizations provide the opportunity for benefits, including group insurance and discount travel rates. There are hundreds of professional health organizations in the United States, and it would be difficult to describe them all here.

Philanthropic Foundations

Philanthropic foundations have made and continue to make significant contributions to community and public health in the United States and throughout the world. These foundations support community health by funding programs and research on the prevention, control, and treatment of many diseases. Foundation directors, sometimes in consultation with a review committee, determine the types of programs that will be funded. Some foundations fund an

Philanthropic foundations endowed institutions that donate money for the good of humankind

array of health projects, whereas others have a much narrower scope of interests. Some foundations, such as the Bill and Melinda Gates Foundation, fund global health projects, whereas others restrict their funding to domestic projects. The geographic scope of domestic foundations can be national, state, or local. Local foundations may restrict their funding only to projects that benefit local citizens.

The activities of these foundations differ from those of the voluntary health agencies in two important ways. First, foundations have money to give away, and; therefore, no effort is spent on fundraising. Second, foundations can afford to fund long-term or innovative research projects, which might be too risky or expensive for voluntary or even government-funded agencies. The development of a vaccine for yellow fever by a scientist funded by the Rockefeller Foundation is an example of one such long-range project.

Some of the larger foundations, in addition to the Bill and Melinda Gates Foundation, that have made significant commitments to community health are the Commonwealth Fund, which has contributed to community health in rural communities, improved hospital facilities, and tried to strengthen mental health services; the Ford Foundation, which has contributed greatly to family planning and youth sexuality efforts throughout the world; the Robert Wood Johnson Foundation, which has worked to improve the culture of health and policies dealing with health-related systems; the Henry J. Kaiser Family Foundation, which has supported the healthcare reform and community health promotion; the W. K. Kellogg Foundation, which has funded many diverse health programs that address human issues and provide a practical solution; and the Milbank Memorial Fund, which has primarily funded projects dealing with the integration of people with disabilities into all aspects of life.

Service, Social, and Religious Organizations

Service, social, and religious organizations have also played a part in community and public health over the years (see **Figure 2.11**). Examples of service and social groups involved in community health are the Jaycees, Kiwanis Club, Fraternal Order of Police, Rotary Club, Elks, Lions, Moose, Shriners, American Legion, and Veterans of Foreign Wars. Members of these groups enjoy social interactions with people of similar interests in addition to fulfilling the groups' primary reason for existence—service to others in their communities. Although health may not be the specific focus of their mission, several of these groups make important contributions in that direction by raising money and funding health-related programs. Sometimes, their contributions are substantial. Examples of such programs include the Shriners' children's hospitals and burn centers; the Lions' contributions to pilot (lead) dog programs and other services for those who are visually impaired, such as the provision of eyeglasses for school-aged children unable to afford them; and the Lions' contributions to social and emotional learning of pre-K–12 children via the educational program, Lions Quest.[36]

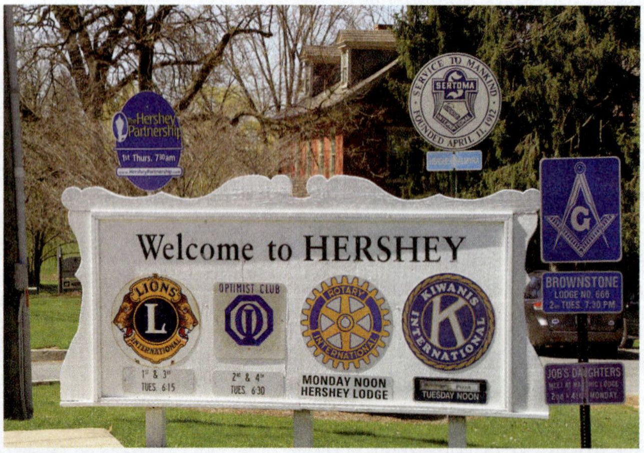

The contributions of religious groups to community and public health have also been substantial. Such groups have also been effective avenues for promoting health programs because (1) they have had a history of volunteerism and pre-existing reinforcement contingencies for volunteerism, (2) they can influence entire families, and (3) they have accessible meeting-room facilities.[39] One way in which these groups contribute is through donations of money for missions for the less fortunate. Examples of religious organizations that solicit donations from their members include the Presbyterian's One Great Hour of Sharing, the Catholics' Relief Services, and the Jewish Relief Agency. Other types of involvement

FIGURE 2.11 Community service groups contribute needed resources for the improvement of the health of the community.

© James F. McKenzie

in community health by religious groups include (1) the donation of space for voluntary health programs, such as blood donations, Alcoholics Anonymous, and other support groups; (2) the sponsorship of food banks and shelters; (3) the sharing of the doctrine of good personal health behavior; and (4) allowing community and public health professionals to deliver their programs through the congregations. This latter contribution has been especially useful in Black American communities because of the importance of churches in the culture of this group of people.

In addition, it should be noted that some religious groups have hindered the work of community and public health workers. Almost every community in the country can provide an example where a religious organization has protested the offering of a school district's sex education program, picketed a public health clinic for providing reproductive information or services to women, or has spoken out against homosexuality.

Corporate Involvement in Community and Public Health

From the way it treats the environment by its use of natural resources and the discharge of wastes, to the safety of the work environment, to the products and services it produces and provides, to the provision of health care benefits for its employees, corporate America is very much involved in community and public health. Although each of these aspects of community and public health is important to the overall health of a community, because of the concern for the "bottom line" in corporate America, it is the provision of health care benefits that often receives the most attention. In fact, many corporations today find that their single largest annual expenditure behind salaries and wages is for employee health care benefits.

In an effort to keep a healthy workforce and reduce the amount paid for health care benefits, many companies support health-related programs both at and away from the worksite. Worksite programs aimed at reducing employee medical bills include such programs as mental health services, nutrition education, smoking cessation, stress management, physical fitness, flu shots, ergonomics, and disease management. Many companies are also implementing health promotion policies and enforcing state and local laws that prohibit (or severely restrict) smoking on company grounds.

Chapter Summary

- Contemporary society is too complex to respond effectively to community and public health problems on either an emergency or a long-term basis. This fact necessitates organizations and planning for health in our communities.

- The different types of organizations that contribute to the promotion, protection, and maintenance of health in a community can be classified into three groups according to their sources of funding and organizational structure—governmental, quasi-governmental, and nongovernmental.

- Governmental health agencies exist at the local, state, federal, and international levels and are funded primarily by tax dollars.

- The World Health Organization is the largest and most visible governmental health agency on the international level.

- The Department of Health and Human Services (HHS) is the U.S. government's principal agency for the protection of the health of all Americans and for providing essential human services, especially for those who are least able to help themselves.

- Public schools are a key component of the community and an essential part of a collaborative and comprehensive approach to addressing health outcomes of young people.

- The core functions of public health include the assessment of information on the health of the community, comprehensive public health policy development, and assurance that public health services are provided to the community. Ten essential services are used to meet these core functions.

- Quasi-governmental agencies, such as the American Red Cross, share attributes with both governmental and nongovernmental agencies.

- Nongovernmental organizations include voluntary and professional associations, philanthropic foundations, and service, social, and religious groups.

- Corporate America has also become more involved in community and public health, both at the worksite and within the community.

Scenario: Analysis and Response

After having read this chapter, please respond to the following questions in reference to the scenario at the beginning of the chapter.

1. What type of health agency do you think will be of the most help to Mary?

2. If this scenario were to happen to someone in your community, what recommendations would you give to them on seeking help from health agencies?

3. The Internet has many sources of information that could help Mary. Use a search engine (e.g., Google, Bing, Yahoo) and enter the word "cancer." Find the website of one governmental health agency at the national level and one voluntary health agency that might be able to help her. Explain how these agencies could be of help.

4. If Mary did not have Internet access, how would you suggest she find out about local health agencies in her area that could help her?

Review Questions

1. What characteristics of modern society necessitate planning and organization for community and public health?

2. What is a governmental health agency?

3. What is the World Health Organization (WHO), and what does it do?

4. Which federal department in the United States is the government's principal agency for protecting the health of all Americans and for providing essential human services, especially to those who are least able to help themselves? What major services does this department provide?

5. What are the three core functions of public health?

6. What are the 10 essential public health services?

7. How do state and local health departments interface?

8. Discuss how public schools are a key component of a comprehensive approach to addressing health outcomes for young people.

9. What is meant by the term *quasi-governmental agency*? Name one such agency.

10. Describe the characteristics of a nongovernmental health agency.

11. What are the major differences between a governmental health organization and a voluntary health agency?

12. Describe the value a health professional gains from being a member of a professional health organization.

13. How do philanthropic foundations contribute to community health? List three well-known foundations.

14. How do service, social, and religious groups contribute to the health of the community?

15. Why has corporate America become involved in community and public health?

Activities

1. Using the Internet, identify 15 health-related organizations that service your community. Divide your list by the three major types of health organizations noted in this chapter.

2. Make an appointment to interview someone at one of the organizations identified in Activity 1. During your visit, find answers to the following questions:

   a. How did the organization begin?

   b. What is its mission?

   c. How is it funded?

   d. How many people (employees and volunteers) work for the organization, and what type of education/training do they have?

   e. What types of programs/services does the organization provide?

3. Obtain organizational charts from the U.S. Department of Health and Human Services (see Figure 2.2),

your state department of health, and your local health department. Compare and contrast these charts and describe their similarities and differences.

4. Call a local voluntary health organization in your community and ask if you could volunteer to work 10 to 15 hours during this academic term. Then, volunteer those hours and keep a journal of your experience.

References

1. Green, L. W. (1990). The revival of community and the public obligation of academic health centers. In R. E. Bulger & S. J. Reiser (Eds.), *Integrity in institutions: Humane environments for teaching, inquiry and health* (pp. 163–180). University of Iowa Press.
2. World Health Organization. (2024). *About WHO.* Available at https://www.who.int/about
3. World Health Organization. (2024). *What we do.* Available at https://www.who.int/about/what-we-do
4. World Health Organization. (2024). *World Health Assembly.* Available at https://www.who.int/about/governance/world-health-assembly
5. World Health Organization. (2024). *Draft fourteenth general programme of work, 2025-2028.* Available at https://www.who.int/about/general-programme-of-work/fourteenth
6. World Health Organization. (2024). *How WHO is funded.* Available at https://www.who.int/about/funding
7. World Health Organization. (2024). *WHO commemorates the 40th anniversary of smallpox eradication.* Available at https://www.who.int/news/item/13-12-2019-who-commemorates-the-40th-anniversary-of-smallpox-eradication
8. World Health Organization. (2024). *World experts and funders set priorities for COVID-19 research.* Available at https://www.who.int/news-room/detail/12-02-2020-world-experts-and-funders-set-priorities-for-covid-19-research
9. World Health Organization. (2024). *Coronavirus disease (COVID-19): Strategy and planning.* Available at https://www.who.int/emergencies/diseases/novel-coronavirus-2019/strategies-and-plans
10. World Health Organization. (2024). *Sustainable development goals.* Available at https://www.un.org/sustainabledevelopment/
11. World Health Organization. (2024). *World health statistics 2024: Monitoring health for the SDGs, sustainable development goals.* Available at https://www.who.int/publications/i/item/9789240094703
12. U.S. Department of Health and Human Services. (2024). *About HHS.* Available at http://www.hhs.gov/about/index.html
13. U.S. Department of Health and Human Services. (2024). *Fiscal year 2024 budget in brief.* Available at https://www.hhs.gov/sites/default/files/fy-2024-budget-in-brief.pdf
14. U.S. Department of Health and Human Services. (2024). *Office of health start.* Available at https://www.acf.hhs.gov/ohs/about
15. U.S. Department of Health and Human Services. (2024). *Administration for community living.* Available at https://acl.gov/about-community-living
16. Agency for Health Care Research and Quality. (2024). *Agency for Healthcare Research and Quality: A profile.* Available at https://www.ahrq.gov/cpi/about/profile/index.html
17. ARPA-H. (2024). *About: Frequently asked questions.* Available at https://arpa-h.gov/about/faqs
18. ARPA-H. (2024). *News and insights.* Available at https://arpa-h.gov/news-and-events
19. Administration for Strategic Preparedness & Response. (2024). *About ASPR.* Available at https://aspr.hhs.gov/AboutASPR/ProgramOffices/Pages/ProgramOffice.aspx
20. Agency for Toxic Substances and Disease Registry. (2024). *Agency for toxic substances and disease registry.* Available at http://www.atsdr.cdc.gov/
21. Centers for Disease Control and Prevention. (2024). *About CDC.* Available at *https://www.cdc.gov/about/cdc/index.html*
22. U.S. Food and Drug Administration. (2023). *What we do.* Available at https://www.fda.gov/about-fda/what-we-do
23. United States Census Bureau. (2023). *Health insurance coverage in the United States: 2022.* Available at https://www.census.gov/library/publications/2023/demo/p60-281.html
24. Health Resources and Services Administration. (2023). *About HRSA.* Available at https://www.hrsa.gov/about
25. Indian Health Service. (2024). *About IHS.* Available at https://www.ihs.gov/aboutihs/
26. National Institutes of Health. (2024). *What we do.* Available at https://www.nih.gov/about-nih/what-we-do/mission-goals
27. Substance Abuse and Mental Health Services Administration. (2024). *SAMSHA: About us.* Available at https://www.samhsa.gov/about-us
28. National Academy of Sciences, Institute of Medicine. (1988). *The future of public health.* National Academies Press.
29. Center for Disease Control and Prevention. (2024). *Public health professionals gateway: 10 Essential public health services.* Available at https://www.cdc.gov/public-health-gateway/php/about/index.html/publichealthservices/essentialhealthservices.html
30. National Association of County and City Health Officials. (2024). *2022 National profile of local health departments.* Available at https://www.naccho.org/resources/lhd-research/national-profile-of-local-health-departments
31. Centers for Disease Control and Prevention. (2023). *CDC healthy schools: Whole School, Whole Community, Whole Child (WSCC).* Available at https://www.cdc.gov/healthyschools/wscc/index.htm
32. Allensworth, D. D., & Kolbe, L. J. (1987). The comprehensive school health program: Exploring an expanded concept. *Journal of School Health, 57*(10), 409–412.
33. American Red Cross. (2024). *About us.* Available at https://www.redcross.org/about-us.html
34. International Committee of the Red Cross. (2024). *History.* Available at https://www.icrc.org/en/who-we-are/history
35. International Committee of the Red Cross. (2005). *An additional emblem—red crystal alongside the red cross and red crescent.* Available at https://www.icrc.org/eng/resources/documents/press-briefing/emblem-press-briefing-081205.htm
36. American Cancer Society. (2024). *Our history.* Available at https://www.cancer.org/about-us/who-we-are/our-history.html
37. American Cancer Society. (2024). *American Cancer Society.* Available at https://www.cancer.org/
38. Lions Clubs International. (2024). *Lions Quest.* Available at https://www.lions-quest.org/
39. Lasater, T. M., Wells, B. L., Carleton, R. A., & Elder, J. P. (1986). The role of churches in disease prevention research studies. *Public Health Report, 101*(2), 123–131.

CHAPTER 3

Epidemiology: The Study of Disease, Injury, and Death in the Community

Chapter Outline

Chapter Objectives

After studying this chapter, you will be able to:

1. Define the terms *epidemic, endemic, pandemic, epidemiology*, and *epidemiologist*, and explain their importance in community and public health.

2. List some diseases that caused epidemics in the past and some that are causing epidemics today.

3. Discuss how the practice of epidemiology has changed since the days of Benjamin Rush and John Snow.

4. Explain why rates are important in epidemiology and list some of the commonly used rates.

5. Define incidence and prevalence rates and provide examples of each.

6. Discuss the importance of disease reporting to a community's health and describe the reporting process.

7. Summarize the following standardized measurements of health status—life expectancy, years of potential life lost (YPLL), disability-adjusted life years (DALYs), and health-adjusted life expectancy (HALE).

8. Identify sources of secondary data used by epidemiologists, community health workers, health officials, and list the types of data available from each source.

9. Describe the two main types of epidemiologic studies.

10. List the criteria used to evaluate whether a risk factor causes a disease.

Scenario

John thought about this afternoon's picnic. Everyone had a great time. For a while, it had seemed almost too warm, but plenty of cold drinks were available, and by late afternoon, it had become quite pleasant. The games were fun, too . . . Frisbee, soccer, softball, and volleyball. Then, there was the picnic itself—turkey, potato salad, bread and butter, milk, and dessert—served at around noon.

It was now 8 P.M. the next night, and instead of studying as he had planned, John was lying on his bed with a bad stomachache. He was experiencing severe diarrhea and had made several hurried trips to the bathroom in the last half-hour.

John received a message from his roommate Michael. He had gone to his girlfriend's house after the picnic to work on a class project with her. He and Caroline were both sick with stomach cramps and diarrhea, and Michael was wondering if John was sick, too. John began to think about what a coincidence it was that all three of them were sick with the same symptoms at about the same time. Could they have become ill from the food they ate at the picnic? There were about 50 people at the picnic; how many others might also be sick? Was it the heat? Was it the food? Was this an epidemic? A half-hour later, John messaged Michael to tell him that he had decided to go to the campus health center.

Elsewhere . . .

This had turned out to be an interesting volunteer experience. As a requirement for her community health class, Kim had agreed to volunteer at the local health department. The spring semester was almost over now, and she was writing a final report of her activities. During the term, she had spent her Friday afternoons accompanying a sanitarian on his inspections of restaurants and retail food stores. She had also helped him complete his reports on substandard housing and malfunctioning septic tanks.

Dr. Turner, the health officer, had given Kim permission to use one of the department's computers to prepare her final report. Because it was late Sunday evening, she was alone in the health department office when the telephone rang. She briefly considered not answering it but finally picked up the receiver. It was Dr. Lee from the University Health Center. He said he was calling in the hope that someone might be there because he needed to reach Dr. Turner immediately. He said that he had admitted six students to the infirmary with severe stomach cramps, vomiting, and diarrhea. The students had been at a picnic the previous day, and he thought they could have a foodborne illness. He called to ask Dr. Turner to investigate this outbreak and asked Kim to try to reach him as soon as possible.

Introduction

When you become ill and visit a doctor, the first thing the physician does is take measurements and collect information. The measurements include your temperature, heart rate, and blood pressure. The information includes time of onset of your illness, where you have traveled, and what you might have eaten. Next, you may be given a physical examination and be asked to provide a specimen, such as urine or blood for laboratory examination. The information gathered helps the physician understand the nature of your illness and prescribe an appropriate treatment.

While a primary-care physician is concerned with the health of an individual patient, an epidemiologist is concerned with the health of a population. Monitoring health at a population level is important to determine when unexpected or unacceptable levels of health events occur, such as illness, injury, or death. When this happens, epidemiologists seek to collect information about the health status of the community. First, epidemiologists want to know how many people are sick. Second, they want to know who is sick—the old? the young? males? females? rich? poor? They also want to know when they became sick, and finally, where the sick people live or have traveled. In summary, epidemiologists are investigators who want to know what commonalities exist among the sick people. For this reason, epidemiology is sometimes referred to as population medicine. Although epidemiology was originally applied to infectious diseases, its application has expanded to other areas, including, but not limited to, chronic diseases (e.g., diabetes and cancer), reproductive health issues (e.g., infertility and preterm birth), environmental health concerns (e.g., pollution), occupational health hazards (e.g., asbestos exposure), and understanding health disparities in disease risk and outcomes.

Epidemiology is one of the community health activities "aimed at protecting or improving the health of a population or community." Information gathered from epidemiologic studies assists community decision makers to make the best use of the community's resources. Data gathered at local, state, and national levels can be used not only to prevent disease outbreaks or control those that are in progress but also to assess whether an ongoing disease prevention program is effective.

Definition of Epidemiology

Before we discuss the types of questions an epidemiologist asks, we need to define the term *epidemiology*. **Epidemiology** is "the study of the distribution and determinants of health-related states or events in specified populations, and the application of this study to control health problems."[1] The term *epidemiology* is derived from the Greek words "epi" "demos," and "logos," whose smooth translation is "the study of what befalls a population." The principles of epidemiology are highlighted in the keywords in its definition:

- *Study*: Epidemiology is a basic science in public health that uses quantitative data and scientific study designs to examine the relationship between exposures and diseases.
- *Distribution*: Epidemiologists search for patterns and the frequency (or occurrence) of diseases in the population.
- *Determinants*: One of the goals of epidemiology is to find risk factors, contributing agents, exposures, or causes of diseases.
- *Health-related states or events*: While epidemiology has focused on infectious and communicable diseases in the past, this science has now extended to look at other diseases, including chronic illnesses, environmental health issues, occupational conditions, genetic diseases, mental conditions, injuries, and other health concerns.
- *Specified population*: Epidemiologists are called "population doctors" because they focus on the total population and not individual patients.
- *Application*: The goal of epidemiology is to find useful information for the purpose of limiting undesirable health events and promoting positive health factors in a community. For example, illness can be limited by identifying the food that is making people sick or determining modifiable risk factors for heart disease. This is accomplished by describing the distribution and determinants of health events to validate new approaches to prevention, control, and treatment. Through these practices, epidemiologists contribute to our knowledge of how diseases begin and spread through populations, and how they can be prevented, controlled, and treated.

The question might be asked, how many cases are required before a disease outbreak is considered an epidemic—10 cases? 100 cases? 1,000 cases? The answer is that it depends on the disease and the population. However, any unexpectedly large number of cases of an illness, specific health-related behavior, or other health-related event in a particular population at a particular time and place can be considered an **epidemic**. Some recent epidemics in the United States are presented in **Table 3.1**.

Although describing the same phenomenon, the term **outbreak** is usually used to describe an epidemic that is limited to a small geographica area. Outbreak examples include food poisoning, enterovirus, norovirus, and seasonal flu.

The question might be asked: What are diseases called that occur regularly in a population but are not epidemic? This type of disease is referred to as an **endemic disease**. Whether a disease is epidemic or endemic depends on the disease and the population. Heart disease is endemic in America, whereas in many regions of equatorial Africa, malaria is endemic.

An **epidemiologist** studies the occurrence of disease or other health-related conditions in specific populations. Some epidemics begin as outbreaks of disease in animals, known as epizootics, and then spread to human populations. Examples are bubonic plague that first affects rodents and West Nile fever virus that first affects birds. Occasionally, an epidemic will spread over a wide area, perhaps even across an entire continent or around the world. Such

Epidemiology the study of the distribution and determinants of health-related states or events in specified populations, and the application of this study to control health problems

Epidemic an unexpectedly large number of cases of an illness, specific health-related behavior, or other health-related event in a particular population

Outbreak an event similar to an epidemic except that it is used for a limited geographic area

Endemic disease a disease that occurs at an expected level in a population or in a certain location

Epidemiologist one who practices epidemiology

TABLE 3.1 Notable Outbreaks and Epidemics in the United States

Disease	Cases in Previous Years	Epidemic Period	Number of Cases
St. Louis encephalitis	5–72	1975	1,815[2]
Legionnaires' disease	Unknown	1976	235[3]
Toxic shock syndrome	11–272	1980	877[4]
HIV/AIDS	Unknown (before 1975)	1981–2012	1,115,215 diagnosed with Stage 3 AIDS,[5] 652,409 deaths[6]
West Nile virus	Unknown in the United States	1999–2022	56,575[7]
Mumps	200–600	2006, 2016–2017	Approximately 6,000-6,5000[8,9]
2009 (H1N1)	This strain was previously unknown in the United States	April 2009–April 2010	An estimated 60.8 million cases and 12,469 deaths[10]
Pertussis	7,580–27,550	2012	48,277 cases[8]
E-cigarette, or vaping, product use-associated lung injury (EVALI)	Unknown	2019–	2,807 hospitalized EVALI cases and 68 deaths (as of February 18, 2020)[11]
COVID-19	0	January, 2020–May 11, 2023; endemic	6,143,551 hospitalizations, 1,127,938 Deaths[12]

Pandemic an outbreak of disease over a wide geographic area, such as a continent or multiple continents

a widespread epidemic is termed a **pandemic**. The influenza pandemic of 1918 is an example (see **Figure 3.1**). This disease spread in Europe, Asia, and North America simultaneously.[13] An estimated 25 million people died over several years as a result of this pandemic. The spread of 2009 H1N1 influenza, which disproportionately affected young people, also reached pandemic status. The outbreak of acquired immunodeficiency syndrome (AIDS) is another example of a pandemic. Worldwide, an estimated 770,000 people died from AIDS in 2018, and approximately 37.9 million people were living with HIV (human immunodeficiency virus). The number of new HIV infections has declined by 40% since its global peak in 1997.[14] More recently, the COVID-19 virus and disease, a concern in early 2020, evolved into a full pandemic within months, and resulted in the infection of tens of millions of people and the death of hundreds of thousands around the world (see **Box 3.1**).[15]

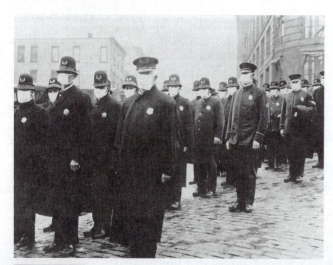

FIGURE 3.1   More than 25 million people died during the influenza pandemic of 1918–1919.

Courtesy of The National Archives.

History of Epidemiology

If one searches diligently, it is possible to trace the roots of epidemiologic thinking back to the "father of medicine," Hippocrates, who as early as 300 BCE, suggested a relationship between the occurrence of disease and the physical environment.[16] For example, cases of a disease fitting the description of malaria were found to occur in the vicinity of marshes and swamps.

With the fall of the classical civilizations of Greece and Rome and the return in Europe to a belief in spiritual causes of disease, few advances were made in the field of epidemiology. As a result, epidemics continued to occur. There were three waves of plague—one in 542 to 543, one in 1348 to 1349, and another in 1664 to 1665.[17] There were also epidemics of leprosy, smallpox, malaria, and, later, syphilis and yellow fever.

Epidemics occurred in the New World as well. One such epidemic of yellow fever struck Philadelphia in 1793, causing fever, body aches, and sometimes bleeding and

BOX 3.1   Novel Coronavirus Disease 2019 (COVID-19): A New Global Pandemic

At the end of December of 2019, the World Health Organization's Country Office in China was notified of an outbreak of an atypical, pneumonia-like illness with a common origin of the Huanan Seafood Wholesale Market, which was swiftly ordered closed on the first day of the new year. By January 7th, 2020, Chinese public health officials were able to identify a novel coronavirus as the source of the outbreak, with the WHO ascribing it the moniker "2019 Novel Coronavirus." By January 19th, there were 282 cases across four countries, with the United States reporting their first case on January 20th. Case counts continued to slowly rise to 180,000 worldwide cases, when the WHO declared COVID-19 a pandemic on March 11, 2020. The United States declared a nationwide emergency on March 13th, with states beginning to implement shutdowns on March 15th. The CDC rolled out masking guidelines on April 3rd. By April 10th, the United States becomes the country with the most reported cases and deaths, prompting the launch of Operation Warp Speed on April 30th, an initiative to fund and produce a vaccine against SARS-CoV-2. On May 28th, the United States' death toll surpassed 100,000. On July 7th, the number of confirmed U.S. cases passed 3 million, and the United States began the process of withdrawing from the WHO, following earlier statements made by the then president of the United States. On August 17, 2020, COVID-19 became the 3rd leading cause of U.S. deaths. Deaths and infections continued to soar, until December 14, when COVID vaccines first became available outside of clinical trials. By the end of the year 2020, 2.8 million Americans have received a COVID-19 vaccine. Early 2021 saw the expansion of monitoring and vaccination rollout, with worldwide cases passing 100 million. The CDC dropped masking recommendations among vaccinated individuals in March of 2021 and U.S. vaccinations surpassed 200 million in April. The Delta variant surged over summer months, prompting increased calls for vaccinations and boosters. In November, the Omicron variant was identified as a potential concern, with cases being detected in the United States into 2022. Infections continued to rise, as the daily average reached over 800,000 new cases throughout January of 2022. By March, 10 billion vaccine doses had been administered globally, and the United States approached 80 million cases. With increasing vaccination rates, infection rates began a long-term downward trend, culminating in the pandemic being declared over in May of 2023, with almost 775 million cumulative cases worldwide and nearly 7 million deaths over the course of 3 years.

According to the WHO, as of January of 2024, global COVID-19 cases and deaths were as follows:

Total COVID-19 Cases

WHO Region	Cases	Deaths
Globally	774,291,287	7,019,704
Africa	9,571,930	175,486
Americas	193,238,351	2,997,127
Eastern Mediterranean	23,410,381	351,878
Europe	278,731,686	2,267429
South-East Asia	61,248,144	808,329
Western Pacific	208,090,031	419,442

Data from World Health Organization 2023 data.who.int, WHO Coronavirus (COVID-19) dashboard > Cases [Dashboard]. https://data.who.int/dashboards/covid19/cases

COVID-19 is highly contagious and spreads rapidly, causing respiratory symptoms similar to those of a cold, flu, or pneumonia. However, it can also affect other parts of the body. While most cases result in mild symptoms, some individuals can become severely ill.

Spread: COVID-19 is transmitted when an infected person releases droplets and tiny particles containing the virus through breathing, speaking, coughing, or sneezing. These particles can be inhaled by others or come into contact with their eyes, nose, or mouth. Additionally, surfaces touched by infected individuals can become contaminated.

Symptoms: Symptoms of COVID-19 vary widely, ranging from mild to severe, and can appear 2 to 14 days after exposure. Common symptoms include fever, cough, shortness of breath, fatigue, muscle aches, headache, loss of taste or smell, sore throat, congestion, nausea, and diarrhea.

Prevention: In addition to standard hygiene practices like handwashing, preventive measures recommended by the CDC include staying updated with COVID-19 vaccines, improving ventilation, getting tested if necessary, following recommendations for exposure, staying home when sick, seeking treatment if at high risk, and avoiding contact with infected individuals.

People at Risk: Certain individuals, such as older adults, immunocompromised individuals, those with specific disabilities, or underlying health conditions, are at higher risk of severe illness if infected with COVID-19.

Data from (1) CDC. (2023, March 15). CDC museum COVID-19 timeline. Centers for Disease Control and Prevention. https://www.cdc.gov/museum/timeline/covid19.html; (2) CDC. (2024, January 16). Coronavirus disease 2019 (COVID-19). Centers for Disease Control and Prevention. https://www.cdc.gov/coronavirus/2019-nCoV/index.html./; (3) World Health Organization 2023 data.who.int, WHO Coronavirus (COVID-19) dashboard > Deaths [Dashboard]. https://data.who.int/dashboards/covid19/deaths

imparting a yellowish tone to the skin (jaundice).[18] This eighteenth-century outbreak also led to the death of 4,044 people. Yellow fever was an epidemic again in Philadelphia in 1797, 1798, and in 1803.[19] Dr. Benjamin Rush, a prominent Philadelphia physician and signatory

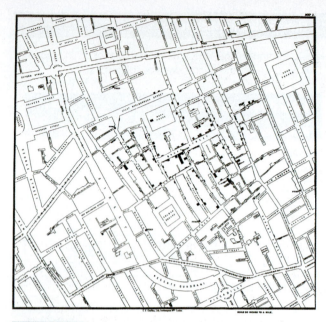

FIGURE 3.2 Cholera map—illustrated by John Snow in 1854.

© Pictorial Press Ltd/Alamy Stock Photo

of the Declaration of Independence, was able to trace the cases of yellow fever to the docks where ships arrived from tropical ports. However, his conclusion that the disease was caused by vapors arising from decaying coffee beans in port warehouses was incorrect. He could not have known that yellow fever is caused by a virus and is carried by the yellow fever mosquito, *Aedes aegypti*. These facts were discovered by Major Walter Reed of the U.S. Army and his associates a century later.

In 1849, some 50 years after the yellow fever outbreaks in Philadelphia, cholera became epidemic in London. A prominent physician, John Snow, investigated the outbreak by interviewing numerous victims and their families experiencing diarrhea, vomiting, and low blood pressure that can lead to shock and even death.[20]

Through the "**natural experiment**" that involved mapping of cholera cases and water sources, John Snow concluded that the epidemic was probably a waterborne disease and not attributable to the "miasma theory," a medical theory positing that "bad airs" entering the human body were the cause of cholera.[21] He concluded that the source of the epidemic was probably water drawn from a particular communal well located on Broad Street. Snow extinguished the epidemic in 1854 when he removed the pump handle from the Broad Street pump, thus forcing people to obtain their water elsewhere[22,23] (see **Figure 3.2**). For his investigative and analytical work, John Snow is widely considered the "father of modern epidemiology."

John Snow's quashing of the London cholera epidemic in 1854 is a classic example of how epidemiologic methods can be used to limit disease and deaths. His achievement was even more remarkable because it occurred 30 years before Louis Pasteur proposed his "germ theory of disease." It was not until 1883 that Robert Koch discovered the organism that causes cholera, *Vibrio cholerae*.

From its early use for the description and investigation of communicable diseases, epidemiology has developed into a sophisticated field of science. John Snow's method of going door to door to collect information is known as "shoe leather" epidemiology. While face-to-face interviewing is still used to collect data, epidemiologists also use other available methods, such as telephones and surveys to collect information. Modern epidemiologists may also use advanced statistical methods and powerful software to describe associations and patterns in the data. Epidemiologic methods are used to evaluate everything from the effectiveness of vaccines to the possible causes of occupational illnesses and unintentional injury deaths.

Knowledge of epidemiology is important to the community health worker who wishes to establish the presence of a set of needs or conditions for a particular health service or program or to justify a request for funding. Likewise, epidemiologic methods are used to evaluate the effectiveness of programs already in existence and to plan to meet anticipated needs for facilities and personnel.

Natural experiment "... naturally occurring circumstances in which subsets of the population have different levels of exposure to a supposed causal factor, in a situation resembling an actual experiment where human subjects would be randomly allocated to groups"[23]

Cases people diagnosed with a disease

Rate the number of events that occur in a given population in a given period of time

The Importance of Rates

Epidemiologists are concerned with numbers. Of prime importance is the number of health-related events, the number of **cases** (people who are sick), and, of course, the number of deaths. These numbers alone, however, are not enough to provide a description of the extent of the disease in a community. Epidemiologists must also know the total number in the susceptible population so that rates can be calculated. A **rate** is the number of events of interest (births,

TABLE 3.2 Deaths and Death Rates for Children Aged 1–4 Years, by Race, 2020

	White	Black
Number of deaths	1,553	917
Number at risk (population)	7,540,986	2,158,900
Death rate (per 100,000 population)	20.6	42.5

Data from Kochanek, K., Murphy, S., Xu, J., & Arias, E. (2023). Deaths: Final Data for 2020. National Center for Health Statistics (U.S.). https://doi.org/10.15620/cdc:131355

cases of disease, or deaths) in a given population over a given period or at a given point in time. Three general categories of rate are **natality (birth) rate**, **morbidity (sickness) rate**, and **mortality (fatality) rate**.

Why are rates important? Why not simply enumerate the sick or dead? The answer is that rates enable one to compare health events that occur at different times or in different places. For example, by using rates, it is possible to determine whether there are more cases of gonorrhea per capita this year than there were last year or whether there are more homicides per capita in City A than in City B. To do this, the population at risk must be considered.

For example, suppose you wish to compare deaths among young children of different races. In 2020, there were 1,553 deaths among White children aged 1 to 4 years and 917 deaths among Black children in the same age group.[24] Without calculating rates, one might assume that deaths were more common among young White children. However, if you knew the population at risk, you could calculate the death rate, the number of deaths divided by the population at risk, for each race (see **Table 3.2**). These rates have greater meaning because they are based on the **population at risk**, those who are susceptible to disease or death from a particular cause. In this case, the death rate is actually higher among Black children aged 1 to 4 years, thus deaths are actually more common among young Black children.

Incidence, Prevalence, and Attack Rates

Two important types of morbidity rates are incidence rates and prevalence rates. An **incidence rate** is defined as the number of *new* health-related events or cases of a disease in a population exposed to that risk in a given time period divided by the total population at risk—the number of new cases of influenza in a community over a week's time, divided by the number of people in the community who were susceptible, for example. Those who became ill with influenza during the previous week and remain ill during the week in question are not counted in an incidence rate. Incidence rates are important in the study of **acute disease**, a disease in which the peak severity of symptoms occurs and subsides within days or weeks. These diseases usually move quickly through a population. Examples of acute diseases are the common cold, influenza, chickenpox, measles, and mumps.

An **attack rate** is a special incidence rate calculated for a particular population for a single disease outbreak and usually expressed as a percentage (see **Table 3.3**). For example, suppose

Natality (birth) rate the number of live births divided by the total population

Morbidity (sickness) rate the number of people who are sick divided by the total population at risk

Mortality (fatality) rate the number of deaths in a population divided by the total population

Population at risk those who are susceptible to a particular disease or condition

Incidence rate the number of new health-related events or cases of a disease divided by the total number in the population at risk

Acute disease a disease with a brief duration of days to a few weeks

Attack rate an incidence rate calculated for a particular population for a single disease outbreak and expressed as a percentage

TABLE 3.3 Incidence Rates, Prevalence Rates, and Attack Rates

Name of Rate	Definition of Rate
Incidence rate =	$\dfrac{\text{Number of } new \text{ health-related events or cases of disease}}{\text{Population at risk during the same time period}}$
Attack rate* =	$\dfrac{\text{Number of people ill}}{\text{Number of people ill + well}} \times 100$ in a specific time period
Prevalence rate =	$\dfrac{\text{Number of individuals with health-related event or cases of a disease}}{\text{Total population at the same time period}}$

*Attack rates are usually given as a percentage.

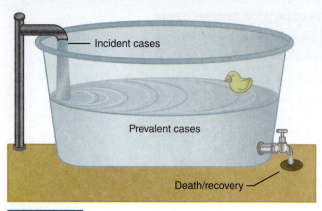

FIGURE 3.3 Analogy of incidence and prevalence.

Image from Alexander, L.K., Lopes, B., Ricchetti-Masterso , K., Yeatts, K.B. (n.d.). *Incident vs. prevalent cases and measures of occurrence*. https://sph.unc.edu/files/2015/07/nciph_ERIC1.pdf

a number of people who traveled on the same airline flight developed a similar illness and epidemiologists suspected that the cause of this illness was associated with the flight itself. An attack rate could be calculated for the passengers on that flight to express the percentage of who became ill. Furthermore, attack rates could be calculated for various subpopulations, such as those seated at various locations in the plane, those who selected specific entrees from the menu, those of particular age groups, or those who boarded the flight at specific stops. Differences in attack rates for different subpopulations might indicate to the epidemiologists the source or cause of the illness.

The **prevalence rate** is calculated by dividing *all current* cases of a disease (old and new) by the total population. Prevalence rates are useful for the study of **chronic disease**, diseases that usually last 3 months or longer. In these cases, it is more important to know how many people are currently suffering from a chronic disease—such as arthritis, heart disease, cancer, or diabetes—than it is to know when they developed it. Furthermore, with many chronic diseases, it is difficult or impossible to determine the date of onset of disease. Because a preponderance of health services and facilities are used for the treatment of persons with chronic diseases and conditions, prevalence rates are more useful than incidence rates for the planning of public health programs, personnel needs, and facilities.

An analogy of incidence and prevalence is demonstrated in **Figure 3.3**. The water from the faucet symbolizes incidence, while the water in the bathtub symbolizes prevalence.

Interpretation of Rates

Incidence and prevalence rates can be expressed in two forms—crude and adjusted. The **crude rate** is that in which the denominator includes the total population. Crude rates are relatively easy to obtain and are useful when comparing similar populations. However, crude rates can be misleading when populations differ in age structure or by some other attribute. For example, crude birth rates are normally higher in younger populations, which have a higher proportion of people of reproductive age, compared to populations with older people. Conversely, crude death rates are normally higher in older populations. This makes it difficult to use crude rates to compare the risk of death in different populations, such as those of the states of Florida and Alaska. To show what the level of mortality would be if the age composition of different populations were the same, epidemiologists use the **age-adjusted rate**. For example, in 2020, because of its larger senior population, Florida had a higher crude death rate (1,102.8 per 100,000) compared with Alaska's (707.1 per 100,000), where the population is younger. To address these differences, the death rates can be altered through mathematical approaches to account for differences in the age makeup of the populations being considered. After doing so, one can see that the death rate in Florida (735.7 per 100,000) compares favorably with the death rate in Alaska (769.4 per 100,000; see **Table 3.4**).[24] There are many types of rates, including those that focus on a particular

Prevalence rate the number of new and old cases of a disease in a population in a given period of time, divided by the total number in that population

Chronic disease a disease or health condition that lasts longer than 3 months

Crude rate a rate in which the denominator includes the total population

Age-adjusted rate a rate used to make comparisons across groups and over time when groups differ in age structure

TABLE 3.4 Crude and Age-Adjusted Mortality Rates for Alaska and Florida, 2020

State	Number of Deaths	Crude Death Rate*	Age-Adjusted Death Rate*
Alaska	5,170	707.1	769.4
Florida	239,685	1,102.8	735.7

*Deaths per 100,000 population.

Data from Kochanek, K., Murphy, S., Xu, J., & Arias, E. (2023). Deaths: Final Data for 2020. National Center for Health Statistics (U.S.). https://doi.org/10.15620/cdc:131355

population or condition. Details about these and methods for calculating various rates can be found in standard epidemiology textbooks.

Reporting of Births, Deaths, and Diseases

It is important to epidemiologists that births, deaths, and cases of diseases be recorded promptly and accurately. Physicians, clinics, and hospitals are required by law to report all births and deaths as well as all cases of certain **reportable diseases** to their local health departments. States determine conditions to designate as reportable diseases that are of local public health concern. Some noninfectious conditions, such as lead poisoning or acute cases of pesticide-related illness, are also included in this monitoring.[25]

At the national level, **notifiable diseases** are conditions that warrant monitoring, such as infectious diseases that can become epidemic and for which health officials maintain weekly records. The CDC oversees the National Notifiable Diseases Surveillance System (NNDSS) and issues a list of notifiable diseases for which it requests reports from each state health department. This list is revised periodically due to changing health concerns. The list is established by the CDC in collaboration with the Council of State and Territorial Epidemiologists (CSTE), although it may not align with state reportable disease lists. In 2023, more than 80 diseases were designated as notifiable at the national level (see **Table 3.5**).[26] The reporting guidelines vary for each condition listed. For example, some conditions warrant immediate/urgent reporting (e.g., anthrax), whereas others only stipulate annual reporting (e.g., cancer). Furthermore, the guidelines also specify which types of cases must be reported for each disease. The CDC website has more information about the national reporting guidelines for each condition.[26]

Local health departments are required by their respective state health departments to summarize all records of births (see **Figure 3.4**), deaths, and reportable diseases. State health

Reportable diseases conditions whose reporting is mandatory when encountered by health providers, hospitals, or laboratories

Notifiable diseases diseases for which health officials request nonidentifiable reporting for public health reasons

TABLE 3.5 Nationally Notifiable Conditions, 2023	
Anthrax	Listeriosis
Arboviral disease[a]	Lyme disease
Babesiosis	Malaria
Botulism	Measles
Brucellosis	Melioidiosis
Campylobacteriosis	Meningococcal disease (*Neisseria meningitides*)
Cancer[b,c]	Mpox virus infection
Candida auris, clinical & screening	Mumps
Carbapenemase Producing Carbapenem-Resistant Enterobacteriaceae (CP-CRE)	Novel influenza A virus infection
Carbon monoxide poisoning[b,c]	Pertussis
Chancroid	Pesticide-related illness, acute (nonoccupational and occupational)
Chlamydia trachomatis infection	Plague
Cholera	Poliomyelitis, paralytic
Coccidioidomycosis	Poliovirus infection, nonparalytic
Congenital spyhilis	Psittacosis

(continues)

TABLE 3.5 Nationally Notifiable Conditions, 2023 *(continued)*

Coronavirus Disease 2019 (COVID-19)	Q fever (acute and chronic)
Cryptosporidiosis	Rabies in a human or animal
Cyclosporiasis	Rickettsiosis, spotted fever
Dengue virus infections[d]	Rubella
Diphtheria	Rubella, congenital syndrome
Ehrlichiosis and anaplasmosis	*Salmonella* Paratyphi infection
Escherichia coli, Shiga toxin-producing (STEC)	*Salmonella* Typhi infection
Foodborne disease outbreaks[e]	Salmonellosis
Giardiasis	SARS-associated coronavirus
Gonorrhea	Shigellosis
Haemophilus influenzae, invasive disease	Silicosis
Hansen's disease	Smallpox
Hantavirus infection, nonhantavirus pulmonary syndrome	*Staphylococcus aureus* infection (Vancomycin-intermediate or vancomycin-resistant)
Hantavirus pulmonary syndrome	Streptococcal toxic-shock syndrome (STSS)
Hemolytic uremic syndrome, post-diarrheal	Syphilis
Hepatitis A, acute	Tetanus
Hepatitis B virus, perinatal infection	Toxic-shock syndrome (non-*Streptococcus*)
Hepatitis B, acute	Trichinellosis (Trichinosis)
Hepatitis B, chronic	Tuberculosis
Hepatitis C, acute	Tularemia
Hepatitis C, chronic	Vancomycin-intermediate and resistant *Staphylococcus aureus*
Hepatitis C, perinatal infection	Varicella and varicella deaths
HIV infection	Vibriosis
Influenza-associated pediatric mortality	Viral hemorrhagic fevers[g]
Invasive pneumococcal disease (IPD)	Waterborne disease outbreaks
Lead, exposure screening test result[f]	Yellow fever
Legionellosis	Zika virus disease and infection
Leptopsirosis	

Note: Approved by the Council of State and Territorial Epidemiologists (CSTE) June 2019, implemented January 2020.

[a]Arboviral diseases: Chikungunya virus disease, Eastern equine encephalitis virus disease (EEE), Jamestown Canyon virus disease, La Crosse virus disease, Powassan virus disease, St. Louis encephalitis virus disease (SLE), Western equine encephalitis virus disease (WEE), West Nile virus disease (WNV).

[b]Notification for all confirmed cases of cancers should be made at least annually.

[c]Noninfectious condition.

[d]Dengue virus infections include dengue, severe dengue, and dengue-like illness.

[e]Outbreaks are defined by state and local health departments, all situations deemed by a local or state health department to be an outbreak are notifiable.

[f]Notification for lead exposure screening results should be submitted quarterly for children and twice a year for adults.

[g]Viral hemorrhagic fever diseases: Crimean-Congo, Ebola, Guanarito, Junín (Argentine), Lassa virus, Lujo virus, Machupo (Bolivian), Marburg virus, or Sabia-associated (Brazilian).

Data from Center for Disease Control and Prevention. (2022, January 1). *Protocol for public health agencies to notify CDC about the occurrence of nationally notifiable conditions, 2022.* Cdc.gov. https://ndc.services.cdc.gov/wp-content/uploads/NNC_2022_Notification_Requirements_By_Timeframe _FINAL_01252022.pdf

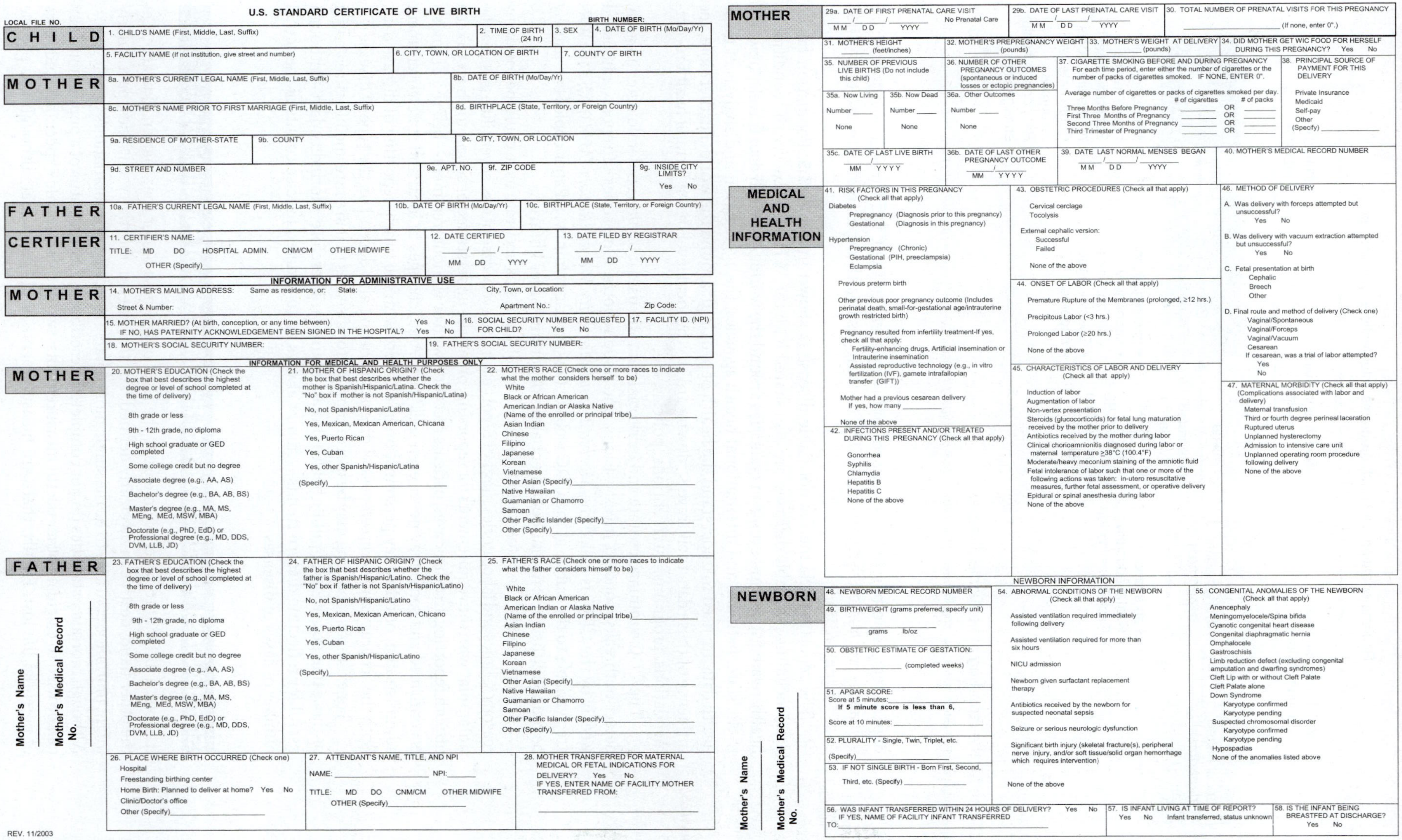

FIGURE 3.4   Birth certificates are issued by local health departments that have jurisdiction where the birth occurred.

Reproduced from Centers for Disease Control and Prevention. (2003). "U.S. Standard Certificate of Live Birth." http://www.cdc.gov/nchs/data/dvs/birth11-03final-acc.pdf

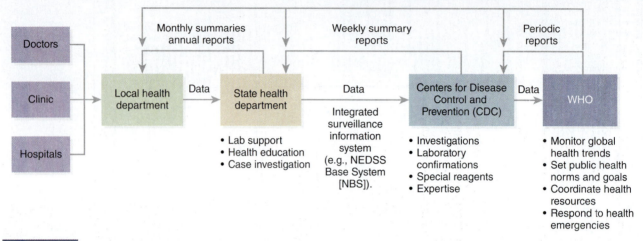

FIGURE 3.5 Scheme for the reporting of notifiable diseases.

Data from Centers for Disease Control and Prevention. *National Notifiable Diseases Surveillance System (NNDSS)*. Available at https://wwwn.cdc.gov/nndss/data-collection.html

---

Integrated surveillance information systems health information systems for the National Notifiable Diseases Surveillance System (NNDSS) that are based on the National Electronic Disease Surveillance System (NEDSS) architectural standards

NEDSS Base System (NBS) information system created by the CDC to record and report notable disease information to the CDC

departments summarize these reports and relay them to the CDC through **integrated surveillance information systems**. The CDC encourages health departments to use the **NEDSS Base System (NBS)**.[25]

The reporting scheme for notifiable disease is shown in **Figure 3.5**. Population health data, including notifiable diseases, are also shared with the WHO, to observe the condition of health-related states and events in countries around the world. As health data travels "upward" to the state, national, and international health agencies, the aggregation and analysis of these health data are used to understand the health of people all around the world. Furthermore, the influence of these data then travels "downward" to the local level in the form of health recommendations, programs, interventions, policies, etc.

The CDC summarizes state and territorial data and uses it to plan epidemiologic research, detect outbreaks, conduct investigations, and issue reports. One series of reports, published weekly by the CDC, is called the *Morbidity and Mortality Weekly Report (MMWR)*. *MMWR*s are available to the public at the CDC website (www.cdc.gov/mmwr). Paper copies can usually be found in the government document areas of certain larger libraries.

Unfortunately, the information reported is not always as accurate as it could be for many reasons. Clinics and laboratories may not report each and every case of less-severe illnesses, may be unfamiliar with the requirements for reporting, or may be understaffed or simply too busy to keep up with reporting. In other cases, patients recover—with or without treatment—before a diagnosis is confirmed and some may never even seek care. Also, changes in local and state government administration or other key personnel often interfere with the timely reporting of disease data. Both the accuracy and completeness of disease reporting also depend on the type of disease.[27]

For example, reporting may be more complete for diseases that are rare and life-threatening or those that pose a larger public health threat or burden. Therefore, morbidity data—although useful for reflecting disease trends—cannot always be considered precise counts of the actual number of cases of diseases.

Standardized Measurements of Health Status of Populations

It is often difficult to precisely measure the level of wellness or, for that matter, ill health. On the other hand, death can be clearly defined. For this reason, mortality statistics, particularly infant mortality, continue to be the single most reliable indicator of a population's health status. Although mortality statistics do not completely describe the health status of a population, they can be used to calculate other useful measurements; two of these are life expectancy and years of potential life lost. Finally, there are measurements of ill health that, although less precise than mortality, can nonetheless be meaningful. Such measurements are disability-adjusted life years and health-adjusted life expectancy.

Mortality Statistics

In 2020, there were 3,383,729 deaths registered in the United States. The crude mortality rate was 1,027.0 per 100,000, while the age-adjusted death rate, which eliminates the effects of the aging population, was 835.4 deaths per 100,000 U.S. standard population. Age-adjusted death rates show what the level of mortality would be if no changes occurred in the age makeup of the population from year to year. Thus, they are a better indicator than unadjusted (crude) death rates for examining changes in the risk of death over a period of time when the age distribution of the population is changing. Death rates and age-adjusted death rates for the 15 leading causes of death in the United States in 2020 are presented in **Table 3.6**.[24]

TABLE 3.6 Number of Deaths, Percentage of Total Deaths, Death Rates, and Age-Adjusted Death Rates for 2020, Percentage Change in Age-Adjusted Death Rates in 2020 from 2019 for the 15 Leading Causes of Death in 2020: United States

Rank[a]	Cause of Death (Based on ICD-10)	Number	Percentage of Total Deaths	Crude Death Rate	2020	Percent Change from 2019 to 2020 from 2019 to 2020
...	All causes	3,383,729	100.0	1,027.0	835.4	16.8
1	Diseases of heart (I00–I09, I11, I13, I20–I51)	696,962	20.6	211.5	168.2	4.1
2	Malignant neoplasms (C00–C97)	602,350	17.8	182.8	144.1	−1.4
3	COVID-19 (U07.1)	350,831	10.4	106.5	85.0	—
4	Accidents (unintentional injuries) (V01–X59, Y85–Y86)	200,955	5.9	61.0	57.6	16.8
5	Cerebrovascular diseases (I60–I69)	160,264	4.7	48.6	38.8	4.9
6	Chronic lower respiratory diseases (J40–J47)	152,657	4.5	46.3	36.4	−4.7
7	Alzheimer's disease (G30)	134,242	4.0	40.7	32.4	8.7
8	Diabetes mellitus (E10–E14)	102,188	3.0	31.0	248.	14.8
9	Influenza and pneumonia (J09–J18)	53,544	1.6	16.3	13.0	5.7
10	Nephritis, nephrotic syndrome and nephrosis (N00–N07, N17–N19, N25–N27)	52,547	1.6	15.9	12.7	0.0
11	Chronic liver disease and cirrhosis (K70, K73–K74)	51,642	1.5	15.7	13.3	17.7
12	Intentional self-harm (suicide) (`U03, X60–X84, Y87.0)	45,979	1.4	14.0	13.5	−2.9
13	Essential hypertension and hypertensive renal disease (I10, I12, I15)	41,907	1.2	12.7	10.1	13.5
14	Parkinson's disease (G20–G21)	40,284	1.2	12.2	9.9	12.5
15	Septicemia (A40–A41)	40,050	1.2	12.2	9.7	2.1
...	All other causes (residual)	657,327	19.4	199.5	...	...

[a]Rank based on number of deaths.

Naturally, morbidity and mortality rates vary greatly, depending on age, sex, race, and ethnicity. For example, as of 2021, whereas heart disease was the leading cause of death for the general population and especially for older adults (those who have reached 65 years of age), COVID-19 was the leading cause of death for the 45–54 age group, cancer is the leading cause of death for the 55- to 64-year-old age group, and unintentional injuries are the leading cause of death for all age groups between 1 and 44 years.[24]

There has been a shift in the leading causes of death since the beginning of the twentieth century. When the century began, communicable diseases, such as pneumonia, tuberculosis, and gastrointestinal infections were the leading causes of death.[28] However, a century of progress in public health practice and in biomedical research resulted in a significant reduction in the proportion of deaths from communicable diseases so that the seven leading causes of death today are noncommunicable diseases (see **Figure 3.6** and **Table 3.7**). Figure 3.6 shows the shift in the causes of death between 1900 and 2021. Table 3.7 shows that in 2021, the five leading causes of death in the United States—heart disease, cancer, COVID-19, unintentional injuries (accidents and adverse effects), and stroke—accounted for

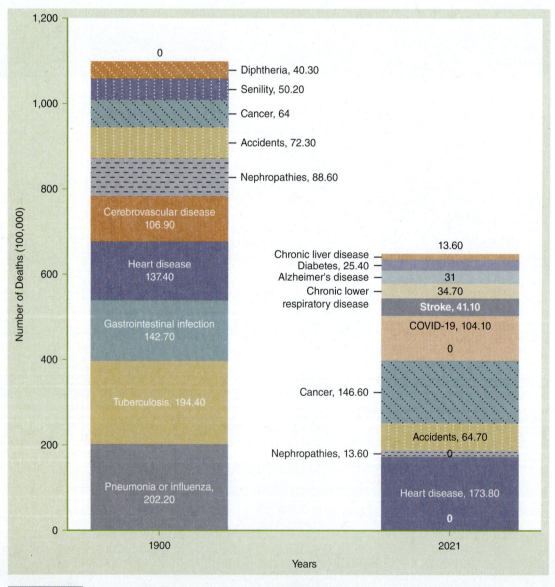

FIGURE 3.6   Death rates in the United States in 1900 and 2021.

TABLE 3.7 Leading Causes of Death in the United States: 1900, 1940, 2021	
1900	
1.	Pneumonia, influenza
2.	Tuberculosis
3.	Diarrhea
4.	Diseases of the heart
5.	Cerebrovascular diseases (stroke)
6.	Nephritis
7.	Unintentional injuries (accidents)
8.	Malignant neoplasms (cancers)
9.	Senility
10.	Diphtheria
1940	
1.	Diseases of the heart
2.	Malignant neoplasms (cancers)
3.	Cerebrovascular diseases (stroke)
4.	Nephritis
5.	Pneumonia, influenza
6.	Unintentional injuries (nonmotor vehicle)
7.	Tuberculosis
8.	Diabetes mellitus
9.	Unintentional injuries (motor vehicle)
10.	Premature birth
2020	
1.	Diseases of the heart
2.	Malignant neoplasms (cancers)
3.	COVID-19
4.	Accidents (unintentional injuries)
5.	Cerebrovascular diseases (stroke)
6.	Chronic lower respiratory diseases
7.	Alzheimer's disease
8.	Diabetes mellitus
9.	Influenza and pneumonia
10.	Nephritis, nephrotic syndrome, and nephrosis

Data from Kochanek, K., Murphy, S., Xu, J., & Arias, E. (2023). *Deaths: Final Data for 2020*. National Center for Health Statistics (U.S.). https://doi.org/10.15620/cdc:131355; Centers for Disease Control and Prevention, National Center for Health Statistics. (1998). *Leading causes of death, 1900–1998*. http://www.cdc.gov/nchs/data/dvs/lead1900_98.pdf

about 60% of all deaths.[24] In 2019, the five leading causes of death worldwide were ischemic heart disease, stroke, chronic obstructive pulmonary disease, lower respiratory infections, and neonatal conditions.[29]

This domination of annual mortality statistics by noncommunicable diseases masks the importance of communicable diseases as causes of death in certain age groups. For example, COVID-19 and pneumonia and influenza account for a larger portion of deaths among young

Life expectancy the average number of years a person from a specific cohort is projected to live from a given point in time

Years of potential life lost (YPLL) the number of years lost when death occurs before the age of 65 or 75

children and older adults compared with other age groups. Thus, it is important to remember that viewing the leading causes of death for the entire population does not provide a clear picture of the health of any one segment of the population.

Life Expectancy

Life expectancy is another standard measurement used to compare the health status of various populations. Also based on mortality, **life expectancy** is defined as the average number of years a person from a specific cohort is projected to live from a given point in time. Whereas life insurance companies are interested in life expectancy at every age, health statisticians are usually concerned with life expectancy at birth, at the age of 65 years, and, more recently, at age 75. It is important to remember that life expectancy is an average for an entire cohort (usually of a single birth year) and is not necessarily a useful prediction for any one individual. Moreover, it certainly cannot describe the quality of one's life. However, the ever-increasing life expectancy for Americans suggests that as a country, we have managed to control some of those factors that contribute to early deaths.

Table 3.8 provides a summary of life expectancy figures for the United States from 1900 to 2021. The data presented indicate that the overall life expectancy at birth, at 65 years, and at 75 years has generally increased since 1900 except following the COVID-19 pandemic. Life expectancies at birth for both sexes rose from 47.3 years in 1900 to 78.7 years in 2018 and have since fallen to 76.4 in 2021 due to COVID-19 pandemic. In 2021, the life expectancy of a newborn baby girl was 79.3 years compared with a newborn baby boy—73.5 years.[30]

Compared with the 2023 life expectancy figures of other countries (see **Table 3.9**), the United States figures (approximately 79 years for both ages combined) roughly correspond with those of other countries with well-developed economies. The highest life expectancy figures are reported in Japan (84 years); whereas the lowest are reported from countries in Africa (53 years in the Central African Republic, Lesotho, and Sierra Leone).[31]

Years of Potential Life Lost

Whereas standard mortality statistics, such as leading causes of death, provide one measure of the importance of various diseases, **years of potential life lost (YPLL)** provides another, different measure. YPLL is calculated by subtracting a person's age at death from a predefined, standard

TABLE 3.8 Life Expectancy at Birth, at 65 Years of Age, and at 75 Years of Age According to Sex: In the United States, During the Selected Years 1900–2021

Year	At Birth			At 65 Years			At 75 Years		
	Both Sexes	Male	Female	Both Sexes	Male	Female	Both Sexes	Male	Female
1900	47.3	46.3	48.3	11.9	11.5	12.2	*	*	*
1950	68.2	65.6	71.1	13.9	12.8	15.0	*	*	*
1960	69.7	66.6	73.1	14.3	12.8	15.8	*	*	*
1970	70.8	67.1	74.7	15.2	13.1	17.0	*	*	*
1980	73.7	70.7	77.4	16.4	14.1	18.3	10.4	8.8	11.5
1990	75.4	71.8	78.8	17.2	15.1	18.9	10.9	9.4	12.0
2000	76.8	74.1	79.3	17.6	16.0	19.0	11.0	9.8	11.8
2010	78.7	76.2	81.0	19.1	17.7	20.3	12.1	11.0	12.9
2021	76.4	73.5	79.3	18.4	17.0	19.7	*	*	*

*Data not available.

**Data for 2017 (data on life expectancy at age 75 for 2018 not available).

Data from Xu, J., Murphy, S., Kochanek, K., & Arias, E. (2022). Mortality in the United States, 2021. National Center for Health Statistics (U.S.). Kochanek, K., Murphy, S., Xu, J., & Arias, E. (2023). Deaths: Final Data for 2020. National Center for Health Statistics (U.S.). https://doi.org/10.15620/cdc:131355

TABLE 3.9 Life Expectancy at Birth for Selected Countries by Sex in 2023

	Male	Female
Central African Republic	50.2	56.3
Ethiopia	66.9	70.5
Malawi	62.3	68.9
India	69.5	72.2
Nicaragua	72.1	77.9
Ecuador	76.4	80.5
Congo	63.8	65.6
Thailand	61.5	67.2
Malaysia	72.6	77.1
South Africa	62.2	68.3
Brazil	72.4	79.4
Latvia	70.6	79.8
Republic of Korea	80.3	86.1
Greece	78.6	83.6
New Zealand	80.4	83.5
United Kingdom	79.8	83.0
United States	76.3	80.7
Sweden	80.8	84.0
Japan	81.5	86.9

Data from World Health Organization. World Health Organization. (2023). World health statistics 2023: monitoring health for the SDGs, Sustainable Development Goals. World Health Organization.

age. Each person may have a different life expectancy at any given time, so the age 75 years is often used in these calculations. For example, for a person who dies at age 59, the YPLL-75 is 16. Although age 75 is conventionally used for calculations, the standard age could be 65, 70, 80, or any other predefined age.

YPLL helps epidemiologists gauge the impact of early death in a population. Using this measure weighs deaths in a way that the death of a very young person counts more than the death of a much older person. **Table 3.10** provides a summary of the age-adjusted YPLL before age 75 (YPLL-75) for the 10 leading causes of death in the United States for 1990 and 2016.[30] In examining this table, note that the number of YPLL-75 per 100,000 population was highest for malignant neoplasms (cancer) and unintentional injuries. This is because unintentional injuries and malignant neoplasms (cancer) are more common causes of death for people who are young. These differences can also be seen in the two pie charts shown in **Figure 3.7**. Also, notice that the YPLL-75 per 100,000 population declined for most of the leading causes of death between 1980 and 2016.

YPLL from specific causes varies depending on the subpopulation under consideration. For example, the YPLL-75 per 100,000 population resulting from unintentional injuries is nearly two and a half times higher for men compared with women. The YPLL-75 per 100,000 for diseases of the heart for Black people is two and a half times more than for White people, and for homicide, it is over six times greater.[30]

Disability-Adjusted Life Years

Mortality does not entirely express the burden of disease. For example, chronic depression and paralysis caused by polio are responsible for great loss of healthy life but are not reflected in mortality tables. Because of this, the World Health Organization (WHO) and the World Bank have developed a measure called the **disability-adjusted life years (DALYs)**.[32,33]

Disability-adjusted life years (DALYs) a measure for the burden of disease that takes into account premature death and loss of healthy life resulting from disability

TABLE 3.10 Age-Adjusted Years of Potential Life Lost Before 75 (YPLL-75) for the 10 Leading Causes of Death, United States, 1990 and 2020

	Population	
	1,990	2,020
Diseases of heart	1,539	995.56
Malignant Neoplasms	1933.8	1,107.1
COVID-19	*	497.54
Accidents (unintentional injuries)	1171.4	1,658.6
Cerebrovascular diseases	246.54	170.28
Chronic lower respiratory diseases	173.14	155.27
Alzheimer's disease	5.46	13.27
Diabetes mellitus	149.50	220.70
Influenza and pneumonia	136.20	90.36
Nephritis, nephrotic syndrome and nephrosis	48.14	72.72

*Comparable data not available.

Data from Centers for Disease Control and Prevention. Web-based Injury Statistics Query and Reporting System (WISQARS) [Online]. (2003). National Center for Injury Prevention and Control, Centers for Disease Control and Prevention (producer). Available from URL: www.cdc.gov/ncipc/wisqars. Accessed 2024, Feb. 24.

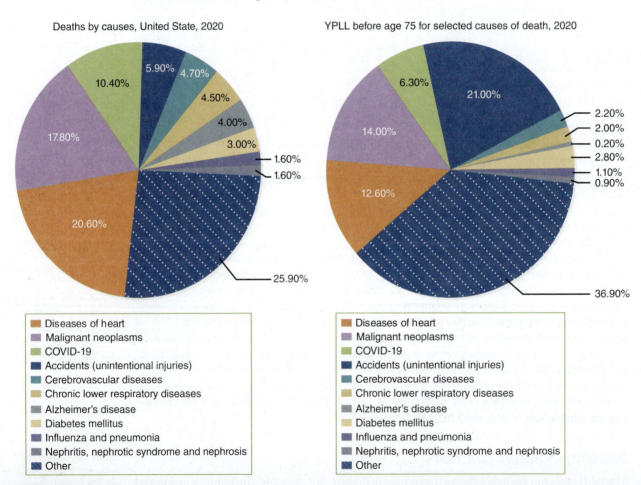

FIGURE 3.7 Deaths by cause in the United States, 2016, and the years of potential life lost before age 75 (YPLL-75) per 100,000 population for selected causes of death within the United States, 2016.

Data from Kochanek, K., Murphy, S., Xu, J., & Arias, E. (2023). *Deaths: Final Data for 2020*. National Center for Health Statistics (U.S.). https://doi.org/10.15620/cdc:131355; Centers for Disease Control and Prevention. (2003). *Web-based Injury Statistics Query and Reporting System (WISQARS)* [Online]. National Center for Injury Prevention and Control, Centers for Disease Control and Prevention (producer). Available from https://wisqars.cdc.gov/about/

One DALY is one lost year of healthy life. Total DALYs for a given condition for a particular population can be calculated by estimating the total years of life lost and the total years of life lived with disability, and then by summing these totals. As an example, the DALYs incurred through firearm injuries in the United States could be calculated by adding the total of YPLL incurred from fatal firearm injuries to the total years of life lived with disabilities by survivors of firearm injuries. **Figure 3.8** illustrates the number of DALYs lost per 100,000 population in 2019 from four income level regions of the world.[34] This figure shows that DALY is calculated by adding both YLL (Years of Life Lost) and YDL (Years lost due to Disability[34]).

Health-Adjusted Life Expectancy

Health-adjusted life expectancy (HALE), sometimes referred to as healthy life expectancy, is the number of years of healthy life expected, on average, in a given population or region of the world. The HALE indicator used by the WHO is similar to the disability-adjusted life expectancy (DALE) first reported in the original Global Burden of Disease study.[35] The methods used to calculate HALE are beyond the scope of this text, but have been described elsewhere.[36] Worldwide, HALE at birth in 2019 was 63.7 years, 9.6 years lower than overall life expectancy at birth. When comparing global regions, HALE in African nations is very low—56.0 years for males and females, compared with around 68 years in Europe and the Western Pacific region (**Figure 3.9**).[37]

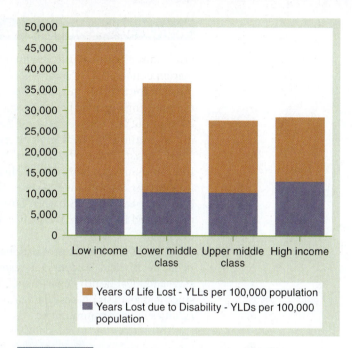

FIGURE 3.8   Burden of disease: years of life lost due to premature mortality (YLL) and years of life lived with a disability (YLD) per one hundred thousand by World Bank Income Groups, 2019. DALYs: disability-adjusted life years.

Data from Global health estimates: Leading causes of DALYs. (2019). Who.int. Retrieved February 26, 2024, from https://www.who.int/data/gho/data/themes/mortality-and-global-health-estimates/global-health-estimates-leading-causes-of-dalys

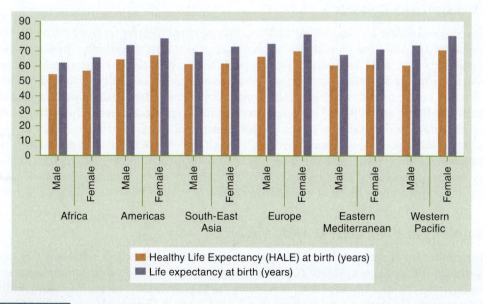

FIGURE 3.9   Life expectancy, health-adjusted life expectancy (HALE), and lost healthy years by region and sex, 2016.

Data from World Health Organization. (2020). *Life expectancy and healthy life expectancy Data by WHO region.* https://apps.who.int/gho/data/view.main.SDG2016LEXREGv?lang=en

Health-adjusted life expectancy (HALE) the number of years of healthy life expected, on average, in a given population

Sources of Secondary Data

Data sources can be either primary or secondary. Primary data consist of original information collected firsthand, whereas secondary data have been collected by someone else, possibly for another purpose. Because demographic and epidemiological data are used in the planning of public health programs and facilities, students of community health should be aware of the sources of these secondary data. Students can obtain secondary data for use in community health work from the following sources: the U.S. Census, *National Vital Statistics Reports, Morbidity and Mortality Weekly Reports*, the National Health Interview Survey, the National Health and Nutrition Examination Survey, the Behavioral Risk Factor Surveillance System, the Youth Risk Behavior Surveillance System, and the National Health Care Surveys. This is only a small selection of secondary data sources commonly used in community health; many more sources of secondary data exist on a variety of topics.

Each of these sources of national data has a specific value and usefulness to those in the public health field. Students interested in studying local health problems can obtain data from state and local health departments, hospitals, volunteer agencies, and disease registries. The study and analysis of these data provide a basis for planning appropriate health programs and facilities in your communities.

The U.S. Census

The **U.S. Census**, taken every 10 years, is an enumeration of the population living in the United States. Following the directive in the U.S. Constitution's Article I, Section 2, George Washington ordered the first census in 1790 for the purpose of apportioning representation to the House of Representatives. Through the years, the census form has become much more complex than the one filled out more than 200 years earlier. Data are gathered about income, employment, family size, education, dwelling type, and many other social indicators. Copies of the U.S. Census results are available in most libraries and online at www.census.gov.

Census data are important to health workers because they are used for calculating disease and death rates and for program planning. The U.S. Census is carried out by the Bureau of the Census, located in the U.S. Department of Commerce.

Vital Statistics Reports

The National Center for Health Statistics (NCHS), one of the Centers for Disease Control and Prevention, provides the most up-to-date national vital statistics available. These statistics appear in the *National Vital Statistics Reports*, published by the NCHS in Hyattsville, Maryland. **Vital statistics** are statistical summaries of vital records, that is, records of major life events. Listed are births, deaths, marriages, and divorces. Detailed reports of data from the birth and death certificates are published in preliminary and final reports each year. The birth reports include data on a wide range of topics, including maternal and infant characteristics as well as details about prenatal care and delivery. The death report includes data on death rates, life expectancy, leading causes of death, and infant mortality. In addition to these reports, four to six reports are published each year on special topics related to vital statistics. *National Vital Statistics Reports* are available at www.cdc.gov/nchs.

Morbidity and Mortality Weekly Report

Reported cases of specified notifiable diseases are reported weekly in the *Morbidity and Mortality Weekly Report (MMWR)*, which lists morbidity and mortality data by state and region of the country. The report is prepared by the CDC based on reports from state health departments. This report is printed and distributed through an agreement with the Massachusetts Medical Society, publishers of the *New England Journal of Medicine*. Each weekly

U.S. Census the enumeration of the population of the United States that is conducted every 10 years

Vital statistics statistical summaries of records of major life events, such as births, deaths, marriages, divorces, and infant deaths

issue also contains several reports of outbreaks of disease, environmental hazards, unusual cases, or other public health problems. The *MMWR* and its annual summary reports are available at www.cdc.gov/mmwr.

National Health Surveys

Another source of secondary data is the national health surveys. These surveys are a result of the National Health Survey Act of 1956, which authorized a continuing survey of the amount, distribution, and effects of illness and disability in the United States. The intent of this Act is currently being fulfilled by three types of surveys: (1) health interviews of people; (2) clinical tests, measurements, and physical examinations of people; and (3) surveys of places where people receive medical care, such as hospitals, clinics, and doctors' offices. The following paragraphs describe these surveys. More information about these surveys and results is available at the National Center for Health Statistics website: www.cdc.gov/nchs.

National Health Interview Survey

In the National Health Interview Survey (NHIS), conducted by the National Center for Health Statistics (NCHS), people are asked numerous questions about their health. One of the questions asks respondents to describe their health status using one of five categories— excellent, very good, good, fair, or poor. About 14.5% of the adult respondents in 2022 described their health status as either fair or poor, while approximately 6 in 10 Americans believe they are in very good or excellent health. College graduates were more likely than persons who had not graduated from high school to describe their health as good, excellent, or very good (93.2%and 65.8%, respectively). Persons with family incomes of $100,000 or more were also more likely than those with incomes of less than the federal poverty level to describe their health as good, excellent, or very good (89.8% and 69.6%, respectively). There were also differences when comparing race, ethnicity, age, marital status, and place of residence.[38]

It is important to remember that these data were generated by self-reported responses to NHIS questions and not by actual examinations objectively generated in a clinic. As such, respondents may over-report good health habits or under-report bad ones. Such reporting is often dependent on the respondent's perceived social stigma or support for a response and the degree to which people's responses are confidential or anonymous. Furthermore, people have widely divergent views on what constitutes poor or good health. For example, many sedentary, cigarette-smoking, high-stress people see themselves as being in good health, whereas "health nuts" may feel their health is deteriorating when they miss a day of exercise. In general, the young assess their health better than the old do, males better than females, White people better than Black people, and those with large family incomes better than those with smaller ones. Other topics covered by the NHIS include limitations and injuries, access to health care, and health insurance coverage.

National Health and Nutrition Examination Survey

Another of the national health surveys is the National Health and Nutrition Examination Survey (NHANES). The purpose of the NHANES is to assess the health and nutritional status of the general U.S. population. Using a mobile examination center (see **Figure 3.10**), the data are collected through direct physical examinations, clinical and laboratory testing, and related procedures on a representative group of Americans. These examinations result in the most authoritative source of standardized clinical, physical, and physiologic data on the American people. Included in the data are the prevalence of specific conditions and diseases and data on blood pressure, serum cholesterol, body measurements, nutritional status and deficiencies, and exposure to environmental toxins.

The first series of these surveys, known as National Health Examination Surveys (NHES), were carried out during the 1960s. Beginning in the 1970s, nutrition was added as a new focus, and the surveys became known as the National Health and Nutrition Examination Survey

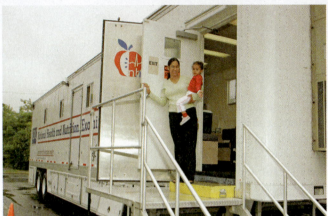 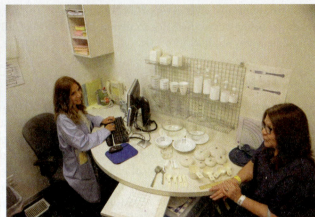

FIGURE 3.10   A National Health and Nutrition Examination Survey (NHANES) mobile examination center.
Courtesy of CDC.

(NHANES). Three cycles of the NHANES were conducted at periodic time intervals by the NCHS, the third ending in 1994. The survey became a continuous, rather than periodic, program in 1999. The focus of the program is on a variety of health and nutrition measurement changes to meet emerging needs.

Results of NHANES benefit people in the United States in important ways. Facts about the distribution of health problems and risk factors in the population give researchers important clues to the causes of disease. Information collected from the current survey is compared with information collected from previous surveys. This allows health planners to detect the extent to which various health problems and risk factors have changed in the U.S. population over time. By identifying the healthcare needs of the population, government agencies and private sector organizations can establish policies and plan research, education, and health promotion programs that help improve present health status and prevent future health problems.[39]

Each year, the survey examines a nationally representative sample of about 5,000 people, located in 15 counties across the country using mobile examination centers.

Behavioral Risk Factor Surveillance System

The Behavioral Risk Factor Surveillance System (BRFSS) is a state-based telephone survey of the civilian, noninstitutionalized, adult population conducted by the Office of Surveillance, Epidemiology, and Laboratory Services at the CDC. This survey seeks to ascertain the prevalence of such high-risk behaviors as cigarette smoking, excessive alcohol consumption, physical inactivity, and the lack of preventive health care such as screening for cancer. These results are published periodically as part of *MMWR's CDC Surveillance Summaries* and are available wherever copies of the CDC *MMWR* are found. Information is also available at www.cdc.gov/brfss.

Youth Risk Behavior Surveillance System

The national Youth Risk Behavior Survey (YRBS) monitors six categories of priority health-risk behaviors among youth and young adults, including behaviors that contribute to unintentional injuries and violence; tobacco use; alcohol and other drug use; sexual behaviors that contribute to unintended pregnancy and sexually transmitted infections (STIs), including human immunodeficiency virus (HIV) infection; unhealthy dietary behaviors; and physical inactivity. In addition, the national YRBS monitors the prevalence of obesity and asthma. The national YRBS is conducted every 2 years during the spring semester and provides data representative of ninth- through twelfth-grade students in public and private schools in the United States.[40]

YRBS includes a national school-based survey conducted by the CDC, and state and local school-based surveys conducted by state and local education and health agencies. The YRBS is conducted by the CDC's Division of Adolescent and School Health. More information about YRBS is available at www.cdc.gov/healthyyouth/yrbs.

National Health Care Surveys

The National Health Care Surveys comprise 11 different national surveys that gather information on the nation's healthcare system. The purpose of these surveys is to help healthcare providers, policymakers, and researchers answer questions about resources, care quality, and disparities in services for care provided in the United States. The surveys are delivered according to settings that include physician offices and community health centers, hospitals, ambulatory surgery centers, long-term care facilities, hospice and home health, and prisons. Summaries of the results of these surveys are published by the NCHS and are available at www.cdc.gov /nchs/dhcs.htm.

Epidemiologic Studies

Epidemiologists conduct investigations to better understand how disease is distributed in the population and what determines who gets sick and who does not. These investigations may be descriptive or analytic (observational or experimental/interventional) in nature, depending on the objectives of the specific study.

Descriptive Studies

Descriptive studies seek to describe the extent of disease with regard to *person, time*, and *place*. These studies are designed to answer the questions who, when, and where. To answer the first question (who), epidemiologists first take a "head count" to determine how many cases of a disease have occurred. At this time, they also try to determine who is ill—children, older adults, men, women, or both. The data they gather should permit them to develop a summary of cases by age, sex, race, marital status, occupation, employer, and other relevant characteristics of the people involved. These data provide important information to identify disparities in health outcomes among different segments of the population.

To answer the second question (when), epidemiologists will characterize health events by time of occurrence. The time period of interest will vary and usually depends on the health condition in question. For example, data for the number of people with cancer may be summarized by year, whereas the onset of illness for an infectious disease may be reported by hour. Two ways of displaying time-related data are secular and seasonal curves. The secular display of a disease shows the distribution of cases over many years (e.g., cases of varicella for the period 1993 to 2015; see **Figure 3.11**). Secular graphs illustrate the long-term trend of a disease. A graph of the case data by season or month is usually prepared to show cyclical changes in the numbers of cases of a disease. Cases of influenza-like illness, for example, peak in the winter months (see **Figure 3.12**). Data for infectious diseases is often characterized using an **epidemic curve**, a graphic display of the cases of disease by the time or date of the onset of symptoms.

Epidemic curves for single epidemics vary in appearance with each disease outbreak; however, two classic types exist. The first is the **common source epidemic curve** (see **Figure 3.13**). In a common source epidemic, each case can be traced to an exposure to the same source—spoiled food, for example. Because an epidemic curve shows cases of disease by time or date of the onset of symptoms, the epidemic curve for a single epidemic can be used to calculate the **incubation period**, the period of time between exposure to an infectious agent and the onset of symptoms. The incubation period, together with the symptoms, can often help epidemiologists determine the cause of the disease. A common source epidemic can be further categorized as a **point source epidemic**, where exposure occurs at a single

Descriptive studies epidemiologic studies that describe a disease with respect to person, time, and place

Epidemic curve a graphic display of the cases of disease according to the time or date of the onset of symptoms

Common source epidemic curve a graphic display of a disease where each case can be traced to a single source of exposure

Incubation period the period between exposure to a disease and the onset of symptoms

Point source epidemic a type of epidemic where all cases were exposed at the same point in time

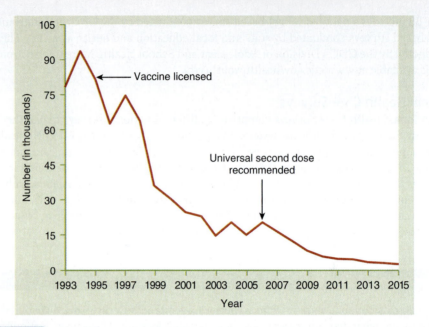

FIGURE 3.11 Varicella (chickenpox). Number of reported cases—Illinois, Michigan, Texas, and West Virginia, 1993–2015.

Reproduced from Adams, D.A., Thomas, K.R., Jajosky, R.A., Foster, L., Baroi, G., Sharp, P., Onweh, D.H., Schley, A.W., Anderson, W.J. (2017). Summary of notifiable infectious diseases and conditions—United States, 2015. *MMWR. Morbidity and mortality weekly report*, 64.

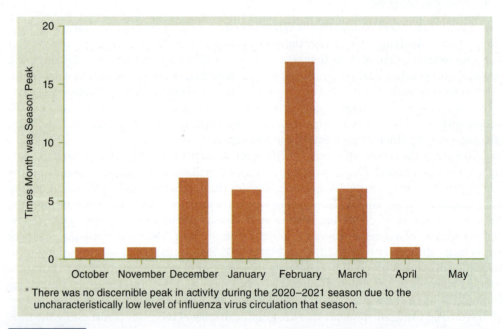

* There was no discernible peak in activity during the 2020–2021 season due to the uncharacteristically low level of influenza virus circulation that season.

FIGURE 3.12 Peak influenza activity, by month—United States, 1982–1983 through 2021–2022 influenza seasons.

Reproduced from Centers for Disease Control and Prevention. (2022). *The flu season.* https://www.cdc.gov/flu/about/season/index.html

Continuous source epidemic a type of epidemic where cases are exposed to a common source over time

point in time, or a **continuous source epidemic**, where exposure is continuous or intermittent. Identifying the source is especially important when exposure is continuous because individuals will continue to be exposed until transmission is interrupted. The cholera epidemic mentioned earlier in this chapter is a classic example of a continuous source epidemic. When

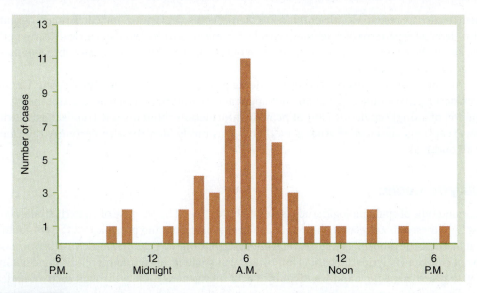

FIGURE 3.13 Point source epidemic curve: cases of gastroenteritis following ingestion of a common food source.

Reproduced from Centers for Disease Control and Prevention.

John Snow determined that the common source was the Broad Street pump, he was able to remove the handle and stop the epidemic.

The second type of epidemic curve for an outbreak is a **propagated epidemic curve**. In this type of epidemic, primary cases appear first at the end of the incubation period following exposure to an infected source. Secondary cases arise after a second incubation period, and they represent exposure to the primary cases; tertiary cases appear even later as a result of exposure to secondary cases, and so on. Because new cases give rise to more new cases, this type of epidemic is termed a propagated epidemic. Epidemics of communicable diseases such as chickenpox follow this pattern (see **Figure 3.14**).

Finally, epidemiologists must determine where the outbreak occurred. To determine where the illnesses may have originated, the residential address and travel history, including restaurants, schools, shopping trips, and vacations, of each case are recorded. This information provides a geographic distribution of cases and helps to delineate the extent of the outbreak. By plotting cases on a map, along with natural features such as streams and human-made structures such as factories, it is sometimes possible to learn something about the source of the disease.

A descriptive study is usually the first epidemiologic study carried out on a disease. Descriptive data provide valuable information to healthcare providers and administrators, enabling

Propagated epidemic curve an epidemic curve depicting a distribution of cases traceable to multiple sources of exposure

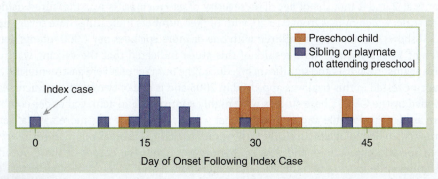

FIGURE 3.14 Propagated epidemic curve: cases of chickenpox during April through June.

Courtesy of CDC.

them to allocate resources efficiently and to plan effective prevention and education programs. Also, detectable patterns of cases may provide investigators with ideas that can lead to a hypothesis about the cause or source of the disease outbreak. This hypothesis can subsequently be tested in an analytic study.

As important and useful as they are, descriptive studies have some limitations. Results from descriptive studies are usually not applicable to outbreaks elsewhere. Also, the investigation of a single epidemic cannot provide information about disease trends. Lastly, with few exceptions, descriptive studies by themselves rarely identify with certainty the cause of an outbreak.

Analytic Studies

A second type of epidemiologic study is the **analytic study**. The purpose of analytic studies is to test hypotheses about relationships between health problems and possible **risk factors**, factors that increase the probability of disease. Although front-line community health workers usually do not conduct analytic studies, it is important that students of community health understand how they are carried out and what kinds of data they generate. Only through such an understanding can those who work in community and public health interpret the findings of these studies for others in the community, who may then apply the knowledge to improve their own health and that of the community.

An example of an analytic study might be one designed to discover whether cigarette smoking (possible risk factor) is associated with lung cancer (health problem) or whether improperly prepared food (possible risk factor) is associated with an outbreak of salmonellosis (health problem). It is important to remember that the associations discovered through analytic epidemiologic studies are not always cause-and-effect associations.

There are two types of analytic studies—observational and experimental (interventional). These differ in the role played by the investigator. In **observational studies**, the investigator simply observes the natural course of events, taking note of who is exposed or unexposed and who has or has not developed the disease of interest. **Experimental (interventional) studies** are carried out to identify risk factors of a disease or to determine the effectiveness of an intervention (vaccine, therapeutic drug, surgical procedure, or behavioral or educational intervention). The central feature of an experimental (interventional) study is that the investigator can manipulate the study factor (intervention, exposure, or variable of interest). For example, groups of study participants could be followed after receiving different medications or being asked to adhere to different diets to see which interventions were most effective.

An example of just such an experiment was performed to see whether or not a vaccine could prevent severe rotavirus gastroenteritis.[41] Rotavirus is the most common cause of severe diarrheal disease among young people worldwide. Participants were assigned to either receive a vaccine (the intervention) or a **placebo**. There were 31,673 children in the vaccine group and 31,552 children in the placebo group. Oral doses of either vaccine or placebo were administered to infants at 2 and 4 months of age. The severity of gastroenteritis was measured using the Vesikari scale, which ranges from 0 to 20, with higher numbers indicating more severe illness. **Table 3.11** shows the number of children with one or more episodes per 1,000 infants per year at different Vesikari scores. The results of this study indicated that the vaccine was highly effective against rotavirus and significantly reduced the number of severe gastroenteritis cases. The vaccine tested in this trial was approved in 2008 and is one of two rotavirus vaccines recommended by the CDC. These studies were highly controlled and achieved under conditions that are as ideal as possible and may not reflect what would occur in a more natural setting. In summary, epidemiologists carefully plan studies to define outbreaks of disease, injury, and death in specific populations and develop hypotheses about the causes of these outbreaks. By designing and carrying out analytic and experimental studies, epidemiologists test these hypotheses. The results of hypothesis tests are assimilated across studies and provide evidence on which to base public health practice.

Analytic study an epidemiologic study aimed at testing hypotheses

Risk factors factors that increase the probability of disease, injury, or death

Observational studies analytic epidemiologic studies in which the investigator observes the natural course of events, noting exposed and unexposed subjects and disease development

Experimental (interventional) studies analytic studies in which the investigator allocates exposure or intervention and follows development of disease

Placebo treatment of no therapeutic effect, usually given to a group within an experimental study to serve as comparison to another group receiving the intervention of interest

TABLE 3.11 Number of Subjects with One or More Episode of Severe Rotavirus Gastroenteritis per 1,000 Infants per Year by Vesikari Score*

Vesikari Score	Vaccine Group	Placebo Group
≥11	1.9	12.2
≥15	1.2	0.3
≥19	0	0.8

*During the time period from 2 weeks after the second dose to 1 year of age.

Data from Ruiz-Palacios, G. M., Perez-Schael, I., Velezquez, F. R., Abate, H., et al., Human Rotavirus Vaccine Study Group. (2006). Safety and efficacy of an attenuated vaccine against severe rotavirus gastroenteritis. *New England Journal of Medicine, 354*(1), 11–22.

Determining Causation

In any scientific discipline, there is an important phrase: "association does not imply causation." Often, even after numerous epidemiologic studies have identified an association between exposure to a suspected risk factor (A) and the development of a specific disease (B), it may not be clear that there is a causal relationship between risk factor (A) and effect (B). Some relationships are quite easy to see, such as the connection between the malaria parasite causing the disease malaria. However, other associations are more difficult to discern, such as looking at pesticide use and cancer cases in a community. In 1965, this problem was addressed by Sir Austin Bradford Hill, who laid out nine criteria that should be considered when deciding whether an association might be one of causation.[43] As he developed a total of nine criteria, he often cited the behavior of cigarette smoking and the development of lung cancer as examples. With minor modifications, the following are some of Hill's criteria:

1. *Strength.* How strong is the association between the exposure and the disease? Are those exposed 3, 5, 10, or 100 times more likely to develop disease than those who are not exposed? How many times more likely are cigarette smokers to get lung cancer than nonsmokers?

2. *Dose-response.* Is there a dose-response relationship? Is it the case that the greater the exposure to a particular risk factor results in a higher rate of disease or death? Are those who smoke more heavily more likely to develop lung cancer than lighter smokers are?

3. *Consistency.* Has the association been reported in a variety of people exposed in a variety of settings? Are the results repeatable by other researchers?

4. *Specificity.* Is the disease or health problem associated with the exposure the only one? When someone becomes ill after exposure, is it always, or almost always, the same disease? When cigarette smokers become ill, is it always, or almost always, lung cancer?

5. *Temporality.* Does A (the exposure) always precede B (the disease)? Does the behavior of cigarette smoking precede the onset of lung cancer, or do those with lung cancer take up the habit of smoking for some reason?

6. *Biological plausibility.* Does the suspected causation make sense with what we know about biology, physiology, and other medical knowledge? Does it make sense, in light of what we know about biology and physiology, that cigarette smoking could produce lung cancer?

These criteria are guidelines rather than rules. They should be considered along with careful interpretation of epidemiologic studies and other evidence. Using these criteria together with analytic epidemiologic data, health researchers often can persuade legislatures and public officials to pass laws or alter public policies that promote health. In the next chapter, we examine how epidemiologic studies can be used to prevent and control diseases and health problems in the community.

Chapter Summary

- Epidemiology is the study of the distribution and determinants of health-related states or events in specified populations, and the application of this study to control health problems.

- Rates of birth, death, injury, and disease are essential tools for epidemiologists.

- Incidence rates are a measurement of the number of new cases of disease, injury, or death in a population over a given period of time. Prevalence rates measure all cases. An attack rate is a special kind of incidence rate used for a single outbreak.

- Cases of certain diseases, called notifiable or reportable diseases, are reported by doctors, clinics, medical laboratories, and hospitals to local health agencies. These agencies then report them to state health agencies, who then forward the data to the CDC. These reports assist epidemiologists who study disease trends.

- The health status of a population or community can be measured in a number of different ways, including mortality statistics, life expectancy, years of potential life lost (YPLL), disability-adjusted life years (DALYs), and health-adjusted life expectancy (HALE).

- Epidemiologists also consult the data available from the U.S. Census, the vital statistics reports, the *Morbidity and Mortality Weekly Report*, and a variety of national health surveys.

- Epidemiologists conduct two general types of studies to learn about disease and injury in populations—descriptive studies and analytic studies.

- Descriptive studies describe the extent of outbreaks with regard to person, time, and place.

- Analytic studies test hypotheses regarding associations between diseases and risk factors.

- Analytic studies can be either observational or experimental.

- Criteria for judging whether an association identified in epidemiologic studies represent a causal relationship include strength of association, consistency, specificity, temporal correctness, and biological plausibility.

- Epidemiologic studies provide the data and information that enable public health officials and policymakers to make decisions and take actions to improve health.

Scenario: Analysis and Response

Assume that you were Kim and you were able to reach Dr. Turner, the local health officer. He then asked whether you would like to help in the investigation of the foodborne outbreak mentioned in the scenario. You agreed to help. So far, you have learned that on Sunday, May 28, 49 people were at a picnic where they had eaten, beginning about noon. People began to report their illnesses later that night. Dr. Turner developed a foodborne outbreak investigation worksheet, which you helped to complete by making numerous phone calls and house visits with the public health nurse. The histories of people attending the picnic appear in **Table 3.12**. Using **Table 3.13**, the Epidemic

TABLE 3.12 Histories Obtained from Persons Eating Picnic Lunch

Person No.	Bread	Butter	Turkey	Potato Salad	Milk	Jell-O	Ill*	Not Ill
1			x	x	x		7:30*	
2	x	x		x	x			x
3	x	x	x	x	x	x	8:00	
4			x		x	x		x
5			x	x	x		9:15	
6			x	x	x		7:40	
7	x	x		x	x			x
8	x	x	x	x	x	x	8:10	
9			x		x	x		x
10			x	x	x	x	10:15	

Person No.	Bread	Butter	Turkey	Potato Salad	Milk	Jell-O	Ill*	Not Ill
11	X			X		X		X
12	X	X	X	X	X	X	8:30	
13			X		X			X
14	X	X	X	X	X	X	9:30	
15	X	X		X	X	X		X
16	X			X		X		X
17	X	X	X	X	X	X	8:35	
18			X		X			X
19	X	X	X	X	X	X	10:05	
20	X	X		X	X	X		X
21			X		X	X	9:15	
22	X	X		X	X	X		X
23	X	X			X	X	8:30	
24	X	X			X	X		X
25	X	X	X	X	X	X	12:30 a.m.	
26			X		X	X	9:20	
27	X	X		X	X	X		X
28	X	X	X		X	X	8:40	
29	X	X			X	X		X
30	X	X	X	X	X		12:15 a.m.	
31			X	X	X		7:30	
32	X	X		X	X			X
33	X	X	X	X	X	X	8:00	
34			X		X	X		X
35			X	X	X		10:30	
36			X	X	X		7:30	
37	X	X		X	X			X
38	X	X	X	X	X	X	8:05	
39			X		X	X		X
40			X	X	X	X	9:45	
41	X			X		X		X
42	X	X	X	X	X	X	8:30	
43			X		X			X
44	X	X	X	X	X	X	9:30	
45	X	X			X	X		X
46	X			X		X		X
47	X	X	X	X	X	X	8:30	
48			X		X	X		X
49	X	X	X	X	X	X	10:10	

*All times are p.m. unless otherwise indicated.

TABLE 3.13 Epidemic Curve Tally Sheet

Time of Onset	Tally	Number	Incubation Period
7:00–7:59			
8:00–8:59			
9:00–9:59			
10:00–10:59			
11:00–11:59			
12:00–12:59			

Curve Tally Sheet, you tally the cases by hour of onset of illness. Using the results of the tally, you establish the incubation period—the range of hours (after the meal) over which symptoms started. Next, you prepare a graph to illustrate the epidemic curve of the outbreak. Try to answer the following questions:

1. What is the incubation period?

2. Does the curve you prepared suggest a single- or multiple-exposure epidemic?

3. Based solely on the incubation period, can you make a guess as to the cause of the outbreak?

Unfortunately, by the time the investigation began, all the picnic food had been discarded, and no samples were available for laboratory testing. To determine which food at the picnic might have caused the outbreak, you need to calculate attack rates for people eating each food as well as for people not eating each food. Using **Table 3.14**, the Attack Rate Worksheet, calculate the attack rates for those who ate and did not eat each food served.

1. Which food would you most suspect of causing the illness?

2. Based on this information, what might the causative agent have been?

3. How could the Internet be of assistance to health department officials in this situation?

TABLE 3.14 Attack Rate Worksheet

Food	Persons Eating Food				Persons Not Eating Food			
	Total	Ill	Not Ill	Attack Rate	Total	Ill	Not Ill	Attack Rate
Bread								
Butter								
Turkey								
Potato salad								
Milk								
Jell-O								

Review Questions

1. What is an epidemic? A pandemic? Name some diseases that caused epidemics in the past. Name some diseases that are epidemic today.

2. Why are epidemiologists sometimes interested in epizootics?

3. What does the term *endemic disease* mean? Give examples of such diseases.

4. What is the difference between natality, morbidity, and mortality?

5. Why are rates important in community health?

6. What is the difference between crude and adjusted rates?

7. Why are prevalence rates more useful than incidence rates for measuring chronic diseases?

8. What is an infant mortality rate? Why is it such an important rate in community health?

9. What are notifiable diseases? Give some examples.

10. In general, contrast the leading causes of death in the United States in 1900 with those in 2013. Comment on the differences.

11. At what ages is life expectancy calculated? What does it tell us about a population? Which country has the longest life expectancy?

12. What are years of potential life lost (YPLL)? How does calculating YPLL change the way we think about the leading causes of death?

13. How would you define disability-adjusted life years (DALYs)? How would you define health-adjusted life expectancy (HALE)?

14. What is the U.S. Census? How often is it conducted? What types of data does it gather?

15. What kinds of data would you expect to find in the Centers for Disease Control and Prevention's *Morbidity and Mortality Weekly Report*?

16. List five important national health surveys that are valuable sources of data about the health and health care of our population.

17. What can be said about the reliability of self-reported health data?

18. What is the National Health and Nutrition Examination Survey? Why is it carried out?

19. In a descriptive epidemiologic study, what types of information does the epidemiologist gather?

20. What is the purpose of an analytic study?

21. How do experimental studies differ from observational studies?

22. What are Hill's criteria for judging whether an association between a risk factor and a disease can be considered causal?

Activities

1. When you hear the word "epidemic," what disease comes to your mind first? Ask this question of 10 people you know, allowing them time to think and give you an answer. Try to find people of different ages as you complete your informal poll. List their answers on paper. Are there any answers that surprise you? Does your list include both classic and contemporary epidemic diseases?

2. Look at the data in **Table 3.15**. What conclusion can you draw about the risk for acquiring tuberculosis for populations in each age group? Write down your answer. Now examine **Table 3.16**. Which age groups exhibit the highest disease rates? Explain why it is important to calculate rates to report disease outbreaks accurately.

3. There are 346 students at Hillside School. During March and April, 56 pupils were absent with chickenpox. What is the attack rate for chickenpox at Hillside School? The 56 pupils who were absent had 88 brothers and sisters at home. Of the 88 siblings, 19 developed chickenpox. What was the attack rate among these children? Of the 75 total cases of chickenpox, one child died. Calculate the case fatality rate for chickenpox in this epidemic.

4. Contact your state or local health department or visit their website. Ask for or determine the total number of birth and death certificates issued for the latest year for which complete data are available. Assuming no migration into or out of your state or county occurred, what is the natural rate of population increase (number of births minus number of deaths)? Try to obtain an estimate of the total population of the state or county for that same year. Calculate a crude birth rate and a crude death rate (number of births and deaths) per 1,000 population.

5. Using the data presented in Table 3.8, estimate (as best you can) the life expectancy of your siblings, parents, and grandparents at birth. If your grandparents are older than 65, determine what their life expectancies were when they turned 65. If you were to fulfill your life expectancy exactly, in what year can you expect to die?

TABLE 3.15 Reported Tuberculosis Cases by Age Group, Low Socioeconomic Area, City of Dixon, 1960

Age Group in Years	Number of Cases	Age Group in Years	Number of Cases
0–4	7	35–44	6
5–14	7	45–54	9
15–24	6	55–64	8
25–34	10	65+	7

Reproduced from Centers for Disease Control and Prevention.

TABLE 3.16 Reported Tuberculosis Cases and Incidence Rates per 100,000, Low Socioeconomic Area, City of Dixon, 1960

Age Group in Years	Number of Cases	Population of Age Group	Rate*
1–4	7	8,638	81.0
5–14	7	13,098	53.4
15–24	6	10,247	58.5
25–34	10	8,680	115.2
35–44	6	7,528	79.7
45–54	9	6,736	133.6
55–64	8	4,534	176.4
65+	7	4,075	171.8
Total	60	63,536	94.4

*Example: 7 cases ÷ 8,638 population × 100,000 = 81.0.

Reproduced from Centers for Disease Control and Prevention.

6. Visit your campus library and locate the *American Journal of Epidemiology*. Examine several recent issues, taking note of the different types of articles as they appear in the table of contents. Select six articles and read the abstracts. On a piece of paper, list the titles of these articles. Were these descriptive, analytic, or experimental studies? After each title that you have listed, put either the letter D (descriptive), A (analytic), or E (experimental) to denote the type of study that you examined.

References

1. Centers for Disease Control and Prevention. (2012). *Principles of epidemiology in public health practice, third edition: An introduction to applied epidemiology and biostatistics*. Available at https://www.cdc.gov/csels/dsepd/ss1978/Lesson1/Section1.html#_ref1

2. Taubenberer, J. K., & Morens, D. M. (2006). 1918 Influenza: The mother of all pandemics. *Emerging Infectious Diseases, 12*(1), 15–22.

3. *UNAIDS warns that after significant reductions, declines in new HIV infections among adults have stalled and are rising in some regions*. (2016). Unaids.org. Retrieved February 26, 2024, from https://www.unaids.org/en/resources/presscentre/pressreleaseandstatementarchive/2016/july/20160712_prevention-gap

4. World Health Organization 2023 data.who.int, WHO Coronavirus (COVID-19) dashboard > Cases [Dashboard]. Available at https://data.who.int/dashboards/covid19/cases

5. Monath, T. P. (1980). *St. Louis encephalitis*. American Public Health Association.

6. Centers for Disease Control and Prevention. (2003). Summary of notifiable diseases—United States, 2001. *Morbidity and Mortality Weekly Report, 50*(53), 1–108.

7. Centers for Disease Control and Prevention. (1981). Toxic shock syndrome—United States, 1970–1980. *Morbidity and Mortality Weekly Report, 30*(3), 25–33.

8. Centers for Disease Control and Prevention. (2014). HIV/AIDS surveillance report: Diagnoses of HIV infection in the United States and dependent areas, 2012. *HIV Surveillance Report, 24*. Available at http://www.cdc.gov/hiv/pdf/statistics_2012_HIV_Surveillance_Report_vol_24.pdf

9. Centers for Disease Control and Prevention. (2015). HIV/AIDS surveillance report: Diagnoses of HIV infection in the United States and dependent areas, 2013. *HIV Surveillance Report, 25*. Available at http://www.cdc.gov/hiv/pdf/library/reports/surveillance/cdc-hiv-surveillance -report-vol-25.pdf

10. CDC. (2023, October 11). *West Nile Virus Historic Data (1999-2022)*. Available at Cdc.gov. https://www.cdc.gov/westnile/statsmaps/historic-data.html

11. Centers for Disease Control and Prevention. (2014). Summary of notifiable diseases—United States, 2012. *Morbidity and Mortality Weekly Report, 61*(53), 1–121.

12. CDC. (2024). *Mumps*. Centers for Disease Control and Prevention. Available at https://www.cdc.gov/mumps/outbreaks.html

13. Shrestha, S. S., Swerdlow, D. L., Borse, R. H., Prabhu, V. S., Finelli, L., Atkins, C. Y., ... Meltzer, M. I. (2011). Estimating the burden of 2009 pandemic influenza A (H1N1) in the United States (April 2009–April 2010). *Clinical Infectious Diseases, 52*(Suppl 1), S75–S82.

14. CDC's Office on Smoking & Health. (2022). *Smoking and tobacco use; electronic cigarettes*. Available at https://www.cdc.gov/tobacco/basic_information/e-cigarettes/severe-lung-disease.html

15. Centers for Disease Control and Prevention. (2023). COVID Data Tracker. Atlanta, GA: US Department of Health and Human Services, CDC; 2023, May 11. Available at https://covid.cdc.gov/covid-data-tracker

16. Markellis, V. C. (December 1985–January 1986). Epidemiology: Cornerstone for health education. *Health Education, 15–17*.

17. Gale, A. H. (1959). *Epidemiologic disease*. Pelican Books; 25.

18. Centers for Disease Control and Prevention. (2019). *Yellow fever*. Available at https://www.cdc.gov/yellowfever/index.html

19. Woodruff, A. W. (1977). Benjamin Rush, his work on yellow fever and his British connections. *American Journal of Tropical Medicine and Hygiene, 26*(5), 1055–1059.

20. Centers for Disease Control and Prevention. (2018). *Cholera-Vibrio cholerae infection: General information*. Available at https://www.cdc.gov/cholera/general/index.html

21. Ruths, M. B. (2009). The lesson of John Snow and the Broad Street pump. *AMA Journal of Ethics, 11*(6), 470–472. doi: 10.1001/virtualmentor.2009.11.6.mhst1-0906

22. Johnson, S. R. (2006). *The Ghost Map: The story of London's most terrifying epidemic—and how it changed science, cities, and the modern world*. Riverhead Books.

23. Snow, J. (1855). *On the mode of communication of cholera*. London: J Churchill.

24. Kochanek, K., Murphy, S., Xu, J., & Arias, E. (2023). *Deaths: Final Data for 2020*. National Center for Health Statistics (U.S.). Available at https://doi.org/10.15620/cdc:131355

25. Centers for Disease Control and Prevention. (n.d.). *National Notifiable Diseases Surveillance System (NNDSS)*. Available at https://wwwn.cdc.gov/nndss/index.html

26. Center for Disease Control and Prevention. (2022). *Protocol for public health agencies to notify CDC about the occurrence of nationally notifiable conditions, 2022*. Cdc.gov. Available at https://ndc.services.cdc.gov/wp-content/uploads/NNC_2022_Notification_Requirements_By_Timeframe_FINAL_01252022.pdf

27. Doyle, T. J., Glynn, M. K., & Groseclose, S. L. (2002). Completeness of notifiable infectious disease reporting in the United States: An analytical literature review. *American Journal of Epidemiology, 155*(9), 866–874.

28. Centers for Disease Control and Prevention, National Center for Health Statistics. (1998). *Leading causes of death, 1900–1998*. Available at http://www.cdc.gov/nchs/data/dvs/lead1900_98.pdf

29. World Health Organization. (2020). *The top 10 causes of death*. Available at https://www.who.int/news-room/fact-sheets/detail/the-top-10-causes-of-death

30. Centers for Disease Control. (2017). *Table 18. Years of potential life lost before age 75 for selected causes of death, by sex, race, and Hispanic origin: United States, selected years 1980–2016. Health, United States, 2017: Trend Tables*. Available at https://www.cdc.gov/nchs/data/hus/2017/018.pdf

31. World Health Organization. (2019). *World health statistics 2019: Monitoring health for the SDGs, sustainable development goals*. Available at https://apps.who.int/iris/handle/10665/324835

32. Murray, D. J. L., & Lopez, A. D. (Eds.). (1996). The global burden of disease: A comprehensive assessment of mortality and disability from diseases, injuries and risk factors in 1990 and projected to 2020. In *Global Burden of Disease and Injury* (Vol. 1). Harvard School of Public Health (on behalf of WHO).

33. World Health Organization. (2008). *The global burden of disease: 2004 update*. Available at https://www.who.int/publications/i/item/9789241563710

34. World Health Organization. (2019). *Global health estimates: Leading causes of DALYs*. Who.int. Retrieved February 26, 2024, from https://www.who.int/data/gho/data/themes/mortality-and-global-health-estimates/global-health-estimates-leading-causes-of-dalys

35. Mathers, C. C., Sdana, R., Salomon, J. A., Murray, C. J. L., & Lopez, A. D. (2000). Healthy life expectancy in 191 countries in the year 2000: Methods and results. In *Global Programme on Evidence for Health Policy Working Paper No. 16*. World Health Organization. Available at http://www.eurohex.eu/bibliography/pdf/Mathers_HLE_2001-3583071490/Mathers_HLE_2001.pdf

36. World Health Organization. (2020). *Life expectancy and healthy life expectancy: Data by WHO region*. Available at https://apps.who.int/gho/data/view.main.SDG2016LEXREGv?lang=en

37. National Center for Health Statistics. Percentage of angina for adults aged 18 and over, United States, 2019—2022. National Health Interview Survey. Generated interactively: Feb 26 2024 from Available at https://wwwn.cdc.gov/NHISDataQueryTool/SHS_adult/index.html

38. Centers for Disease Control and Prevention. (2023). *National Health and Nutrition Examination Survey: About the National Health and Nutrition Examination Survey*. Available at https://www.cdc.gov/nchs/nhanes/about_nhanes.htm

39. Centers for Disease Control and Prevention. (2021). *Youth Risk Behavior Surveillance System (YRBSS) overview*. Available at https://www.cdc.gov/healthyyouth/data/yrbs/index.htm

40. Ruiz-Palacios, G. M., Pérez-Schael, I., Velázquez, F. R., Abate, H., Breuer, T., Clemens, S. C., ... Human Rotavirus Vaccine Study Group. (2006). Safety and efficacy of an attenuated vaccine against severe rotavirus gastroenteritis. *New England Journal of Medicine, 354*(1), 11–22.

41. Hill, A. B. (1965). The environment and disease: Association or causation? *Proceeding of the Royal Society of Medicine, 58*, 295–300.

CHAPTER 4

Communicable and Noncommunicable Diseases: Prevention and Control of Diseases and Health Conditions

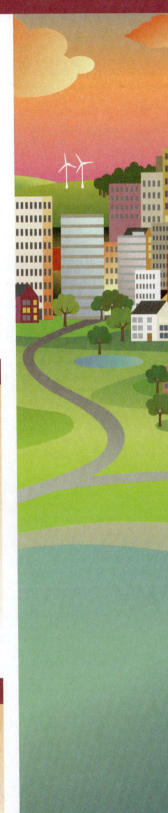

Chapter Objectives

After studying this chapter, you will be able to:

1. Discuss the differences between communicable (infectious) and noncommunicable (noninfectious) diseases and between acute and chronic diseases and provide examples of each.

2. Describe and explain communicable and multicausation disease models.

3. Explain how communicable diseases are transmitted in a community using the chain-of-infection model, and use a specific communicable disease to illustrate your explanation.

4. Identify why noncommunicable diseases are a community and public health concern, and provide some examples of important noncommunicable diseases.

5. Compare and contrast between primary, secondary, and tertiary prevention of disease, and provide examples of each.

Chapter Objectives   *(continued)*

6. State and describe the various criteria that communities might use to prioritize their health problems in preparation for the allocation of prevention and control resources.

7. List and discuss important measures for preventing and controlling the spread of communicable diseases in a community.

8. List and discuss approaches to noncommunicable disease control in the community.

9. Define and explain the purpose and importance of health screenings.

10. Outline a chronic, noncommunicable disease control program that includes primary, secondary, and tertiary disease prevention components.

Scenario

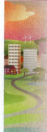

Bob and Susan have been married for 43 years. Their two daughters, Shawna and Emily, are also married, with school-age children of their own. Susan has been fastidious about regular health screenings, including biennial mammograms and Pap smears. Her routine mammogram, originally scheduled for April of 2020 was cancelled due to COVID-19 restrictions on routine care. In 2021, although COVID-19 mitigating policies were in place at the hospital, Susan was hesitant to go for routine testing.

When Susan's 2022 mammogram was reviewed by the radiologist, a suspicious area was identified. She was immediately scheduled for a biopsy. The clinic managing Susan's care requested that she be tested for the presence of the BRCA gene mutations.

Introduction

Elsewhere in the text, we discussed the measurement and reporting of disease and the use of incidence and prevalence to describe disease occurrence. We also explained how epidemiologists describe disease outbreaks by person, place, and time and how they search for associations through analytic and experimental studies.

In this chapter, we extend our discussion of epidemiology. We begin by describing the different ways to classify diseases and other health conditions. Then, we explain models of communicable and noncommunicable diseases, which are conceptual frameworks used by epidemiologists to develop prevention and control strategies.

We also discuss criteria used by communities to prioritize their health problems and allocate health resources. Finally, we discuss some approaches to disease prevention and control; introduce the concepts of primary, secondary, and tertiary prevention; and provide examples of their application to a communicable and noncommunicable disease.

Classification of Diseases and Health Problems

Diseases and health problems can be classified in several meaningful ways. The public often classifies diseases by organ or organ system, such as kidney disease, heart disease, respiratory infection, and so on. Another method of classification is by causative agent—viral disease, chemical poisoning, physical injury, and so forth. In this scheme, causative agents may be biological, chemical, or physical. Biological agents include viruses, rickettsiae, bacteria, protozoa, fungi, and metazoa (multicellular organisms). Chemical agents include drugs, pesticides, industrial chemicals, food additives, air pollutants, and cigarette smoke. Physical agents that can cause injury or disease include various forms of energy, such as heat, ultraviolet light, radiation, noise vibrations, and speeding or falling objects (see **Table 4.1**). In community health, diseases are usually classified as acute or chronic, and as communicable (infectious) or noncommunicable (noninfectious).

TABLE 4.1 Causative Agents for Diseases and Injuries

Biological Agents	Chemical Agents	Physical Agents
Viruses	Pesticides	Heat
Rickettsiae	Food additives	Light
Bacteria	Pharmacologics	Radiation
Fungi	Industrial chemicals	Noise
Protozoa	Air pollutants	Vibration
Metazoa	Cigarette smoke	Speeding objects

Communicable versus Noncommunicable Diseases

A **communicable (infectious) disease** is a disease for which biological agents or their products are the cause, and that is transmissible from one individual to another. The disease process begins when the agent is able to enter and grow or reproduce within the body of the host. The establishment of a communicable disease agent in a host organism is called an *infection*.

A **noncommunicable (noninfectious) disease** or illness is one that cannot be transmitted from one person to another. Delineating the causes of noncommunicable diseases is often more difficult because several, or even many, factors may contribute to the development of a given noncommunicable health condition. These contributing factors may be genetic, environmental, or behavioral in nature. For this reason, many noncommunicable health conditions are called multicausation diseases; an example of which is heart disease. Genetics, environmental factors such as stress, and behavioral choices such as poor diet and lack of exercise can all contribute to heart disease.

Communicable (infectious) disease an illness caused by some specific biological agent or its toxic products that can be transmitted from an infected person, animal, or inanimate reservoir to a susceptible host

Noncommunicable (noninfectious) disease a disease that cannot be transmitted from infected host to susceptible host

Acute versus Chronic Diseases and Illnesses

In the acute/chronic classification scheme, diseases are classified by their duration of symptoms. Acute diseases are diseases in which the peak severity of symptoms occurs and subsides within 3 months (usually sooner) and the recovery of those who survive is usually complete. Examples of acute communicable diseases include the common cold, influenza (flu), chickenpox, measles, mumps, Rocky Mountain spotted fever, and COVID-19. Examples of acute noncommunicable illnesses are appendicitis, injuries from motor vehicle crashes, acute alcohol intoxication or drug overdose, and sprained ankles (see **Table 4.2**).

Chronic diseases or conditions are those in which symptoms continue longer than 3 months and, in some cases, for the remainder of one's life (see **Figure 4.1**). Recovery is slow and sometimes incomplete. These diseases can be either communicable or noncommunicable.

TABLE 4.2 Classification of Diseases

Types of Diseases	Examples
Acute diseases	
Communicable	Common cold, pneumonia, mumps, measles, pertussis, typhoid fever, cholera, COVID-19
Noncommunicable	Appendicitis, poisoning, injury (due to motor vehicle crash, fire, gunshot, etc.)
Chronic diseases	
Communicable	AIDS, Lyme disease, tuberculosis, syphilis, rheumatic fever following streptococcal infections, hepatitis B
Noncommunicable	Diabetes, coronary heart disease, osteoarthritis, cirrhosis of the liver due to alcoholism

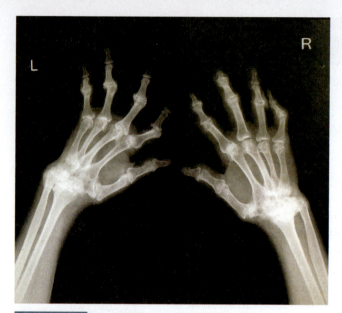

L

R

FIGURE 4.1 Arthritis is a noninfectious chronic condition that can persist for one's entire life.

Examples of chronic communicable diseases are AIDS, tuberculosis, herpes virus infections, syphilis, and Lyme disease. Chronic noncommunicable illnesses include hypertension, hypercholesterolemia, coronary heart disease, diabetes, and many types of arthritis and cancer.

Communicable Diseases

Whereas **infectivity** refers to the ability of a biological agent to enter and grow in a host, the term **pathogenicity** refers to an infectious disease agent's ability to produce disease. Selected pathogenic agents and the diseases they cause are listed in **Table 4.3**. Under certain conditions, pathogenic biologic agents can be transmitted from an infected individual in the community to an uninfected, susceptible one. Communicable disease agents may be further classified according to the manner in which they are transmitted.

The elements of a simplified **communicable disease model**—agent, host, and environment—are presented in **Figure 4.2**. These three factors are the minimal requirements for the occurrence and spread of communicable diseases in a population. In this model, the **agent (pathogenic agent)** is the element that must be present for disease to occur. For example, the influenza virus must be present for a person to become ill with the flu.

The **host** is any susceptible organism—a single-celled organism, a plant, an animal, or a human—invaded by an infectious agent. The environment includes all other factors—physical, biologic, or social—that inhibit or promote disease transmission. Communicable disease transmission occurs when a susceptible host and a pathogenic agent exist in an environment conducive to disease transmission.

Infectivity the ability of a biological agent to enter and grow in the host

Pathogenicity the capability of a communicable disease agent to cause disease in a susceptible host

Communicable disease model the minimal requirements for the occurrence and spread of communicable diseases in a population—agent, host, and environment

Agent (pathogenic agent) the cause of the disease or health problem

Host a person or other living organism that affords subsistence or lodgment to a communicable agent under natural conditions

TABLE 4.3 Biological Agents of Disease

Type of Agent	Name of Agent	Disease
Viruses	Varicella virus	Chickenpox
	Human immunodeficiency virus (HIV)	Acquired immunodeficiency syndrome (AIDS)
	SARS-CoV-2	COVID-19
Rickettsiae	*Rickettsia rickettsii*	Rocky Mountain spotted fever
Bacteria	*Vibrio cholerae*	Cholera
	Clostridium tetani	Tetanus
	Yersinia pestis	Plague
	Borrelia burgdorferi	Lyme disease
Protozoa	*Entamoeba histolytica*	Amebic dysentery
	Plasmodium falciparum	Malaria
	Trypanosoma gambiense	African sleeping sickness
Fungi and yeasts	*Tinea cruris*	Jock itch
	Tinea pedis	Athlete's foot
Nematoda (worms)	*Wuchereria bancrofti*	Filariasis (elephantiasis)
	Onchocerca volvulus	Onchocerciasis (river blindness)

Chain of Infection

Communicable disease transmission is a complicated but well-studied process that is best understood through a conceptual model known as the **chain of infection** (see **Figure 4.3**). Using the chain of infection model, one can visualize the step-by-step process by which communicable diseases spread from an infected person to an uninfected person in the community. The pathogenic (disease-producing) agent leaves its reservoir (infected host) via a portal of exit. Transmission occurs in either a direct or indirect manner, and the pathogenic agent enters a susceptible host through a portal of entry to establish infection. For example, let us follow the common cold through the chain of infection. The agent (the cold virus) leaves its reservoir (the throat of an infected person), perhaps when the host sneezes. The portals of exit are the nose and mouth. Transmission may be direct if saliva droplets enter the respiratory tract of a susceptible host at close range (someone standing nearby breathes in the droplets), or it may be indirect if droplets dry and become airborne. The portal of entry could be the nose or mouth of a susceptible host. The agent enters, and a new infection is established.

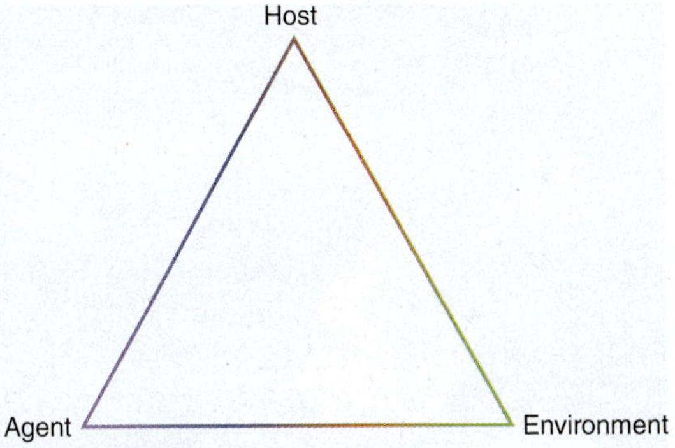

There are many variations in the chain of infection, depending on the disease agent, environmental conditions, infectivity, and host susceptibility. For example, the reservoir for a disease may be a **case**—a person who has the disease—or a **carrier**—one who is well but infected and is capable of serving as a source of infection. A carrier could be someone who is incubating the disease, such as a person who is HIV positive but has no signs of AIDS, or someone who has recovered from the disease (is asymptomatic) but still infectious, as is sometimes the case with typhoid fever. For some diseases, the reservoir is not humans but animals. A disease for which the reservoir resides in animal populations is called a **zoonosis**. Plague, rabies, Rocky Mountain spotted fever, and Lyme disease are zoonoses. A disease for which humans are the only known reservoir, like measles, is known as an **anthroponosis**.

Portals of exit (see **Figure 4.4**) and entry vary from disease to disease. Natural portals of exit and examples of diseases that use them are the respiratory tract (cold, influenza, measles, tuberculosis, COVID-19, and whooping cough), urogenital tract (gonorrhea, syphilis, herpes, and AIDS), digestive tract (amebic dysentery, shigellosis, polio, typhoid fever, and cholera), and skin (ringworm and jock itch). The skin is actually a good barrier to infection, but it can be bypassed by a hypodermic needle or when there is an open wound. Blood-sucking insects and ticks make their own portals of entry with mouth parts that penetrate the skin. Finally, many pathogenic agents can cross the placenta from mother to fetus (for example, rubella virus, syphilis spirochetes, and hepatitis B virus).

Modes of Transmission

As noted in the previous paragraphs, communicable disease transmission may be direct or indirect. **Direct transmission** implies the immediate transfer of the disease agent between the infected and the susceptible individuals by direct contact, "such as touching, biting, kissing, sexual intercourse, or by direct projection (droplet spread) of droplet spray onto the conjunctiva or mucous membranes of the eye, nose, or mouth during sneezing, coughing, spitting, singing or talking (usually limited to a distance of one meter or less)."[1] Examples of diseases for which transmission is usually direct are AIDS, syphilis, gonorrhea, rabies, and the common cold.

FIGURE 4.2   Communicable disease model.

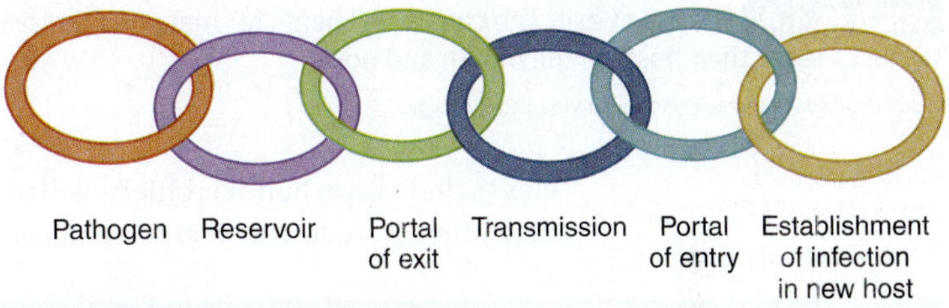

Pathogen   Reservoir   Portal of exit   Transmission   Portal of entry   Establishment of infection in new host

FIGURE 4.3   Chain of infection.

Chain of infection a model to conceptualize the transmission of a communicable disease from its source to a susceptible host

Case a person who is sick with a disease

Carrier a person or animal that harbors a specific communicable agent in the absence of discernible clinical disease and serves as a potential source of infection to others

Zoonosis a communicable disease transmissible under natural conditions from vertebrate animals to humans

Anthroponosis a disease that infects only humans

Direct transmission the immediate transfer of an infectious agent by direct contact between infected and susceptible individuals

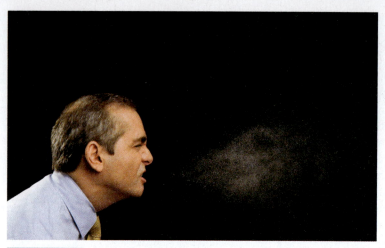

FIGURE 4.4   Portal of exit: The causative agents for many respiratory diseases leave their host via the mouth and nose.

© John M Lund Photography Inc/DigitalVision/Getty Images

Indirect transmission may be one of three types—airborne, vehicleborne, or vectorborne. Airborne transmission is the dissemination of microbial aerosols to a suitable portal of entry, usually the respiratory tract. Microbial aerosols are suspensions of dust or droplet nuclei made up wholly or in part of micro-organisms. In contrast to droplets, which spread no more than several feet, airborne particles may remain suspended and infective for long periods of time. Tuberculosis, influenza, histoplasmosis, legionellosis, and measles (see **Box 4.1**) are examples of airborne diseases.

In vehicleborne transmission, contaminated materials or objects (fomites) serve as **vehicles**—nonliving objects by which communicable agents are transferred to a susceptible host. The agent may or may not have multiplied or developed on the vehicle. Examples of vehicles include toys, handkerchiefs, soiled clothes, bedding, food service utensils, and surgical instruments. Also considered vehicles are water, milk, food, or biological products, such as

---

BOX 4.1   Preventing Transmission of Communicable Diseases

Interrupting the spread of disease requires information about the symptoms, what causes the disease, how it is diagnosed, the reservoir, the incubation period, how it is transmitted, who may be at risk, prevention measures, and how to manage an ill patient and their surroundings.[1]

For example, to understand the spread of COVID-19, we would want to know the following:

- **Symptoms**: COVID-19 is a contagious disease, and symptoms include fever, conjunctivitis, cough, difficulty breathing, fatigue, muscle and body aches, headache, new loss of taste or smell, sore throat, congestion or runny nose, nausea or vomiting, and diarrhea.
- **Causative agent**: SARS-CoV-2 virus.
- **Diagnosis**: Diagnosis is based on symptoms, laboratory testing, and history of contact with infected persons.
- **Occurrence**: COVID-19 is short for Coronavirus Disease 2019. It was first identified in Wuhan, China, in 2019. It was recognized as a worldwide pandemic in 2020.
- **Reservoir**: Humans.
- **Incubation period**: Symptoms may appear 2 to 14 days after exposure.
- **Transmission**: Between people in close contact with one another; through respiratory droplets produced when the infected person coughs, sneezes, or talks. It may be spread by people who are asymptomatic.
- **Risk groups**: All age groups are susceptible to infection but the symptoms vary. Older adults and individuals with comorbidities, such as heart disease, lung disease, high blood pressure, and obesity are at a higher risk for more serious complications.

- **Prevention**: Vaccination is key. Mitigation efforts to prevent the spread include hand hygiene, disinfection of frequently touched surfaces, social distancing (keeping at least 6 feet away from others), wearing face masks, paying attention to symptoms, and self-quarantine following exposure.
- **Management of the patient**: Individuals with COVID-19 should be isolated from others while ill to prevent spread to others. Treatment depends on the severity of the symptoms. Hospitalized patients may require ventilator therapy and intensive care management.
- **Management of contacts and the immediate environment**: Household contacts of infected individuals are at the greatest risk, especially if they have underlying medical conditions or are of advanced age. The individual who is sick should have a separate bedroom and bathroom, if possible. If rooms are shared, individuals should keep at least 6 feet of distance, use ventilating fans to increase circulation in the home, and disinfect common areas frequently. Guidance for isolation and quarantine is updated by the Centers for Disease Control and Prevention (CDC) depending upon the pathogenicity and infectivity of the predominant strain of the virus. In 2020, COVID-19 infection was a nationally notifiable disease, meaning it must be reported by state and territorial jurisdictions to the CDC. Health professionals conducted investigations to identify contacts and ensure that measures were taken to prevent spread. Effective May 1, 2024, this strict reporting was no longer required. The most recent recommendations for isolation and quarantine can be found at the CDC website.

Data from Centers for Disease Control and Prevention. (2020). Coronavirus Disease 2019. Available at https://www.cdc.gov/coronavirus/2019-nCoV/index.html

blood, serum, plasma, organs, and tissues. Almost any disease can be transmitted by vehicles, including those for which the primary mode of transmission is direct, such as dysentery and hepatitis.

Vectorborne transmission is the transfer of disease by a living organism, such as a mosquito, fly, or tick. Transmission may be mechanical, via the contaminated mouth parts or feet of the **vector**, or biological, which involves multiplication or developmental changes of the agent in the vector before transmission occurs. In mechanical transmission, multiplication and development of the disease organism usually do not occur. For example, organisms that cause dysentery, polio, cholera, and typhoid fever have been isolated from insects, such as cockroaches and houseflies and could presumably be deposited on food prepared for human consumption.

In biological transmission, multiplication and/or developmental changes of the disease agent occur in the vector before transmission occurs. Biological transmission is much more important than mechanical transmission in terms of its impact on community health. Examples of biological vectors include mosquitoes, fleas, lice, ticks, flies, and other insects. Mosquitoes are by far the most important vectors of human disease. They transmit the viruses that cause yellow fever, dengue fever, West Nile fever, and more than 200 other viruses, including Zika virus (see **Figure 4.5**). They also transmit malaria, which infected an estimated 247 million people in 2021, and led to 619,000 deaths. These values are higher than those prior to the COVID-19 pandemic. The increase is attributed to limited resources, conflict leading to global economy imbalance, and disruption in services due to the pandemic.[2]

Ticks, another important vector, transmit Rocky Mountain spotted fever, relapsing fever, and Lyme disease. Other insect vectors (and the diseases they transmit) are flies (African sleeping sickness, onchocerciasis, loiasis, and leishmaniasis), fleas (plague and murine typhus), lice (epidemic typhus and trench fever), and kissing bugs (Chagas' disease).

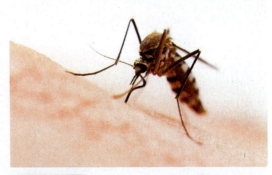

FIGURE 4.5   The *Aedes aegypti* mosquito is the vector of Zika virus.

© Frank60/Shutterstock

Noncommunicable Diseases

Although communicable diseases remain an important concern for communities, certain noncommunicable diseases, such as heart disease, stroke, and cancer, continue to rank high among the nation's leading causes of death. Although these diseases are not infectious, they nonetheless can occur in epidemic proportions. Furthermore, the chronic nature of many of these diseases means that they can deplete a community's resources quite rapidly.

The model showing agent, host, and environment is specific to communicable diseases but can be adapted for noncommunicable diseases where *agent* is the population and their characteristics, *hosts* are the factors that may cause disease, and *environment* is the physical environment, behaviors, cultural factors, physiology, and other external factors that impact disease.[3] Because the **etiology** (cause) of many noncommunicable diseases, such as coronary heart disease, is very complex, it is often illustrated using a **multicausation disease model** (see **Figure 4.6**). In this model, the human host is pictured in the center of the environment in which they live. Within the host, there exists a unique genetic endowment that is inalterable. The host exists in a complex environment that includes exposures to a multitude of risk factors that can contribute to the disease process. These environmental risk factors may be physical, chemical, biological, or social in nature.

Physical factors include the latitude, climate, and physical geography of where one lives. The major health risks in the tropics—communicable and parasitic diseases—are different from those in temperate regions with cold winters—difficulty in finding food and remaining warm. Chemical factors not only include natural chemical hazards of polluted water and air but also the added pollutants of our modern, industrial society. Biological hazards include

Indirect transmission communicable disease transmission involving an intermediate step

Vehicle an inanimate material or object that can serve as a source of infection

Vector a living organism, usually an arthropod (e.g., mosquito, tick, louse, or flea), that can transmit a communicable agent to susceptible hosts

Etiology the cause of a disease

Multicausation disease model a visual representation of the host together with various internal and external factors that promote and protect against disease

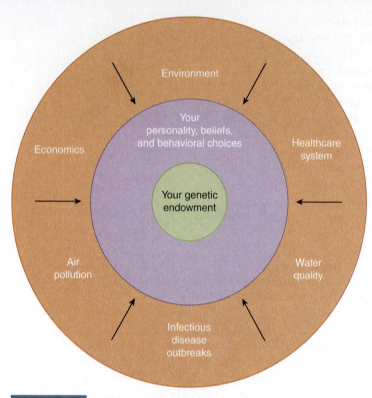

FIGURE 4.6 Multicausation disease model.

communicable disease agents, such as pathogenic viruses, bacteria, and fungi. Social factors include one's occupation, recreational activities, and living arrangements. Poor choices in life can increase the number and severity of one's risk factors and be detrimental to one's health.

Diseases of the Heart and Blood Vessels

Disease of the heart and blood vessels, cardiovascular disease (CVD), is a leading cause of death in the United States. **Coronary heart disease (CHD)** is the number one killer of Americans. In 2022 alone, 699,659 people died of heart disease in the United States, accounting for 21% of deaths that year. This was an increase compared with 2021.[4,5] The prevalence of CVD in adults in the United States is 49.2%.[6]

The American Heart Association classifies the leading causes of death from CVD in order as CHD (41.3%), stroke (17.2%), high blood pressure (11.7%), heart failure (9.9%), diseases of the arteries (2.8%), and other (17.3%).[6]

Sometimes called coronary artery disease, CHD is characterized by damage to the coronary arteries, the blood vessels that carry oxygen-rich blood to the heart muscle. Damage to the coronary arteries usually evolves from the condition known as atherosclerosis, a narrowing of the blood vessels. This narrowing usually results from the buildup of fatty deposits on the inner walls of arteries. When blood flow to the heart muscle is severely reduced or interrupted, a heart attack can occur. If heart damage is severe, the heart may stop beating—a condition known as cardiac arrest.

Heart disease became the leading cause of death in 1921, and stroke was the third leading cause of death beginning in 1938. The age-adjusted death rates from CVD declined dramatically during the twentieth century, representing a significant public health achievement of that time.[7] Further reductions in cardiovascular disease were also noted as an important public health achievement in the first decade of the twenty-first century.[8] This trend has reversed in recent years (see **Box 4.2**).

Numerous risk factors for coronary artery disease have been identified. Whereas some of these risk factors cannot be altered by changes in lifestyle or behavior, others can. Factors that cannot be altered include one's age, sex, race, and the genetic tendency toward developing the disease. Factors that can be modified include cigarette smoking, high blood pressure, high blood cholesterol, physical inactivity, obesity, diabetes, and stress.

Cerebrovascular disease (stroke) is the fifth leading cause of death in the United States.[4] Strokes killed 150,005 individuals in the United States in 2019.[6] During a stroke, or cerebrovascular accident, the blood supply to the brain is interrupted. The risk factors for developing cerebrovascular disease are similar to those for CHD and include hereditary, behavioral, and environmental factors. Hypertension and cigarette smoking are especially important risk factors for cerebrovascular disease. Prevalence of stroke increases with increasing age.

Malignant Neoplasms (Cancer)

An estimated 609,820 people died from malignant neoplasms (cancer) in 2023, making it the second leading cause of death in the United States.[9] A malignant neoplasm occurs when cells lose control over their growth and division. Normal cells are inhibited from continual growth

Coronary heart disease (CHD) a chronic disease characterized by damage to the coronary arteries in the heart

Cerebrovascular disease (stroke) a chronic disease characterized by damage to blood vessels of the brain, resulting in disruption of circulation to the brain

BOX 4.2   Improved Trends in Mortality from Heart Disease and Stroke Reversed During COVID-19 Pandemic

You Gotta Have Heart

The decline in cardiovascular disease death rates that began in the twentieth century continued from 2001 to 2010, making the list of important public health achievements. Age-adjusted death rates for coronary heart disease declined from 195 to 126 per 100,000 population from 2001 to 2010.[10] From 2010 to 2019, the age-adjusted mortality rate (AAMR) for CVD in adults 35 and older declined by 8.9%. A global health emergency due to COVID-19 was declared in March of 2020. From 2019 to 2022, the CVD AAMR increased by 9.3%. The rate of CVD in 2022 was similar to the rate in 2011. The AAMR for stroke increased an average of 4.0% per year in 2020, 2021, and 2022. The rate of stroke mortality in 2022 was higher than the rate in 2010. The estimated excess stroke deaths during this 3-year period was 45,236.[5]

Advances in Prevention, Treatment, and Quality of Care

Prevention efforts resulting in lower prevalence of risk factors, such as hypertension, high cholesterol, smoking, and improvements in treatment, medications, and care contributed to declines in CVD and stroke prior to 2020. Cardiac events associated with acute infection and long-term COVID sequelae may account for some of the increased deaths. Disrupted access to health care, hesitancy to seek care, and changes in healthy habits account for this decline as well.

---

and division by virtue of their contact with adjacent cells. Malignant (cancerous) cells are not so inhibited; they continue to grow and divide, eventually piling up in a "new growth," a neoplasm, or tumor. Early-stage tumors, sometimes called in situ cancers, are more treatable than later-stage cancers because they are confined to the location where they started and have not spread to other parts of the body. As tumor growth continues, parts of the neoplasm can break off and be carried to distant parts of the body, where they can lodge and continue to grow. When this occurs, the cancer is said to have undergone **metastasis**, or to have metastasized. When **malignant neoplasms** have spread beyond the original cell layer where they developed, the cancer is said to be invasive.[9] The more the malignancy spreads, the more difficult it is to treat and the lower the survival rates. For more information on the staging of cancer, see **Box 4.3**.

Common cancer sites, in order of frequency of reported cases and deaths for both men and women, are shown in **Figure 4.7**. In the United States, the cancer sites with the highest number of new cases are the prostate gland (men) and breast (women), but cancer frequently occurs in other sites, including the lung, colon and rectum, pancreas, uterus, ovaries, mouth, bladder, and skin. The highest mortality rates are seen in non-Hispanic Black men and women. Lung cancer is the leading cause of cancer deaths in both sexes. An estimated 238,340 new cases of lung cancer and an estimated 127,070 lung cancer deaths were expected to occur in 2023 alone. Cigarette smoking is the most important risk factor for developing lung cancer. Tobacco is a modifiable risk factor for cancers of the colon and rectum, kidney, lung and bronchus, oral cavity and pharynx, breast, ovary, leukemia, urinary bladder, and pancreas. Excess body weight, physical inactivity, excess alcohol consumption, and poor nutrition also increase the risk for cancer.[9]

> **Metastasis** the spread of cancer cells to distant parts of the body by the circulatory or lymphatic system
>
> **Malignant neoplasm** uncontrolled new tissue growth resulting from cells that have lost control over their growth and division

---

BOX 4.3   How Is Cancer Staged?

According to the American Cancer Society, "staging describes the extent or spread of the disease." A number of different staging systems exist. One of the most popular is the TNM staging system, which assesses tumors in three ways: the extent of the primary tumor (T), absence or presence of regional lymph node involvement (N), and absence or presence of distant metastases (M). Once the T, N, and M are determined, a stage of I, II, III, or IV is assigned, with stage I being early stage and stage IV being the most advanced.

A different system of summary staging (in situ, local, regional, and distant) is used for descriptive and statistical analysis of tumor registry data. If cancer cells are present only in the layer of cells where they developed and have not spread, the stage is in situ. If the cancer has spread beyond the original layer of tissue, the cancer is invasive.

Data from American Cancer Society. (2023). Cancer Facts & Figures 2023. https://www.cancer.org/content/dam/cancer-org/research/cancer-facts-and-statistics/annual-cancer-facts-and-figures/2023/2023-cancer-facts-and-figures.pdf

Estimated New Cases

Male

Prostate	299,010	29%
Lung & bronchus	116,310	11%
Colon & rectum	81,540	8%
Urinary bladder	63,070	6%
Melanoma of the skin	59,170	6%
Kidney & renal pelvis	52,380	5%
Non-Hodgkin lymphoma	44,590	4%
Oral cavity & pharynx	41,510	4%
Leukemia	36,450	4%
Pancreas	34,530	3%
All sites	**1,029,080**	

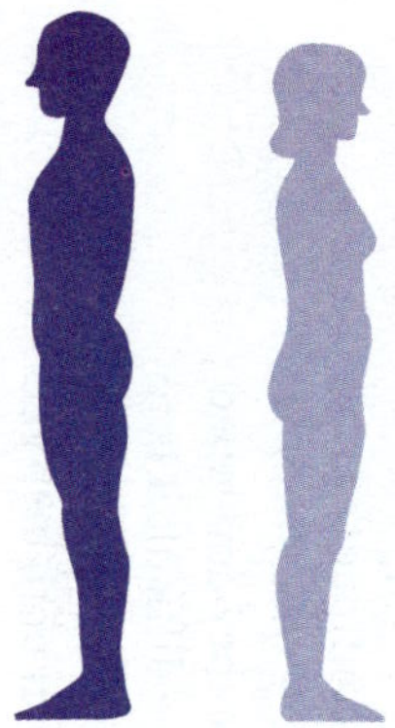

Female

Breast	310,720	32%
Lung & bronchus	118,270	12%
Colon & rectum	71,270	7%
Uterine corpus	67,880	7%
Melanoma of the skin	41,470	4%
Non-Hodgkin lymphoma	36,030	4%
Pancreas	31,910	3%
Thyroid	31,520	3%
Kidney & renal pelvis	29,230	3%
Leukemia	26,320	3%
All sites	**972,060**	

Estimated Deaths

Male

Lung & bronchus	65,790	20%
Prostate	35,250	11%
Colon & rectum	28,700	9%
Pancreas	27,270	8%
Liver & intrahepatic bile duct	19,120	6%
Leukemia	13,640	4%
Esophagus	12,880	4%
Urinary bladder	12,290	4%
Non-Hodgkin lymphoma	11,780	4%
Brain & other nervous system	10,690	3%
All sites	**322,800**	

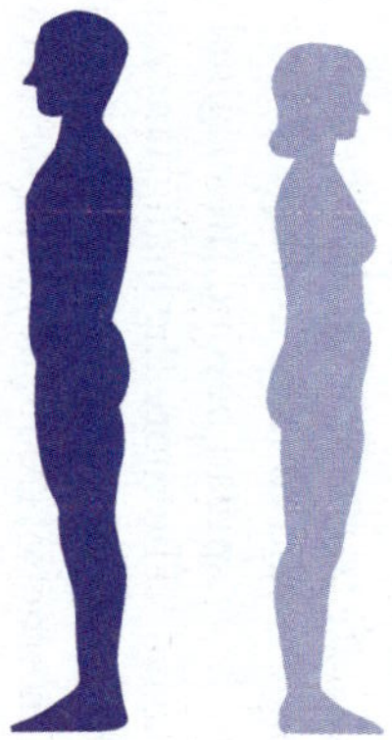

Female

Lung & bronchus	59,280	21%
Breast	42,250	15%
Pancreas	24,480	8%
Colon & rectum	24,310	8%
Uterine corpus	13,250	5%
Ovary	12,740	4%
Liver & intrahepatic bile duct	10,720	4%
Leukemia	10,030	3%
Non-Hodgkin lymphoma	8,360	3%
Brain & other nervous system	8,070	3%
All sites	**288,920**	

FIGURE 4.7 Leading sites of new cancer cases and deaths—United States, 2023 estimates. Ranking is based on modeled projections and may differ from the most recent observed data.

Estimates are rounded to the nearest 10, and cases exclude basal cell and squamous cell skin cancers and in situ carcinoma except urinary bladder. Estimates do not include Puerto Rico or other US territories. Excludes basal and squamous cell skin cancer and in situ carcinomas except urinary bladder.

TABLE 4.4 Some Noncommunicable Health Conditions That Affect Americans

Allergic disorders	Endogenous depression	Multiple sclerosis
Alzheimer's disease	Epilepsy	Osteoporosis
Arthritis	Fibrocystic breast condition	Premenstrual syndrome
Cerebral palsy	Low back pain	Sickle cell trait and sickle cell disease

Skin cancer is the most commonly diagnosed cancer in the United States. It is estimated that 5.4 million new cases of basal cell or squamous cell skin cancer were diagnosed among 3.3 million people in the United States in 2012. Actual numbers are not available because these types of cancer are not reported to cancer registries. Melanoma is reportable even though it causes a small percentage of skin cancers; the number of estimated new cases was 97,610 in 2023, with the estimated number of deaths at 7,990. It is highly curable when detected early.[9] Most skin cancers are attributable to exposure to ultraviolet (UV) light, light skin color is a risk factor. Measures to prevent skin cancer include wearing protective clothing and hats, using of sunscreen with a sun protection factor of at least 30, and avoiding excessive sun exposure.[9]

Other Noncommunicable Disease Problems

Other noncommunicable diseases of major concern are chronic lower respiratory diseases (the sixth leading cause of death in 2022), Alzheimer's disease (the seventh leading cause of death), and diabetes mellitus (the eighth leading cause of death).[9]

Each of these chronic noncommunicable diseases and those listed in **Table 4.4** not only place a burden on the afflicted individuals and their families but also on the community's health resources.

Prioritizing Prevention and Control Efforts

Communities are confronted with a multitude of health problems—communicable and non-communicable diseases, unintentional injuries, violence, substance use disorders, and so on. How can health officials make logical and responsible choices about the allocation of community resources to prevent or control these problems? Which problems are indeed the most urgent? Which problems will benefit the most from a timely intervention? Many criteria can be used to judge the importance of a particular disease to a community. Among these are (1) the number of people who die from a disease, (2) the number of years of potential life lost attributable to a particular cause, and (3) the economic costs associated with a particular disease or health condition. Communities may collect primary data or use secondary sources to inform prioritization of community health issues. Other useful sources of secondary data include Kaiser State Health Facts (www.statehealthfacts.org), Kids Count (https://datacenter.aecf.org), and County Health Rankings (www.countyhealthrankings.org). Each of these sources provides data on numerous health, social, economic, and environmental factors. These tools also allow comparison of geographic areas, which is useful if a community wants to show how they compare with either other communities, the state, or the nation.

Leading Causes of Death

The National Center for Health Statistics (NCHS) regularly publishes a list of the leading causes of death. For more than 80 years, the leading cause of death in America has been heart disease. Cancers (malignant neoplasms) represent the second leading killer. Unintentional injuries rank third. COVID-19 was a newcomer to the leading causes of death beginning in 2020, and its rank has varied. Stroke, chronic lower respiratory disease and Alzheimer's disease are followed by diabetes, kidney disease, and chronic liver disease and cirrhosis.[11]

One might prioritize expenditures of healthcare resources solely on the basis of the number of deaths, but in doing so, one would spend about two-thirds of the entire health budget on the four leading health problems alone. Very little or perhaps none of the resources would be available for infant and childhood nutrition programs, for example, which have been shown to prevent more serious health problems in later life. Nor would there be any funds available for the treatment of those with debilitating, but usually nonfatal, diseases such as chronic arthritis or mental illness.

Years of Potential Life Lost

Another approach to prioritizing a community's healthcare problems is by using the years of potential life lost before the age of 65 (YPLL-65) statistic. Using this approach, conditions that kill people of all ages become as important as those that primarily kill older adults. In the United States, unintentional injuries are the leading cause of YPLL-65, accounting for 24.9% of the total YPLL. This category showed a substantial increase beginning in 2020. Unintentional poisoning, which includes drug overdose, accounted for 58.9% of unintentional injuries. COVID-19 accounted for 10.6% of the YPLL-65 in 2021. Malignant neoplasms (cancers) are the third leading cause, accounting for approximately 10.0% of age-adjusted YPLL-65, and diseases of the heart account for 9.7% of the total YPLL-65.[12] There is a racial bias to YPLL data. Unintentional injuries are the leading cause for White people, Black people, and American Indians and Alaskan Natives. Cancer remains the leading cause of YPLL-65 for Asians, and in 2021, COVID-19 was the leading cause of YPLL for Pacific Islanders.[12]

Economic Cost to Society

Still another way to evaluate the impact of a particular disease or health problem is to estimate the economic cost to the country or community. Economic cost data are hard to come by, and sometimes even experts cannot agree on the estimates obtained. An example of such an estimate is the cost to our federal, state, and local governments' spending resulting from the use and abuse of drugs. The President's FY 2023 National Drug Control Budget Request increased by nearly $3.2 billion from 2022, to $42.5 billion. Spending includes treatment, prevention, law enforcement, interdiction, and international operations.[13] This cost estimate does not include state and local community efforts.

Prevention, Intervention, Control, and Eradication of Diseases

The goals of epidemiology are to prevent, control, and in rare cases, to eradicate diseases and injuries. **Prevention** implies the planning for and taking of action to prevent or forestall the occurrence of an undesirable event, and is, therefore, more desirable than **intervention**, the taking of action during an event. For example, immunizing to prevent a disease is preferable to taking an antibiotic to cure one.

Control is a general term for the containment of a disease and can include both prevention and intervention measures. The term *control* is often used to mean the limiting of transmission of a communicable disease in a population. **Eradication** is the uprooting or total elimination of a disease from the human population. It is an elusive goal, one that is rarely achieved in public health. Smallpox is the only communicable disease that has been eradicated in humans (see **Box 4.4**). Several characteristics of smallpox made eradication possible: Humans are the only reservoir, the disease is visible shortly after infection so individuals can be identified before infecting a large number of other people, and infection results in lifelong immunity. After intense identification and vaccination efforts, the last case of naturally occurring human smallpox was in 1977.

Prevention the planning for and taking of action to forestall the onset of a disease or other health problem

Intervention efforts to control a disease in progress

Eradication the complete elimination or uprooting of a disease (e.g., smallpox)

BOX 4.4   Community Health in Your World: Smallpox Eradication

October of 2023 marked 46 years since the last naturally acquired case of smallpox in the world. This last case occurred in Somalia in October of 1977.[1] Although two cases of smallpox were reported in the United Kingdom in 1978, these were associated with a research laboratory and did not represent a natural recurrence.

Smallpox is caused by the variola virus. In its severest form, it is a disfiguring and deadly disease. Manifestations of the disease include fever, headache, malaise, and prostration. A rash appears and covers the body, and there is bleeding into the skin, mucous linings, and genital tract. The circulatory system is also severely affected. Between 15% and 40% of cases die, usually within 2 weeks. Survivors are terribly scarred for life and are sometimes blinded.

Mass vaccinations and case-finding measures by the World Health Organization (WHO), with financial support from the United States, led to the eradication of smallpox from the world. Why was it possible to eradicate smallpox? Why have we been unable to eradicate any other diseases since 1977? Do you think we will ever be able to do so? If so, what disease will be eliminated next? How could a personal or religious opinion affect this goal?

Levels of Prevention

There are three levels of application of preventive measures in disease control—primary, secondary, and tertiary. The purpose of **primary prevention** is to forestall the onset of illness or injury during the prepathogenesis period (before the disease process begins). Examples of primary prevention include health education and health promotion programs, safe-housing projects, and character-building and personality development programs. Other examples are the use of immunizations against specific diseases, the practice of personal hygiene, such as handwashing, the use of rubber gloves, and the chlorination of the community's water supply. These are illustrated in **Figure 4.8**. During the COVID-19 pandemic, mitigation efforts to "flatten the curve," or lower the rate of new infections, included vaccination, social distancing, limiting the number of individuals at a common gathering, and the wearing of personal protective equipment (PPE), such as face masks.

Unfortunately, disease or injury cannot always be avoided. Chronic diseases in particular sometimes cause considerable disability before they are detected and treated. In these cases, prompt intervention can prevent death or limit disability. **Secondary prevention** is the early diagnosis and prompt treatment of diseases before the disease becomes advanced and disability becomes severe.

One of the most important secondary prevention measures is health screenings. The goal of these screenings is not to prevent the onset of disease but rather to detect its presence during early pathogenesis, thus permitting early intervention (treatment) and limiting disability. It is important to note that the purpose of a health screening is not to diagnose disease. Instead, the purpose is to economically and efficiently sort those who are probably healthy from those who could possibly be positive for a disease. Those who screen positively can then be referred for more specific diagnostic procedures. Those who screen negatively are rescreened at prescribed intervals. Screenings for diabetes and high blood pressure are popular examples of health screenings for noncommunicable diseases, as are Pap smears, mammograms, and testicular self-examination.

Secondary prevention efforts related to the spread of COVID-19 include isolation for individuals with the disease and self-quarantine for individuals who had been exposed to the disease. Diagnostic testing performed with nasal swabs identifies those with an active viral infection and/or carrier status for the virus. Antibody testing, performed with a blood sample, identifies individuals with prior exposure and is not used to determine if someone is infectious. Antibody testing is used for epidemiologic purposes.

The goal of **tertiary prevention** is to retrain, re-educate, and rehabilitate the patient who has already incurred a disability. Tertiary preventive measures include those that are applied after significant pathogenesis has occurred. Therapy for a heart patient is an example of tertiary prevention.

Primary prevention preventive measures that forestall the onset of illness or injury during the prepathogenesis period

Secondary prevention preventive measures that lead to an early diagnosis and prompt treatment of a disease or injury to limit disability and prevent more severe pathogenesis

Tertiary prevention measures aimed at rehabilitation following significant pathogenesis

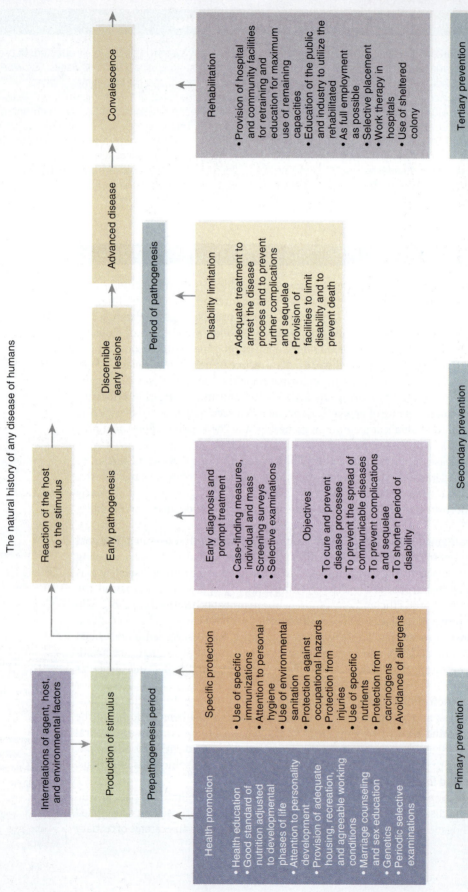

FIGURE 4.8   Applications of levels of prevention.

Prevention of Communicable Diseases

Prevention and control efforts for communicable diseases include primary, secondary, and tertiary approaches. Successful application of these approaches, particularly primary prevention, resulting in unprecedented declines in morbidity and mortality from communicable diseases, has been one of the outstanding achievements in public health in the first part of this century (see **Box 4.5**).

BOX 4.5   The Vaccination Response to the COVID-19 Pandemic

Coronavirus Disease Detected in 2019

Coronavirus Disease 2019 (COVID-19) is caused by the SARS-CoV-2 virus. Symptoms appear 2 to 14 days after exposure, and include fever, conjunctivitis, cough, difficulty breathing, fatigue, muscle and body aches, headache, new loss of taste or smell, sore throat, congestion or runny nose, nausea or vomiting, pneumonia, and diarrhea. It can be fatal. Humans are the reservoir, and transmission is airborne. COVID-19 can be spread by asymptomatic carriers. All age groups are susceptible. Older adults and individuals with comorbidities, such as heart disease, high blood pressure, and obesity are at higher risk for more serious complications.[14]

The novel virus COVID-19 originated in Wuhan China in 2019 and rapidly spread worldwide. The COVID-19 pandemic affected everyone. In February of 2020, the World Health Organization declared a Global Health Emergency, and the United States followed suit. By March of that year, the crisis was declared a pandemic by WHO. The same month travel, businesses, and schools shut down. States issued Stay-at-Home orders except for essential workers and shopping for essential needs. Measures to flatten the curve of transmission included masking, hand hygiene, quarantine, and social distancing. Operation Warp Speed was a U.S. project to rapidly develop and deploy a COVID-19 vaccine.[15]

The Pandemic Continues

In 2020, COVID-19 infected over 20 million people in the United States and was the third leading cause of death, with more than 346,000 deaths.[15] Hospitals and health professionals worked overtime as they cared for the sick. The first vaccines available to fight COVID-19 received emergency use authorization (EUA) from the FDA in December of 2020 and were distributed to specific subpopulations, e.g., military, healthcare workers, skilled nursing, and long-term care facility residents, on a tiered basis. Immunizations were procured and distributed by the federal government, with no cost to the individual. By the end of 2020, an estimated 2.8 million people had received one vaccination dose.[15] Special storage temperatures and winter storms affected the transportation of vaccines, leading to delays in vaccinations. Variants of the original strain led to a drop in the efficacy of the vaccine in neutralizing the virus. Manufacturing and side-effect complications associated with two vaccine manufacturers resulted in the CDC and FDA pausing their use, and consequently, the overall availability of vaccines. In a poll in February of 2021,

vaccination hesitancy was noted along party lines, with 91% of Democrats and only 51% of Republicans indicating their intent to be vaccinated (poll by CNN). This bias was reiterated in March (poll by PBS).[15]

Vaccination Mandates and Recommendations

By April 19, 2021, all 50 states expanded vaccine eligibility to all adults. At the same time, the number of new cases increased compared with the previous week. Data from the CDC showed that the risk of COVID-19 infection among those who were fully vaccinated was 0.01%. In June of 2021, the Equal Employment Opportunity Commission (EEOC) allowed employers to mandate that their workers receive a COVID vaccine.[16] In July, mandatory vaccination was required for municipal and state workers in California and New York City, and the Department of Veterans Affairs required the vaccine for its healthcare workers. Civilian federal workers were required to be vaccinated or obey strict testing, social distancing, restricted travel, and masking. Medicaid and Medicare participating nursing homes were required to vaccinate their staff. By August of 2021, 90% of Americans aged 60 and older had received at least one dose of the COVID-19 vaccine. After the Pfizer/BioNTech vaccine received full FDA approval, several large organizations issued vaccine mandates for employees. In October of 2021, President Joe Biden announced a plan that all companies with over 100 employees mandate vaccines or require weekly testing. The mandate was challenged by several lawsuits, and in November, the mandate was put on hold.[17] Two anti-viral oral medications for at-home use received FDA emergency use authorization in December of 2021. COVID-19 was the third leading cause of death in the United States, the second year in a row.[18] COVID-19 was listed on the death certificates of 463,267 people, and for at least 90% of these, it was the underlying cause of death.[19] The death rates were much higher in individuals 65 and older (**Figure 4.9**).[20]

Public Health Emergency Due to COVID-19 Ended in the United States

Requirements for testing, quarantine, and isolation were modified over time as more of the population was vaccinated. State and local governments adjusted their recommendations for public gatherings, referring to the COVID-19 community transmission levels for guidance. U.S. state, and local dashboards were updated regularly

(continues)

BOX 4.5   The Vaccination Response to the COVID-19 Pandemic   *(continued)*

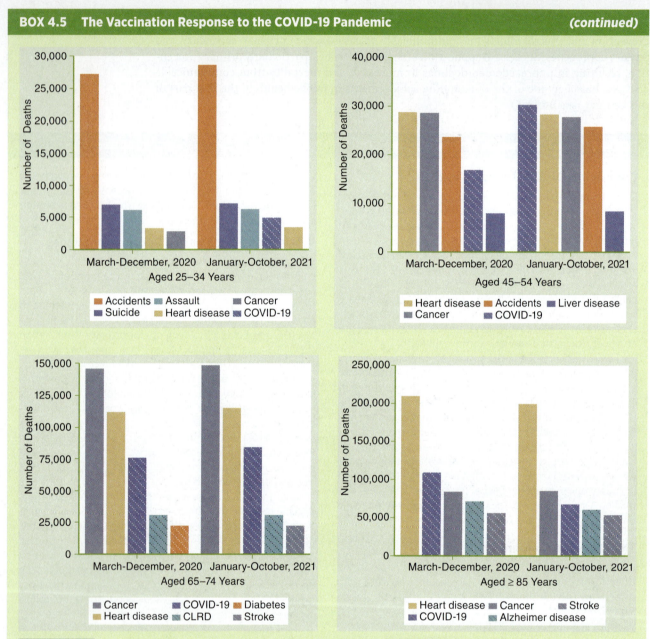

FIGURE 4.9   Leading Causes of Death in the US, March to December 2020 and January to October 2021.

Data from Shiels, M. S., Haque, A. T., de González, A. B., & Freedman, N. D. (August 2022). Leading causes of death in the US during the COVID-19 pandemic, March 2020 to October 2021. JAMA Internal Medicine, 182, 883–885.

to show where transmission was highest. Identification of COVID-19 variants led to updated booster vaccine recommendations.

In January of 2022, the Moderna vaccine was FDA approved for adults 18 and older. Two years after the COVID-19 pandemic began, the CDC showed that more than 98% of the U.S. population was in a location with either low or medium community transmission. In June, the United States marked the grim total of 1,003,571 deaths from COVID-19. Vaccination was recommended for infants by the Advisory Committee on Immunization Practices, making

it recommended for all individuals 6 months and older.[18,21] COVID-19 was the fourth leading cause of death in 2022, accounting for 186,702 (5.7%) of all deaths that year.[4]

In May of 2023, President Joe Biden announced the end of the national and public health emergency declarations in the United States. COVID-19 was less prevalent; from January to July 22 of that year, 28,140 individuals died from COVID-19. The virus continued to mutate. In September of 2023, the SARS-CoV-2- XBB variant was the predominant strain in the United States, and COVID-19 vaccines based on the ancestral strain were no longer effective, so FDA authorization was rescinded. Updated vaccines were created in response to this strain. The cost for COVID-19 vaccines transitioned into the commercial marketplace in the fall of 2023, and insurers became responsible for the cost of immunizations, without cost sharing requirements.[21]

Figure 4.9 compares the five leading causes of death in the United States from the start of the pandemic through October of 2021. COVID-19 is the sole communicable disease in the data. Each set of graphs represents a different age demographic; note that the scales differ. Two time-points demonstrate the spread of infection in different age groups and suggest the positive effects of early preferential vaccination in the older adults.[20] CLRD: chronic lower respiratory disease.

Data from Centers for Disease Control and Prevention. (2022). Provisional Mortality Data — United States, 2022. Morbidity and Mortality Weekly Report 2023;72:488–492. http://dx.doi.org/10.15585/mmwr.mm7218a3; Centers for Disease Control and Prevention. (2020). Coronavirus Disease 2019. https://www.cdc.gov/coronavirus/2019-nCoV/index.html; AJMC Staff. A Timeline of COVID-19 Developments in 2020. https://www.ajmc.com/view/a-timeline-of-covid19-developments-in-2020; AJMC Staff. A Timeline of COVID-19 Vaccine Developments in 2021. https://www.ajmc.com/view/a-timeline-of-covid-19-vaccine-developments-in-2021; AJMC Staff. A Timeline of COVID-19 Vaccine Developments for the Second Half of 2021. https://www.ajmc.com/view/a-timeline-of-covid-19-vaccine-developments-for-the-second-half-of-2021; Centers for Disease Control and Prevention. (2022). CDC Museum COVID-19 Timeline. https://www.cdc.gov/museum/timeline/covid19.html; Centers for Disease Control and Prevention (2023). COVID-19 Mortality Overview. Provisional Death Counts for COVID-19. https://www.cdc.gov/nchs/covid19/mortality-overview.htm; Shiels, M.S., Haque, A.T., Berrington de Gonzalez, A., Freedman, N.D. (2022). Leading Causes of Death in the US During the COVID-19 Pandemic, March 2020 to October 2021. JAMA Internal Medicine. 182, (8) 883–885; Centers for Disease Control and Prevention (2023). Use of Updated COVID-19 Vaccines 2023–2024 Formula for Persons Aged ≥6 Months: Recommendations of the Advisory Committee on Immunization Practices — United States, September 2023. Morbidity and Mortality Weekly Report 2023;72:1140–1146. http://dx.doi.org/10.15585/mmwr.mm7242e1

Primary Prevention of Communicable Diseases

The primary prevention measures for communicable diseases can best be visualized using the chain of infection (see **Figure 4.10**). In this model, prevention strategies are evident at each link in the chain. Successful application of each strategy can be seen as weakening a link, with the ultimate goal of breaking the chain of infection, or interrupting the disease transmission cycle. Examples of community measures include chlorination of the water supply, the inspection of restaurants and retail food markets, immunization programs that reach all citizens, the maintenance of a well-functioning sewer system, the proper disposal of solid waste, and the control of vectors and rodents. To these can be added personal efforts at primary prevention, including handwashing, the proper cooking of food, adequate clothing and housing, wearing PPE, the use of condoms, and obtaining all of the available immunizations against specific diseases.

Immunity can be developed actively or passively. **Active immunity** happens when a person is exposed to an organism that causes disease and their body develops antibodies that know how to fight off that disease. A person can be exposed to a disease-causing organism through an infection or through a vaccine (see **Figure 4.11**). **Passive immunity** is where people receive the antibodies rather than their own body making them. For example, newborn babies receive antibodies from their mothers, which helps their immune systems fight off infections early in

Active immunity occurs when exposure to a disease-causing organism prompts the immune system to develop antibodies against that disease

Passive immunity occurs when people receive antibodies against a disease rather than their own immune system producing them

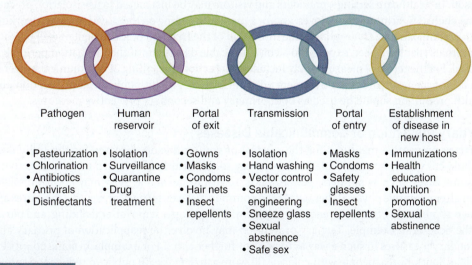

FIGURE 4.10   Chain of infection model showing disease prevention and control strategies.

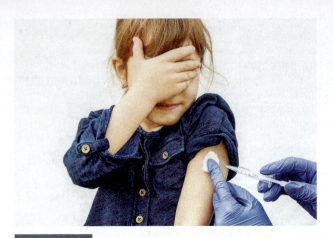

FIGURE 4.11   Child receiving a vaccination.

© Tatevosian Yana/Shutterstock

life. It is difficult to overstate the importance of vaccines or immunizations to community and public health. Vaccines prevent disease and save lives. They prevent disease in those who receive them and also protect those who come into contact with them. Many serious infectious diseases that were common as recently as the middle of the last century are rare now, including polio, measles, diphtheria, pertussis (whooping cough), rubella (German measles), mumps, tetanus, and *Haemophilus influenzae* type b (Hib).[22] Vaccines help the body fight off these diseases and help protect those members of the community who are unable to be vaccinated, namely, infants, those with certain diseases, such as childhood leukemia, and those unable to respond to an immunization. The Advisory Committee on Immunization Practices (ACIP), a group of medical and public health experts, issues recommendations for immunizations for children, for teens and college students, and for adults. These recommendations include immunizations for about 15 different disease agents and often indicate the need for a series of doses to acquire adequate protection. Infants are immunized against several agents during their first year. Immunization against human papillomavirus (HPV) is started in the preteen years. HPV is spread through intimate contact and is linked to six types of cancer. The current recommendations and timetables can be accessed through the website: www.cdc.gov/vaccines/acip/.

Secondary Prevention of Communicable Diseases

Secondary preventive measures against communicable diseases for the individual involve either (1) self-diagnosis and self-treatment with nonprescription medications or home remedies, or (2) diagnosis and treatment with an antibiotic or antiviral prescribed by a physician. Secondary preventive measures undertaken by the community against infectious diseases are usually aimed at controlling or limiting the extent of an epidemic. Examples include carefully maintaining records of cases and complying with the regulations requiring the reporting of notifiable diseases and investigating cases and contacts—those who may have become infected through close contact with known cases.

Occasionally, secondary disease control measures may include isolation and quarantine. These two practices are quite different from one another and are often confused. **Isolation** is the separation, for the period of communicability, of infected persons or animals from others so as to prevent the direct or indirect transmission of the communicable agent to a susceptible person. In healthcare settings, providers and visitors may be instructed to use isolation precautions, such as wearing a gown, gloves, and/or a mask (depending on the situation), when working with certain patients. **Quarantine** is the limitation of the freedom of movement of well persons or animals that have been exposed to a communicable disease until the incubation period has passed. Further control measures may include **disinfection**, the killing of communicable agents outside of the host, and mass treatment with antibiotics. Finally, public health education and health promotion should be used as both primary and secondary preventive measures.

Tertiary Prevention of Communicable Diseases

Tertiary preventive measures for the control of communicable diseases for the individual include convalescence from infection, recovery to full health, and return to normal activity. In some cases, such as paralytic poliomyelitis, return to normal activity may not be possible, even after extensive physical therapy. At the community level, tertiary preventive measures are aimed at preventing the recurrence of an epidemic. The proper removal, embalming, and burial of the dead is an example. Tertiary prevention may involve the reapplication of primary and secondary measures in such a way as to prevent further cases. For example, in some countries, such as South Korea, people with colds or flu wore gauze masks in public to reduce the spread of disease even before the COVID-19 pandemic.

Isolation the separation of infected persons from those who are susceptible

Quarantine limitation of freedom of movement of those who have been exposed to a disease and may be incubating it

Disinfection the killing of communicable disease agents outside of the host, on countertops, for example

Application of Prevention Measures in the Control of a Communicable Disease: HIV Infection and AIDS

Acquired immunodeficiency syndrome (AIDS) is the late stage of an infection with the human immunodeficiency virus (HIV). HIV destroys specific blood cells (CD4+ T cells) that are crucial in fighting diseases. People can become infected when they come into contact with the virus through unprotected sexual activity, intravenous drug use, or exposure to the blood of an infected person. Most people have flu-like symptoms within a few weeks after exposure. This initial stage is called acute HIV infection. The next stage, chronic HIV infection, is asymptomatic and can last for several years. One reason to test asymptomatic individuals for HIV is that a person can spread HIV, even if they feel well. Another reason to test is that HIV treatment may prevent an infected person from progressing to the most severe stage, AIDS. People with AIDS have a difficult time fighting other communicable diseases and certain cancers. In the past, it took only a few years for someone infected to develop AIDS. With the development of antiretroviral therapy (ART), a person with HIV can expect to live nearly as long as a person without HIV.[23] Between 2000 and 2022, the number of new infections and HIV-related deaths have decreased significantly.[24]

Despite advances in the diagnosis and treatment, HIV infections and AIDS are still epidemic in the United States and in the world. The WHO estimated that 39 (33.1–45.7) million people were living with HIV/AIDS worldwide at the end of 2022. In the same year, 1.3 million people were newly infected with HIV and 630,000 people died of HIV-related causes. From the beginning of the epidemic through 2022, approximately 40.4 million people had died from AIDS-related causes.[24] The estimated number of people living with HIV in the United States was 1.2 million in 2021, the last year that data were complete. Of these, only 87% knew of their positive status.[23]

The reservoir for HIV is the infected human population; there are no known animal or insect reservoirs. Referring to the chain of infection, HIV normally leaves its infected host (reservoir) during sexual activity or pregnancy. The portal of exit is the urogenital tract. Transmission is direct and occurs when reproductive fluids or blood are exchanged with the susceptible host. The portal of entry is usually either genital, oral, or anal in direct (sexual) transmission. Transmission can occur between a pregnant woman and her fetus. Transmission can also occur to healthcare providers during medical procedures if there is an accidental needlestick, or significant exposure to infected blood or other potentially infectious material. Blood-to-blood transmission can occur using shared needles, such as in the case of injection drug users. Blood banks screen donor blood units for HIV using multiple methods and discard contaminated units.

A closer examination of the chain of infection reveals that prevention or control measures can be identified for each link. The pathogen in the diseased host can be held in check by the appropriate drug. Outside of the host, measures such as sterilizing medical equipment and other possible vehicles readily kill the virus and reduce the likelihood of transmission by contamination. The infected host (reservoir) can be identified through blood tests and educated to take precautions against the careless transmission of live virus through unsafe sex and needle sharing. Condoms can be used to reduce the likelihood of transmission through portals of exit (and entry). There are effective medications that can be taken daily by individuals at a high risk of acquiring HIV from sex and IV drug use. These are referred to as pre-exposure prophylaxis (PrEP). Government programs exist to provide PrEP at no cost to individuals who lack prescription coverage, currently test negative for HIV, and have a prescription for PrEP.[25]

For injection drug users, abstinence from such drug use would preclude transmission by needles and syringes. A more realistic and proven approach to reducing the transmission of HIV/AIDS in this population is a syringe (and needle) exchange policy. Needle exchange programs also prevent the spread of other infections, such as hepatitis. Syringe service programs (SSPs) are regulated at the state and local level, but not all states support them. Communities that meet certain requirements are eligible for federal funding for SSPs, exclusive of providing needles, syringes, and equipment used solely for illicit drug use. In addition, SSPs provide referrals to drug treatment programs and provide training on overdose prevention and overdose reversal by the use of naloxone. Furthermore, SSPs provide safe disposal of used needles, which minimizes the risk of accidental needlestick to first responders and family members.[26] One set of *Healthy People 2030* objectives focuses on reducing the rate of HIV transmission and, thus, the number of new cases of AIDS. One way to do this is to increase condom use, particularly among high-risk populations. Another way is to increase the number of persons living with HIV who know their serostatus (if they are negative or positive for antibodies to HIV). Finally, one objective aim is to increase the proportion of adolescents and adults who have been tested for HIV in the past 12 months. These goals are incorporated into the plan, Ending the HIV Epidemic: A Plan for America (see **Box 4.6**).

BOX 4.6   The Plan to End the HIV Epidemic in the United States

In the State of the Union Address in 2019, President Donald Trump announced a plan and his support to end the HIV epidemic. He requested $291 million for fiscal year 2020 in the Department of Health and Human Services (HHS) budget to begin the work. The initiative is coordinated by the Office of the Assistant Secretary for Health (OASH) and involves state and local health departments and community feedback to create plans that are specific to each location.

The goal has two timelines, a 75% reduction in new HIV infections in 5 years and at least 90% reduction in 10 years.

The four strategies of the plan are similar to the goals of Healthy People 2030. They are as follows:

- **Diagnose:** Provide an early diagnosis for all individuals with HIV.
- **Treat:** Treat HIV infection rapidly and effectively to achieve sustained viral suppression.

- **Prevent:** Protect at-risk individuals from acquiring HIV infections using proven interventions, including PrEP and SSPs.
- **Respond:** Rapidly detect and take action on emerging HIV clusters and prevent new infections.

A major difference in this initiative compared with the past is the targeted approach to geographic areas called "hotspots," which have the highest numbers of new HIV cases. These locations will be the focus in the early years of the program. The program will be implemented across the entire United States within 10 years. **Figure 4.12** shows the targeted areas for year 1. The blue dots are the 48 counties with the highest burden of new HIV infection, Washington, DC, and San Juan, Puerto Rico. The states highlighted in blue have a substantial rural burden and are also first-year targets. New infections are more frequent in men having sex with men; minorities,

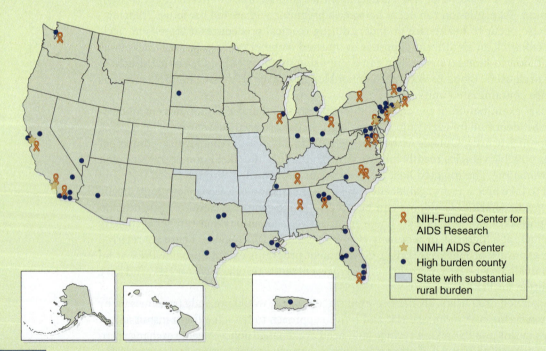

Legend:
- NIH-Funded Center for AIDS Research
- NIMH AIDS Center
- High burden county
- State with substantial rural burden

FIGURE 4.12   Geographical hotspots in the United States and Puerto Rico to be targeted to end the HIV epidemic.

Reproduced from National Institutes of Health, Office of AIDS Research. (2019). *A new plan to end the HIV epidemic in the United States*. https://oar.nih.gov/about/directors-corner/new-plan-end-hiv-epidemic-united-states

especially African American people, Hispanic/Latino people, Native American people, and Alaska Native people; and those living in the southern United States.

The initiative builds on strengths from many public health organizations as well as state and community efforts. The national organizations involved are the CDC, Health Resources and Services Administration (HRSA), Indian Health Service (IHS), National Institutes of Health (NIH), OASH, Substance Abuse and Mental Health Services Administration (SAMHSA), HIV.gov, and the U.S. Public Health Service (USPHS).

For Further Thought

Reducing the rate of HIV transmission is the best way to decrease both the number of persons living with HIV infection and the number of new AIDS cases. Reducing the number of new HIV cases decreases the number of deaths from AIDS. Is your community one of the geographic hotspots? What community resources exist in your county?

Data from National Institutes of Health, Office of AIDS Research. (2019). A New Plan to End the HIV Epidemic in the United States. Available at https://oar.nih.gov/about/directors-corner/new-plan-end-hiv-epidemic-united-states

For those working in the health professions, the risk of acquiring an HIV infection in the workplace is of particular concern. The Occupational Safety and Health Administration (OSHA) estimates that 5.6 million workers in the healthcare industry and related occupations are at risk of occupational exposure to **bloodborne pathogens**, including HIV, hepatitis B virus (HBV), hepatitis C virus (HCV), and others. The risk occurs mostly in the handling and disposal of contaminated needles.[27] In 1991, OSHA, recognizing that workers in the healthcare industry were at risk of occupational exposure to bloodborne pathogens, issued the **Bloodborne Pathogens Standard**.

In November of 2000, Congress, acknowledging the estimates of 600,000 to 800,000 needlestick and other percutaneous injuries occurring among healthcare workers annually, passed the Needlestick Safety and Prevention Act.[28] In 2001, in response to the Needlestick Safety and Prevention Act, OSHA revised its Bloodborne Pathogens Standard. This revised standard, currently in effect, added requirements for employers to select safer needle devices when available, seek employee input on choosing those devices, and maintain a log of injuries from contaminated sharps.[29] The goal of all of these regulations and standards is to reduce the number of HIV/AIDS cases, as well as cases of other bloodborne diseases, resulting from workplace exposure.

Bloodborne pathogens disease agents, such as HIV, that are transmissible in blood and other body fluids

Bloodborne Pathogens Standard a set of regulations promulgated by OSHA that sets forth the responsibilities of employers and employees with regard to precautions to be taken concerning bloodborne pathogens in the workplace

Prevention of Noncommunicable Diseases

Both the individual and the community can contribute substantially to the prevention and control of multicausation diseases. The community can provide a pro-health environment—physical, economic, and social—in which it becomes easier for individuals to achieve a high level of health.

Primary Prevention of Noncommunicable Diseases

Primary preventive measures for noncommunicable diseases include adequate food and energy supplies; good opportunities for education, employment, and housing; and efficient community services. Beyond this foundation, a community should provide health promotion and health education programs, health and medical services, and protection from environmental and occupational hazards.

Individuals can practice primary prevention by obtaining an education that includes knowledge about health and disease and the history of disease of others in one's family. In particular, the individual should take responsibility for eating properly, exercising adequately, maintaining appropriate weight, limiting alcohol use, and avoiding nonessential drugs. Individuals can also protect themselves from injury by adopting behaviors that reduce their risk of injuries. These behaviors include driving safely and wearing a safety belt at all times while traveling in a vehicle. Examples of primary prevention also include avoiding overexposure to the sun and limiting one's environmental pollutants that might cause cancer.

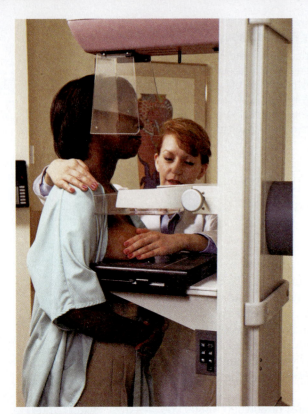

FIGURE 4.13 Mammography, used for screening and early detection of breast cancer, is an example of secondary prevention.

© Photodisc

Secondary Prevention of Noncommunicable Diseases

Secondary preventive measures undertaken by the community can include the provision of mass screenings for chronic diseases (see **Figure 4.13**), case-finding measures, and the provision of adequate health personnel, equipment, and facilities for the community. Secondary prevention responsibilities of individual citizens include personal screenings, such as self-examination of skin for abnormal moles and testicles for lumps that could be cancerous, the hemoccult test (for colorectal cancer), and medical screenings, such as the HPV test (for cervical cancer), the PSA test (for prostate cancer), mammography (for breast cancer), and screenings for diabetes, glaucoma, or hypertension. Participating in such health screenings and having regular medical and dental checkups represent only the first step in the secondary prevention of noncommunicable diseases. This must be followed by the pursuit of definitive diagnosis and prompt treatment if any diseases are detected.

Tertiary Prevention of Noncommunicable Diseases

Tertiary preventive measures for a community include adequate emergency medical personnel, services, and facilities to meet the needs of those citizens for whom primary and secondary preventive measures were unsuccessful. Examples include ambulance services, hospitals, physicians and surgeons, nurses, and other allied health professionals. Health care in the United States focuses mostly on tertiary prevention, and many experts feel that America should reallocate resources from tertiary prevention to primary and secondary preventive measures.

Tertiary prevention for the individual often requires significant behavioral or lifestyle changes. Examples include strict adherence to prescribed medications, exercise programs, and diet. For example, a heart attack patient could receive nutrition education and counseling and be encouraged to participate in a supervised exercise program, thus maximizing the use of remaining capabilities. This could lead to a resumption of employment and the prevention of a second heart attack. For certain types of noncommunicable health problems, such as those involving substance use disorders, regular attendance at support group meetings or counseling sessions may constitute an important part of a tertiary prevention program. Naloxone is a medication that can be used to reverse an opioid overdose. The CDC encourages individuals who struggle with opioid use disorders and their close contacts to carry naloxone. It is available without a prescription in most states.[30]

Application of Preventive Measures in the Control of a Noncommunicable Disease: Cancer

One set of *Healthy People 2030* objectives aims at reducing risk factors and deaths from cancer (see **Box 4.7**). There are many types of cancer, and several risk factors. Behavioral changes and early detection are important for lowering the risk of morbidity and mortality from cancer. Both the community and the individual can contribute to the prevention of cancer. The Healthy People Objectives that start with "C" pertain to cancer targets.

The Community's Role

The community must recognize the importance of preventing chronic disease. Intervention following a diagnosis, such as a suspicious lung X-ray, is the least effective and most expensive way to provide help to individuals. Individual behavioral changes hold the best prospects for reducing the prevalence of cancer in this country, and communities can provide a supporting environment for these behavioral changes. For example, the community can support restricting smoking areas and can provide a clear message to youth that smoking is damaging to health.

BOX 4.7   *Healthy People 2030*: Objectives to Reduce Cancer Death Rates

Target setting method: Projection

Data source: National Vital Statistics System-Mortality (NVSS-M), CDC/NCHS, Population Estimates Census

Objective	Baseline 2018	Interim Data 2021	2030 Target
Objective C-01: Reduce the overall cancer death rate			
Cancer deaths per 100,000 population			
Status: improving	149.1	146.6	122.7
Objective C-02: Reduce the lung cancer death rate			
Lung cancer deaths per 100,000 population			
Status: improving	34.8	31.7	25.1

Female specific

Objective	Baseline 2018	Interim Data 2021	2030 Target
Objective C-04: Reduce the female breast cancer rate			
Breast cancer deaths per 100,000 females			
Status: improving	19.7	19.4*	15.3

*Breast cancer death in 2020 was 19.1 per 100,000 females

Objective	Baseline 2018	Interim Data 2021	2030 Target
Objective C-05: Increase the proportion of females who get screened for breast cancer; measured as the percent of women 50 to 74 who received a breast cancer screening. Baseline in 2019.			
Status: Little or no detectable change	76.2%	75.6%	80.3%

Male specific

Objective	Baseline 2018	Interim Data 2021	2030 Target
Objective C-08: Reduce the prostate cancer death rate			
Prostate cancer deaths per 100,000 males			
Status: Little or no detectable change	18.8	19.0	16.9

For Further Thought

Cancer is the second leading cause of death in the United States. Risk factors for cancer include smoking, obesity, and family history (genetics). Interestingly, these are also risk factors for heart disease and stroke. Early detection of cancer increases the likelihood of a cure. Data from Healthy People 2030 shows improvement in some of its cancer objectives but little or no detectable change in others. What can individuals and communities do to reduce the incidence of cancer? October is appointed as Breast Cancer Awareness month. How does that help?

Data from U.S. Department of Health and Human Services, Office of Disease Prevention and Health Promotion. (2023). *Healthy People 2030*. https://health.gov/healthypeople

Communities also can provide adequate opportunity for health screening such as mammograms for women and prostate-specific antigen (PSA) screening for men. Schools can permit the administration of Youth Risk Behavior Surveillance System surveys and use these occasions as opportunities to teach students about the importance of healthy behavioral choices. Communities also can promote and assist in the development of areas for recreation and exercise, such as safe paths for jogging or cycling and lighted sidewalks for walking. Exercise reduces obesity, thereby lowering risk for cancer, diabetes, and heart disease. Finally, access to nutritious foods is critical, including providing healthy menus in schools and ensuring that communities have access to grocery stores with nutritious and affordable food selections.

Unmodifiable risk factors contributing to the development of a noncommunicable disease that cannot be altered by modifying one's behavior or environment

Modifiable risk factors contributing to a noncommunicable disease that can be altered by modifying one's behavior or environment

The Individual's Role

In addition to community-level factors, each individual has responsibility for their health. For example, women can perform self-examination of their breasts, and men can perform self-examination of their testes. There are age recommendations for routine screening for cervical, breast, prostate, and skin cancer. Colon cancer screening can be initiated at home or via a colonoscopy. Oral cancer screenings are part of routine dental care.

Each person is endowed with a unique genetic code. An individual's innate resistance or susceptibility to cancer is encoded in the genes. For example, mutations in the BRCA1 or BRCA2 gene can make an individual more susceptible to breast and ovarian cancer. **Unmodifiable risk factors** for cancer include one's race, gender, and age.

Modifiable risk factors for cancer include environmental and behavioral factors over which an individual has some control. Modifiable risk factors that would increase the likelihood of cancer include smoking, poor nutrition, lack of exercise, obesity, unprotected exposure to ultraviolet or sun light, and alcohol use.

Chapter Summary

- Diseases can be classified as communicable (infectious) or noncommunicable (noninfectious), and acute or chronic.

- Acute diseases last for less than 3 months, whereas chronic diseases continue for longer than 3 months.

- Communicable diseases are caused by biological agents and are transmissible from a source of infection to a susceptible host.

- The process of communicable disease transmission is best understood by the chain of infection model, in which the interruption of disease transmission can be visualized as the breaking of one or more links in the chain.

- Noncommunicable diseases are often the result of multiple risk factors that can be genetic, behavioral, and environmental in origin.

- Several of the noncommunicable diseases rank among the leading causes of death in the United States.

- There are three levels of disease prevention—primary, secondary, and tertiary.

- Primary prevention includes measures that forestall the onset of disease or injury, whereas secondary prevention encompasses efforts aimed at early detection and intervention to limit disease and disability. Tertiary prevention includes measures aimed at re-education and rehabilitation after significant pathogenesis has occurred.

- Both the spread of communicable diseases and the prevalence of noncommunicable diseases can best be reduced by the appropriate application of primary, secondary, and tertiary preventive measures by the community and the individual.

- The prevention and control of noncommunicable diseases require both individual and community efforts.

Scenario: Analysis and Response

1. Search the American Cancer Society website for information about breast cancer (www.cancer.org). What are the screening recommendations for women with an average breast cancer risk?

2. Susan was positive for the BRCA1 mutation. What types of cancer does she have an increased risk for?

3. Are Shawna and Emily considered high risk for breast cancer? Why or why not? For women at high risk, what are the screening recommendations? Are these considered primary, secondary, or tertiary preventive measures?

4. Susan encouraged Bob to make an appointment for a complete physical and to get a PSA test. What type of cancer does the PSA screen for? What are the two leading causes of cancer death in men?

Review Questions

1. What are some of the ways in which diseases and health problems are classified in community health?

2. Contrast the terms *acute disease* and *chronic disease*. Provide three examples of each type of disease.

3. Contrast the terms *communicable disease* and *noncommunicable disease*. Provide three examples of each type of disease.

4. What is the difference between a communicable agent and a pathogenic agent?

5. What are the components of a simplified communicable disease model?

6. List some examples of environmental factors that can influence the occurrence and spread of disease.

7. Draw and explain the model for multicausation diseases.

8. What is the difference between prevention and intervention?

9. Explain the difference between primary, secondary, and tertiary prevention and provide an example of each.

10. What is the chain of infection model of disease transmission? Draw the model and label its parts.

11. Again referring to the chain of infection, indicate how prevention and control strategies can be implemented to interrupt the transmission of COVID-19. Classify these strategies as primary, secondary, or tertiary prevention measures.

12. Define the following terms—*case, carrier, vector, vehicle*.

13. List three examples each of vectorborne diseases and nonvectorborne diseases.

14. Explain the difference between the public health practices of isolation and quarantine.

15. Explain the importance of vaccinations or immunizations in preventing diseases in the community.

16. Apply the principles of prevention and the examples given in this chapter to outline a prevention strategy for diabetes mellitus that includes primary, secondary, and tertiary prevention components.

Activities

1. The COVID-19 pandemic was first recognized in the United States in the spring of 2020. Many people worked from home, but essential workers did not have that luxury. What primary and secondary preventive measures were taken at the time to prevent the spread of COVID-19 infections? The CDC recommended specific time intervals for isolation and quarantine. How are these activities different? What is the purpose of quarantine?

2. List some of the infections you have had. How were these infections transmitted to you—directly, by vehicle, or by vector? Talk to an older adult about chicken pox, measles, and polio. Ask if these diseases affected them and their families. Take notes on the response and hand them in or share them orally in class.

3. Look up the disease tuberculosis (TB) on the Internet. After reading about the disease, see if you can complete a chain of infection model for TB. Identify the causative agent, the vector (if there is one), the reservoir, and the mode of transmission. Why is it called consumption? What types of prevention and control strategies are used to stop the spread of this disease? What populations are most at risk?

4. Unintentional injury was the third leading cause of death in 2022. Unintentional poisoning (drug overdose) exceeds all other types of injuries. List some primary, secondary, and tertiary preventive measures that the community can take to reduce the number of lethal drug overdoses. What preventive measures have you observed in your community?

5. Americans living in rural areas have a lower level of health and access to health care than their urban counterparts. Check the CDC.gov website and one other website for a description of rural and urban health. What factors contribute to this health disparity?

6. The success of Ending the HIV Epidemic is displayed on the AHEAD dashboard, found at https://ahead.hiv.gov. What is the purpose of the dashboard? The six indicators used to monitor progress are incidence, knowledge of status, diagnoses, linkage to HIV medical care, viral suppression, and PrEP coverage. Which indicator(s) do you feel are the most significant in ending the HIV epidemic? Explain your choice. Evaluate the current success toward those goals nationwide by selecting "National" as the base population. Drill down to the region that is closest to you. Select the "Stratified Data" option. Compare the incidence of HIV in your region to the five indicators. Explain why data from 2020 should be interpreted with caution. This activity should take about 20 minutes to complete.

References

1. Heymann, D. L. (Ed.). (2014). *Control of communicable diseases manual* (20th ed.). American Public Health Association.
2. World Health Organization. (2022). *World Malaria Report 2022.* Available from https://www.who.int/teams/global-malaria-programme/reports/world-malaria-report-2022
3. Merrill, R. M. (2012). *Introduction to Epidemiology* (6th ed.). Jones & Bartlett Learning; 13–14.
4. Centers for Disease Control and Prevention. (2022). *Provisional Mortality Data — United States, 2022. Morbidity and Mortality Weekly Report, 2023, 72,* 488–492. Available from http://dx.doi.org/10.15585/mmwr.mm7218a3
5. Woodruff, R. C., Tong, X., Khan, S. S., Shah, N. S., Jackson, S. L., Loustalot, F., & Vaughan, A. S. (2023). Trends in Cardiovascular Disease Mortality Rates and Excess Deaths, 2010–2022. *American Journal of Preventive Medicine,* S0749-3797(23)00465-8. doi: 10.1016/j.amepre.2023.11.009. Epub ahead of print. PMID: 37972797
6. American Heart Association Council on Epidemiology and Prevention Statistics Committee and Stroke Statistics Subcommittee. (2022). AHA Statistical Update. Heart Disease and Stroke Statistics—2022 Update: A Report from the American Heart Association. *Circulation, 145,* e153–e639.
7. Centers for Disease Control and Prevention. (1999). Ten great public health achievements—United States, 1900–1999. *Morbidity and Mortality Weekly Report, 48,* 241–242. Available from https://www.cdc.gov/mmwr/PDF/wk/mm4812.pdf
8. Centers for Disease Control and Prevention. (2011). Ten great public health achievements—United States, 2001–2010. *Morbidity and Mortality Weekly Report, 60,* 619–623. http://www.cdc.gov/mmwr/preview/mmwrhtml/mm6019a5.htm
9. American Cancer Society. *Cancer Facts & Figures 2023.* Atlanta: American Cancer Society. (2023). Available from https://www.cancer.org/content/dam/cancer-org/research/cancer-facts-and-statistics/annual-cancer-facts-and-figures/2023/2023-cancer-facts-and-figures.pdf
10. Centers for Disease Control and Prevention, National Center for Health Statistics. (2019). Number of deaths, percentage of total deaths, and age-adjusted death rates for the 10 leading causes of death in 2018: United States, 2016 and 2017. National Vital Statistics System Mortality Tables. Available from https://www.cdc.gov/nchs/data/databriefs/db328_tables-508.pdf#4
11. Xu, J., Murphy, S. L., Kochanek, K. D., & Arias E. (2022). Mortality in the United States, 2021. *NCHS Data Brief,* No. 456.
12. Centers for Disease Control and Prevention. *WISQARS Leading Causes of Death. Years of Potential Life Lost before age 65 for 10 ALL 2021, United States.* Available from https://wisqars.cdc.gov/.
13. White House. *National drug control budget FY 2023 Funding Highlights.* Available from https://www.whitehouse.gov/wp-content/uploads/2022/03/FY-2023-Budget-Highlights.pdf
14. Centers for Disease Control and Prevention. (2020). *Coronavirus Disease 2019.* Available from https://www.cdc.gov/coronavirus/2019-nCoV/index.html
15. AJMC Staff. *A Timeline of COVID-19 Developments in 2020.* Available from https://www.ajmc.com/view/a-timeline-of-covid19-developments-in-2020
16. AJMC Staff. *A Timeline of COVID-19 Vaccine Developments in 2021.* Available from https://www.ajmc.com/view/a-timeline-of-covid-19-vaccine-developments-in-2021
17. AJMC Staff. (2021). *A Timeline of COVID-19 Vaccine Developments for the Second Half of 2021.* Available from https://www.ajmc.com/view/a-timeline-of-covid-19-vaccine-developments-for-the-second-half-of-2021
18. Centers for Disease Control and Prevention. (2022). *CDC Museum COVID-19 Timeline.* Available from https://www.cdc.gov/museum/timeline/covid19.html
19. Centers for Disease Control and Prevention. (2023). *COVID-19 Mortality Overview. Provisional Death Counts for COVID-19.* Available from https://www.cdc.gov/nchs/covid19/mortality-overview.htm
20. Shiels, M. S., Haque, A. T., Berrington de Gonzalez, A., & Freedman, N. D. (2022). Leading causes of death in the US during the COVID-19 pandemic, March 2020 to October 2021. *JAMA Internal Medicine, 182,* 883–885.
21. Centers for Disease Control and Prevention. (2023). Use of updated COVID-19 vaccines 2023–2024 formula for persons aged ≥6 months: Recommendations of the Advisory Committee on Immunization Practices — United States, September 2023. *Morbidity and Mortality Weekly Report, 72,* 1140–1146. Available from http://dx.doi.org/10.15585/mmwr.mm7242e1
22. Centers for Disease Control and Prevention. (2019). *Vaccines and immunizations.* Available from http://www.cdc.gov/vaccines/.
23. Centers for Disease Control and Prevention. (2023). *HIV basic statistics.* Available from https://www.cdc.gov/hiv/basics/statistics.html Accessed 11/5/2023.
24. World Health Organization. (2023) *HIV statistics, globally and by WHO region,* 2023. Epidemiological fact sheet. Available from https://cdn.who.int/media/docs/default-source/hq-hiv-hepatitis-and-stis-library/j0294-who-hiv-epi-factsheet-v7.pdf. Accessed 10/31/2023.
25. Centers for Disease Control and Prevention. (2023). *HIV Basics. PrEP.* Available from https://www.cdc.gov/hiv/basics/prep.html Accessed 11/5/2023.
26. Centers for Disease Control and Prevention. (2023). *Syringe Services Program Fact Sheet.* Accessed 11/5/2023. Available from https://www.cdc.gov/ssp/
27. Occupational Safety and Health Administration. (2023). *Bloodborne Pathogens and Needlestick Prevention. Hazard Recognition.* Available from https://www.osha.gov/bloodborne-pathogens/hazards
28. U.S. Congress. (2000). An Act to Require Changes in the Bloodborne Pathogens Standard in Effect under the Occupational Safety and Health Act of 1970. *Congressional Record,* 146.
29. U.S. Department of Labor. (2001). *Revision to OSHA's bloodborne pathogens standard: Technical background and summary.* Available from https://www.osha.gov/needlesticks/needlefact.html
30. Centers for Disease Control and Prevention. (2023). *Stop Overdose. Lifesaving Naloxone.* Available from https://www.cdc.gov/stop-overdose/caring/naloxone.html

CHAPTER 5

Community Organizing/ Building and Health Promotion Programming

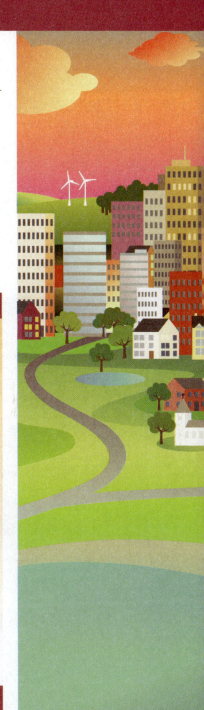

Chapter Objectives

After studying this chapter, you will be able to:

1. Explain the terms *evidence, evidence-based practice*, and *socioecological perspective*.

2. Define community organizing, community capacity, community participation, and empowered community.

3. Identify the assumptions that underlie the process of community organization.

4. Briefly explain the differences among planning and policy practice, community capacity development, and social advocacy strategies to community organization.

5. Illustrate the difference between needs-based and strengths-based community organizing models.

6. List the steps for a generalized model for community organizing/ building.

Chapter Objectives   *(continued)*

7. Explain what community building means.
8. Describe the difference between health education and health promotion.
9. Summarize the steps involved in creating a health promotion program.
10. Define the term *needs assessment*.
11. Briefly explain the six steps used in assessing needs.
12. Discuss the difference between goals and objectives.
13. List the different types of intervention strategies.
14. Demonstrate the differences among best practices, best experiences, and best processes.
15. Explain the purposes of pilot testing in program development.
16. State the difference between formative and summative evaluation.

Scenario

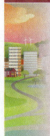

It was becoming obvious to many that the suburb of Kenzington now had a drug problem, but few wanted to admit it. The community's residents liked their quiet neighborhoods, and most never thought that drugs would be a problem. In fact, the problem really sneaked up on everyone. The town had only one bar, and although occasionally someone drank too much, the bar's patrons usually controlled their drinking and didn't bother anyone. Occasionally, two or three high school seniors would be caught drinking beer given to them by their older friends. Yet these isolated incidents gave no indication of Kenzington's impending drug problem.

Within the past year, the climate of the town had changed considerably. Incidents of teenagers being arrested for possession of alcohol or even other drugs, such as marijuana and heroin, were being reported more regularly. There seemed to be more reports of burglaries, too. There had even been a robbery and two assaults reported within the last month. The population of young adults in the community seemed to be increasing, and many of these seemed to be driving impressive cars, using the hottest new digital devices, and wearing the latest clothes. All of these signs were obvious to a group of concerned citizens in Kenzington and suggested the possibility of a drug problem. So the citizens decided to take their concerns to the city council.

Introduction

To deal with the health issues that face many communities, community and public health professionals must possess specific knowledge and skills. They need to be able to identify problems, develop a plan to attack each problem, gather the resources necessary to carry out that plan, implement that plan, and then evaluate the results to determine the degree of progress that has been achieved. Elsewhere in the text, we described epidemiologic methods as essential tools of the community and public health professionals. In this chapter, we present two other important tools that each successful community and public health worker must master—the skills to organize/build a community and to plan a health promotion program.

Inherent in the community organizing/building and health promotion programming processes is behavior change. That is, for community organizing/building and health promotion programming efforts to be successful, people must change their behavior. Some of the behaviors that need to change as part of these processes are health related and others are not. To be able to better understand the behavior change associated with community organizing/building and health promotion programming, we need to introduce two important concepts. The first is evidence-based practice and the second is the socioecological approach.

To understand evidence-based practice, one first needs to be clear on the meaning of evidence. **Evidence** is the body of data that can be used to make decisions. When community

Evidence the body of data that can be used to make decisions and public health workers systematically find, appraise, and use evidence as the basis for decision making related to community organizing/building and health promotion programming, it is referred to as **evidence-based practice**.[1] **Evidence-based interventions (evidence-based programs)** originated from evidence-based medicine, and they are now used in community and public health as practices whose effectiveness has been proven or informed by research and evaluation.[2] Evidence comes in many different forms ranging from objective evidence, derived from science (e.g., systematic reviews of science-based research), to subjective evidence that can come from personal experiences and observations. Because objective evidence comes from the scientific process, it is usually seen as a higher quality of evidence.[3] Community and public health workers should strive to use the best evidence possible, but they should also understand that scientific evidence associated with some health problems may not be available or even exist, and thus they may be faced with using the best evidence available.[4]

The underlying foundation of the **socioecological approach (ecological perspective)** is that behavior has multiple levels of influence. There are levels of influence that include family, community, and societal factors that can influence individual behavior.[5] In other words, the health behavior of individuals is shaped in part by the social context in which they live. Scholars who study and write about the levels of influence have used various labels to describe them. For many years, the commonly used labels for the levels included intrapersonal, interpersonal, institutional or organizational, community, and public policy.[6] More recently, two additional levels—physical environment and culture—have been added (see **Figure 5.1**).[7]

An application of the socioecological approach can be seen in the efforts that have been put forth to encourage adults in the United States to exercise regularly. At the intrapersonal (or individual) level, most adults know that regular exercise is good for them, but many have found it difficult to start and maintain such a program. At the interpersonal level, adults are often encouraged by people close to them, such as their physician and/or family and friends, to start an exercise program. After such encouragement, some may attempt to get active on their own, while others may join a formal exercise group at a fitness facility. At the institutional (or organizational) level, a number of employers have developed worksite health promotion programs that include incentives (e.g., extra pay, reduced healthcare premiums, fitness facility memberships) to encourage their employees to engage in regular exercise to get healthier and reduce healthcare costs. At the community level, some towns, cities, and counties have passed ordinances to include bicycle lanes on the roads in order to make

Evidence-based practice systematically finding, appraising, and using evidence as the basis for decision making

Evidence-based interventions (evidence-based programs) programs or practices that are peer reviewed and based on empirical evidence of effectiveness

Socio-ecological approach (ecological perspective) individuals' influence and are influenced by their families, social networks, the organizations in which they participate (workplaces, schools, religious organizations), the communities of which they are a part, and the society in which they live

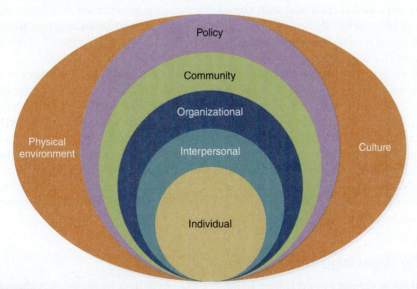

FIGURE 5.1 Socio-ecological model.

Data from CDC, Health Equity Toolkit. Retrieved from https://www.cdc.gov/nccdphp/dnpao/state-local-programs/health-equity/index.html

it easier to exercise. At the public policy level, many states and the U.S. government have spent lots of dollars on public service announcements (PSAs) and other forms of media advertising to encourage regular exercise. At the physical environment level, a number of communities have built new structures, such as walking paths to make it more convenient to exercise. And, at the cultural level, a focus has been placed on getting and reinforcing regular exercise as the cultural norm. As can be seen by these examples, a central conclusion of the socioecological approach is that it takes multilevel interventions to achieve substantial changes in health behavior.[8]

As you read the rest of this chapter, consider the impact that evidence-based practice and the socioecological approach have on both community organizing and health promotion programming.

Community Organizing/Building

Community and public health problems can range from small and simple to large and complex. Small, simple problems that are local and involve few people can often be solved with the effort of a small group of people and a minimal amount of organization. Large, complex problems that involve whole communities require significant skills and resources for their solutions. For these larger problems, a considerable effort must be expended to organize the citizens of the community to work together to implement a lasting solution to their problem. For example, a trained smoking cessation facilitator could help a single person or a small group of people to stop smoking. But to reduce the smoking rates community wide, community collaboration is needed. The same smoking cessation facilitators are needed to work with individuals, but others are also needed. Schools are needed to provide appropriate tobacco education programs to youth, organizations (e.g., worksites) and institutions (e.g., religious communities) are needed to create smoking policies, government agencies are needed to enforce the laws associated with the sale of tobacco, and cities, counties, and states are needed to create clean indoor air ordinances or laws. This more comprehensive approach to reducing smoking rates needs to bring together, in an organized and coordinated effort, the people and groups interested in the issue and the resources necessary for change. In other words, a community organization effort is needed. Community organizing for large, complex problems reached a whole new level when the novel human coronavirus disease (COVID-19) spread worldwide in 2020. Organizing community members in response to the pandemic on a global scale and with constantly evolving information was unprecedented. COVID-19 affected health, healthcare systems, behavior, and attitudes, and was impacted by constant global media coverage and public policy. COVID-19 will be covered in more depth throughout this textbook.

"The term community organization was coined by American social workers in the late 1880s to describe their efforts to coordinate services for newly arrived immigrants and the poor."[9] More recently, community organization has been used by a variety of professionals, including community and public health workers, and refers to various methods of interventions to deal with social problems. More formally, **community organizing** has been defined as "the process by which community groups are helped to identify common problems or change targets, mobilize resources, and develop and implement strategies for reaching their collective goals."[9] Community organizing is not a science but an art of consensus building within a democratic process.[10] (See **Table 5.1** for terms associated with community organizing/building.)

Need for Organizing Communities

In recent years, the need to organize communities seems to have increased. Advances in electronics (e.g., handheld digital devices) and communications (e.g., multifunction cell phones and the Internet), household upgrades (e.g., energy efficiency), and increased mobility (i.e., frequency

Community organizing a process by which community groups are helped to identify common problems or change targets, mobilize resources, and develop and implement strategies for reaching their collective goals

TABLE 5.1 Terms Associated with Community Organizing/Building

Community capacity	"Community characteristics affecting its ability to identify, mobilize, and address problems"[9]
Empowerment	"Social action process for people to gain mastery over their lives and the lives of their communities"[9]
Grassroots participation	"Bottom-up efforts of people taking collective actions on their own behalf, and they involve the use of a sophisticated blend of confrontation and cooperation in order to achieve their ends"[11]
Macro practice	The methods of professional change that deal with issues beyond the individual, family, and small group level
Participation and relevance	"Community organizing should 'start where the people are' and engage community members as equals"[9]
Social capital	"Social capital refers to the social norms and networks that build trust and enable individuals to pursue shared objectives; it can vary considerably between communities and across time."[12]
Systems change	"A change in organizational or legislative policies or in environmental supports that encourages and channels improvement(s) in systems, community, and individual-level health outcomes"[13]

of moving and ease of worldwide travel) have resulted in a loss of a sense of community. Individuals are much more independent than ever before. The days when people knew everyone on their block are past. Today, it is not uncommon for people to never meet their neighbors (see **Figure 5.2**). In other cases, people see or talk to their neighbors only a few times each year. Because of these changes in community social structure, it now takes specific skills to organize a community to act together for the collective good. Note that the usefulness of community organizing skills extends beyond community health.

Community Organizing Methods

Although there is no single, preferred method for organizing a community, a careful review reveals that several different approaches have been successful.[14]

The early approaches to community organization used by social workers emphasized the use of consensus and cooperation to deal with community problems.[15] However, Rothman created an original typology of three primary methods of community organization: locality development, social planning, and social action.[16] More recently, the strategies have been renamed *planning and policy practice, community capacity development,* and *social advocacy.*[14] At the heart of the *planning and policy practice* strategy are data. By using data, community and public health workers generate persuasive rationales that lead toward proposing and enacting particular solutions.[17]

The *community capacity development* strategy is based on empowering those impacted by a problem with knowledge and skills to understand the problem and then work cooperatively together to deal with the problem. Group consensus and social solidarity are important components of this strategy.[17] The third strategy, *social advocacy*, is used to address a problem through the application of pressure, including confrontation, on those who have created the problem or stand as a barrier to a solution to the problem. This strategy creates conflict.[17]

Although each of these strategies has unique components, each strategy can be combined with the others to deal with a community problem. In fact, Rothman has offered a 3 × 3 matrix to help explain

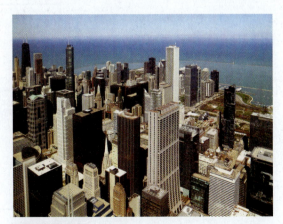

FIGURE 5.2 In today's complex communities, it is not uncommon for people never to meet their neighbors.

© Hal_P/Shutterstock

the combinations.[17] Whatever strategy is used, they all revolve around a common theme: The work and resources of many have a much better chance of solving a problem than the work and resources of a few.

Minkler and Wallerstein have done a nice job of summarizing the models, old and new, by presenting a typology that incorporates both needs- and strengths-based approaches (see **Figure 5.3**).[9] Their typology is divided into four quadrants, with strengths-based and needs-based on the vertical axis and consensus and conflict on the horizontal axis. Although this typology separates and categorizes the various methods of community organizing and building, Minkler and Wallerstein point out that when they

> . . . look at primary strategies, we see that the consensus approaches, whether needs based or strengths based, primarily use collaboration strategies, whereas conflict approaches use advocacy strategies and ally building to support advocacy efforts. Several concepts span these two strength-based approaches, such as community competence, leadership development, and multiple perspectives on gaining power. Again, as with the Rothman model, many organizing efforts use a combination of these strategies at different times throughout the life of an organizing campaign and community building process.[9]

No matter what community organizing/building approach is used, they all incorporate some fundamental principles. These include "strengths-based approaches; the principle of relevance, or starting where the people are; the principle of participatory issue selection

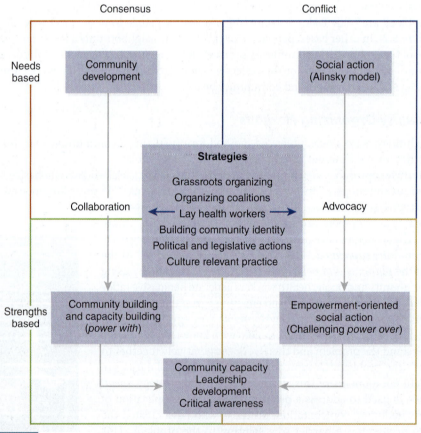

FIGURE 5.3   Community organization and community building typology.

Reproduced from Minkler, M., and N. Wallerstein. (2012). "Improving Health through Community Organization and Community Building: Perspectives from Health Education and Social Work." In M. Minkler, ed., *Community Organizing and Community Building for Health and Welfare*, 3rd ed. New Brunswick, NJ: Rutgers University Press, 44. Reprinted with permission.

and choice of actions; and the importance of creating environments in which individuals and communities can become empowered as they increase their community capacity or problem-solving ability."[9]

The Process of Community Organizing/Building

It is beyond the scope of this textbook to explain all of the approaches to community organizing/building in detail. Instead, we will present a generic approach created by McKenzie, Neiger, and Thackeray that draws upon many of the other approaches.[3] The 10 steps of this generic approach are briefly reviewed in the sections that follow.

Recognizing the Issue

The process of community organizing/building begins when someone recognizes that a problem exists in a community and decides to do something about it. This person (or persons) is referred to as the initial organizer. This individual may not be the primary organizer throughout the community organizing/building process; however, they are the ones who get things started. For the purposes of this discussion, let us assume the problem is violence. People in most communities would like to have a violence-free community, but it would be most unusual to live in a community that was without at least some level of violence. How much violence is too much? What is the tipping point? At what point is a community willing to organize to deal with the problem? In a small-town community, an acceptable level of violence would be very low, while in a large city, an acceptable level would be much higher.

The people, or organizers, who first recognize a problem in the community and decide to act, can be members of the community, or they can be individuals from outside the community. If those who initiate community organization are members of the community, the movement is referred to as being **grassroots**, citizen initiated, or organized from the bottom up. Typically, grassroots organizations are built where no community group or leadership exists.[18] Community members who might recognize that violence is a problem could include teachers, police officers, or other concerned citizens. When individuals from outside the community initiate community organization, it is referred to as *top-down organization*. Individuals from outside the community who might initiate organization could include a judge who presides over cases involving violence, a state social worker who handles cases of family violence, or a politically active group that is against violent behavior wherever it happens. In cases where the person who recognizes the community problem is not a community member, great care must be taken when notifying those in the community that a problem exists.

Gaining Entry into the Community

This second step in the community-organizing process may or may not be needed, depending on whether the issue in Step 1 was identified by someone from within the community or outside. If the issue is identified by someone outside the community, this step becomes a critical step in the process.[3] Gaining entry may seem like a relatively easy matter, but an error by organizers at this step could ruin the chances of successfully organizing the community. This may be the most crucial step in the whole process.

Braithwaite and colleagues have stressed the importance of tactfully negotiating entry into a community with the individuals who control, both formally and informally, the "political climate" of the community.[19] These people are referred to as the **gatekeepers**. Thus, the term indicates that you must pass through this "gate" to get to your priority population.[20] These "power brokers" know their community, how it functions, and how to accomplish tasks within it. Long-time residents are usually able to identify the

Grassroots a process that begins with those who are affected by the problem/concern

Gatekeepers those who control, both formally and informally, the political climate of the community

gatekeepers of their community. A gatekeeper can be a representative of an intermediary organization—such as a church or school—that has direct contact with your priority population.[20] Examples include politicians, leaders of activist groups, business and education leaders, and clergy, to name a few.

Organizers must approach such figures on the gatekeepers' own terms and play the gatekeepers' ball game. However, before approaching these important individuals, organizers must study the community well. They must be culturally sensitive and work toward cultural competence. That is, they must be aware of the cultural differences within a community and effectively work with the cultural context of the community. Tervalon and Garcia have stated the need for cultural humility—openness to others' culture.[21] Organizers need to know where the power lies, the community power dynamics, what type of politics must be used to solve a problem, and whether the particular problem they wish to solve has ever been dealt with before in the community.[11] In the violence example, organizers need to know (1) who is causing the violence and why, (2) how the problem has been addressed in the past, (3) who supports and who opposes the idea of addressing the problem, and (4) who could provide more insight into the problem. This is a critical step in the community organization process because failure to study the community carefully in the beginning may lead to a delay in organizing it later, a subsequent waste of time and resources, and possibly the inability to organize at all.

Once the organizers have a good understanding of the community, they are then ready to approach the gatekeepers. In keeping with the violence example, the gatekeepers would probably include the police department, elected officials, school board members, social service personnel, members of the judicial system, and possibly some of those who are creating the violence.

When the top-down approach is being used, organizers might find it advantageous to enter the community through a well-respected organization or institution that is already established in the community, such as a religious organization, a service group, or another successful local group. If those who make up such an organization/institution can be convinced that the problem exists and needs to be solved, it can help smooth the way for gaining entry and achieving the remaining steps in the process.

Organizing the People

Obtaining the support of community members to deal with the problem is the next step in the process. It is best to begin by organizing those who are already interested in seeing that the problem is solved. This core group of community members, sometimes referred to as "executive participants,"[22] will become the backbone of the workforce and will end up doing the majority of the work. For our example of community violence, the core group could include law enforcement personnel, former victims of violence and their families (or victims' support groups), parent–teacher organizations, and public health officials. It is also important to recruit people from the subpopulation that is most directly affected by the problem. For example, if most of the violence in a community is directed toward teenagers, teenagers need to be included in the core group. If older persons are affected, they need to be included.

Among the core group, it is important to identify a leader, preferably a person from the community with knowledge of the health issue, familiar with the dynamics of the community, and who possesses leadership skills.[3] The skillset for a leader ideally includes a vision for change, the ability to analyze the pertinent issues and develop strategies for change, and interpersonal skills working with individuals and organizations.[3]

Although the formation of the core group is essential, this group is usually not large enough to do all the work itself. Therefore, one of the core group's tasks is to recruit more members of the community to the cause. This step can take place via a networking process, which is when organizers make personal contacts with others who might be interested. Or, the organizers can call an organizing meeting at a local school, community center, or religious organization. By broadening the constituency, the core group can spread out the workload and generate additional resources to deal with the problem. However, recruiting additional workers can often be difficult. Over the last 30 years, the number of people in many communities interested in volunteering their time has decreased. Today, if you ask someone to volunteer, you may hear the reply, "I'm already too busy." There are two primary reasons for this response. First, there are many families in which both husband and wife work outside the home. Second, there are more single-parent households.

Therefore, when organizers are expanding their constituencies, they should be sure to (1) identify people who are affected by the problem that they are trying to solve, (2) provide "perks" for or otherwise reward volunteers, (3) keep volunteer time short, (4) match volunteer assignments with the abilities and expertise of the volunteers, and (5) consider providing appropriate training to make sure volunteers are comfortable with their tasks. For example, if the organizers need someone to talk with law enforcement groups, it would probably be a good idea to solicit the help of someone who feels comfortable around such groups and who is respected by them, such as another law enforcement person.

When the core group has been expanded to include these other volunteers, the larger group is sometimes referred to as a task force. A **task force** has been defined as "a self-contained group of 'doers' that is not ongoing. It is convened for a narrow purpose over a defined time frame at the request of another body or committee."[23] There may even be an occasion where a coalition is formed. A **coalition** is "a formal alliance of organizations that come together to work for a common goal,"[18] often, to compensate for deficits in power, resources, and expertise. A larger group with more resources, people, and energy has a greater chance of solving a community problem than a smaller, less powerful group (see **Figure 5.4**). "Building and maintaining effective coalitions have increasingly been recognized as vital components of much effective community organizing and community building."[24]

Assessing the Community

Earlier in this chapter, we noted that there are a number of strategies that have been used for community organizing. Many of those strategies operate from the point of view that there is a deficiency (or a need) in the community and, if that deficiency can be dealt with, the community problem can be solved. In contrast to these strategies is community building. **Community building** is focused on establishing and fostering community capacity, not developing solutions to community issues.[22] Thus, one of the major differences between community organizing and the newer ideas of community building is the type of assessment that is used to determine where to focus the community's efforts. In the community organizing approach, the assessment is focused on the needs of the community, while in community building, the assessment focuses on the assets and capabilities of the community. It is assumed that a clearer picture of the community will be revealed and a stronger base will be developed for change if the assessment includes the identification of both needs and assets/capacities and involves those who live in the community. It is from these capacities and assets that communities are built.[25]

To determine the needs and assets/capacities of a community, an assessment must be completed. There are two reasons for completing an effective and comprehensive assessment: Information is needed for change, and it is also needed for empowerment.[26] This could include a traditional needs assessment and/or a newer technique called mapping community capacity. A *needs assessment* is a process by which data about the issues of concern are collected and analyzed. From the analyzed data, concerns or problems emerge and are prioritized so that strategies can be created to tackle them.

Task force a temporary group that is brought together for dealing with a specific problem

Coalition formal alliance of organizations that come together to work for a common goal

Community building an orientation to practice focused on community, rather than a strategic framework or approach, and on building capacities, not fixing problems

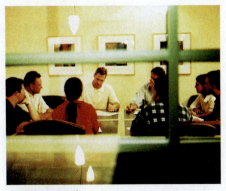

FIGURE 5.4 Coalition building is often an important step in successful community organization.

© Jack Hollingsworth/Photodisc/Getty Images

Traditional forms of data collection for needs assessments have included techniques, such as completing written questionnaires or interviewing people in the community. Because of the importance of getting participation from community members and "starting where the people are,"[27] some organizers have used participatory data collection processes. Such processes get those from whom the data are to be collected to help with data collection. Photovoice[28,29] and videovoice are two newer techniques that have been used to do this. With these techniques, community members are provided with cameras and skills training, and then they use the cameras to convey their own images of community problems and strengths.[30] After the images have been collected, participants work together to select the images that best capture their collective thoughts and feelings and use them to tell their stories and to stimulate change through community organizing and building. Another contemporary community assessment is the "windshield survey" or walking survey, which are systematic observations made from a moving vehicle or on foot. For example, a windshield or walking survey can be used to estimate the poverty level of certain neighborhoods.[31] Needs assessment is discussed at greater length in the second half of this chapter, with regard to program planning.

Mapping community capacity, on the other hand, is a process of identifying community assets, not concerns or problems. It is a process by which organizers literally use a map to identify the different assets of a community. McKnight and Kretzmann[25] have categorized assets and capacities into three different groups based on their availability to the community and refer to them as building blocks. Primary building blocks are the most accessible assets and capacities. They are located in the neighborhood and are controlled by those who live in the neighborhood. Primary building blocks can be organized into the assets and capacities of individuals (e.g., skills, talents, and incomes) and those of organizations or associations (e.g., faith-based and citizen organizations). The next most accessible building blocks are secondary building blocks. Secondary building blocks are assets located in the neighborhood but are largely controlled by people outside (e.g., social service agencies, schools, hospitals, and housing structures). The least accessible assets are referred to as potential building blocks. Potential building blocks are resources originating outside the neighborhood and controlled by people outside (e.g., welfare expenditures and public information). By knowing the needs, assets, and capacities of the community, organizers can work to identify the true concerns or problems of the community and use the assets of the community as a foundation for dealing with the concerns or problems.

Determining the Priorities and Setting Goals

An analysis of the community assessment data should result in the identification of the problems to be addressed. However, more often than not, the resources needed to solve all identified problems are not available. Therefore, the problems that have been identified must be prioritized. This prioritization is best achieved through general agreement or consensus of those who have been organized so that "ownership" can take hold. It is critical that all those working with the process feel that they "own" the problem and want to see it solved. Without this sense of ownership, they will be unwilling to give of their time and energy to solve it. For example, if a few highly vocal participants intimidate people into voting for certain activities to be the top priorities before a consensus is actually reached, it is unlikely that those who disagreed on this assignment of priorities will work enthusiastically to help solve the problem. They may even drop out of the process because they feel they have no ownership in the decision-making process.

Miller[32] has identified five criteria that community organizers need to consider when selecting a priority issue or problem. The issue or problem (1) must be winnable, ensuring that working on it does not simply reinforce fatalistic attitudes and beliefs that things cannot be improved; (2) must be simple and specific, so that any member of the organizing group can explain it clearly in a sentence or two; (3) must unite members of the organizing group and involve them in a meaningful way in achieving resolution of the issue or problem; (4) should affect many people and build up the community; and (5) should be a part of a larger plan or strategy to enhance the community.

Once the problems have been prioritized, goals—the hoped-for results—need to be identified and written to serve as guides for problem solving. The practice of consensus building should again be employed during the setting of goals. These goals, which will become the foundation for all of the work that follows, can be thought of as the "hoped-for end result." In other words, once community action has occurred, what will have changed? In the community where violence is a problem, the goal may be to reduce the number of violent crimes or eliminate them altogether. Sometimes at this point in the process, some members of the larger group drop out because they do not see their priorities or goals included on consensus lists. Unable to feel ownership, they are unwilling to expend their resources on this process. Because there is strength in numbers, efforts should be made to keep members engaged. One strategy for doing so is to keep the goal list as long as possible.

Arriving at a Solution and Selecting Intervention Strategies

There are alternative solutions for every community problem. The group should examine the alternatives in terms of probable outcomes, acceptability to the community, probable long- and short-term effects on the community, and the cost of resources to solve the problem.[33] A solution involves selecting one or more intervention strategies (see **Table 5.2**). Each type of intervention strategy has advantages and disadvantages. The group must try to agree on the best strategy and then select the most advantageous intervention activity or activities. Again, the group must work toward consensus through compromise. If the educators in the group were asked to provide a recommended strategy, they might suggest offering more preventive-education programs; law enforcement personnel might recommend more enforceable laws; judges might want more space in the jails and prisons. The protectionism of the subgroups within the larger

TABLE 5.2 Intervention Strategies and Example Activities
1. *Health communication strategies*: Mass media, social media, billboards, booklets, bulletin boards, flyers, direct mail, newsletters, pamphlets, posters, and video and audio materials
2. *Health education strategies*: Educational methods (such as lecture, discussion, and group work) as well as audiovisual materials, computerized instruction, laboratory exercises, and written materials (books and periodicals)
3. *Health policy/enforcement strategies*: Executive orders, laws, ordinances, judicial decisions, policies, position statements, regulations, and formal and informal rules
4. *Environmental change strategies*: Activities designed to change the structure of services, systems of care, or the built environment to improve health promotion services, such as removing physical or financial barriers to access, safety belts and air bags in cars, speed bumps in parking lots, or environmental cues such as *No Smoking* signs
5. *Health-related community services*: The use of health risk appraisals (HRAs), clinical screenings for health problems (e.g., hypertension), and immunization clinics
6. Other strategies: • *Behavior modification activities*: Modifying behavior to stop smoking, start to exercise, manage stress, and regulate diet   • *Community advocacy activities*: Mass mobilization, social action, community planning, community service development, community education, and community advocacy (such as a letter-writing campaign)   • *Organizational culture activities*: Activities that work to change norms and traditions within an organization   • *Incentives and disincentives*: Items that can either encourage or discourage people to behave a certain way, which may include money and other material items or fines   • *Social intervention activities*: Support groups, social activities, and social networks   • *Technology-delivered activities*: Educating or informing people by using technology (e.g., social media, computers, and cell phones)

Data from McKenzie, J. F., Neiger, B. L., & Thackeray, R. (2017). *Planning, implementing, and evaluating health promotion programs: A primer* (7th ed., pp. 194–225). Pearson Education.

group is often referred to as *turfism*. It is not uncommon to have turf struggles when trying to build consensus.

The Final Steps in the Community Organizing/Building Process: Implementing, Evaluating, Maintaining, and Looping Back

The last four steps in this generalized approach to organizing/building a community include implementing the intervention strategy and activities that were selected in the previous step, evaluating the outcomes of the plans of action, maintaining the outcomes over time, and if necessary, going back to a previous step in the process—"looping back"—to modify or restructure the work plan to organize the community.

Implementation of the intervention strategy includes identifying and collecting the necessary resources for implementation and creating the appropriate timeline for implementation. Often the resources can be found within a community, and thus, horizontal relationships, the interaction of local units with one another, are needed. Other times, the resources must be obtained from units located outside the community; in this case, vertical relationships, those where local units interact with extra community systems, are needed. An example of this latter relationship is the interaction between a local nonprofit organization and a state agency with which it has contact.

Evaluation of the process often involves comparing the long-term health and social outcomes of the process to the goals that were set in an earlier step. Some scholars have indicated that such traditional evaluations of community organizing efforts are not easy to carry out and have some limitations.[9] There are times when evaluations are not well planned or funded. As such, they may fail to capture the shorter term, system-level effects with which community organizing is heavily concerned, such as improvements in organizational collaboration, community involvement, capacity, and healthier public policies or environments.

Maintaining or sustaining the outcomes may be one of the most difficult steps in the entire process. It is at this point that organizers need to seriously consider the need for a long-term capacity for problem solving. Finally, through the steps of implementation, evaluation, and maintenance of the outcomes, organizers may see the need to loop back to a previous step in the process to rethink or rework before proceeding onward in their plan.

A Special Note About Community Organizing/Building

Before we leave the processes of community organizing/building, it should be noted that no matter what approach or strategy is used in organizing/building a community, not all problems can be solved. In other cases, repeated attempts may be necessary before a solution is reached. In addition, it is important to remember that if a problem exists in a community, there are probably some people who benefit from its existence and who may work toward preventing a successful solution to the problem. Whether or not the problem is solved, the final decision facing the organized group is whether to disband the group or to reorganize in order to take on a new problem or attack the first problem from a different direction.

Health Promotion Programming

Elsewhere in the text, we discuss how communities describe, analyze, and intervene to solve existing health problems, such as disease outbreaks or other community problems. However, the 1979 U.S. Surgeon General's report on health promotion and disease prevention, *Healthy People* (see **Figure 5.5**), charted a new course for community and public health—away from curing diseases and toward preventing diseases and promoting health. Health promotion programming has now become an important tool of community and public health professionals. The second half of this chapter presents the process of health promotion programming.

Basic Understanding of Program Planning

Prior to discussing the process of program planning, two relationships must be presented. These are the relationships between health education and health promotion, and program planning and community organizing/building.

Health education and *health promotion* are terms that are sometimes used interchangeably. This is incorrect because health education is only a part of health promotion. The Joint Committee on Health Education and Promotion Terminology defines the process of **health education** as "any combination of planned learning experiences using evidence-based practices and/or sound theories that provide the opportunity to acquire knowledge, attitudes, and skills needed to adopt and maintain health behaviors."[34] The committee defines **health promotion** as "any planned combination of educational, political, environmental, regulatory, or organizational mechanisms that support actions and conditions of living conducive to the health of individuals, groups, and communities."[34] From these definitions, it is obvious that the terms are not the same and that health promotion is a much more encompassing term than health education.

The first half of this chapter described the process of community organizing/building—the process by which individuals, groups, and organizations engage in planned action to influence social problems. Program planning may or may not be associated with community organizing/building. **Program planning** is a process in which an intervention is planned to help meet the needs of a specific group of people. It may take a community organizing/building effort to be able to plan such an intervention. The antiviolence campaign used earlier in the chapter is such an example, where many resources of the community were brought together to create interventions (programs) to deal with the violence problem. However, program planning need not be connected to community organizing/building. For example, a community organizing/building effort is not needed before a company offers a smoking cessation program for its employees or a religious organization offers a stress management class for its members. In such cases, only the steps of the program planning process need to be carried out. These steps are described in the following section.

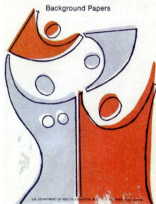

HEALTHY PEOPLE

The Surgeon General's Report On Health Promotion And Disease Prevention

Background Papers

FIGURE 5.5 *Healthy People*, the 1979 U.S. Surgeon General's report on health promotion and disease prevention, charted a new course for community health.

Courtesy of U.S. Surgeon General's Office.

Creating a Health Promotion Program

The process of developing a health promotion program, like the process of community organizing/building, involves a series of steps. Success depends on many factors, including the assistance of a professional experienced in program planning.

Experienced program planners use models to guide their work. Planning models are the means by which structure and organization are given to the planning process. Many different planning models exist, some of which are used more often than others. Some of the more frequently used models include the PRECEDE/PROCEED model,[35] Mobilizing Action through Planning and Partnerships (MAPP),[36] Intervention Mapping,[37] and the more recently developed consumer-based planning models that are based on health communication and social marketing, such as CDCynergy[38] and Social Marketing Assessment and Response Tool (SMART).[39] Each of these planning models has its strengths and weaknesses, and each has distinctive components that make it unique. In addition, each of the models has been used to plan health promotion programs in a variety of settings, with many successes.

It is not absolutely necessary that the student studying community and public health for the first time have a thorough understanding of the models mentioned here, but it is important to know the basic steps in the planning process. Therefore, we present the Generalized model[3] that draws on the major components of these other models.

Prior to undertaking the first step in the Generalized model, it is important to do some preplanning.[3] Preplanning is a quasi-step that allows program planners to gather answers to key

Health education any combination of planned learning experiences using evidence-based practices and/or sound theories that provide the opportunity to acquire knowledge, attitudes, and skills needed to adopt and maintain health behaviors

Health promotion any planned combination of educational, political, environmental, regulatory, or organizational mechanisms that support actions and conditions of living conducive to the health of individuals, groups, and communities

Program planning a process by which an intervention is planned to help meet the needs of a priority population

Priority population (audience) those whom a program is intended to serve

Needs assessment the process of identifying, analyzing, and prioritizing the needs of a priority population

questions, which will help them to understand the community and engage the **priority population (audience)**, those whom the health promotion program is intended to serve. Understanding the community means finding out as much as possible about the priority population and the environment in which it exists. Engaging the priority population means getting those in the population involved in the early stages of the health promotion program planning process. If the priority population was composed of the employees of a corporation, the planners would want to read all the material they could find about the company, spend time talking with various individuals and subgroups in the company (e.g., new employees, employees who had been with the company for a long time, management, clerical staff, and labor representatives) to find out what they wanted from a health promotion program, and review old documents of the company (e.g., health insurance records, labor agreements, written history of the company). In addition, the planners should consider forming a program planning committee with representation from the various subgroups of the workforce (e.g., management, labor, and clerical staff). The planning committee can help ensure that all segments of the priority population will be engaged in the planning process.

Assessing the Needs of the Priority Population

To create a useful and effective program for the priority population, planners, with the assistance of the planning committee, must determine the needs and wants of the priority population. This procedural step is referred to as a needs assessment. A **needs assessment** is "the process of identifying, analyzing, and prioritizing the needs of a priority population. Other terms that have been used to describe the process of determining needs include *community analysis, community diagnosis,* and *community assessment*"[35] (see **Box 5.1**). A needs assessment may be the most important part of the planning process in that it not only identifies and prioritizes health problems but it also establishes a baseline for evaluating program impact.[40] For those interested in a detailed explanation of the process of conducting a needs assessment, extensive accounts are available.[41,42] The following is a six-step approach that can be used to conduct a needs assessment.[2]

Step 1: Determining the Purpose and Scope of the Needs Assessment

The first step in the needs assessment process is to determine the purpose and the scope of the needs assessment. That is: What is the goal of the needs assessment? What does the planning committee hope to gain from the needs assessment? How extensive will the assessment be? What kind of resources will be available to conduct the needs assessment? Once these questions are answered, the planners are ready to begin gathering data.

BOX 5.1   Increased Emphasis on Needs Assessment

Although a needs assessment has long been an important part of program planning, two actions made the needs assessment process more visible to the public. The first dealt with the establishment of the Public Health Accreditation Board (PHAB) in 2007 to develop an accreditation process for health departments operated by tribes, states, local jurisdictions, and territories.[43] In 2011, the PHAB released the *Accreditation Standards and Measures.* The standards and measures, spread over 12 domains, outline what criteria a health department must meet in order to be accredited. Domain 1 is "Conduct and Disseminate Assessments Focused on Population Health Status and Public Health Issues Facing the Community."[44]

The second action was the passing of the Patient Protection and Affordable Care Act (generally referred to as the Affordable Care Act, or ACA) that added section 501(r) to the Internal Revenue Code. Under this section of the code, 501(c)(3) organizations that operate one or more hospitals (i.e., nonprofit hospitals) must meet four general requirements in order to maintain their tax-exempt status. One of those four requirements is to conduct, at least once every 3 years, a community health needs assessment (CHNA) and to adopt an implementation strategy for addressing the identified needs.[45] In addition, the Internal Revenue Service guidelines require that the 501(c)(3) organizations partner with a public health agency in conducting the CHNA.

Step 2: Gathering Data

The second step in the process is gathering the data that will help to identify the true needs of the priority population. Such data are categorized into two groups—primary and secondary. **Primary data** are those that are collected specifically for use in this process. An example is having those in the priority population complete a needs assessment questionnaire about their health behavior. The completion of the questionnaire may be in a traditional paper–pencil format, as an online survey, or via face-to-face or telephone interviews (see **Figure 5.6**). **Secondary data** are data that have already been collected for some other purpose, such as health insurance claims records or Behavioral Risk Factor Surveillance System (BRFSS) data. Using both primary and secondary data usually presents the clearest picture of the priority population's needs.

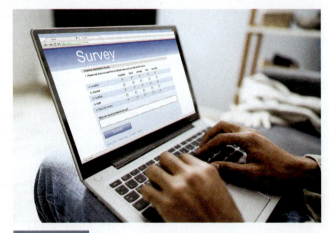

FIGURE 5.6   An online survey is a common form of data collection for a health needs assessment.

© Andrey_Popov/Shutterstock

Step 3: Analyzing the Data

Collected data can be analyzed in one of two ways—formally or informally. Formal analysis consists of some type of statistical analysis, assuming that the appropriate statistical criteria have been met to collect the data. However, a more common means of analysis is an informal technique referred to as "eyeballing the data." With this technique, program planners look for the obvious differences between the health status or conditions of the priority population and the health behaviors, and programs and services available to close the gap between what is and what ought to be. Regardless of the method used, data analysis should yield a list of the problems that exist, with a description of the nature and extent of each.

The final part of the needs assessment process is prioritizing the list of problems. Prioritization must take place because, although all needs are important, seldom are there enough resources (personnel, money, and time) available to deal with all of the problems identified. When prioritizing, planners should consider (1) the importance of the need,[35] (2) how changeable[35] the need is, and (3) whether adequate resources are available to address the problem.

Step 4: Identifying the Risk Factors Linked to the Health Problem

In this step of the process, planners need to identify and prioritize the genetic, behavioral, and environmental risk factors that are associated with the health problem. Thus, if the prioritized health problem identified in Step 3 is heart disease, planners must analyze the genetic, behavioral, and environmental conditions of the priority population for known risk factors of heart disease. For example, higher than expected obesity and smoking behavior may be present in the priority population, in addition to a community that lacks recreational facilities and areas for exercise. Once these risk factors are identified, they also need to be prioritized using the same three criteria noted in Step 3.

Step 5: Identifying the Program Focus

With risk factors identified and prioritized, planners need to identify those predisposing, enabling, and reinforcing factors that seem to have a direct impact on the targeted risk factors. In the heart disease example, those in the priority population may not (1) have the knowledge and skills to begin an exercise program (predisposing factors), (2) have access to recreational facilities (enabling factor), or (3) have people around them who value the benefits of exercise (reinforcing factor). Once the predisposing, enabling, and reinforcing factors have been identified, like in steps 2 and 3, they too need to be prioritized. The resulting prioritized list provides the program focus.

Primary data original data collected by the planners

Secondary data information that has been collected by someone else and is available for use by the planners

Step 6: Validating the Prioritized Need

The final step in this process is to double-check or to confirm that the identified need and resulting program focus indeed need to be addressed in the priority population. For example, a limited amount of data may indicate the primary need of the priority group to be one thing—knowledge about heart disease, for example. However, more extensive data or more comprehensive networking may identify another problem, such as lack of free or inexpensive recreational facilities. Before Step 6 is completed, planners must make sure they have indeed identified a true need. In short, all work should be double-checked.

At the conclusion of a needs assessment, planners should be able to answer the following questions:

1. Who is the priority population?[42]
2. What are the needs of the priority population?[42]
3. Which subgroups within the priority population have the greatest need?[42]
4. Where are the subgroups located geographically?[42]
5. What is currently being done to resolve identified needs?[42]
6. How well have the identified needs been addressed in the past?[42]
7. What is the capacity of the community to deal with the needs?
8. What are the assets in a community on which a program can be built?

Setting Appropriate Goals and Objectives

Once the problem has been well defined and the needs prioritized, the planners can set goals and develop objectives for the program. The goals and objectives should be thought of as the foundation of the program and for the evaluation. The remaining portions of the programming process—intervention development, implementation, and evaluation—will be designed to achieve the goals by meeting the objectives.

The words goals and objectives are often used interchangeably, but there is really a significant difference between the two. "A goal is a future event toward which a committed endeavor is directed; objectives are the steps taken in pursuit of a goal."[46] Goals are broad statements describing expected outcomes, while objectives are more specific statements of the intended outcomes.[3] Goals are easy to write and include two basic components—who will be affected and what will change because of the program. Here are some examples of program goals:

1. To help employees learn how to manage their stress
2. To reduce the number of teenage pregnancies in the community
3. To help cardiac patients and their families deal with the lifestyle changes that occur after a heart attack

Objectives are more precise and, as noted earlier, can be considered the steps to achieve the program goals. Because some program goals are more complex than others, the number and type of objectives will vary from program to program. For example, the process of getting a group of people to exercise is a more complex activity than trying to get people to identify their risk factors for heart disease. The more complex a program, the greater the number of objectives needed. To deal with these different types of programs, McKenzie and colleagues[3] adapted a hierarchy of program objectives first developed by Deeds[47] and later updated by Cleary and Neiger.[48] **Table 5.3** presents the hierarchy and an example of an objective at each of the levels within the hierarchy.

From the examples presented in Table 5.3, it should be obvious that the hierarchy goes from less complex to more complex levels. Thus, it takes less time and fewer resources to increase awareness in the priority population than to improve its health status. Close examination of the example objectives reveals that the objectives are written in specific terms. They

TABLE 5.3   Hierarchy of Objectives and Examples of Each

Type of Objective	Program Outcomes	Possible Evaluation Measures	Type of Evaluation	Example Objective
Process objectives	Activities presented and tasks completed	Number of sessions held, exposure, attendance, participation, staff performance, appropriate materials, adequacy of resources, tasks on schedule	Process (form of formative)	During the next 6 months, a breast cancer brochure will be distributed to all female customers over the age of 18 at the Ross grocery store.
Impact objectives				
Learning objectives	Change in awareness, knowledge, attitudes, and skills	Increase in awareness, knowledge, attitudes, and skill development/acquisition	Impact (form of summative)	When asked in class, 50% of the students will be able to list the four principles of cardiovascular conditioning.
Behavioral objectives	Change in behavior	Current behavior modified or discontinued, or new behavior adopted	Impact (form of summative)	During a telephone interview, 35% of the residents will report having had their blood cholesterol checked in the last 6 months.
Environmental objectives	Change in the environment	Measures associated with economic, service, physical, social, psychological, or political environments, e.g., protection added to, or hazards or barriers removed from, the environment	Impact (form of summative)	By the end of the year, all persons over 65 who requested transportation to the congregate meals will have received it.
Outcome objectives	Change in quality of life (QOL), health status, or risk, and social benefits	QOL measures, morbidity data, mortality data, measures of risk (e.g., HRA)	Outcome (form of summative)	By the year 2030, infant mortality rates will be reduced to no more than 7 per 1,000 in Franklin County.

Data from Deeds, S. G. (1992). *The health education specialist: Self-study for professional competence.* Loose Cannon Publications; Cleary, M. J., & Neiger, B. L. (1998). *The certified health education specialist: A self-study guide for professional competence* (3rd ed.). National Commission for Health Education Credentialing; McKenzie, J. F., Neiger, B. L., & Thackeray, R. (2017). *Planning, implementing, and evaluating health promotion programs: A primer* (7th ed.). Pearson Education.

are composed of four parts (who, what, when, and how much) and outline changes that should result from the implementation of the program.[3] Objectives that include these four parts are referred to as **SMART objectives**. SMART stands for specific, measurable, achievable, realistic, and time-phased.[38] Every objective written for a program should be SMART!

One final note about objectives: Elsewhere in the text, *Healthy People 2030*, the national health goals and objectives of the nation, are discussed. Selected objectives from this publication are presented in boxes throughout this text (see **Box 5.2**). These goals and objectives provide a good model for a new program. In fact, these goals and objectives can be adapted for use in most community and public health promotion programs.

Creating an Intervention

The next step in the program planning process is to design activities that will help the priority population meet the objectives and, in the process, achieve the program goals. These activities are collectively referred to as an **intervention**, or treatment. This intervention is the planned action designed to prevent disease or injury or promote health in the priority population.

SMART objectives those that are specific, measurable, achievable, realistic, and time-phased

Intervention an activity or activities designed to create change in people

The number of activities in an intervention may be many or only a few. Although no minimum number has been established, it has been shown that multiple activities are often more effective than a single activity. For example, if the planners wanted to change the attitudes of community members toward a new landfill, they would have a greater chance of doing so by distributing pamphlets door to door, writing articles for the local newspaper, and speaking to local service groups, than by performing any one of these activities by itself. In other words, the size and amount of intervention are important in health promotion programming. Few people change an attitude or behavior based on a single exposure; instead, multiple exposures are generally needed to create change. It stands to reason that "hitting" the priority population from several angles or through multiple channels should increase the chances of making an impact.[3]

Two terms that relate to the size and amount of an intervention are *multiplicity* and *dose*. **Multiplicity** refers to the number of components or activities that make up the intervention, whereas **dose** refers to the number of program units delivered. Thus, if an intervention has two activities—say, an educational workshop and the release of a public service announcement via social networking sites—they define multiplicity, and the number of times each of the activities is presented defines the dose.[3]

The actual creation of the intervention should begin by asking and answering a series of questions.[3] The first two are: What needs to change? and, Where is change needed? The answers to these questions come from the needs assessment and the resulting goals and objectives. The third question is: At what level of prevention (i.e., primary, secondary, or tertiary) will the program be aimed? The approach taken to a primary prevention need, that is, preventing a problem before it begins, would be different from a tertiary prevention need of managing a problem after it has existed for a while. The fourth question asks: At what level of influence will the intervention be focused? The various levels of influence (i.e., intrapersonal, interpersonal, institutional or organizational, community, public policy, physical environment, and culture) that were presented earlier in this chapter as part of the socioecological approach need to be considered. These levels provide the planners with a framework from which to think about how they will "attack" the needs of the priority population. For example, if the goal of a program is to reduce the prevalence of smoking in a community, the intervention could attack the problem by focusing the intervention on individuals through one-on-one counseling, via groups by offering smoking cessation classes, by trying to change policy by enacting a state

Multiplicity the number of components or activities that make up the intervention

Dose the number of program units delivered as part of the intervention

law prohibiting smoking in public places, or by attacking the problem using more than one of these strategies.

The fifth question asks: Has an effective intervention strategy to deal with the focus of the problem already been created? There are three sources of guidance for selecting intervention strategies—best practices, best experiences, and best processes.[35] **Best practices** refers to "recommendations for an intervention, based on a critical review of multiple research and evaluation studies that substantiate the efficacy of the intervention in the populations and circumstances in which the studies were done, if not its effectiveness in other populations and situations where it might be implemented."[35] Examples of best practices related to health promotion programs are provided in *The Guide to Community Preventive Services: What Works to Promote Health*,[49] also known as *The Community Guide* (see **Box 5.3** for other sources of evidence-based practices).

When best practice recommendations are not available for use, planners need to look for information on best experiences. **Best experience** intervention strategies are those of prior or existing programs that have not gone through the critical research and evaluation studies and thus fall short of best practice criteria but nonetheless show promise in being effective. Best experiences can often be found by networking with other professionals and by reviewing the literature.

If neither best practices nor best experiences are available to planners, the third source of guidance for selecting an intervention strategy is using best processes. **Best processes** intervention strategies are original interventions that the planners create based on their knowledge and skills of good planning processes, including the involvement of those in the priority population and the theories and models used to change behaviors, such as Social Cognitive theory[50] or the Transtheoretical Model of Change.[51]

Once it is known whether best practices, best experiences, or best processes will be used, three more questions need to be asked. The sixth question asks: Is the intervention an appropriate fit for the priority population? In other words, does the planned intervention meet the specific characteristics of the priority population, such as the educational level, developmental stages, or the specific cultural characteristics of the people being served?

The seventh question that needs to be asked is: Are the resources available to implement the intervention selected? Planners need to evaluate the amount of money, time, personnel, and/or space that is needed to carry out the various interventions and make a determination if such resources are available to implement the intervention.

The eighth and final question that needs to be asked is: Would it be better to use an intervention that consists of a single strategy or one that is made up of multiple strategies? A single strategy would probably be less expensive and time consuming, but multiple strategies would probably have a greater chance for change in the priority population.

Best practices recommendations for interventions based on critical review of multiple research and evaluation studies that substantiate the efficacy of the intervention

Best experience intervention strategies used in prior or existing programs that have not gone through the critical research and evaluation studies and thus fall short of best practice criteria

Best processes original intervention strategies that the planners create based on their knowledge and skills of good planning processes, including the involvement of those in the priority population and the use of theories and models

---

BOX 5.3   Sources of Evidence-Based Practices

Agency for Healthcare Research and Quality
www.ahrq.gov/programs/index.html?search_api_views_fulltext=&field_program_topics=14175
The Campbell Collaboration
www.campbellcollaboration.org/
Centre for Reviews and Dissemination, University of York
www.york.ac.uk/crd/
The Cochrane Collaboration
www.cochrane.org
Canadian Task Force on Preventive Health Care
www.canadiantaskforce.ca
Health Evidence, McMaster University, Canada
http://healthevidence.org

National Cancer Institute, Evidence-Based Cancer Control Programs (EBCCP)
https://ebccp.cancercontrol.cancer.gov/index.do
National Institutes of Health, Evidence-Based Practices and Programs
https://prevention.nih.gov/research-priorities/dissemination-implementation/evidence-based-practices-programs
Substance Abuse and Mental Health Services, Evidence-Based Practices Resource Center
www.samhsa.gov/ebp-resource-center

Implementing the Intervention

The moment of truth is when the intervention is implemented. **Implementation** is the actual carrying out or putting into practice the activity or activities that make up the intervention. More formally, implementation has been defined as "the act of converting planning, goals, and objectives into action through administrative structure, management activities, policies, procedures, regulations, and organizational actions of new programs."[52]

To ensure a smooth-flowing implementation of the intervention, it is wise to pilot test it at least once and sometimes more than once. A **pilot test** is a trial run. It is when the intervention is presented to just a few individuals who are either from the intended priority population or from a very similar population. For example, if the intervention is being developed for fifth graders in a particular school, it might be pilot tested on fifth graders with similar educational backgrounds and demographic characteristics but from a different school.

The purpose of pilot testing an intervention is to determine whether there are any problems with it. Some of the more common problems that pop up are those dealing with the design or delivery of the intervention; however, any part of it could be flawed. For example, it could be determined during pilot testing that there is a lack of resources to carry out the intervention as planned or that those implementing the intervention need more training. When minor flaws are detected and corrected easily, the intervention is then ready for full implementation. However, if a major problem surfaces—one that requires much time and many resources to correct—it is recommended that the intervention be pilot tested again with the improvements in place before implementation.

An integral part of the piloting process is collecting feedback from those in the pilot group. By surveying the pilot group, planners can identify popular and unpopular aspects of the intervention, how the intervention might be changed or improved, and whether the program activities were effective. This information can be useful in fine-tuning this intervention or in developing future programs.

Once the intervention has been pilot tested and corrected as necessary, it is ready to be disseminated and implemented. If the planned program is being implemented with a large priority population and there is a lot at stake with the implementation, it is advisable that the intervention be implemented gradually rather than all at once. One way of doing so is by phasing in the intervention. **Phasing in** refers to a step-by-step implementation in which the intervention is introduced first to smaller groups instead of the entire priority population. Common criteria used for selecting participating groups for phasing in include participant ability, number of participants, program offerings, and program location.[2]

The following is an example of phasing in by location. Assume that a local health department wants to provide smoking cessation programs for all the smokers in the community (priority population). Instead of initiating one big intervention for all, planners could divide the priority population by residence location. Facilitators would begin implementation by offering the smoking cessation classes on the south side of town during the first month. During the second month, they would continue the classes on the south side and begin implementation on the west side of town. They would continue to implement this intervention until all sections of the town were included.

Evaluating the Results

The final step in the generalized planning model is the evaluation. Although evaluation is the last step in this model, it really takes place in all steps of program planning. It is very important that planning for evaluation occurs during the first stages of program development, not just at the end because the purpose of the evaluation is twofold—to improve the quality of programs and to measure their effectiveness.

Evaluation is the process in which planners determine the value or worth of the object of interest by comparing it against a **standard of acceptability**.[53] Common standards of acceptability include, but are not limited to, mandates (policies, statutes, and laws), values, norms, comparison/control groups, and the "how much" in an objective for the program.

Evaluation can be categorized further into summative and formative evaluation. **Formative evaluation** is done during the planning and implementing processes to improve or refine the program. Validating the needs assessment and pilot testing are both forms of formative evaluation. **Summative evaluation** begins with the development of goals and objectives and is conducted after implementation of the intervention to determine the program's effect on the priority population. Often, the summative evaluation is broken down into two categories—impact and outcome evaluation. **Impact evaluation** focuses on immediate, observable effects of a program, such as changes in awareness, knowledge, attitudes, skills, environmental surroundings, and behavior of those in the priority population, whereas **outcome evaluation** focuses on the end result of the program and is generally measured by improvements in morbidity, mortality, or vital measures of symptoms, signs, or physiologic indicators.[53]

Like other steps in the planning model, the evaluation step can be broken down into smaller steps. The Centers for Disease Control and Prevention (CDC) has developed a framework for program evaluation (see **Figure 5.7**) that includes these six steps: (1) engage stakeholders, (2) describe the program, (3) focus on the evaluation design, (4) gather credible data, (5) justify conclusions, and (6) ensure use and share lessons learned. Prior to engaging in this six-step process, it should be determined who will conduct the evaluation—an internal evaluator (one who is already involved in the program) or an external evaluator (one from outside the program).[54]

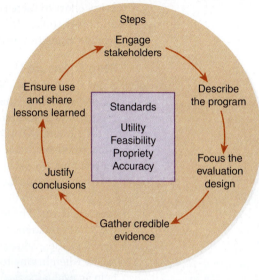

FIGURE 5.7   Framework for program evaluation.

Reproduced from Centers for Disease Control and Prevention. (1999). Framework for program evaluation in public health. *Morbidity and Mortality Weekly Report, 48*(RR-11), 1–40.

Step 1: Engage Stakeholders

Stakeholders include (1) those involved in the creation and delivery of the program, (2) those in the priority population or affected by the program in some other way, and (3) those who will be the primary users of the evaluation results.[3] These individuals must be engaged to ensure that their perspectives are understood and that the evaluation results meet their expectations. If stakeholders are not engaged, evaluation findings may be ignored, criticized, or resisted.[54]

Step 2: Describe the Program

A clear program description helps to clarify program components and the intended outcomes. Therefore, well-written goals and objectives and a well-conceived intervention are important steps in describing the program. A clear program description helps to focus the evaluation on the central and important questions to be answered.[55]

Step 3: Focus the Evaluation Design

This step of the evaluation process includes stating the purpose of the evaluation (i.e., improving the quality of the program or assessing its effects, or both) and formulating the questions to be answered by the evaluation. Once those things have been completed, a specific evaluation design (i.e., qualitative, quantitative, or both) and the type of data analysis can be determined.

Step 4: Gather Credible Data

Gathering credible data includes deciding what type of data need to be collected, determining how to collect the data (e.g., with an online survey, from existing records, by observation), determining who will collect the data, pilot testing the procedures, and performing the actual data collection. "Having credible evidence strengthens evaluation judgments and the recommendations that follow from them."[54]

Step 5: Justify Conclusions

Once the data are in hand, they must be analyzed and interpreted. This means that the evaluator will compare the collected data against the standards of acceptability to determine effectiveness, and ultimately, the value of the program.[3] In conducting this step, the evaluator must make

Formative evaluation the evaluation that is conducted during the planning and implementing processes to improve or refine the program

Summative evaluation the evaluation that determines the effect of a program on the priority population

Impact evaluation the evaluation that focuses on immediate, observable effects of a program

Outcome evaluation the evaluation that focuses on the end result of the program

every effort to increase objectivity and decrease subjectivity.[3] "When agencies, communities, and other stakeholders agree that the conclusions are justified, they will be more inclined to use the evaluation results for program improvement."[55]

Step 6: Ensure Use and Share Lessons Learned

After the data have been analyzed and interpreted, the evaluation report should be written. Decisions must be made (if they have not been made already) regarding who should write the report, who should receive the report, in what form it should be distributed, and when it should be distributed. With the findings in hand, it then must be decided how they will be used. When time, resources, and effort are spent on an evaluation, it is important that the results be useful for reaching a constructive end. This is a time when a decision can be made to modify, continue, or discontinue the intervention based on the evaluation data.[2]

In addition to the six steps just presented, the framework for program evaluation also has four standards. The four standards of utility (i.e., needs of the stakeholders are met), feasibility (i.e., the evaluation is viable and pragmatic), propriety (i.e., the evaluation is ethical), and accuracy (i.e., the evaluation findings are correct) provide practical guidelines for an evaluator to follow when having to decide among evaluation options.[3,54] For example, these standards can help an evaluator avoid evaluations that may be accurate and feasible but not useful.[54]

Over the last several decades, the National Commission for Health Education Credentialing (NCHEC) has developed a set of core responsibilities and competencies in the field of health education and promotion (see **Table 5.4**). The list of responsibilities was developed as a result of an extensive project called the Health Education Specialist Practice Analysis (HESPA),

TABLE 5.4　National Commission for Health Education Credentialing			
Areas of Responsibility for Health Education Specialists			
Area	**2010**	**2015**	**2020**
Area 1	Assess needs, assets, and capacity for health education	Assess needs, resources, and capacity for health education/promotion	Assessment of needs and capacity
Area 2	Plan health education	Plan health education/promotion	Planning
Area 3	Implement health education	Implement health education/promotion	Implementation
Area 4	Conduct evaluation and research related to health education	Conduct evaluation and research related to health education/promotion	Evaluation and research
Area 5	Administer and manage health education	Administer and manage health education/promotion	Advocacy
Area 6	Serve as a health education resource person	Serve as a health education/promotion resource person	Communication
Area 7	Communicate and advocate for health and health education	Communicate, promote, and advocate for health, health education/promotion, and the profession	Leadership and management
Area 8	(only seven areas)	(only seven areas)	Ethics and professionalism

Changes from 2010 to 2015: Terminology changes from "health education" to "health education/health promotion"; added clarity to the scope of the role of the health education specialist.

Changes from 2015 to 2020: Addition of an eighth area of responsibility: ethics and professionalism. Advocacy and communication became stand-alone areas of responsibility. New competencies and subcompetencies were developed to reflect the increasing role of social media.

Data from National Commission for Health Education Credentialing. (2020). *Responsibilities and competencies.* Available at https://www.nchec.org/responsibilities-and-competencies

conducted every 5 years. The areas of responsibilities represent the required skills and expertise needed to work successfully in community and public health. The roles are updated to reflect current professional practices; however, it is important to note that the essential skills of assessing, planning, implementing, and evaluation have stayed constant through every revision.[56]

Chapter Summary

- A knowledge of community organizing/building and program planning is essential for community and public health workers whose job it is to promote and protect the health of the community.

- When conducting community organizing/building and program planning processes, community and public health workers must keep in mind the concepts of the socioecological approach and evidence-based practice.

- Community organizing is a process by which community groups are helped to identify common problems or change targets, mobilize resources, and develop and implement strategies for reaching their collective goals.

- Community building is an orientation to practice focused on community, rather than a strategic framework or approach, and on building capacities, not fixing problems.

- The steps of the general model for community organizing/building include recognizing the issue, gaining entry into the community, organizing the people, assessing the community, determining the priorities and setting goals, arriving at a solution and selecting the intervention strategies, implementing the plan, evaluating the outcomes of the plan of action, maintaining the outcomes in the community, and, if necessary, looping back.

- Program planning is a process in which an intervention is planned to help meet the needs of a priority population.

- The steps in the program planning process include assessing the needs of the priority population, setting appropriate goals and objectives, creating an intervention that considers the peculiarities of the setting, implementing the intervention, and evaluating the results. In addition, the quasi-step of preplanning must also be addressed.

Scenario: Analysis and Response

The town of Kenzington sounds like a good candidate for a community organizing/building effort. Assume that Kenzington is the town in which you now live and you belong to the group that has taken the issue to the city council. Based on what you know about the problem in the scenario and what you know about your town, answer the following questions.

1. What is the real problem?

2. Who do you think the gatekeepers are in the community?

3. What groups of people in the community might be most interested in solving this problem?

4. What groups might have a vested interest in seeing the problem remain unsolved?

5. What interventions do you believe would be useful in dealing with the problem? What sources of evidence might you use to help with deciding on an intervention?

6. How would you evaluate your efforts to solve the problem?

7. What strategies might you recommend to make the solution lasting?

8. If you were to look for help on the Internet to deal with this problem, what keywords would you use to search the web for help?

Review Questions

1. Briefly explain the concepts of the socioecological approach and evidence-based practice.

2. What is community organizing?

3. What are the assumptions (identified by Ross) under which organizers work when bringing a community together to solve a problem?

4. What is the difference between top-down and grass-roots community organizing?

5. What does the term *gatekeepers* mean? Who would they be in your home community?

6. Identify the steps in the generalized approach to community organizing/building presented in this chapter.

7. What does community building mean?

8. What is a needs assessment? Why is it important in the health promotion programming process?

9. What are the five major steps and one quasi-step in program development?

10. What are the differences between goals and objectives?

11. What are intervention strategies? Provide five examples.

12. What are best practices, best experiences, and best processes? How are they different?

13. What does the term *pilot testing* mean? How is it useful when developing an intervention?

14. What is the difference between formative and summative evaluation? What are impact and outcome evaluation?

15. Name and briefly describe the six steps of the Centers for Disease Control and Prevention's framework for program evaluation.

Activities

1. From your knowledge of the community in which you live (or the use of the Internet), generate a list of seven to 10 agencies that might be interested in creating a coalition to deal with community drug problems. Provide a one-sentence rationale for each regarding why it might want to be involved.

2. Identify community organizing/building efforts in a local community. If you are able to identify such an effort, make an appointment—either by yourself or with some of your classmates—to meet with the person who is leading the effort and ask the following questions:
   - What is the problem the community faces?
   - What is the goal of the group?
   - What steps have been taken so far to organize/build the community, and what steps are yet to be taken?
   - Who is active in the core group?
   - Did the group conduct a community assessment?
   - What intervention will be/has been used?
   - Is it anticipated that the problem will be solved?

3. Using the socioecological approach, explain how a local health department could create a childhood immunization program by intervening at a minimum of four levels of influence.

4. Using a nutrition education program for college students, write one program goal and one objective for each of the levels presented in Table 5.3.

5. Visit a voluntary health agency in your community, either by yourself or with classmates. Ask employees if you may review a written report of a recent program evaluation of one of their programs. Examine the report and compare its content to the six-step framework of evaluation of the Centers for Disease Control and Prevention's framework for program evaluation presented in this chapter. Then, in a two-page paper, briefly summarize how the agency dealt with each of the steps.

6. Prepare a community assessment of a selected community where you live or work using the following resource for a windshield survey as a guide: https://ctb.ku.edu/en/table-of-contents/assessment/assessing-community-needs-and-resources/windshield-walking-surveys/main

References

1. Cottrell, R. R., & McKenzie, J. F. (2011). *Health promotion & education research: Using the five-chapter thesis/dissertation model* (2nd ed.). Jones & Bartlett Publishers.

2. Hailemariam, M., Bustos, T., Montgomery, B. Bsrajas, R., Evans, L. B., & Drahota, A. (2019). Evidence-based intervention sustainability strategies: A systematic review. *Implementation Science, 14,* 57. https://doi.org/10.1186/s13012-019-0910-6

3. McKenzie, J. F., Neiger, B. L., & Thackeray, R. (2023). *Planning, implementing, and evaluating health promotion programs* (8th ed.). Jones & Bartlett Learning.

4. Muir Gray, J. A. (1997). *Evidence-based health care: How to make health policy and management decisions.* Churchill Livingstone.

5. Institute of Medicine (IOM). (2001). *Health and behavior: The interplay of biological, behavioral, and societal influences.* National Academies Press.

6. McLeroy, K. R., Bibeau, D., Steckler, A., & Glanz, K. (1988). An ecological perspective for health promotion programs. *Health Education Quarterly, 15*(4), 351–378.

7. Simons-Morton, B. G., McLeroy, K. R., & Wendel, M. L. (2012). *Behavior theory in health promotion practice and research.* Jones & Bartlett Learning.

8. Sallis, J. F., Owen, N., & Fisher, E. B. (2008). Ecological models of health behavior. In K. Glanz, B. K. Rimer, & K. Viswanath (Eds.), *Health behavior and health education practice: Theory, research, and practice* (4th ed., pp. 465–485). Jossey-Bass.

9. Minkler, M., & Wallerstein, N. (2012). Improving health through community organization and community building: Perspectives from health education and social work. *Community organizing and community building for health and welfare* Edited by Meredith Minkler. New Brunswick: Rutgers University Press, 2012. Copyright © 2012 by Meredith Minkler. Reprinted by permission of Rutgers University Press.

10. Ross, M. G. (1967). *Community organization: Theory, principles, and practice* (pp. 86–92). Harper and Row.

11. Perlman, J. (1978). Grassroots participation from neighborhood to nation. In S. Langton (Ed.), *Citizen participation in America* (pp. 65–79). Lexington Books.

12. Cronin, C. E., Franz, B., & Garlington, S. (2021). *Population health partnerships and social capital: Facilitating hospital-community partnerships.* SSM - Population Health, 13, 100739. https://doi.org/10.1016/j.ssmph.2021.100739

13. Centers for Disease Control and Prevention. (2020). *A guide to facilitating health systems change.* Retrieved from www.cdc.gov/dhdsp/programs/spha/docs/guide_facilitating_hs_change.pdf

14. Rothman, J., & Tropman, J. E. (1987). Models of community organization and macro practice perspectives: Their mixing and phasing. In F. M. Cox, J. L. Erlich, J. Rothman, & J. E. Tropman (Eds.), *Strategies of community organization: Macro practice* (pp. 3–26). Peacock Publishers.

15. Garvin, C. D., & Cox, F. M. (2001). A history of community organizing since the Civil War with special reference to oppressed communities. In J. Rothman, J. L. Erlich, & J. E. Tropman (Eds.), *Strategies of community intervention* (5th ed., pp. 65–100). Peacock Publishers.

16. Rothman, J. (2001). Approaches to community intervention. In J. Rothman, J. L. Erlich, & J. E. Tropman (Eds.), *Strategies of community intervention* (6th ed.). Peacock Publishers.

17. Rothman, J. (2007). Multi modes of intervention at the macro level. *Journal of Community Practice, 15*(4), 11–40.

18. Butterfoss, F. D. (2007). *Coalitions and partnerships in community health.* Jossey-Bass.

19. Braithwaite, R. L., Murphy, F., Lythcott, N., & Blumenthal, D. S. (1989). Community organization and development for health promotion within an urban black community: A conceptual model. *Health Education, 20*(5), 56–60.

20. Wright, P. A. (1994). *A key step in developing prevention materials is to obtain expert and gatekeepers' reviews* [Technical assistance bulletin]. Bethesda, MD: Center for Substance Abuse Prevention (CASP) Communications Team; 1–6.

21. Tervalon, M., & Garcia, J. (1998). Cultural humility versus cultural competence: A critical distinction in defining physician training outcomes in multicultural education. *Journal of Health Care for the Poor and Underserved, 9*(2), 117–125.

22. Brager, G., Specht, H., & Torczyner, J. L. (1987). *Community organizing* (pp. 55). Columbia University Press.

23. Butterfoss, F. D. (2013). *Ignite! Getting your community coalition fired up for change.* AuthorHouse.

24. Minkler, M. (2012). Introduction to community organizing and community building. In M. Minkler (Ed.), *Community organizing and community building for health and welfare* (3rd ed., pp. 5–26). Rutgers University Press.

25. McKnight, J. L., & Kretzmann, J. P. (2012). Mapping community capacity. In M. Minkler (Ed.), *Community organizing and community building for health and welfare* (3rd ed., pp. 171–186). Rutgers University Press.

26. Hancock, T., & Minkler, M. (2012). Community health assessment or healthy community assessment: Whose community? Whose health? Whose assessment? In M. Minkler (Ed.), *Community organizing and community building for health and welfare* (3rd ed., pp. 153–170). Rutgers University Press.

27. Nyswander, D. B. (1956). Education for health: Some principles and their application. *Health Education Monographs, 14,* 65–70.

28. Wang, C. C., & Burris, M. A. (1994). Empowerment through photovoice: Portraits of participation. *Health Education Quarterly, 21*(2), 171–186.

29. Wang, C. C., & Burris, M. A. (1997). Photovoice: Concept, methodology, and use for participatory needs assessment. *Health Education and Behavior, 24*(3), 369–387.

30. Kramer, L., Schwartz, P., Cheadle, A., Borton, J. E., Wright, M., Chase, C., & Lindley, C. (2010). Promoting policy and environmental change using photovoice in Kaiser Permanente Community Health Initiative. *Health Promotion Practice, 11*(3), 332–339.

31. Community Toolbox. (2020). *Section 21. Windshield and walking surveys.* Retrieved from https://ctb.ku.edu/en/table-of-contents/assessment/assessing-community-needs-and-resources/windshield-walking-surveys/main

32. Miller, M. (1986). Turning problems into actionable issues [Unpublished paper]. Organize Training Center.

33. Archer, S. E., & Fleshman, R. P. (1985). *Community health nursing.* Wadsworth Health Sciences.

34. Joint Committee on Health Education and Promotion Terminology. (2012). Report of the 2011 Joint Committee on Health Education and Promotion Terminology. *American Journal of Health Education, 43*(2), 1–19.

35. Green, L. W., & Kreuter, M. W. (2005). *Health program planning: An educational and ecological approach* (4th ed.). McGraw-Hill.

36. National Association of County and City Health Officials. (2001). *Mobilizing for Action through Planning and Partnerships (MAPP).* Washington, DC: Author.

37. Bartholomew, L. K., Parcel, G. S., Kok, G., Gottlieb, N. H., & Fernandez, M. E. (2011). *Planning health promotion programs: An intervention mapping approach* (3rd ed.). Jossey-Bass.

38. Centers for Disease Control and Prevention, U.S. Department of Health and Human Services (CDC). (2003). *CDCynergy 3.0: Your guide to effective health communication* [CD-ROM Version 3.0]. CDC.

39. Neiger, B. L., & Thackeray, R. (1998). Social marketing: Making public health sense. Paper presented at the annual meeting of the Utah Public Health Association, Provo, UT.

40. Grunbaum, J. A., Gingiss, P., Orpinas, P., Batey, L. S., & Parcel, G. S. (1995). A comprehensive approach to school health program needs assessment. *Journal of School Health, 65*(2), 54–59.

41. Gilmore, G. D. (2012). *Needs and capacity assessment strategies for health education and health promotion* (4th ed.). Jones & Bartlett Learning.

42. Peterson, D. J., & Alexander, G. R. (2001). *Needs assessment in public health: A practical guide for students and professionals.* Kluwer Academic/Plenum Publishers.

43. Public Health Accreditation Board. (2024). *About.* Retrieved from https://phaboard.org/about/#:~:text=2007,implement%20and%20oversee%20national%20accreditation

44. Public Health Accreditation Board. (2013). *Standards and measures: An overview.* Retrieved from https://www.phaboard.org/wp-content/uploads/2019/01/PHAB-Standards-Overview-Version-1.5.pdf

45. Centers for Disease Control and Prevention (CDC). (n.d.). *Summary of the Internal Revenue Service's April 5, 2013, Notice of Proposed Rule Making on Community Health Needs Assessments for Charitable Hospitals.* Retrieved from https://www.cdc.gov/phlp/docs/summary-irs-rule.pdf

46. Ross, H. S., & Mico, P. R. (1980). *Theory and practice in health education* (pp. 219). Mayfield Press.

47. Deeds, S. G. (1992). *The health education specialist: Self-study for professional competence.* Loose Cannon Publications.

48. Cleary, M. J., & Neiger, B. L. (1998). *The certified health education specialist: A self-study guide for professional competence* (3rd ed.). National Commission for Health Education Credentialing.

49. Centers for Disease Control and Prevention (CDC). (2016). *The guide to community preventive services—the community guide: what works to promote health.* Retrieved from https://www.thecommunity guide.org

50. Crosby, R. A., Salazar, L. F., & DiClemente, R. J. (2013). Social cognitive theory applied to health behavior. In R. J. DiClemente, L. F. Salazar, & R. A. Crosby (Eds.), *Health behavior theory in public health* (pp. 163–185). Jones & Bartlett Learning.

51. DiClemente, R. J., Redding, C. A., Crosby, R. A., & Salazar, L. F. (2013). Stage models for health promotion. In R. J. DiClemente, L. F. Salazar, & R. A. Crosby (Eds.), *Health behavior theory in public health* (pp. 105–129). Jones & Bartlett Learning.

52. Timmreck, T. C. (1997). *Health services cyclopedic dictionary* (3rd ed.). Jones & Bartlett Learning.

53. Green, L. W., & Lewis, F. M. (1986). *Measurement and evaluation in health education and health promotion.* Mayfield Press.

54. Centers for Disease Control and Prevention. (1999). Framework for program evaluation in public health. *Morbidity and Mortality Weekly Report, 48*(RR-11), 1–40.

55. Centers for Disease Control and Prevention. (2011). *Introduction to program evaluation for public health programs: A self-study guide.* Retrieved from http://www.cdc.gov/eval/guide

56. National Commission for Health Education Credentialing. (2020). *Responsibilities and competencies.* Retrieved from https://www .nchec.org/responsibilities-and-competencies

CHAPTER 6

The School Health Program: A Component of Community and Public Health

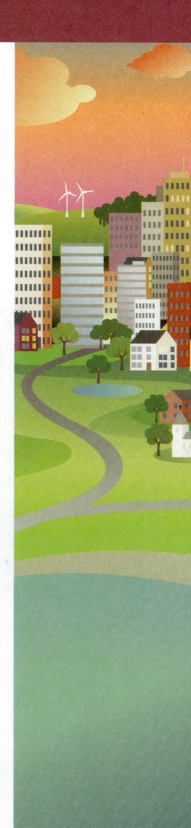

Chapter Objectives

After studying this chapter, you will be able to:

1. Describe the Whole School, Whole Community, Whole Child model.
2. List the ideal members of a school health advisory council.
3. Illustrate why a school health program is important.
4. Summarize written school health policies and explain their importance to the school health program.

Chapter Objectives *(continued)*

5. Discuss processes for developing and implementing school health policies.
6. State the 10 components of the Whole School, Whole Community, Whole Child model.
7. Describe the role of the school health coordinator.
8. Identify those services offered as part of school health services and explain why schools are logical places to offer such services.
9. Explain what is meant by a healthy school environment and discuss the two major environments.
10. Define school health education.
11. Identify the eight National Health Education Standards.
12. Demonstrate how a health education specialist could locate credible health education curricula.
13. Discuss and briefly explain four issues that school health advocates face.

Scenario

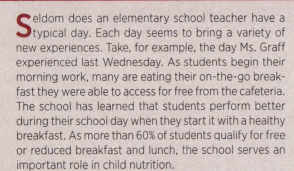

Seldom does an elementary school teacher have a typical day. Each day seems to bring a variety of new experiences. Take, for example, the day Ms. Graff experienced last Wednesday. As students begin their morning work, many are eating their on-the-go breakfast they were able to access for free from the cafeteria. The school has learned that students perform better during their school day when they start it with a healthy breakfast. As more than 60% of students qualify for free or reduced breakfast and lunch, the school serves an important role in child nutrition.

Math class was disrupted when a student brought a gun to school. Police were called and students were locked into their classrooms to ensure that everyone was safe while police investigated the situation. While it was determined the gun was a BB gun, safety is of the utmost importance at this school, so extreme precautions were taken, and learning was disrupted.

After lunch, Ms. Graff began her writing lesson—students are practicing writing an essay with a beginning, middle, and end. She wasn't 10 minutes into her lesson when the school nurse stuck her head in the door and asked if Ms. Graff could send five students for their annual vision and hearing screenings. Reluctantly, Ms. Graff excused the students.

During the last half-hour of the school day, students were engaged in success time—focused instruction in preparation for standardized testing. Just before the last bell was to ring, Annie came up to Ms. Graff's desk and told her she was worried about her classmate, Joseph—he had not been in school the entire week and Annie had heard that his mom got a new job working nights.

A variety of issues impact the success of students in Ms. Graff's class; there is no "typical day" in an elementary school that serves a population of high-risk students and families.

Introduction

The school health program is an important component of community and public health. Although the primary responsibility for the health of school-aged children lies with their parents/guardians, the schools have immeasurable potential for affecting the health of children, their families, and the health of the community. As former U.S. Surgeon General David Satcher stated, "The school setting is a great equalizer, providing all students and families—regardless of ethnicity, socioeconomic status, or level of education—with the same access to good nutrition and physical activity. Because children also teach their parents, important lessons learned at school can help the entire family,"[1] thus improving the health of the entire community. Full-service community schools provide a good example of the link between school health and community health. These schools, using an integrated approach, offer a variety of educational, counseling, social, and health services to families in one location, resulting in improved educational outcomes. Such schools focus on the well-being of the child and family. These school buildings serve as neighborhood hubs and institutions that are safe, attentive, and comfortable.[2]

In this chapter, we describe the Whole School, Whole Community, Whole Child (WSCC) model, explain who is involved in school health programs, explore the reasons why school health is important, discuss the components of the WSCC model, and present some of the issues facing school health programs today.

Whole School, Whole Community, Whole Child: A Collaborative Approach to Learning and Health

The **Whole School, Whole Community, Whole Child (WSCC)** model focuses on addressing the educational and health needs of children within the context of the school setting, which is a critical component of the local community. As a result, community strengths not only boost the role of the school in addressing child health and learning needs but also can reflect areas of need in the community.[3] "Each child, in each school, in each of our communities deserves to be healthy, safe, engaged, supported, and challenged. That's what a whole child approach to learning, teaching, and community engagement really is about."[3] This model includes 10 components. The components of WSCC include (1) physical education and physical activity; (2) nutrition environment and services; (3) health education; (4) social and emotional school climate; (5) physical environment; (6) health services; (7) counseling, psychological, and social services; (8) employee wellness; (9) community involvement; and (10) family engagement. WSCC provides a shared framework and approach for schools and the community to work together to provide a systematic, integrated, and collaborative approach to health and learning[4] (see **Figure 6.1**).

Whole School, Whole Community, Whole Child (WSCC) model that focuses on addressing the educational and health needs of children within the context of the school setting

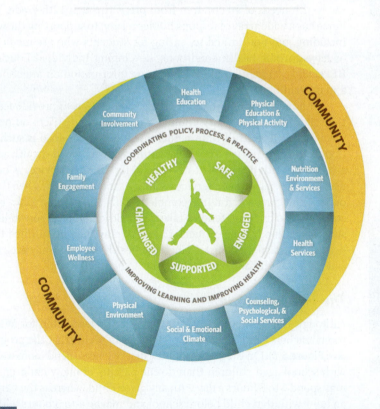

FIGURE 6.1   Whole School, Whole Community, Whole Child model: a collaborative approach to learning and health.

Reproduced from Centers for Disease Control and Prevention, *Whole School, Whole Community, Whole Child*, https://www.cdc.gov/healthyschools/wscc/index.htm.

The School Health Advisory Council

For WSCC efforts to be effective, a great deal of time and effort must be expended by individuals in schools with an investment in the health of students. When these individuals work together to plan and implement a school health program, they are referred to as the **school health advisory council**, sometimes called a school wellness council. The primary role of this council is to provide coordination of the various components of WSCC to help students improve health and learning outcomes. An ideal council would include representation from each of the WSCC components and district administrators, parents, students, and community representatives involved in the health and well-being of students. For the successful implementation of the work of this group, a full-time or part-time school health coordinator is critical to maintain active school health advisory councils and facilitate health programming in the district. The American School Health Association describes the ideal school health coordinator as a key facilitator and program evaluator. They are the individual responsible for operationalizing the WSCC model at the school level.[5] The school health coordinator should ideally have a formal educational background in school health or in a related field, such as physical education, public health, or nursing.

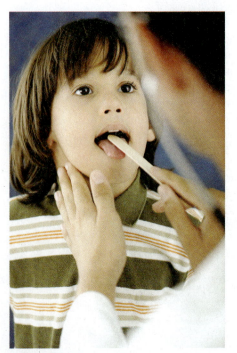

FIGURE 6.2 The school nurse is in a good position to guide the school health efforts.

© ZouZou/Shutterstock

The School Nurse

The field of school nursing has a long history of providing health care to students to improve academic and health outcomes for students. The school nurse is one of several people who is positioned to provide leadership for WSCC efforts (see **Figure 6.2**). The nurse not only has medical knowledge but should also have formal training in health education and an understanding of the health needs of all children from pre-K through 12th grade. The school nurse has a wide array of responsibilities related to supporting the whole child, including, but not limited to, caring for students who are medically fragile or have chronic health conditions, developing Individual Education Plans (IEPs) and 504 Plans, and disseminating information on infectious diseases and prevention.[6]

Although school nurses are in a good position to provide leadership to the school health advisory council, many school districts do not have the resources to hire a full-time school nurse or the caseload is such that additional duties are not feasible. Contracting with an outside health agency, such as a local health department or hospital for nursing services is one strategy used for securing nursing services within a school district. When this scenario occurs, the contracted nurse completes only the nursing tasks required by state law and does not tend to take on the leadership responsibilities for the school health advisory council. This task may then be fulfilled by a school health education specialist. In fact, the health educator may even be responsible when a full-time nurse is present.

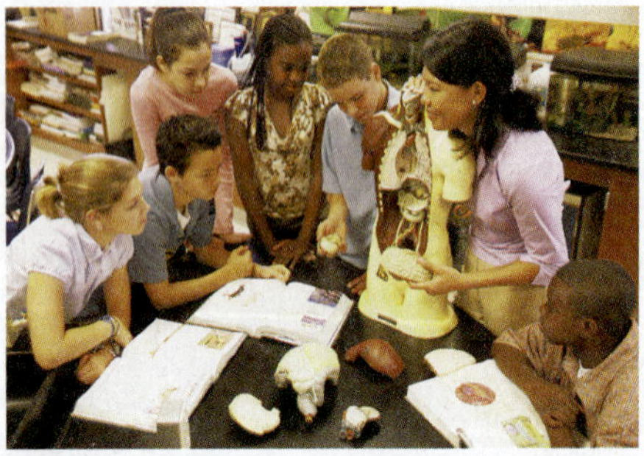

The Teacher's Role

Although the school nurse might provide the leadership for WSSC, classroom teachers carry a heavy responsibility in seeing that the program works (see **Figure 6.3**). On the average school day, teachers spend more waking hours with school-aged children than do the parents of many children. A teacher may spend 6 to 8 hours a day with any given child, whereas the parents spend an hour with that child before school and maybe 4 to 5 hours with the child after school and before bedtime. Teachers are also in a position to make observations on typical behaviors and conditions of children because they are able

FIGURE 6.3 The classroom teacher's participation is essential for a successful school health program.

© Arthur Tilley/Stockbyte/Getty Images

TABLE 6.1 Health Education Teacher Preparation Standards
Standard 1: Functional Knowledge. Possess functional health education knowledge.
Standard 2: Assessing Needs. Assess needs and assets of learners, learning, and the learning community.
Standard 3: Planning. Use needs assessment data, health education standards, and principles of learning to plan cohesive, sequential lessons and units.
Standard 4: Implementation. Employ a variety of research-based instructional strategies.
Standard 5: Evaluation. Use multiple assessment methods.
Standard 6: Professionalism. Demonstrate professionalism and ethical practices.

Data from SOPHE. (2019). 2019 health education teacher preparation standards: Guidelines for initial licensure programs. https://www.sophe.org/wp-content/uploads/2020/04/Health-Ed-Stds-for-CAEP_v3-3.pdf

to compare the students in their classroom each day. Furthermore, many health teachers are receiving leadership training regarding WSCC in their undergraduate or postgraduate coursework, thus, making them ideal individuals to lead the coordination. **Table 6.1** summarizes the competencies for teachers who expect to be involved in school health education and WSCC leadership.

The Need for School Health

The primary role of schools is to educate. However, an unhealthy child has a difficult time learning. Consider, for example, a student who arrives at school without having breakfast, with poor hygiene, and without adequate sleep. This student will be unable to concentrate on schoolwork and may distract others. As a reader, you know how difficult it is to study for a test or even to read this textbook when you do not feel well or are depressed or hungry (see **Box 6.1**).

"Health and success in school are interrelated. Schools cannot achieve their primary mission of education if students and staff are not healthy and fit physically, mentally, and socially."[7] These barriers to student learning acutely impact students from low-income households and racial and ethnic minority students. Reduction of health barriers can help both health and academic outcomes. The WSCC model provides the integration of education and health.

The importance of the school health program is also evident by its inclusion in the national health objectives for the year 2030. Of all of the objectives listed in the publication *Healthy People 2030*, a significant number can either be directly attained by schools or their attainment can be influenced in important ways by schools, especially by those who follow the WSCC model (see **Box 6.2**).

Nevertheless, WSCC is not a cure-all. There are no quick and easy solutions to improving the overall health of a community. However, WSCC provides a strong base on which to build.

Foundations of the School Health Program

The true foundations of any school health program are (1) a school administration that supports such an effort; (2) a well-organized school health advisory council that is genuinely interested in providing a coordinated program for the students, families, and staff; and (3) written school health policies. A highly supportive administration is a must for quality WSCC. In almost all organizations—and schools are no different—the administration controls resources. Without

BOX 6.1   It Is Harder to Learn If You Are Not Healthy! A Look at the Impact of Childhood Obesity

It stands to reason that if children are not healthy, it is harder for them to concentrate and in turn to have a meaningful learning experience. One such example that is significantly affecting students and schools is the obesity epidemic. Childhood obesity has more than doubled in children and quadrupled in adolescents in the past 30 years, with the prevalence affecting one in five children and adolescents. Experts have determined that body mass index (BMI) is the most practical tool available to define and screen for obesity.

Childhood obesity is often accompanied by numerous other health conditions, such as increased rates of type 2 diabetes, cardiovascular problems, sleep apnea, and bone and joint problems. The reasons for the obesity epidemic are varied but are slowly becoming understood. Many environments make it difficult for children to make healthy food choices and get enough physical activity. Advertising of less healthy foods, limited access to healthy affordable foods, availability of energy-dense food and sugar-sweetened beverages, and increasing portion sizes have been shown to contribute to the challenges youth experience with healthy eating. A lack of safe places to play or be active makes it difficult or unsafe to be physically active. Half of the children in the United States do not have a park, community center, or sidewalk in their neighborhood.

Researchers are now reporting some of the social, psychological, and educational consequences of obesity. A review of the literature determined that overweight and obese children are more likely to have low self-esteem, higher rates of anxiety disorders, and depression. Severely obese kids report many more missed days of school than the general student population. What is yet to be understood is why these kids miss more school—are they embarrassed to participate in physical activity? Are health conditions keeping them from school? Are they experiencing bullying or teasing? Although there is no known reason, the consequences are significant.

One way that schools addressed concerns about overweight children was by establishing policies related to improved nutritional offerings in the cafeteria, school parties and events, and vending machines, as well as increasing nutrition education and physical activity. The Child Nutrition and WIC Reauthorization Act of 2004 (Public Law 108-265) required all schools participating in the federally funded school feeding programs to establish a local wellness policy by the first day of the 2006–2007 school year. This law helped many districts begin the process of improving the school environment, not only to improve the obesity problem but also to make school a healthier place for all. With the passage of the 2010 Healthy Hunger-Free Kids Act (Public Law 111-296), greater emphasis has been placed on implementation, evaluation, and public reporting of local school wellness policies.

The issue of childhood obesity was a priority in the Obama White House with First Lady Michelle Obama's Let's Move! campaign. The Let's Move! initiative was dedicated to "solving the problem of obesity within a generation, so that children born today will grow up healthier and able to pursue their dreams." The campaign included a comprehensive approach that provided schools, families, and communities with simple tools to help kids be more active, eat better, and get healthy.

In June of 2013, the federal government announced its Smart Snacks in Schools nutrition standards for competitive foods. Competitive foods are those foods that are not part of the regular school meal programs. The standards set limits for calories, fat, sugar, and sodium. High-calorie sports drinks and candy bars are some of the items that were removed from school vending machines and cafeteria lines as a result of these new standards. Many policies and programs have been successfully implemented over the years to address childhood obesity.

Outside of the federal government, local communities and schools are focused on making improvements to the school health environment using tools provided through voluntary health organizations, such as Action for Healthy Kids and The Alliance for a Healthier Generation.

Data from Taras, H., & Potts-Datema, W. (2005). Obesity and student performance at school. *Journal of School Health, 75*(8), 291–295; Centers for Disease Control and Prevention. (2024). *Childhood obesity facts.* Available at https://www.cdc.gov/obesity/php/data-research/childhood-obesity-facts.html; Centers for Disease Control and Prevention. (2022). *Consequences of obesity.* Available at https://www.cdc.gov/obesity/basics/consequences.html; Centers for Disease Control and Prevention. (2024). *Obesity.* https://www.cdc.gov/obesity/index.html

leadership and support from top school administrators, it will be an ongoing struggle to provide a quality program. Furthermore, every effort should be made to employ personnel who are appropriately trained to carry out their responsibilities as members of the school health advisory council. For example, the National Association of School Nurses has taken the position that "every school-age child should have access to a registered professional school nurse, who has a *minimum of* a baccalaureate degree in nursing from an accredited college or university and is licensed as a registered nurse through a board of nursing,"[6] yet many school nurses without college degrees and training in health education are asked to provide health education. Conversely, certified teachers who lack preparation in school health are required to teach health to secure a job.[8] Qualified personnel are a must.

BOX 6.2   Select *Healthy People 2030* Objectives Related to School Health

Objective		Baseline (year)	Most Recent Data	2030 Target
AH-03	Increase the proportion of adolescents who have an adult in their lives with whom they can talk about serious problems	79.0% (2018)	78.3% (2019)	82.9%
AH-04	Increase the proportion of students participating in the School Breakfast Program	30.2% (2017–2018)	21.0% (2020–2021)	34.9%
AH-07	Reduce chronic school absence among early adolescents	20.3% (2017)	32.0% (2022)	16.4%
FP-08	Increase the proportion of adolescents who get formal sex education before age 18 years	52.8% (2015–2017)	54.5% (2017–2019)	59.1%
LGBT-05	Reduce bullying of lesbian, gay, or bisexual high school students	24.9% (2021)	24.9% (2021)	20.7%
PA-09	Increase the proportion of children who do enough aerobic physical activity	25.9% (2016–2017)	23.6% (2020–2021)	30.4%

Data from U.S. Department of Health and Human Services, Office of Disease Prevention and Health Promotion. (2024). *Healthy People 2030*. Available at https://www.healthypeople.gov/

School Health Policies

School health policies, which include laws, regulations, procedures, standards, and guidelines that provide a foundation for school district practices and procedures. The written policy describes credibility and the program and procedure for its implementation to those outside of the program.[9] Well-written school health policies provide a sense of direction and a means of accountability and credibility, and strengthen the possibility that a school health program will become "an institutionalized part of the school culture."[10] Steps for creating local health-related policies include the following[11]:

1. Build a policy development team.
2. Assess the environment.
3. Draft the policy.
4. Adopt the policy.
5. Implement the policy.
6. Measure and evaluate.
7. Communicate the results.

> **School health policies**
> written statements that describe the nature and procedures of a school health program

Policy Development

The development of a set of written policies is not an easy task. The school health advisory council should execute this challenging and time-consuming task because the council includes those most knowledgeable about the school health program, in addition to representing many different constituencies in the school community.

The policies should cover all facets of the school health program, such as storage and access to prescription medications, bullying, use or restriction of physical activity as punishment, and foods permitted at school parties, in addition to policies associated with curriculum, health services, and maintaining a safe learning environment. Several professional associations that have an interest in school health programs have written policy statements relating to school health issues and provide guidance for providing current policy statements. A few such associations are the American Academy of Pediatrics (AAP; www.aap.org), the National Association of State Boards of Education (NASBE; http://nasbe.org), and ASCD (ASCD; www.ascd.org).

Once the policies have been written, it is important that they receive approval from key stakeholders. Although the school board is the final authority that adopts policies, approval from school administrators, school-based committees, parents, and other key stakeholders can aid in the implementation process.[11] The approval process provides credibility to the policies as well as legal protection for those who must implement the policies.[10]

Policy Implementation

The development of written policies is an important step in building a solid base for WSCC efforts. However, if the policies are never implemented, the school district will be no better off than before their development.

Implementation begins with the distribution of the policies to those who will be affected by them—faculty, staff, students, and parents. Some ideas for carrying out this process include (1) distributing the policies with a memorandum of explanation, (2) placing the policies in both faculty/staff and student handbooks, (3) presenting them at a gathering of the different groups (e.g., at staff or parent–teacher organization [PTO] meetings or an open house), (4) holding a special meeting for the specific purpose of explaining the policies, and (5) placing them in the school district communication. News releases might even be considered if the policies include major changes. Each school district must decide the best way to disseminate its school health policies.

Policy Development Resources

Because of the requirements of the Child Nutrition and WIC Reauthorization Act of 2004 to implement a school wellness policy by districts,[12] numerous resources have become available to help schools develop, maintain, and revise policies. Action for Healthy Kids (AFHK) is one such organization that is advocating and providing support for creating healthier schools. AFHK has created a large partner network of organizations, corporations, and government agencies concerned with the health and academic success of youth. They have a variety of free online tools to help communities and schools adopt policies and practices that promote healthier learning environments.[13] Tools to assist schools in conducting needs assessments related to WSCC include the School Health Index, available free from the Centers for Disease Control and Prevention (CDC; https://www.cdc.gov/healthyschools/shi/) and the ASCD School Improvement Tool, available from ASCD (https://ascd.org/whole-child).

Monitoring the Status of School Health Policy in the United States

Because school health policy is an important foundation for WSCC, the Division of Adolescent and School Health at the CDC conducts a national survey to assess school health policies and practices in states, school districts, territories, and tribes. The survey, which is titled the School Health Profiles, is conducted biennially by education and health agencies among middle and high school principals and lead health education teachers. The survey data are used to do the following[14]:

- Monitor the current status of various school health policies and practices (e.g., school health education requirements and content, practices related to bullying, school-based mental health services, family engagement).

- Show progress in the use of school policies and practices to improve the health of school-aged youth.
- Identify gaps in school health policies and practices that can impact student health and academic performance.

Components of the Whole School, Whole Community, Whole Child Model

If implemented appropriately, a coordinated approach to child health and learning can have a significant positive impact on the overall health status of students, staff, and the community, which, in turn, can be linked to higher academic achievement for students. To do so, the 10 WSCC components need to be provided in a coordinated fashion. Because of space limitations, we will focus on providing the following: a discussion of the importance of the administration and organization; an overview of three of the traditional components of the school health program: (1) school health services, (2) healthy school environment, and (3) health education; and a brief explanation of the remaining components.

Administration and Organization

Effective administration and organization of the school health program ensure that the people and activities that constitute the program work in a coordinated manner to meet the program's goals. Additionally, a dedicated coordinator is critical to maximizing existing resources and championing student health and wellness within the school, community, and district.[15] As previously noted, the responsibility for coordinating the program in each school district should be delegated to a properly trained and knowledgeable individual. Logical choices for this position of **school health coordinator** would be a trained school nurse or a health education specialist. Nationwide, more than 85% of school districts in the United States have someone who oversees/coordinates school health and safety programs.[14]

The following are responsibilities common to school health coordinators[16,17]:

- Ensuring that the instruction and services provided through various components of the school health program are mutually reinforcing and present consistent messages
- Facilitating collaboration among school health program personnel and between them and other school staff
- Assisting the superintendent/school principal and other administrative staff with the integration, management, and supervision of the school health program
- Providing or arranging for necessary technical assistance
- Identifying necessary resources
- Facilitating collaboration between the district/school and other agencies and organizations in the community that have an interest in the health and well-being of children and their families
- Conducting evaluation activities that assess the implementation and results of the school health program, as well as assisting with reporting evaluation results

School Health Services

School health services "intervene with actual and potential health problems, including providing first aid, emergency care and assessment, and planning for management of chronic conditions."[18] School health services also include wellness promotion, preventive services, and education; access and/or referrals to the medical home or private healthcare provider; support connecting school staff, students, families, community, and healthcare providers to promote the health care of students and a healthy and safe school environment; and remediation of detected health problems within the limits of state laws through referral and follow-up by the school nurse and teachers.[18] Originally, the intent of school health services was to supplement rather

School health coordinator
a trained professional at the state, district, or school level who is responsible for managing, coordinating, planning, implementing, and evaluating school health policies, programs, and resources

School health services
health services provided by school health workers to appraise, protect, and promote the health of students

than to supplant the family's responsibility for meeting the healthcare needs of its children. However, because of the poorer health status of youth, the involvement of youth in high-risk behaviors (such as vaping, drinking, substance use, and unprotected sexual intercourse), and such barriers to health care as inadequate health insurance and lack of providers, there has been a broadening of the role of schools in providing health care.

Because school attendance is required throughout the United States, schools represent the best opportunity to reach many of those children in need of proper health care. More than 95% of all youths aged 5 to 17 years are enrolled in schools.[19] "The school's ability to reach children and youth slipping through the cracks of the healthcare system and at highest risk for poor health and potentially health-threatening behaviors is unmatched."[20] With more than 40% of school-aged children and teens having at least one chronic health condition, like asthma, diabetes, or food allergies, the health services provided by schools are critical.[21] Some of the benefits of having school health services, and specifically a full-time nurse, include[21,22]:

- Students are less likely to visit the emergency room.
- Students are more likely to visit an appropriate healthcare provider if they have a medical referral from the school nurse.
- Students are less likely to miss school due to illness.
- The achievement gap that students with chronic health conditions face can be reduced.

Each school district is unique, from the demographics of its students to the availability of its health resources. The National Association of School Nurses has taken leadership in providing recommendations for evidence-based school nursing practice. The School Nursing Practice Framework™ calls for student-centered nursing care focused on the key principles of care coordination, leadership, quality improvement, and community/public health with standards of practice as the foundation[23] (see **Figure 6.4**).

Expanded services are increasingly being offered through school-based, school-linked programs. School-based health centers (SBHCs) are exactly what the name implies, placing health care where students spend most of their time—in school. Typically, these are partnerships between schools and community health organizations that offer a variety of services, such as primary care, mental health, oral health, and vision services.[24] The idea of young people receiving more comprehensive health care within the context of the school setting is gaining momentum throughout the country and is discussed in greater detail later in this chapter.

Healthy School Environment

The term *healthy school environment* designates the part of WSCC that provides for a safe—both physically and emotionally—learning environment. If children are not placed in a safe environment, learning becomes difficult at best. The most comprehensive definition of **healthy school environment** was provided by the 1972–1973 Joint Committee on Health Education Terminology. They stated that providing a healthy school environment includes "the promotion, maintenance, and utilization of safe and wholesome surroundings, organization of day-by-day experiences and planned learning procedures to influence favorable emotional, physical and social health."[25] Within the WSCC model, the school environment includes the physical environment as well as the social and emotional school climate.

By law, school districts are required to provide a safe school environment. However, the responsibility for maintaining this safe environment should rest with all who use it. Everyone, including those on the board of education, administrators, teachers, custodial staff, and students, must contribute to make a school a safer place through their daily actions. An unsafe school environment can exist only if those responsible for it and those who use it allow it to exist.

The Physical Environment

The physical environment encompasses the school building and its contents, the land on which the school is located, and the area surrounding it. A healthy school environment addresses the school's physical condition, including ventilation, temperature, noise, and

Healthy school environment the promotion, maintenance, and utilization of safe and wholesome surroundings in a school

School Nursing Practice Framework™

Supporting Students to be Healthy, Safe and Ready to Learn

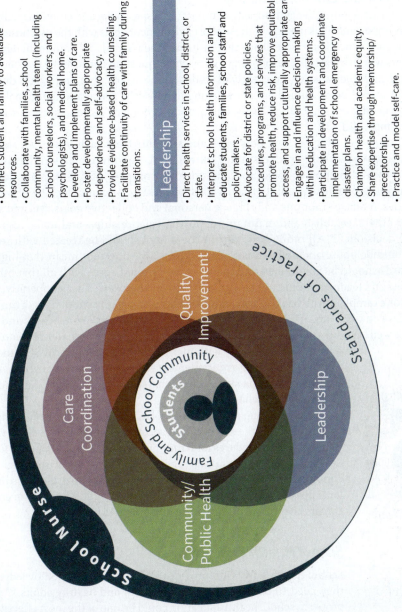

Care Coordination

- Provide direct care for emergent, episodic, and chronic mental and physical health needs.
- Connect student and family to available resources.
- Collaborate with families, school community, mental health team (including school counselors, social workers, and psychologists), and medical home.
- Develop and implement plans of care.
- Foster developmentally appropriate independence and self-advocacy.
- Provide evidence-based health counseling.
- Facilitate continuity of care with family during transitions.

Leadership

- Direct health services in school, district, or state.
- Interpret school health information and educate students, families, school staff, and policymakers.
- Advocate for district or state policies, procedures, programs, and services that promote health, reduce risk, improve equitable access, and support culturally appropriate care.
- Engage in and influence decision-making within education and health systems.
- Participate in development and coordinate implementation of school emergency or disaster plans.
- Champion health and academic equity.
- Share expertise through mentorship/ preceptorship.
- Practice and model self-care.

Quality Improvement

- Participate in data collection for local, state, and national standardized data sets and initiatives.
- Transform practice and make decisions using data, technology, and standardized documentation.
- Use data to identify individual and population level student needs, monitor student health and academic outcomes, and communicate outcomes.
- Engage in ongoing evaluation, performance appraisal, goal setting, and learning to professionalize practice.
- Identify questions in practice that may be resolved through research and evidence-based practice processes.

Community/Public Health

- Provide culturally sensitive, inclusive, holistic care.
- Conduct health screenings, surveillance, outreach, and immunization compliance activities.
- Collaborate with community partners to develop and implement plans that address the needs of school communities and diverse student populations.
- Teach health promotion, health literacy, and disease prevention.
- Provide health expertise in key roles in school, work, and community committees/ councils/coalitions.
- Assess school and community for social and environmental determinants of health.

Standards of Practice

- Ensure practice consistent with the scope and standards of school nursing practice, health and education laws (consider the Individuals with Disabilities Education Act, Section 504 of the Rehabilitation Act of 1973, Nurse Practice Act, state laws regarding school nursing practice and delegation), federal/state/local policies and regulations, and NASN position statements and code of ethics.
- Employ clinical judgment and critical thinking outlined in nursing process and prioritization.
- Integrate evidence and best/promising practices (consider multi-tiered systems of support, clinical practice guidelines).
- Safeguard privacy of students and data (consider Health Insurance Portability & Accountability Act, Family Educational Rights and Privacy Act).

FIGURE 6.4 School Nursing Practice Framework: Supporting Students to be Healthy, Safe, and Ready to Learn.

Reproduced from National Association of School Nurses. (2024). A contemporary Framework update for today's school nursing landscape: Introducing the School Nursing Practice Framework™. *NASN School Nurse, 39*(3). doi:10.1177/19426023X241241092. https://www.nasn.org/nasn-resources/framework

lighting, and it protects occupants from physical threats, such as crime, violence, traffic, and injuries, and from biological and chemical agents in the air, water, and soil.[18] Each school district should have an appropriate protocol for dealing with and maintaining these aspects of the physical environment.

The behavior of both the school personnel and students in the school environment also affects the safety of the environment. Each year a significant number of students throughout the country are injured on their way to, at, or on their way home from school. Some of these injuries occur from an unsafe physical plant that needs repair, but many occur from inappropriate behavior. Unsafe behavior that is observed too frequently in schools includes acts of violence between students and lack of proper supervision by school employees. However, most do not worry about a safe environment until they are faced with a problem. Every school building in the United States could become a safer environment if greater attention were given to prevention than to a cure.

The Social and Emotional Climate

Although a safe physical environment is important, a safe social and emotional environment is equally important. This portion of the school environment deals with the psychosocial elements of "students' educational experience that influence their social and emotional development."[18] Students who are fearful of responding to a teacher's question because the teacher might make fun of them if they answer incorrectly or students who avoid being in the halls during passing time for fear of being bullied are not learning in a healthy social and emotional climate. For many, learning does not come easily, and anxiety-producing factors, such as these can only make it more difficult.

The ways in which school personnel and students treat each other can also add much to the teaching/learning process (see **Figure 6.5**). A trend in education that is growing in popularity and support is social and emotional learning, or SEL. SEL is a process through which young people and adults learn knowledge, skills, and attitudes to "develop healthy identities, manage emotions and achieve personal and collective goals, feel and show empathy for others, establish and maintain supportive relationships, and make responsible and caring decisions."[26] All individuals within the school should be treated with respect. People should be polite and courteous to each other. This does not mean that high academic standards should be abandoned and that everyone should agree with all that others do, but students and teachers should not be afraid to express themselves in a cooperative, respectful way. For example, think back to your middle school and high school days. Think about the teachers you liked best. Did you like them because they were great teachers and knew their subject well? Or did you like them because of the way they treated and respected you? SEL overlaps considerably with many components of the WSCC model. When SEL interventions are implemented in schools, they can have large and lasting impacts on students, teachers, and the overall social and emotional climate of the school.

Implementing a school crisis plan can assist with addressing situations that affect both the physical and social environments. A clear, written plan that includes procedures for handling various emergencies (e.g., fire, tornado, death of a student or staff member, mass illness, terrorism, suicide attempt), communication procedures, staff training, practice drills, coordination with local public safety agencies, among other procedures, can help ensure that if threats occur, safe practices are implemented.[27]

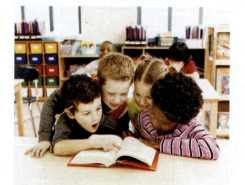

FIGURE 6.5   A healthy social environment that is conducive to learning is an important component of good school health.

© Digital Vision/Photodisc/Getty Images

School Health Education

School health education provides students with "the knowledge and skills they need to become successful learners and healthy adults."[28] If designed properly, school health education could be one of the most effective means to reduce serious health problems in the United States, including cardiovascular disease, cancer, motor vehicle crashes, homicide, and suicide.[29] Such a curriculum should focus on promoting the following priority health content[28]:

- Alcohol and other drugs
- Food and nutrition
- Mental and emotional health
- Personal health and wellness
- Physical activity
- Safety
- Sexual health
- Tobacco
- Violence prevention

School health education includes health education that takes place in the classroom as well as any other activities designed to positively influence the health knowledge and skills of students, parents, and school staff. For example, health education can take place when the school nurse gives a vision-screening test to a student or when coaches talk with their teams about concussion safety.

For health education to be effective, it should be well conceived and carefully planned. The written plan for school health education is referred to as the health **curriculum**. The curriculum not only outlines the **scope** (what will be taught) and the **sequence** (when it will be taught) but also provides (1) learning objectives, (2) standards (see **Box 6.3**), (3) learning experiences leading to the adoption and maintenance of specific health-enhancing behaviors, (4) possible instructional resources, and (5) methods for assessment to determine the extent to which the objectives and standards are met. If health instruction is to be effective, the health curriculum should include lessons of appropriate scope and sequence for all grades from pre-K through 12th grade.

Results from CDC's School Health Profiles show that best practice school health education is not widespread. To enhance the state of health education in schools, National Health Education Standards have been developed. The National Health Education Standards delineate the essential knowledge and skills that every student should know and be able to perform following the completion of quality school health education. The standards are neither a federal mandate nor a national curriculum, but rather provide a foundation for curriculum development, instructional delivery, and assessment of student knowledge and skills for students in grades pre-K through 12.[30] There are eight standards (see Box 6.3), and each standard has grade-level performance indicators set for grades pre-K–2, 3–5, 6–8, and 9–12. "The standards evolved from the health education profession's current thinking about what constitutes grade-appropriate and challenging content and performance expectations for students."[31] Individual states are free to adopt their own health education standards. Many states have used the National Health Education Standards as the framework for the development of their state level health education standards.

Curriculum a written plan for instruction

Scope part of the curriculum that outlines what will be taught

Sequence part of the curriculum that states the order in which the content will be taught

---

BOX 6.3   National Health Education Standards

1. Students comprehend functional health knowledge to enhance health.
2. Students analyze the influence of family, peers, culture, social media, technology, and other determinants on health behaviors.
3. Students demonstrate health literacy by accessing valid and reliable health information, products, and services to enhance health.
4. Students demonstrate effective interpersonal communication skills to enhance health.
5. Students demonstrate effective decision-making skills to enhance health.
6. Students demonstrate effective goal-setting skills to enhance health.
7. Students demonstrate observable health and safety practices.
8. Students advocate for behaviors that support personal, family, peer, school, and community health.

Reproduced from National Consensus for School Health Education. (2022). *National Health Education Standards: Model Guidance for Curriculum and Instruction (3rd Edition)*. www.schoolhealtheducation.org.

Development and Sources of Health Education Curricula

Each year, many school districts throughout the United States are faced with the task of developing a curriculum to guide health education. Such a task can be completed in one of several ways. First, a school district could obtain a prepackaged curriculum that has been developed by nationally recognized specialists. Some of these are prepared and sold by for-profit organizations, and others are available free of charge from nonprofit agencies (i.e., voluntary health agencies). A second means is to use the approved curriculum of either the state departments of education or health. A third method is to adopt a new health textbook series and consider the series as a district's curricular guide. And fourth, some districts may even develop their own in-house curriculum. Each of these approaches has its strengths and weaknesses, and school districts have to decide which approach best suits their particular situation.

Determining what is and what is not an effective curriculum can be a difficult process. The CDC has developed the Health Education Curriculum Analysis Tool (HECAT), a resource that school districts, schools, and others involved in the curriculum process can use to conduct their own analysis of health curricula. The HECAT, which is based on the National Health Education Standards and the CDC's *Characteristics of Effective Health Education Curriculum*, can help in the selection or development of appropriate and effective health education curricula and improve the delivery of health education.[28] See **Box 6.4** for a summary of characteristics of effective health education curricula, which can serve as a guide when evaluating and selecting materials.

In addition to the previously mentioned options, there are a number of additional sources available for obtaining health education curricula. Some of them may be comprehensive (include a variety of topics and for every grade level, K–12), and others may be topic and/or grade-level specific. These other sources include the following:

- *State departments of education or health.* Many states have either recommended or required a particular curriculum. Some states do not have comprehensive curricula but require instruction in some health topics, such as substance use and abuse and sexuality education.
- *Health agencies and associations.* Many of the voluntary health agencies (e.g., American Heart Association and American Lung Association) and other health-related organizations (e.g., National Dairy Council, Hazelden Foundation [cyberbullying], and Donate Life) have developed curricula for grades K–12. Most of these are not comprehensive, but they are

---

BOX 6.4   Characteristics of Effective Health Education Curricula

- Focuses on clear health goals and related behavioral outcomes
- Is research-based and theory-driven
- Addresses individual values, attitudes, and beliefs
- Addresses individual and group norms that support health-enhancing behaviors
- Focuses on reinforcing protective factors and increasing perceptions of personal risk and harmfulness of engaging in specific unhealthy practices and behaviors
- Addresses social pressures and influences
- Builds personal competence, social competence, and self-efficacy by addressing skills
- Provides functional health knowledge that is basic, accurate, and directly contributes to health-promoting decisions and behaviors

- Uses strategies designed to personalize information and engage students
- Provides age-appropriate and developmentally appropriate information, learning strategies, teaching methods, and materials
- Incorporates learning strategies, teaching methods, and materials that are culturally inclusive
- Provides adequate time for instruction and learning
- Provides opportunities to reinforce skills and positive health behaviors
- Provides opportunities to make positive connections with influential others
- Includes teacher information and plans for professional development and training that enhances effectiveness of instruction and student learning

Data from Centers for Disease Control and Prevention. (2021). *Health education curriculum analysis tool* (pp. OV4-OV5). Atlanta, GA: Author. https://www.cdc.gov/healthyyouth/hecat/index.htm

usually well done, supported by audiovisuals and handouts, and available either at very low or no cost.

- *Commercially produced curricula.* These curricula have been developed by private corporations for schools.

Counseling, Psychological, and Social Services

Counseling, psychological, and social services are services provided to support students' mental, behavioral, and social-emotional health. These services can include individual and group assessments, interventions, and referrals. Professionals, such as certified school counselors, psychologists, and social workers provide these services.[4]

Physical Education and Physical Activity

The opportunity for students to be physically active throughout the school day is the goal of a comprehensive school physical activity program, which includes coordination of physical education and physical activity during school, physical activity before and after school, staff involvement, and family and community engagement.[4] Physical education serves as an academic subject and is characterized by a planned, sequential K–12 curriculum based on national standards for physical education. Emphasis is placed on physical fitness and skill development that lead to lifelong physical activity. Physical education should be taught by qualified teachers.[4]

Nutrition Environment and Services

The nutrition environment provides students with opportunities to learn about and practice healthy eating through available food choices, nutrition education, and messages about food. School nutrition services includes the cafeteria, vending machines, grab-and-go kiosks, school stores, concession stands, classroom rewards and parties, school celebrations, and fundraisers. School nutrition services provide access to a variety of nutritious and appealing meals that accommodate the health and nutrition needs of all students in a school district.[4]

Community Involvement

Community groups, organizations, health clinics, and local businesses can be critical partners in improving health and learning for students, thus positively impacting families and the community. Sharing resources and volunteering to support student learning and health are some of the ways the community can strengthen schools and those whom schools serve. Reciprocally, schools, students, and their families can enhance the community through service-learning opportunities and by sharing school facilities with the community.[4]

Family Engagement

Family engagement efforts include families and school staff working together to support and improve the learning, development, and health of students.[4]

Employee Wellness

Schools, in addition to being a place of learning, are also worksites. Fostering school employees' physical and mental health results in positive role models, and employees who are more productive and less likely to be absent.[4] Employee wellness programs includes programs, policies, benefits, and environmental supports that can ultimately result in reduced employee health insurance premiums, improved employee retention, and fewer substitutes.[4]

Issues and Concerns Facing School Health

Like most other community and public health programs, the school health program is not without its issues and concerns. Many of the leading school discipline problems are related to health, such as food insecurity, bullying and other forms of violence, drug use, and mental health challenges. In the remainder of this chapter, we summarize a few of the challenges that lie ahead for those who work in school health.

Lack of Support for School Health Initiatives

Schools are one of the most efficient systems for reaching children and youth to provide health services and programs yet, ironically, school health advocates have had limited success in getting coordinated school health or WSCC implemented in school districts across the country.

We have already pointed out that healthy children are better learners and that WSCC can contribute to the health of children. Coordinated school health efforts, like WSCC, help mobilize professionals and resources in schools and the local community to ensure efforts are systematic and intentional so that all students, not just those with health challenges, receive the support needed to promote health and school success.

Although many Americans support the idea that everyone is entitled to good health, we have not supported through legislation the notion that everyone is entitled to WSCC efforts in our schools. Obviously, getting legislation passed is a complicated process and is dependent on a number of different circumstances, including, but not limited to, economics, social action, and politics. Additionally, limited resources, lack of buy-in and investment, inability of schools to demonstrate competence and effectiveness to stakeholders, lack of organizational capacity, leadership support, and continued emphasis on high-stakes testing have made it difficult for school districts to make WSCC efforts a priority.[32,33] This difficult task should not deter those who feel WSCC is vital. It is becoming more and more clear that many of the answers to current and future health problems lie with the resources found in the school—the one institution of society through which all of us must pass.

The need for coordinated school health efforts should be obvious. We have taken the liberty to rephrase a quote from a group of school health experts who say it best: Society should not be as concerned with what happens when we implement WSCC as about what is likely to happen if we do not.[34] Although garnering support for coordinated school health and WSCC has been an uphill battle, we are moving in the right direction. For example, with the passing of the Child Nutrition and WIC Reauthorization Act of 2004,[12] school districts are required to institute local wellness policies promoting better nutrition, physical activity, and wellness. With the more recent passing of the Healthy, Hunger-Free Kids Act of 2010, school districts have greater accountability for implementation, evaluation, and public reporting related to local wellness policies.[35] Some states have taken this one step further by passing state legislation requiring districts to institute coordinated school health advisory councils.[36] While more work needs to be done, these concrete steps, which add a level of accountability, are moving school health efforts in the right direction.

School Health Curriculum Challenges

Controversy

The words sexual intercourse, suicide, substance use and abuse, sexually transmitted diseases, dating violence, contraception, death and dying, and even abstinence get attention. The very nature of the topics covered in a school health education curriculum today continues to create controversy in some districts and in different parts of the country. Yet, controversy is not new to school health education; it has followed health education ever since it first attempted to deal with the many issues that face youth (see **Figure 6.6**).

Controversy continues to be a challenge for health education for a number of reasons. Part of it deals with the pressure that has been applied to schools by conservative groups.

These groups are interested in discouraging health instruction that includes values-clarification activities and open-ended decision-making processes.[37] Others believe that controversy exists because of the differences in family value systems and religious beliefs. Questions, such as (1) Do students really need to learn in school how to use a condom? (2) Doesn't talk of suicide lead some students to think that it might be the best alternative for them? (3) Aren't chiropractors just health quacks? and (4) Why do students need to know about funeral preplanning in high school? These questions create legitimate concerns, but they are also issues that today's adolescents face. Lack of awareness, knowledge, and skills is not an excuse for undesirable health behavior. If the students do not get this information at school, where will they get it? Studies have shown that the institutions of church and family have taught little about the controversial topics included in health curricula.

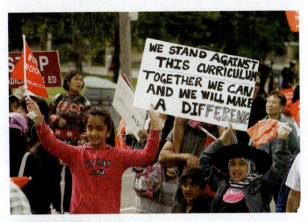

FIGURE 6.6   There are still many controversial issues that surround school health.
© igor kisselev/Alamy Stock Photo

Improper Implementation

Improper implementation of the curriculum is another challenge to school health (see **Box 6.5**). In 2015, the Every Student Succeeds Act (ESSA) replaced No Child Left Behind (NCLB) as the federal legislation that funds elementary and secondary education. One positive shift that came from this change in legislation was the removal of the term "core academic subjects." Instead, the law promotes a "well rounded education." This change allows for health and physical education to be eligible for federal funding that was previously restricted to "core academic subjects" under NCLB. Despite this change, school health still struggles to receive the attention it deserves. In many school districts throughout the United States, the low priority given to health has meant that individuals other than formerly trained heath education teachers provide much of the instruction. These people are not incapable of teaching health, but they have not been educated

---

BOX 6.5   Barriers to Comprehensive School Health Education

Although the importance of school health education is being recognized more and more, there are several barriers to its implementation. Research by various authors has informed health education specialists of barriers to establishing effective health instruction. Those barriers include the following:

1. Lack of local administrative commitment
2. Lack of adequately prepared teachers
3. Lack of time in the school day/year
4. Lack of money/funds
5. Health education's lack of credibility as an academic subject
6. Lack of community/parental support for controversial topics
7. Policy constraints
8. Teacher priorities
9. Pressure to focus on subjects included in high-stakes tests
10. General lack of reinforcement by state and local education policymakers

The top three barriers tend to be seen as the most significant. Recommendations to address them include the following:

1. Inviting administrators to workshops and conferences dealing with current health issues
2. Conducting quality in-service programs
3. Advocacy to school administrators and professors of education

Bender, S. J., Neutens, J. J., Skonie-Hardin, S., & Sorochan, W. D. (1997). *Teaching health science: Elementary and middle school* (4th ed., pp. 32). Jones & Bartlett Learning; Butler, S. C. (1993). Chief state school officers rank barriers to implementing comprehensive school health education. *Journal of School Health, 63*(3), 130–132; Telljohann, S. K., Symons, C. W., Pateman, B., & Seabert, D. (2023). *Health education: Elementary and middle school applications* (10th ed.). McGraw-Hill; Thackeray, R., Neiger, B. L., Bartle, H., Hill, S. C., & Barnes, M. D. (2002). Elementary school teachers' perspectives on health instruction: Implications for health education. *American Journal of Health Education, 33*(2), 77–82; Sy, A., & Glanz, K. (2008). Factors influencing teachers' implementation of an innovative tobacco prevention curriculum for multiethnic youth: Project SPLASH. *Journal of School Health, 78*(5), 264–273; Mann, M. J., & Lohrmann, D. K. (2019). Addressing challenges to the reliable, large-scale implementation of effective school health education. *Health Promotion Practice, 20*(6), 834–844; Birch, D. A., Goekler, S., Auld, M. E., Lohrmann, D. K., & Lyde, A. (2019). Quality assurance in teaching K-12 health education: Paving a new path forward. *Health Promotion Practice, 20*(6), 845–857.

to do so.[38] Reliance on a textbook as the curriculum, lack of awareness/implementation of state or national standards, an emphasis on content rather than skills, and limited, if any, coverage of topics that cause discomfort are some of the outcomes of improperly prepared teachers in the health classroom. The long-term result is that young people do not learn the information and skills necessary to live a healthy lifestyle.

School districts can help reduce controversy and improve the quality of health instruction by (1) implementing age-appropriate curricula, (2) using effective teaching methods, (3) gaining parent/guardian approval of curricula, (4) developing a school policy that enables parents/guardians to review the curricula and to withdraw their children from lessons that go against family or religious beliefs, (5) implementing a school policy that provides for the handling of concern by parents/guardians,[39] and (6) making sure qualified and interested teachers teach health.

School-Based Health Centers

Earlier in the chapter, we mentioned that a number of school districts across the country have opened school-based or linked health centers (SLHCs) to help meet the health needs of their students. In 1970, only one U.S. school had an SBHC/SLHC.[40] By 1984, that number had jumped to 31; by 1989, it had increased to 150.[41] Currently, there are approximately 3,900 school-based health centers operating nationwide.[42] SBHCs operate in four main delivery models: traditional school-based approach, school-linked, mobile, and telehealth-exclusive. The majority of SBHCs follow the traditional delivery model where the SBHC is located on school property. A growing trend is for traditional, school-linked, and mobile models supplementing in-person care with telehealth services.

Although there is no single model for SBHCs, this set of seven core competencies can be used to guide the delivery of health care in a school setting[43]:

- **Access:** SBHC assures students' access to health care and support services to help them thrive.
- **Student focus:** SBHC team and services are organized around student well-being and academic success.
- **High-quality care:** SBHC delivers high-quality, comprehensive care to achieve optimal outcomes for students.
- **Collaborative student partnership:** SBCH is typically governed and administered separately from the school, and works collaboratively with the educational environment to support the school's mission of student success.
- **School wellness:** SBHC engages with the school to participate, support, and improve a culture of health across the school community.
- **Systems coordination:** SBHC coordinates across relevant systems of care that share in the well-being of its patients.
- **Sustainability:** SBHC employs sound management practices to ensure a sustainable business.

As mentioned earlier in the chapter, there are a number of sound reasons why health centers should be based in schools—the primary reason being the ability to reach, in a cost-effective manner, a large segment of the population that is otherwise without primary health care.[44] Yet, SBHCs have not experienced the level of implementation that might be expected of a program that could make such a positive impact on the health of young people. Early on, SBHCs were frequent targets of intense criticism at the local and national levels by political and religious groups.[45-47] Much of the controversy surrounding SBHCs centered around cultural wars and partisan politics.[48] The issue of cultural wars revolved around the views of conservatives versus liberals, and how and where people should receive their health care. Whereas some people who support SBHCs would want their child treated as quickly and effectively as possible for a health problem, others who oppose the centers can see nothing but the "image of a condom on a cafeteria tray."[48] The key to working through the "cultural wars" problem is compromise. That is, recognition that each area of the country is different, and what are reasonable health services provided in an SBHC in one area are unacceptable in another. Thus, advocates of the centers say that the services provided by SBHCs are so badly needed that a single issue, such as reproductive health care should not keep an SBHC from existing.[48]

SBHCs offer an opportunity to address the growing mental health needs of adolescents. Currently, approximately 17% of SBHCs do not offer any form of behavioral health services. Additionally, SBHCs do not limit services to students enrolled in their schools. Seventy-two percent of SBHCs now serve students from other schools, which is an increase of 44% from 2016–2017. Fifty-nine percent serve school staff, which further supports the WSCC employee wellness efforts discussed earlier in this chapter. Family members (47%) and community members (33%) also are often able to seek services at a SBHC.[43]

Since their inception, funding for SBHCs has been an issue. Therefore, most of the SBHCs receive sponsorship from a variety of health system partnerships, such as a community health center, local health department, or hospital/medical center. Funding can often be more challenging, requiring multiple sources of support, such as billing/third party revenue; federal, state, and local grants and contracts; lead sponsor organization resources; private donations; and school system resources.[43]

Another one of the challenges facing SBHCs is the pressure for schools and school-related programs to be accountable for demonstrating their impact on improving the learning environment and academic outcomes.[49] Research studies have explored the link between SBHCs and health outcomes, resulting in positive findings. For example, there is a correlation between asthma and lower student attendance. For those students with asthma attending a school with an SBHC, there were fewer hospitalization days and school absences compared with children at control schools without an SBHC.[50] Much of the research shows positive outcomes; however, more research is needed to fill gaps in the understanding of the impact of SBHCs on adolescent health and academic outcomes. In this current climate of accountability within the educational system, indirect links do not provide enough evidence that SBHCs positively affect academic outcomes. Research demonstrating the specific correlation between SBHCs and health and academic outcomes is needed for SBHCs to gain greater implementation.[51]

Youth Health Issues in Schools

Violence

Over the years, schools have been viewed as safe havens for teaching and learning. But in recent years, there have been a number of high-profile incidents of violence in schools (e.g., Uvalde, Texas; Parkland, Florida; Newtown, Connecticut) that have continued to keep the concerns about violence in schools at the forefront in the minds of the general public. CDC Youth Risk Behavior data indicate that more than one in eight (13.0%) U.S. high school students had missed at least 1 day of school in the preceding month because that student felt unsafe either being at school or going to and from school and one of 11 (9.0%) students had been threatened or injured with a weapon on school property during the preceding year.[52]

We know that males are involved in more violent acts than females.[52] We also know that certain racial and ethnic groups participate in and are victims of violence at school more often than other students are.[52] Yet, it is close to impossible to predict who will be next to commit a violent act in a school.

Another form of violence that has received significant attention recently is bullying. Bullying can be defined as "unwanted, aggressive behavior among school-aged children that involves a real or perceived power imbalance."[53] Bullying can take many forms, such as physical (hitting); verbal (teasing or name calling); social (social exclusion or spreading rumors); and cyber (sending insulting messages or pictures by mobile phone or using the Internet).[53] Research indicates that nearly one in five high school students reported being bullied at school, with more than one in six reporting being bullied electronically in the past year[53,54] Being bullied can affect academic achievement and self-esteem. Bullying can also affect bystanders by creating a climate of fear and disrespect in schools. Furthermore, bullying behavior can be a sign of other serious antisocial or violent behavior by those who bully their peers.[53]

Like most other health problems, risk factors need to be identified and steps taken to reduce the risk of violent acts occurring in the schools. The CDC makes the following recommendations for schools to support teens, prevent violence, and improve the school climate as it relates to violence, bullying, and electronic aggression[55]:

- *Adopt policies and practices that create safe and supportive environments.*
- *Teach teens skills to navigate social and emotional challenges.*
- *Connect students to health and mental health services.*
- *Build strong bonds between staff and students to improve connectedness to school.*

It has become clear that violence is not a problem that will soon go away. Although many school personnel do not believe it is a problem in their schools, life has shown us that it can happen anywhere. Violence is an issue that all schools need to face and something for which they need to plan to reduce the risks to school children and personnel. "We send our children out into the world every day to explore and learn, and we hope that they will approach a trusted adult if they encounter a challenge; now, we need to apply this message to the virtual world."[56]

Mental Health

The CDC has declared, "our nation's youth are experiencing a mental health crisis."[57] There was concern about youth mental health prior to the COVID-19 pandemic, but those concerns grew exponentially as young people experienced profound disruptions at a critical period in their psychosocial development.[58] The percentage of high school students feeling sad and hopeless has gone from 28% in 2011 to 40% in 2023. When we dig deeper into these data, we learn that students who identify as female (53%) and LGBQ+ (65%) are more likely than other demographic groups to report persistent feelings of sadness or hopelessness.[57]

Many wonder how we got here. There is no one answer. What is known is that youth have been suffering for a long time. As stated, more than one in four high school students reported persistent sadness and hopeless since 2011.[57] The social isolation, academic disruption, death of loved ones due to COVID-19, parental job loss, and the sheer unknown are a few of the significant challenges young people across the country experienced.[59]

There are emerging data demonstrating the impact of social media on youth mental health. Nearly all adolescents aged 13 to 17 (95%) use social media and a large number of pre-adolescents aged 8 to 12 (40%) are also active on social media.[60] According to a report from the Office of the Surgeon General, "Scientific evidence suggests that harmful content exposure as well as excessive and problematic social media use are primary areas for concern."[61] While there are benefits to social media, such as helping youth access information and establish community and connection with peers, there is growing concern that social media interaction may negatively impact brain development and lead to increased harm for young people, especially those who are already experiencing poor mental health.[61]

Shortages in the behavioral health workforce were projected long before the COVID-19 pandemic with a 2013 report projecting a significant shortage of behavioral health providers in 2025, including more than 13,000 school counselors and more than 16,000 mental health and substance use social workers, among others, nationwide.[62] For context, according to the American School Counselor Association, the recommended student-to-school counselor ratio is 250:1. In 2022–2023, the national student-to-school-counselor ratio was 385:1.[63] There is little evidence that the mental health needs of our youth will be met any time soon.

In response to this health crisis, the Centers for Disease Control and Prevention developed an action guide to support school leaders in ensuring that schools can implement best practice prevention efforts and interventions now and in the future (see **Table 6.2**).[64] Given the many barriers families experience in accessing mental health services (e.g., provider

TABLE 6.2   Strategies for Promoting Mental Health in Schools

Strategy	Approach
Increase Students' Mental Health Literacy	• Deliver classroom-based mental health education curricula • Implement peer-modeling programs
Promote Mindfulness	• Deliver classroom-based mindfulness education • Dedicate time for students to independently practice mindfulness • Offer small group mindfulness activities
Promote Social, Emotional, and Behavioral Learning	• Provide classroom instruction focused on building social skills and emotional development • Offer targeted education focused on teaching social skills and emotional development
Enhance Connectedness Among Students, Staff, and Families	• Provide relationship-building programs
Provide Psychosocial Skills Training and Cognitive Behavioral Interventions	• Promote acceptance and commitment to change • Provide cognitive behavioral interventions • Engage students in coping skills training groups
Support School Staff Well-Being	• Offer mindfulness-based training programs • Provide therapeutic resources

Reproduced from Centers for Disease Control and Prevention. (2023). Promoting mental health and well-being in schools: An action guide for school and district leaders. https://www.cdc.gov/healthyyouth/mental-health-action-guide/pdf/DASH_MH_Action_Guide_508.pdf

shortages, insufficient or no insurance, transportation), schools can help families overcome these barriers by:

• Helping link students and families and providers offering mental health services via telehealth
• Using multiple funding streams for school-based mental health services
• Embedding mental health supports in school-based health centers

Schools are key in helping address the mental health crisis our young people are experiencing as they are well positioned to reach a large number of youths with strategies that can lessen the impact of negative experiences and improve students' health and well-being. The school is a safe and supportive environment that connects students to caring adults. Improved classroom behavior, school engagement, and positive peer relationships are a few of the benefits we can anticipate when intentional mental health education, prevention, and early interventions are provided through schools.[64]

Chapter Summary

• The potential impact of the Whole School, Whole Community, Whole Child (WSCC) effort on the health of children, their families, and the community is great because the school is the one institution through which we all must pass.

• To date, the full potential of school health has not been reached because of lack of support and interest.

• If implemented properly, WSCC can improve access to health services, educate students about pressing health issues, and provide a safe and healthy environment in which students can learn and grow.

• The foundations of the school health program include (1) a school administration that supports such an effort, (2) a well-organized school health advisory council that is genuinely interested in providing a coordinated program for the students, and (3) written school health policies.

• School health policies are critical for ensuring accountability, credibility, and the institutionalization of programs and efforts to make schools a healthy learning environment.

• The components of WSCC include (1) physical education and physical activity; (2) nutrition environment and

Scenario

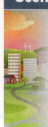

Joan is 18 years old and a recent high school graduate. She lives in a small town of about 2,700 people. Most of the town's residents rely on a larger city nearby for shopping, recreation, and health care. Joan had dated Dave for the past 2 years, but there was never any talk of marriage. Just before graduation, Joan learned that she was pregnant. At Thanksgiving, just as she was completing her seventh month of pregnancy, she went into premature labor. An ambulance rushed her to the emergency room of the hospital in the nearby city for what became the premature birth of her baby. While Joan was in recovery, doctors determined that her baby was not only premature, it also appeared to have other "developmental abnormalities." When asked whether she had received any prenatal care, Joan replied, "No, I couldn't afford it; besides, I didn't know where to go to get help."

Introduction

Creating a health profile of Americans requires a clear understanding of the health-related problems and opportunities of all Americans. Elsewhere in the text, we discussed the role of descriptive epidemiology in understanding the health of populations. In describing the personal characteristics of a population, age is the first and perhaps the most important population characteristic to consider when describing the occurrence of disease, injury, and/or death in a population. Because health and age are related, community and public health professionals look at rates for specific age groups when comparing the amount of disease between populations. When they analyze data by age, they use groups that are narrow enough to detect any age-related patterns, which may be present as a result of either the natural life cycle or behavioral patterns. Viewing age-group profiles in this manner enables community and public health workers to identify risk factors for specific age groups within the population and to develop interventions aimed at reducing these risk factors. Health promotion and disease prevention programs that are successful in reducing exposure to such risk factors within specific age groups can improve the health status of the entire population.

In this chapter, we present a health profile of mothers, infants (younger than 1 year), and children (ages 1–9 years). In the following two chapters, the health profiles will be presented for adolescents and young adults (10–24), adults (25–64), and older adults (65 and older). Various sources may group ages differently to describe and measure health status. In this book, we will consider children as those ages 1–9, which is consistent with how the World Health Organization and many public health professionals define the child age group.

Maternal, infant, and child health encompasses the health of women of childbearing age from prepregnancy through pregnancy, labor, delivery, and the postpartum period, and the health of the child prior to birth up to adolescence.[1] In this chapter, we define and discuss commonly used indicators for measuring maternal, infant, and child health; examine the risk factors associated with maternal, infant, and child morbidity and mortality; and review selected community programs aimed at improving the health of women of childbearing age, infants, and children in the United States.

Maternal, infant, and child health is important to a community for several reasons. First, maternal, infant, and child health statistics are regarded as important indicators of the effectiveness of disease prevention and health promotion services in a community. It is known that unintended pregnancies, late or no prenatal care, poor maternal and child nutrition, maternal drug use, low immunization rates, poverty, limited education, and insufficient child care—combined with a lack of access to healthcare services in a community—are precursors to high rates of maternal, infant, and childhood morbidity and mortality. Second, we now know that many of the risk factors specified can be reduced or prevented with the early intervention of educational programs and preventive medical services for women, infants, and children.

Maternal, infant, and child health the health of women of childbearing age and that of the child up to adolescence

These early community efforts provide a positive environment that supports the physical and emotional needs of the family and reduces the need for more costly medical or social assistance to these same members of society later in their lives (see **Figure 7.1**).

During the past several decades, the United States has made important progress in reducing infant and maternal mortality. Yet, in 2022, we saw a 3% increase over 2021, the first rise in the infant mortality rate in 20 years. Mortality rates increased significantly among infants of American Indian and Alaska Native women, as well as White, non-Hispanic women. Nevertheless, the substantial disparity between mortality rates for White and Black infants and mothers continues to be of concern. The mortality rate among infants of non-Hispanic Black mothers (10.86 per 1,000 live births) was over two times the rate among infants of non-Hispanic White mothers (4.52 per 1,000 live births) and infants of Hispanic mothers (4.88 per 1,000 live births) in 2022 (see **Figure 7.2**).[2] The pregnancy-related deaths (a maternal death occurred during pregnancy, delivery, or up to 1 year post-partum) was greatest among non-Hispanic White mothers (46.6%) followed by non-Hispanic Black mothers (31.4%), and Hispanic mothers (14.4%).[3] These data demonstrate that disparities may not be directly attributable to race or ethnicity, although certain diseases do occur more often among individuals of certain races or ethnicities. Often, race and ethnicity are proxy measures for other factors, such as socioeconomic status that may actually be at the root of observed disparities. For example, research indicates that low income and limited education correlate highly with poor health status.[4] The United States has a higher infant mortality rate than other industrialized nations; it ranked 33 out of 38 countries in 2019 based on the rate of deaths at birth (see **Figure 7.3**).[5] These differences among industrialized nations mirror differences in the health status of women before and during pregnancy; availability of preventive care; and ease of access, quantity, and quality of medical care for pregnant women and their infants.

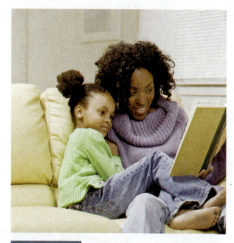

FIGURE 7.1   The health of a nation is often judged by the health of its mothers and children.

© Anthony Harris/Shutterstock

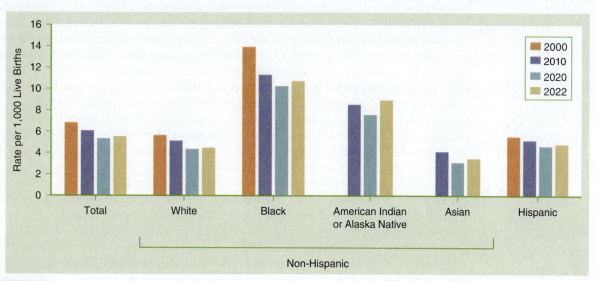

FIGURE 7.2   Infant mortality rates, by race and Hispanic origin of mother, United States, 2000, 2010, 2020, and 2022.

Note: *2000 data not available for American Indian or Alaska Native or Asian populations.*

Data from (1) Ely, D. M. & Driscoll, A. K. (2023). Infant mortality in the United States: Provisional data from the 2022 period linked birth/infant death file. National Vital Statistics Rapid Release, Report No. 33. https://www.cdc.gov/nchs/data/vsrr/vsrr033.pdf; (2) Ely, D.M. & Driscoll, A.K. (2023). Infant Mortality in the United States, 2021: Data from the Period Linked Birth/Infant Death File. National Vital Statistics Reports, Vol 72, No. 11. https://www.cdc.gov/nchs/data/nvsr/nvsr72/nvsr72-11.pdf; (3) National Center for Health Statistics. Health, United States, 2017: Figure 22: Infant mortality rates, by race and Hispanic origin of mother and leading causes of death: United States, 2005–2015. Hyattsville, MD. [2017]. Available from https://www.cdc.gov/nchs/hus/data-finder.htm

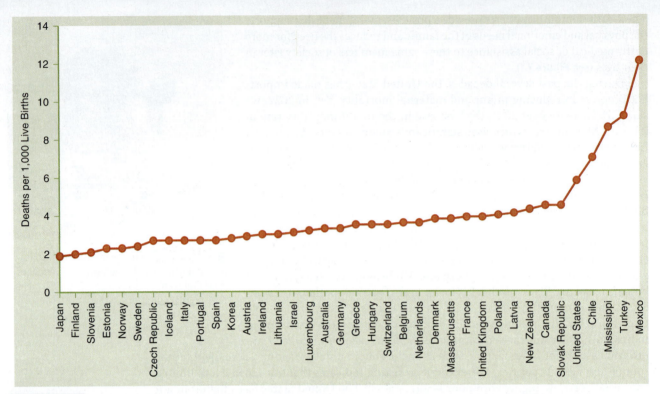

FIGURE 7.3 Infant mortality rates by OECD member countries and top- and bottom-ranking U.S. states, 2019.

Data from United Health Foundation. (2019). *America's Health Rankings® Annual Report.* https://assets.americashealthrankings.org/app/uploads/ahr_2019annualreport.pdf

Similar to the decline in infant and maternal mortality rates, the mortality rates of children and young adolescents (ages 1–14) have gone down significantly in the past few decades. The death rate declined from 64 to 28.0 per 100,000 population among 1- to 4-year-old children and 31 to 15.3 per 100,000 population among 5- to 14-year-old children between 1980 and 2022. Although the rates have declined over time, disparities between races and ethnicities persist (see **Figure 7.4**).[6]

Even with these improvements in child mortality rates, there is still much to be done to improve the health of American children. First, we must recognize that children today face other concerns that can put them at risk for poor health. These concerns have been referred to as the "new morbidities" and include their family and social environments, behaviors, economic security, and education (see **Box 7.1**).[7] Second, we must be concerned about the difference in mortality rates between races and socioeconomic status. If the young are indeed the hope for the future, the United States must continue to work hard to ensure the health of each infant and child, regardless of race or socioeconomic status.

Whereas numerous factors affect the health of both infant and child, many reflect or are related to the health status of the mother and her immediate environment. One of the first steps to ensure healthy children is to ensure that pregnant women have access to prenatal care early in pregnancy and that they receive proper care throughout. There is nothing more dependent than a fetus relying on a mother to eat nutritiously and to avoid drugs or a newborn that is reliant on an adult to survive and develop into a healthy child. Therefore, we begin by looking at the health status of mothers and the family structure.

Family and Reproductive Health

The family is one of society's most treasured foundations. It represents a primary social group that influences and is influenced by other people and establishments. Moreover, families are the primary unit in which infants and children are nurtured and supported regarding their healthy

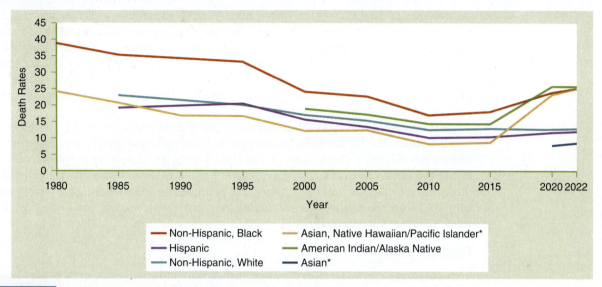

FIGURE 7.4 Death rates among children ages 5 to 14 by race and Hispanic origin: Selected years, 1980–2022.

*Data for Asian population for 1980–2015 is grouped with Native Hawaiian/Pacific Islander population. Data for Asian population is separate from Native Hawaiian/Pacific Islander for 2020 and 2022. Data for American Indian/Alaska Native not available before 2000.

Data from (1) Child Trends. (2019). *Infant, child, and teen mortality.* Available at https://www.childtrends.org/indicators/infant-child-and-teen-mortality; (2) Centers for Disease Control and Prevention, National Center for Health Statistics. (2024). *CDC Wonder Online Database.* https://wonder.cdc.gov/

development.[1] The U.S. Census Bureau defines a family as "a group of any two or more people (not necessarily, including a householder) residing together, and related by birth, marriage, or adoption."[8] This definition does not include a variety of cultural styles and optional family structures that exist in our society today. Friedman broadens the definition of family to include "two or more persons who are joined together by bonds of sharing and emotional closeness and who identify themselves as being part of the family."[9] It is important to remember that the concept of family has changed over time, varies greatly depending on social and cultural norms and values, and may be conceptualized differently on an individual basis.

With delays in childbearing, increases in cohabitation, and changes in societal norms related to having children outside of marriage, the percentage of births to unmarried women has risen over the past several decades. In 2022, the percentage of births to unmarried women was 39.8%, or more than double the 18.4% of live births to unmarried women that occurred in 1980.[10] Historically, nonmarital births were associated with teen childbearing, given that half of all unmarried women giving birth were under 20 years of age. However, the distribution of unmarried childbearing has shifted with more births to older unmarried women.[10] Births to unmarried teenagers have dropped and births to unmarried women in their 20s and 30s have increased.[10]

BOX 7.1   Each Day in America for All Children

5 children are killed by abuse or neglect.
8 children or teens die by suicide.
9 children or teens are killed with a gun.
20 children or teens die from accidents.
46 children or teens are injured with a gun.
59 babies die before their first birthday.
121 children are arrested for violent crimes.
223 children are arrested for drug crimes.
514 public school students are corporally punished.*

678 babies are born without health insurance.
827 babies are born into extreme poverty.
860 babies are born with low birthweight.
1,541 babies are born into poverty.
1,785 children are confirmed as abused or neglected.
1,909 children are arrested.
2,906 high school students drop out.*
14,206 public school students are suspended.*

*Based on 180 school days per year.

Reproduced from Children's Defense Fund. (2021). *The state of America's children 2021.* Available at https://www.childrensdefense.org/wp-content/uploads/2023/08/The-State-of-Americas-Children-2021.pdf

Nonmarital births also vary among other population subgroups. For example, in 2022, 27.1% of births to non-Hispanic White women were not married, whereas 69.3% of births to non-Hispanic Black women were not married.[10] Unmarried women are more likely than married women to experience negative birth outcomes, including low birth weight, preterm birth, small for gestational age, and fetal and infant death.[11–13] These associations are likely due to differences in social and financial support, as well as maternal education level and father acknowledgement and engagement, among other factors.[14]

It is important to keep in mind that within the marital status categories, women are still very heterogeneous. For example, "unmarried" includes both women who are single and those who are cohabiting with the father of their child. For the risk factors and pregnancy outcomes mentioned earlier, cohabiting women generally fall in between those who are married and those who are single but not cohabiting. For example, the odds of having a low birth weight baby are lowest for married women, higher for cohabiting women, and highest for single women who are not cohabiting.[11]

Teenage Births

Teen pregnancy and birth rates have declined steadily in recent years, in large part because of effective community and public health campaigns aimed at reducing teenage pregnancies. Between 1991 and 2021, the teenage birth rate (births per 1,000 females aged 15–19 years) in the United States has declined by 78% from 61.8 to 13.6 births per 1,000 teenagers.[10] Despite the recently declining rates, the United States still leads the industrialized world in teen pregnancy and birth rates by a large margin.[15]

The motivations for and the outcomes of teen pregnancies in the United States are varied and complex. No single narrative can explain all teenage pregnancies. While it has not always been viewed this way, teenage childbearing in the United States is generally seen as placing a social and financial burden on both the family and the community.[13] Teenage pregnancy and childbearing also have substantial economic consequences for society. Teenagers who become pregnant and have a child are more likely than their peers who are not mothers to drop out of school, rely on public assistance, and live in poverty.[16] The burden of teen childbearing is felt by taxpayers and communities due to the costs of health care, foster care, incarceration, and welfare. However, with the declining birth rate, evidence suggests that teen pregnancy prevention efforts result in significant annual savings for taxpayers (federal, state, and local).[16]

Teenage pregnancies are more likely to result in serious health consequences for these women and their babies compared with those who delay childbearing until their 20s.[11] A teenage mother is at greater risk for many pregnancy complications, including low birth weight and infant mortality.[17] Early and adequate prenatal care is critical for identifying and managing health and social issues early in the pregnancy to increase the likelihood of having a safe pregnancy and a healthy child.

Unfortunately, the adverse consequences related to teen pregnancy do not end when the child is born. It is difficult to determine the actual impact of teen pregnancy because the women who face educational, economic, and social hardships may be more likely to experience a teen pregnancy in the first place.[13] Although teen childbearing may not be the sole cause of these hardships, it does make it more difficult to overcome them. Children born to teenage mothers have higher rates of foster care placement, lower school achievement, rely more heavily on publicly funded health care, and daughters are more likely to become teenage mothers themselves compared with children born to older mothers.[17]

As stated in the introduction, the future of our nation depends on our children. The extent to which we actually believe this can be measured by the degree to which we plan, provide for, educate, and protect our children. Yet, on average, 1,599 children are abused or neglected every day, one in five children under the age of 5 relies on WIC to support their development, and one in six children lives in food-insecure households.[7] The need to plan a pregnancy and thereby place children first in families and in communities must be re-emphasized. Unwanted and unplanned childbearing has long been linked with adverse consequences for mothers, couples, and families as well as for the children themselves.[17]

The choice to become a parent is a critical decision that affects the individual and the community. People who become parents acquire the major responsibility for another human being.

They must provide an environment conducive to child development—one that protects and promotes health. However, the broader community also contributes to this growth and development. This is best illustrated by an African proverb, "it takes an entire village to educate and raise a child."[18] Therefore, the community must also make provisions for a child's care, nurture, and socialization.

Family Planning

Family planning gives individuals and couples the ability to determine if they wish to have children, and if so, the number and spacing of their children. Deciding whether to become a parent is an important and consequential decision. Parenthood requires enormous amounts of time, energy, and financial commitment, but most notably, it requires the willingness to take full responsibility for a child's growth and development. Planning a pregnancy is the first step to ensuring the best health for the mother and fetus during the pregnancy. In 2019, approximately 42% of pregnancies in the United States were unintended.[19]

An unintended pregnancy is a pregnancy that at the time of conception is either mistimed (occurred earlier than desired) or unwanted (occurred when no children or no more children were desired).[20] Unintended pregnancy is associated with a range of behaviors that can adversely affect the health of mothers and their babies. Maternal depression, maternal experience of interpersonal violence, and preterm birth and infant low birth weight are some of the significant health outcomes associated with unintended pregnancy. Additionally, delayed entry into prenatal care and the use of harmful substances, such as tobacco, alcohol, or other drugs can occur due to failure to recognize the pregnancy as early as if it had been planned.[21] Planning for pregnancy affords opportunities to address health issues and to adopt healthy practices, such as taking folic acid, that will help to increase the likelihood of a healthy pregnancy and delivery. The rate of unintended births is highest among women ages 15 to 24 years, unmarried women, (particularly those who are cohabitating), low-income women, those with lower educational attainment, and women of racial and ethnic minorities.[22]

The National Survey of Family Growth collects information to better understand unintended pregnancy. Using a 10-point scale, with 1 being "very unhappy to be pregnant" and 10 being "very happy to be pregnant," women were asked to report how they felt upon learning that they were pregnant. The average mean rating was 9.4 for intended pregnancies and 4.8 for unwanted pregnancies.[23] These indicators re-emphasize the importance of community health education programs for family planning.

Family planning is critical for reducing unwanted pregnancies and their adverse consequences. **Family planning** is defined as the process of determining the preferred number and spacing of children in one's family and choosing the appropriate means to achieve this preference. Although many maternal, infant, and child morbidity and mortality outcomes cannot be completely prevented by effective family planning, the frequency of occurrence can be reduced. Thus, preconception education and good gynecologic and maternal health care are required for effective family planning. Given that more than 40% of pregnancies are unintended, achieving and maintaining a good health status during the reproductive years is critical.[19]

Preconception care focuses on the health of partners, even before they are considering having children. For women, this includes making healthy choices and working with a healthcare provider for education and early identification of any health issues. The goal is for a woman to be as healthy as possible before getting pregnant. For example, a woman may work with her healthcare provider to stop smoking, start taking folic acid, or achieve a healthy weight. Partners should also focus on preconception health, as they need to maintain a healthy lifestyle and support healthy choices for their partner.

Community involvement in family planning programs has historically included both governmental and nongovernmental health organizations in the United States. The federal and state governments provide funding assistance through myriad family planning services, including Title X of the Public Health Service Act, Medicaid, state funds, the Maternal and Child Health Bureau, and social service block grants. Of these, Title X, or the Family Planning Act, is the only federal program dedicated solely to funding family planning and related reproductive healthcare services through the National Family Planning Program (Public Law 91-572).[24] **Title X** of the Public Health Service Act was signed into law by President Nixon in

Family planning determining the preferred number and spacing of children and choosing the appropriate means to accomplish it

Title X portion of the Public Health Service Act of 1970 that provides funds for family planning services for low-income people

1970 to provide family planning services to all who wanted but could not afford them. For over 4 decades, Title X has been this nation's major program to reduce unintended pregnancy by providing contraceptive and other reproductive healthcare services, such as screening for sexually transmitted infections, to low-income women. Currently, it provides funding support to a network of more than 4,100 family planning centers nationwide. Every year, 2.60 million family planning users receive healthcare services at family planning clinics funded by Title X. Those served are predominantly female, poor, uninsured, and younger than age 30. In 2022, 14% of all Title X users were male. Most male users were in their 20s or 30s and primarily sought contraceptive and STI testing services.[25]

Family planning services are provided through state, county, and local health departments, community centers, clinics, and hospital-, school-, and faith-based organizations.[25] The administration of all Title X grants is through state health departments or regional agencies that subcontract with local agencies and clinics. In 2022, slightly less than half of the grantees were state and local health departments (49%), and the rest were nonprofit family planning clinics and community health agencies.[25]

For clinics to receive funding under the Title X program, they must offer a broad range of acceptable family planning methods (e.g., oral contraceptives, condoms, sterilization, and abstinence); they must encourage family participation; they must give priority to low-income families; and they must not use abortion as a method of family planning.[26] In addition to family planning methods, clinics also provide a comprehensive group of other health services critical to their clients' sexual and reproductive health, including cervical cancer screenings and STI testing.[25] In 2019, major changes were made to Title X, prompting many former Title X grantees such as Planned Parenthood to withdraw. Although Title X funding has never funded abortion, the 2019 regulations required a physical separation between abortion services and other services covered by the Title X funding, as well as prohibiting referring clients for abortion services. These changes resulted in almost one-third of Title X sites leaving the program. Under the current administration, the regulation was reversed and the Title X network has even more sites than prior to the 2019 regulation changes.[27]

In 1981, family planning clinics that received federal funds were required to provide counseling on all options open to a pregnant woman, including abortion, as outlined in Title X. These facilities were not, however, allowed to perform abortions. In 1984, the "**gag rule**" regulations were enacted. These regulations barred physicians and nurses in clinics from receiving federal funds from counseling clients about abortions. Family planning providers challenged this legislation on the grounds that it denied women the right to information that was needed to make an informed decision. Many healthcare providers believed that the gag rule restricted their right to counsel a client even when childbirth could be detrimental to her health.[28] Supporters of the gag rule regulation felt that Title X was created to help prevent unwanted pregnancy by providing education and contraception services and was not intended to provide services related to pregnancy options.

In 1992, congressional action loosened the gag rule and allowed for abortion options to be discussed between a client and her physician at Title X facilities. Although this may appear to be a reasonable compromise, in reality, most women who visit family planning clinics are served by a nurse or nurse-practitioner and never see a physician; therefore, this change in the gag rule still did not permit the free exchange of information among clients and all professionals in the clinic. Presidents William Clinton, George W. Bush, Barack Obama, Donald Trump, and Joe Biden each reversed the regulations regarding the gag rule set by their predecessor.

Controversy regarding acceptable family planning methods is not new in our country. In the early 1900s, a maternity nurse by the name of Margaret Sanger delivered babies in the homes of poor, mostly immigrant women.[29] Sanger began to write articles about sex education and women's health to address the lack of information she saw in her work. However, she faced challenges disseminating this information because of the "Comstock Laws," which made it a federal offense to provide information, devices, or medications related to contraception and unlawful abortion through the mail. Sanger faced many obstacles, including numerous stays in prison, to spread her message during a time when birth control and sexual health were very controversial.

Gag rule regulations that barred physicians and nurses in clinics receiving federal funds from counseling clients about abortions

In 1921, Margaret Sanger, with the help of funds from numerous supporters worldwide, founded the National Birth Control League. The establishment of this organization is credited with starting the birth control movement in the United States. The purpose of this organization was to win greater public support for birth control by demonstrating the association between a woman's ability to control her fertility and the improvement of both her health and the health of children. In addition, Sanger also challenged the morality of the times by declaring that women had the right to experience sexual pleasure and that freeing them from the fear of pregnancy would assist women in achieving this. In 1942, the National Birth Control League joined with hundreds of family planning clinics nationwide and formed the Planned Parenthood Federation of America.[29]

Today, Planned Parenthood Federation of America, Inc. has grown to be the largest reproductive healthcare organization in the world and is committed to providing high-quality inclusive and comprehensive sexual and reproductive healthcare services no matter the income, insurance, gender identity, sexual orientation, race, or immigrant status of an individual.[30] This not-for-profit organization serves 2.05 million patients each year. Currently, Planned Parenthood operates approximately 600 health centers; it is estimated that their services avert an estimated 325,000 unintended pregnancies each year.[31]

Evaluating the Success of Community Health Family Planning Programs

The establishment of local family planning clinics, many of which receive funding through Title X, has resulted in an improvement in maternal and child health indicators for the communities served. Many people in need of family planning services are uninsured and rely on family planning clinics that may provide contraception at minimal or no cost. Title X funding enables the support network of more than 4,100 clinics that provide comprehensive family planning services to approximately 2.60 million clients each year, 80% of whom are low income, and 15% of whom are under the age of 20.[25] By providing access to contraceptive materials, instructions on how to use contraception effectively, and counseling about reproductive health matters, community family planning clinics are able to show large reductions in unintended pregnancies, abortions, and births. Publicly subsidized family planning services help postpone or avoid 2 million unplanned pregnancies, which would otherwise have resulted in some 1 million births and 700,000 abortions.[32] Publicly funded family planning services are vital to enabling low-income women to avoid unintended pregnancy. From an economic perspective, each dollar invested in publicly funded family planning services saved $4.83 in Medicaid expenditures needed to pay the medical costs of pregnancy, delivery, and early childhood care.[32]

The Affordable Care Act (ACA)'s expanded regulations required new private health plans written on or after August 1, 2012, to cover contraceptive counseling, services, and prescriptions at no out-of-pocket cost to patients. Since that time, the changes have led to millions of women having guaranteed access to free preventive women's health services, despite some inconsistencies in the implementation of the law.[33, 34] However, despite the increase in health insurance coverage through the ACA, 31% of visits to Title X-funded clinics were by patients without insurance coverage, which is three times the national uninsured rate for U.S. adults,[25] and many insured persons still depended on these clinics to provide access to care.[35] While many women take advantage of the free preventive services, including birth control cost coverage afforded through the ACA, a significant number of women (43%) are still unaware of these free preventive women's health services.[34]

Abortion

Abortion has been legal throughout the United States since 1973 when the Supreme Court ruled in the **Roe v. Wade** case that women, in consultation with their physician, have a constitutionally protected right to have an abortion in the first trimester of pregnancy, free from government interference.[36] As a result of the *Roe v. Wade* decision, the number of women dying from illegal abortions has diminished sharply during the last 3 decades in the United States. In June of 2022, the U.S. Supreme Court overturned the federal constitutional right to abortion in *Dobbs v. Jackson*, which left the legality of abortion to individual states.[37]

Since 1969, the Centers for Disease Control and Prevention (CDC) have been documenting the number and characteristics of women obtaining legal, induced abortions to monitor

Roe v. Wade 1973 Supreme Court decision that made it unconstitutional for state laws to prohibit abortions in the first trimester for any reason and placed restrictions on the conditions under which states could regulate them in the second and third trimesters

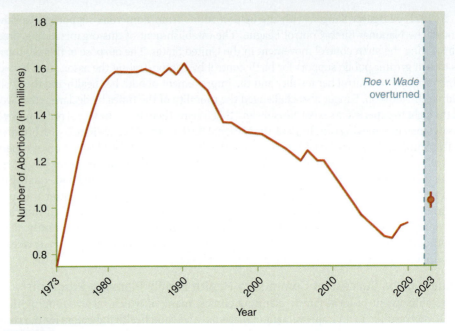

FIGURE 7.5 Number of clinician-provided abortions, United States 1973–2023.

Reproduced from Guttmacher Institute. (2024). Abortion in the United States. https://www.guttmacher.org/fact-sheet/induced-abortion-united-states

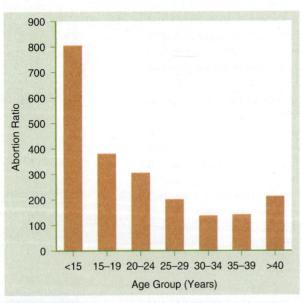

FIGURE 7.6 Abortion ratio, by age group in selected reporting areas—United States, 2021.

Note: Ratio is calculated by the number of abortions obtained by women in a specific age group per 1,000 live births to women in that same age group. For the total abortion ratio only, abortions for women of unknown age were distributed according to the distribution of abortions among women of known age.

Data from Kortsmit, K., Nguyen, A. T., Mandel, M. G., Hollier, L. M., Ramer, S., Rodenhizer, J., Whiteman, M. K. (2023). Abortion surveillance—United States, 2021. *Morbidity and Mortality Weekly Report, 72*(9):1-29. https://www.cdc.gov/mmwr/volumes/72/ss/ss7209a1.htm

unintended pregnancy and to assist with efforts to identify and reduce preventable causes of morbidity and mortality associated with abortions. The number, rate (number of abortions per 1,000 women 15–44 years of age), and ratio (number of abortions per 1,000 live births) of abortions in 2021 was 625,978, 11.6, and 204, respectively (see **Figure 7.5**).[38] Women aged 20 to 29 years make up the largest percentage of abortions (57.0%) and have the highest abortion rate compared with other age groups (**Figure 7.6**). A much higher percentage of abortions are to unmarried women (87.3%) compared with married women (12.7%).[38] Non-Hispanic White and non-Hispanic Black women accounted for the highest percentage of all abortions (30.2 and 41.5%, respectively). White women had the lowest abortion rate (6.4 abortions per 1,000 women aged 15–44 years) and ratio (116 abortions per 1,000 live births). Black women had the highest abortion rate (28.6 abortions per 1,000 women aged 15–44 years) and ratio (498 abortions per 1,000 live births).[38]

With the June 2022 Supreme Court decision in **Dobbs v. Jackson Women's Health Organization**, the U.S. abortion policy landscape continues to evolve. The fate of legalized abortion is as unclear as the right of a client to discuss abortion options in federally funded clinics. The Hyde Amendment of 1976 made it illegal to use federal funds to perform an abortion except in cases where the woman's life was in danger. The *Roe v. Wade* Supreme Court ruling made it unconstitutional for state laws to prohibit abortions. The *Dobbs v Jackson Women's Health Organization* Supreme Court ruling overturned *Roe v. Wade* and, as a result, state laws and policies have been changing rapidly. Nine states immediately banned abortion under "trigger" laws that took effect once

Roe v. Wade no longer applied. One year post-*Roe v. Wade*, abortion legality in the country includes[39]:

- Abortion is completely banned in 13 states (Alabama, Arkansas, Idaho, Kentucky, Louisiana, Mississippi, Missouri, North Dakota, Oklahoma, South Dakota, Tennessee, Texas, and West Virginia).
- Abortion is unavailable in Wisconsin because of ongoing legal complexities.
- In Arizona, a court clarified that an 1864 abortion ban, predating statehood, will not be repealed, but doctors will not be prosecuted for providing abortions. A ban on abortion at 15 weeks of pregnancy is in effect.
- In Georgia, a 6-week abortion ban (passed in 2019) was allowed to take effect in November of 2022 while litigation continues.
- Ohio's 6-week abortion ban (passed in 2019) is also in litigation and abortion remains legal in the state up to 22 weeks after the last menstrual period.
- In Utah, the state's trigger ban remains blocked and an 18-week abortion ban is in effect.
- In Wyoming, the state's trigger ban originally went into effect shortly after the *Dobbs* ruling but has since been blocked in court.

The issue of abortion has become a hotly debated topic. Political appointments can be won or lost, depending on a candidate's stance as "pro-life" or "pro-choice" on the abortion issue (see **Figure 7.7**).

Pro-life groups believe that life begins at conception and that an embryo is a person. Therefore, they conclude that performing an abortion is an act of murder. The **pro-choice** position is that women have a right to reproductive freedom. Pro-choice advocates think that the government should not be allowed to force a woman to carry to term and give birth to an unwanted child. Evidence shows that laws against abortion do not correspond with lower rates of abortion. In fact, the highest rates of abortion occur in countries where the practice is illegal, and the lowest rates are in countries where it is legal and access to contraception is high. This suggests that access to contraception and corresponding declines in unintended pregnancy are the most effective means to reducing abortions. In countries where abortion is illegal, women may resort to dangerous methods to terminate the pregnancy.[40] Unsafe abortions are a significant contributor to maternal death. There are also extenuating circumstances, such as rape or danger to the mother if she continues to carry the child, which make the issue less clear. There is no easy solution to the question of abortion; determining when life begins can only be decided by each individual based on their own values and beliefs.

Pro-life a medical/ethical position that holds that performing an abortion is an act of murder

Pro-choice a medical/ethical position that holds that women have a right to reproductive freedom

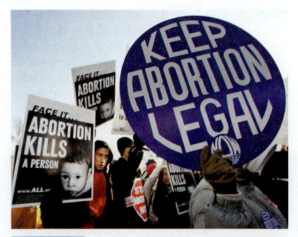

FIGURE 7.7   Political appointments and elections can be won or lost on the issue of abortion.
© Manuel Balce Ceneta/AP/Shutterstock

Maternal Health

Maternal health encompasses the health of women in the childbearing years, including those in the prepregnancy period, those who are pregnant, and those who are caring for young children (see **Figure 7.8**). The effect of pregnancy and childbirth on women is an important indicator of their health. Pregnancy and delivery can lead to serious health problems. Maternal mortality rates are the most severe measure of ill health for pregnant women.

The World Health Organization defines a maternal death (maternal mortality) as "the death of a woman while pregnant

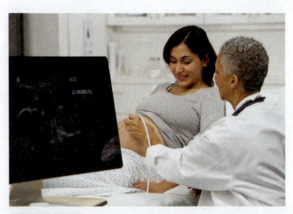

FIGURE 7.8   Maternal health encompasses the health of women in the childbearing years.
© Ariel Skelley/DigitalVision/Getty Images

or within 42 days of termination of pregnancy, irrespective of the duration and site of the pregnancy, from any cause related to or aggravated by the pregnancy or its management but not from accidental or incidental causes."[41] The maternal mortality rate is the number of maternal deaths per 100,000 live births in a given year. Birth certificates can be used to determine the number of total live births, whereas the total number of pregnant women is unknown; therefore, the number of live births is used as the denominator even though maternal mortality includes women who died without having a live birth.

In the United States, the maternal mortality ratio has increased over time from 7.2 deaths per 100,000 live births in 1987 to 24.9 deaths per 100,000 live births in 2020. The reason for this increase is unclear and is likely due, in part, to changes in reporting.[42] The maternal mortality ratio, however, has remained relatively stable prior to this year.[42] Causes of maternal death vary greatly by geographic region, likely due to differences in medical care throughout pregnancy and delivery. Infection or sepsis, including COVID-19, accounts for the increased ratio in 2020 as the percent of associated pregnancy deaths is two times the next leading cause of maternal death. The increase in the 2020 maternal mortality ratios can be greatly attributed to the COVID-19 pandemic as other federal surveillance data systems report mortality rates similar to pre-pandemic.[41] Aside from COVID-19, cardiovascular conditions and thrombotic pulmonary and other embolisms account for the largest proportion of maternal deaths in the United States. An increased number of pregnant women with chronic diseases, such as hypertension and diabetes may be contributing to mortality in the United States (see **Figure 7.9**).[43]

Of all maternal deaths, almost 95% occur in low or lower-middle income countries, and most could have been prevented. The maternal mortality ratio is 430 deaths per 100,000 live births in low-income countries, compared with 13 per 100,000 live births in high-income countries.[44] Most maternal deaths are preventable. Preventing unintended pregnancies and ensuring early initiation of skilled prenatal care, and care during and post childbirth greatly contributes to reductions in perinatal illness, disability, and death for both the mother and the infant.[44] In addition, a number of underlying causes of high maternal morbidity and mortality rates include poverty, sociocultural factors, and limited education.

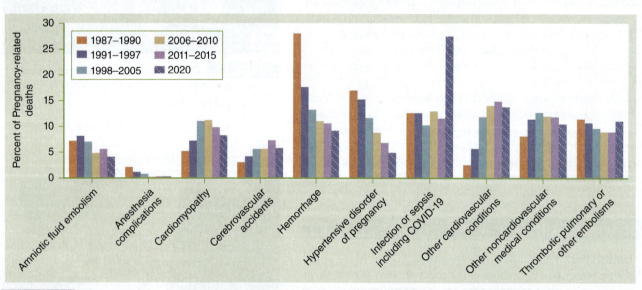

FIGURE 7.9 Cause-specific proportionate pregnancy-related mortality: United States, 1987–2020.

Data from (1) Creanga, A. A., Berg, C. J., Syverson, C., Seed, K., Bruce, F. C., & Callaghan, W. M. (2015). Pregnancy-related mortality in the United States, 2006–2010. *Obstetrics and Gynecology, 125(1)*, 5–12. Available at http://dx.doi.org/10.1097/AOG.0000000000000564; (2) Petersen, E. E., Davis, N. L., Goodman, D., Cox, S., Mayes, N., Johnston, E., Syverson, C., Seed, K., Shapiro-Mendoza, C. K., Callaghan, W. M., & Barfield, W. (2019). Vital signs: Pregnancy-related deaths, United States, 2011–2015, and strategies for prevention, 13 States, 2013–2017. *Morbidity and Mortality Weekly Report, 68(18)*, 423–429. Available at https://www.cdc.gov/mmwr/volumes/68/wr/mm6818e1.htm?s_cid=mm6818e1_w#T1_down. (3) Centers for Disease Control and Prevention. (2024). Pregnancy mortality surveillance system. https://www.cdc.gov/reproductivehealth/maternal-mortality/pregnancy-mortality-surveillance-system.htm

Preconception and Prenatal Health Care

Preconception health care and **prenatal health care** are essential for improving outcomes for mothers and infants. *Preconception care* is individualized care for partners that is designed to reduce maternal and fetal illness and mortality, increase the success of conception when pregnancy is desired, and to provide contraceptive education to prevent undesired pregnancy.[45] Often, medical and behavioral risk factors that can lead to negative pregnancy outcomes can be identified and modified before conception.[46] Ideally, a woman will obtain preconception care prior to pregnancy and can transition into prenatal health care once her pregnancy begins. The CDC encourages all women to develop a reproductive health plan and outlines steps that women can take to be ready for a healthy pregnancy (see **Box 7.2**).[47]

During prenatal visits, tests are performed on both the mother and fetus to assess any potential risks, to treat any maternal or fetal complications, and to monitor the growth and development of the fetus. In addition, counseling and guidance are provided regarding the various aspects of pregnancy, including weight gain, exercise, nutrition, and overall health. The woman and her provider will also discuss what to expect and options for the delivery. Nutrition counseling is especially critical early in pregnancy (and ideally would occur during preconception counseling), as many nutritional deficits can increase the risk for birth defects that develop in the first trimester. For example, pregnant women should have at least 400 micrograms of folic acid intake daily, which is often difficult to achieve through food sources alone, making prenatal vitamins an essential tool for prenatal nutritional health. Use of a multivitamin containing folic acid has been shown to reduce the risk of neural tube defects like spina bifida by two-thirds.[47]

Prenatal care is crucial to maternal and infant health. Women who receive early and continuous prenatal health care have better pregnancy outcomes than women who do not. A pregnant woman who receives no prenatal care is three times more likely to give birth to a **low birth weight infant** (one who weighs less than 5.5 pounds or 2,500 grams) as one who receives the appropriate care, and she is five times more likely to have her baby die in infancy.[48] Getting pregnant women into prenatal care early (during the first 3 months of pregnancy) is the main policy goal of most publicly funded programs designed to reduce the incidence of low birth weight and infant mortality in the United States. However, barriers to receiving prenatal care are complex and difficult to address. Barriers reported by women receiving late or no prenatal care included a lack of insurance coverage for visits, an inability to receive an appointment when desired, the mother being too busy or not having transportation; not knowing she was pregnant, and not wanting others to know she was pregnant.[49]

While most (97.9%) U.S. women receive some level of prenatal care, there is still a significant gap in the adequacy of prenatal care as only 75.5% of women are currently receiving care designated as adequate by federal designation standards.[50] The target goal for Healthy People 2030 is for 80.5% of pregnant women to receive early and adequate prenatal care.[51] Like many aspects of maternal health, disparities exist. Non-Hispanic Black and Hispanic women are not receiving prenatal care at the same rate as White women. Not receiving prenatal care in the first trimester, delaying care to the fifth month or later, and receiving fewer than the recommended number of prenatal care visits are some of the specific prenatal recommendations where racial

---

Preconception health care medical care provided to men and women to promote health prior to conception

Prenatal health care medical care provided to a pregnant woman from the time of conception until the birth process occurs

Low birth weight infant newborn who weighs less than 2,500 grams, or 5.5 pounds, at birth

---

BOX 7.2   Checklist for Preconception Health

1. Talk to your medical provider—discuss current medical conditions, lifestyle and behaviors, medications, and vaccines.
2. Take 400 micrograms of folic acid every day.
3. Stop drinking alcohol, smoking, and using certain drugs.
4. Avoid toxic substances and environmental contaminants.
5. Reach and maintain a healthy weight.
6. Learn your family history.
7. Get mentally healthy, including support if in a stressful or abusive environment.

Modified from Centers for Disease Control and Prevention. (2024). *About planning for pregnancy.* Available at https://www.cdc.gov/pregnancy/about/index.html

disparities exist.[50,51] Educational attainment is also associated with prenatal care—women with less than a high school education are the least likely to receive late or no prenatal care).[51]

Infant Health

An infant's health depends on many factors, which include the mother's health and her health behavior prior to and during pregnancy, genetic characteristics, level of prenatal care, the quality of her delivery, and the infant's environment after birth. The infant's environment includes not only the home and family environment but also the availability of essential medical services, such as a postnatal physical examination, regular visits to a physician, and the appropriate immunizations. The infant's health also depends on proper nutrition and other nurturing care in the home environment. Shortcomings in these areas can result in illness, developmental problems, and even the death of the child.

Infant Mortality

Infant mortality is an important measure of a nation's health because it is associated with a variety of factors, such as maternal health, access to quality medical care, socioeconomic conditions, and public health practices.[23] An infant death (infant mortality) is the death of a child younger than 1 year (see **Figure 7.10**). The infant mortality rate is expressed as the number of deaths of children younger than 1 year per 1,000 live births.

The infant mortality rate has decreased substantially from the early 1900s.[4] Decreases in the infant mortality rate during this period have been attributed to economic growth, improved sanitation, advanced clinical care, improved access to health care, and better nutrition. Improvements made in the 1990s were attributed particularly to the availability of better treatment for respiratory distress syndrome and the recommendation that infants be placed on their backs when sleeping.[4] Between 2000 and 2022, infant mortality rates have been fairly consistent at a current rate of 5.60 deaths per 1,0000 live births.[52] The leading causes of infant death include congenital malformations, preterm birth/low birth weight, sudden infant death syndrome (SIDS), accidents, and maternal complications of pregnancy.[52]

Infant deaths, or infant mortality, can be further divided into neonatal mortality and postneonatal mortality. Neonatal mortality includes deaths that occur during the first 28 days after birth. Approximately two-thirds of all infant deaths take place during this period.[4] The most common causes of neonatal death are disorders related to short gestation (premature births) and low birth weight, congenital malformations, and complications of pregnancy.[53] Postneonatal mortality includes deaths that occur between 28 days and 365 days after birth. The most common causes of postneonatal deaths are SIDS, accidents, and congenital malformations.[53]

Disparities in infant mortality by race and ethnicity are both great and persistent. In 2022, the infant mortality rate was highest for non-Hispanic Black mothers (10.86 per 1,000 live births). This is more than twice the rate for non-Hispanic White mothers (4.88 per 1,000 live births).[52] These disparities are believed to be rooted in broader societal inequities associated with racism and discrimination, such as differences in insurance coverage and access to care.[54]

Improving Infant Health

In part because of medical research and public health and social services supported by both public and private organizations, infant mortality has declined considerably during the past few decades. However, there are many opportunities for decreasing infant deaths and improving infant health even further through reducing risk factors associated with these conditions.

Premature Births

The average length of gestation is 40 weeks, and premature (or preterm) babies are those born prior to 37 weeks of gestation. In 2022, preterm birth affected about one of every 10 infants born in the United States. While the preterm birth rate has remained fairly consistent over the past

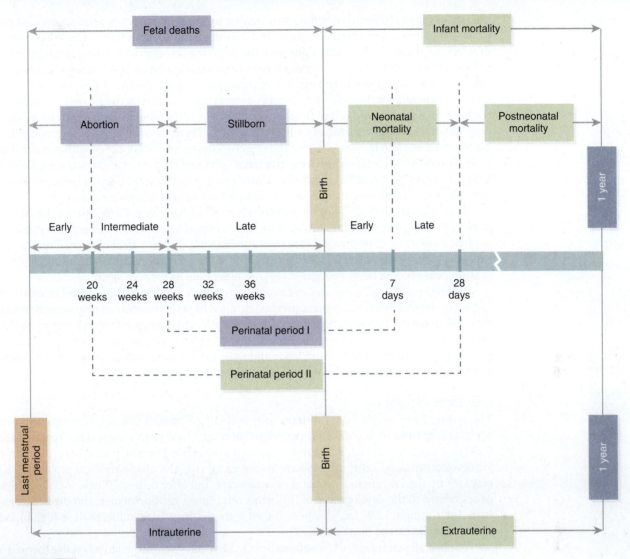

FIGURE 7.10   Important early-life mortality time periods.

decade there continue to be disparities by race, which can also be associated with maternal age and education level.[54] Disorders related to short gestation and low birth weight are the leading causes of neonatal death in the United States.[53] Because premature babies usually have less developed organs than full-term babies, they are more likely to face multiple serious health problems following delivery. Premature babies often require neonatal intensive care, which uses specialized medical personnel and equipment. In the United States, preterm birth costs the healthcare system are estimated at $2.52 billion per year.[55] The majority of the expense is for medical care provided in infancy. Other factors that contribute to the economic burden are maternal care services, early intervention services, special education for preterm infants with learning difficulties, and lost labor productivity.[56] Although it is well established that babies born before 37 weeks have a higher risk of negative outcomes, development of key organs, such as the brain, lungs, and liver, occurs up until 39 weeks. In fact, the brain at 35 weeks only weighs two-thirds of what it will at 39 to 40 weeks. Infants born 39 weeks or later are less likely to have problems with vision and hearing, are more likely to gain adequate weight before delivery, and are more likely to be able to suck and swallow appropriately.[57] Although labor occurs naturally for many women, some women decide with their doctors to have labor induced. This is where the doctor starts labor using medications or other methods, such as "breaking the woman's water." Inductions increase the risk of many problems, including stronger, more painful contractions; infection; changes in the baby's heart rate; uterine rupture; and needing a cesarean section.[57] There has been a dramatic increase in labor inductions over the past two decades, with rates increasing from 9.6% in 1990 to 27.1% in 2018.[10] Although inductions are sometimes done for medical reasons, there has been an increase in the number of inductions that are elective.[58] This means there is no medical reason for the induction, but it is done as a matter of convenience (e.g., scheduling the birth for a particular day and time) or preference (e.g., the woman is uncomfortable being pregnant or wants a certain doctor to deliver the baby). There are many reasons a woman or her doctor could want an induction. Given the negative consequences associated with preterm and early-term deliveries, an increase in elective inductions, and elective cesarean section deliveries before 39 weeks' gestation has resulted in a nationwide effort to reduce births before 39 weeks through provider and patient education, and implementation of quality measures.[57,58]

Approximately half of all premature births have no known cause. Known major risk factors associated with preterm labor and birth include a woman's past history of preterm delivery, multiple fetuses, late or no prenatal care, cigarette smoking, drinking alcohol, using illegal drugs, exposure to domestic violence, lack of social support, low income, diabetes, anemia, high blood pressure, obesity, and being younger than 17 or older than 35 years of age.[56]

Therefore, although a number of causes of premature birth may have eluded researchers and are currently beyond our control, prenatal care and lifestyle changes can help women reduce their risk of having a premature delivery. Consequently, there is much that community health programs can do to assist a woman in reducing her risk of having a premature baby—specifically, educating parents about premature labor and what can be done to prevent it and expanding access to healthcare coverage so that more women can get prenatal care.

Low Birth Weight

The average birth weight for a full-term baby is about 7.5 pounds (3.5 kg), although between 5.5 lb. (2.5 kg.) and 10 lb. (4.5 kg.) is considered normal.[59] Low birth weight (LBW) infants are those that weigh less than 2,500 grams, or about 5.8 pounds.[10] The fetal period is a critical time for development, and LBW infants have an increased risk of multiple medical problems and may require special care in a neonatal intensive care unit after delivery. These include health issues related to the development of the baby's respiratory, cardiovascular, and digestive systems. Interestingly, LBW has also been linked with problems later in life, such as high blood pressure, diabetes, and heart disease.[60]

The overall percentage of U.S. infants born at LBW has remained relatively stable (between 6.97% and 8.28%) in the last 2 decades (see **Figure 7.11**).[10] However, LBW must continue to be aggressively targeted, especially among non-Hispanic Black mothers, who have almost twice the rate of LBW babies.[10] Two factors generally recognized to govern infant birth weight are the duration of gestation (premature births) and intrauterine growth rate. Approximately two-thirds of LBW infants are born premature. Therefore, reduction in premature births holds the most potential for overall reduction in LBW. Intrauterine growth restriction (IUGR), or small for gestational age, is when a baby's weight is below the tenth percentile for their gestational age. Causes of IUGR include low maternal weight; poor nutrition during pregnancy; birth defects; use of drugs, cigarettes, or alcohol; maternal health problems; placental or umbilical cord abnormalities; and having multiples (i.e., twins, triplets, etc.).[61] Therefore, all pregnant women should (1) get early and regular prenatal care; (2) eat a balanced diet, including adequate amounts of folic acid; (3) gain the appropriate amount of weight based on Institute of Medicine (IOM) guidelines; and (4) avoid smoking and drinking alcohol.[60,62]

Cigarette Smoking

Research has shown that maternal cigarette smoking during pregnancy was one of the most common causes of infant morbidity and mortality in the United States, therefore making it an ideal target for intervention. The percentage of women who smoked during pregnancy has decreased significantly over time, from 13.2% in 2010 to 4.6% in 2021[10], exceeding the Healthy People 2030 target of 95.7% of females giving birth reporting not smoking during pregnancy.[63]

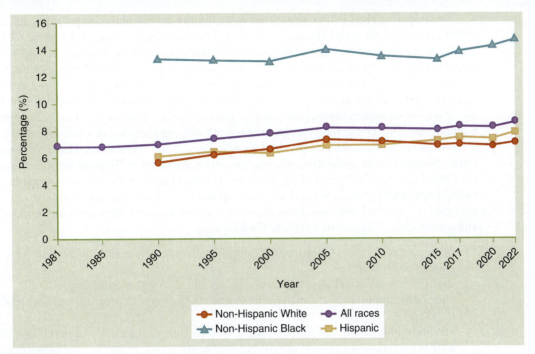

FIGURE 7.11   Percentage of infants born at low birth weight by race and Hispanic origin of the mother, select years 1981–2022.

Note: Persons of Hispanic origin may be of any race. "All races" includes races other than non-Hispanic White, non-Hispanic Black, and Hispanic.

Data from Osterman, M. J., Hamilton, B. E., Martin, J. A., Driscoll, A. K., Valenzuela, C. P. (2024). *Births: Final data for 2022. National Vital Statistics Reports, 73*, 2. Hyattsville, MD: National Center for Health Statistics. doi: https://dx.doi.org/10.15620/cdc:145588

Alcohol and Other Drugs

Prenatal exposure to alcohol can cause a range of disorders, known as fetal alcohol spectrum disorders (FASDs). FASD refers to conditions, such as **fetal alcohol syndrome (FAS)**, fetal alcohol effects (FAE), alcohol-related neurodevelopmental disorder (ARND), and alcohol-related birth defects (ARBD). No level of alcohol during pregnancy is known to be safe. Adverse effects are strongly associated with heavy consumption during the first few months of pregnancy, but alcohol at any time during pregnancy can be harmful.[64] Abstaining from alcohol altogether during pregnancy is highly recommended; however, data from the 2015 to 2017 Behavioral Risk Factor Surveillance System indicated that 13.5% of pregnant women reported current drinking and 5.2% reported binge drinking during the past 30 days.[65]

Other drug use can also result in a number of deleterious effects on the developing fetus, including impaired fetal growth, increased risk for preterm birth, birth defects, withdrawal symptoms, and learning or behavioral problems.[66] Because women who use illicit drugs during pregnancy are also more likely to engage in other risky behaviors, it is difficult to determine what specific effects various substances have on the developing fetus. Furthermore, the impact of the drug(s) depends on when they were used during pregnancy and in what quantity. By understanding how the fetus develops throughout pregnancy, it is possible to determine how exposures at certain times may impact the fetus.

Breastfeeding

The American Academy of Pediatrics (AAP) recommends exclusive breastfeeding for the first 6 months of life and continuing breastfeeding for the first year.[67] Breast milk is the ideal food for babies and has many advantages for both baby and mother. Breast milk contains substances that help babies resist infections and other diseases. As a result, breastfed babies have fewer ear infections and stomach bugs, and lower risk of asthma, obesity, type 1 diabetes, and (SIDS). In addition, breastfeeding has been shown to improve maternal health by reducing postpartum bleeding, and reducing risk of breast and ovarian cancer, type 2 diabetes, and high blood pressure.[67,68]

Fetal alcohol syndrome (FAS) a condition in babies born to mothers who have consumed heavy amounts of alcohol during their pregnancies; affected babies may experience abnormal facial features, growth problems, central nervous system problems, and have problems with learning, memory, attention span, communication, vision, or hearing

Breastfeeding rates demonstrate that most infants receive some breast milk, yet most infants are not exclusively breastfed or continue to breastfeed as long as recommended. In 2020, it was estimated that nationally, 83.1% of infants have ever been breastfed, 58.2% were breastfeeding at 6 months of age, and 37.6% were breastfeeding at 1 year.[69] There continue to be various barriers to breastfeeding and disparities persist in breastfeeding duration and exclusivity rates by race, ethnicity, and socioeconomic status. The *Healthy People 2030* objectives for breastfeeding are to increase the proportion of infants who are breastfed exclusively through age 6 months and to increase the proportion of infants who are breastfed at 1 year (see **Box 7.3**).[63] Two voluntary community groups, the La Leche League and the Nursing Mother's Council, are good sources for breastfeeding information, advice, and support. To promote breastfeeding, the United Nations Children's Emergency Fund (UNICEF) and the World Health Organization (WHO) implemented the Baby Friendly Hospital initiative. This program includes 10 steps at the organization level that have been shown to increase breastfeeding initiation, exclusivity, and continuation.[70] These steps include the following:

- Have a written infant breastfeeding policy that is routinely communicated to staff and parents and monitored.
- Train healthcare staff to implement the policy and support breastfeeding.
- Discuss the importance and management of breastfeeding with pregnant women and their families.
- Facilitate immediate and uninterrupted skin-to-skin contact and support mothers to initiate breastfeeding as soon as possible after birth.
- Support mothers to initiate and maintain breastfeeding and manage common difficulties.
- Do not provide breastfed newborns any food or fluids other than breast milk, unless medically indicated.
- Enable mothers and their infants to remain together and to practice rooming-in 24 hours a day.
- Support mothers to recognize and respond to their infants' cues for feeding.
- Counsel mothers on the use and risks of feeding bottles, artificial nipples (teats), and pacifiers.
- Coordinate discharge so that parents and their infants have timely access to ongoing support and care.

BOX 7.3   *Healthy People 2030* Breastfeeding Objectives

Objective MICH-15: Increase the proportion of infants who are breastfed exclusively through age 6 months
Objective MICH-16: Increase the proportion of infants who are breastfed at 1 year
Target and baseline:

Objective	Increase Proportion of Infants who are Breastfed	2015 Baseline	2020 Status Percent	2030 Target
MICH-15	Exclusively through 6 months of age*	24.9%	25.4%	42.4%
MICH-16	At 1 year	35.9%	37.6%	54.1%

*Exclusive breastfeeding is defined as only human breast milk; no solids, water, or other liquids.

Data from U.S. Department of Health and Human Services. (2024). *Healthy People 2030: Objectives and data.* Available at https://health.gov/healthypeople/objectives-and-data

For Further Thought
An important public health goal is to increase the proportion of infants who are breastfed. Human milk is acknowledged by the American Academy of Pediatrics as the most complete form of nutrition for infants, with a broad realm of benefits for infants' growth and development. What types of programs would you recommend to educate new mothers and their partners as well as educate healthcare providers?

Data from U.S. Department of Health and Human Services. (2024). Healthy People 2030: *Objectives and data.* https://health.gov/healthypeople/objectives-and-data

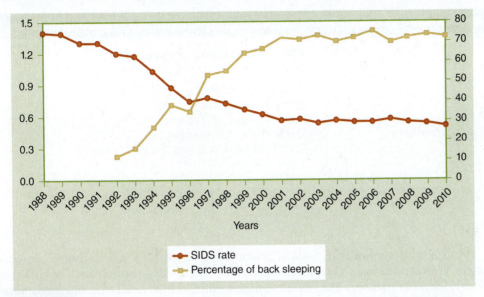

FIGURE 7.12   Rate of sudden infant death syndrome and sleep position: 1988–2010. Deaths are per 1,000 live births.

Reproduced from National Institutes of Health, Eunice Kennedy Shriver National Institute of Child Health and Human Development (NICHD), Safe to Sleep Public Education Campaign. (2015). *About SIDS and safe infant sleep.* Available at https://www.nichd.nih.gov/sts/about/Pages /default.aspx

Sudden Infant Death Syndrome

Sudden infant death syndrome (SIDS) was listed as a cause of death for nearly 1,400 infants in the United States in 2020. There were probably even more deaths caused by SIDS, but issues with correctly classifying infant causes of death result in under-reporting.[53] SIDS is defined as the sudden unanticipated death of an infant in whom, after examination, there is no recognizable cause of death.[71] Because most cases of SIDS occur when a baby is sleeping in a crib, SIDS has been referred to as crib death. SIDS is the third-leading cause of infant death. Moreover, after the first month of life, it is a leading cause of postneonatal mortality.[52] SIDS is just one type of sudden unexpected infant death (SUID), which also includes death due to unknown cause and accidental suffocation or strangulation in bed.[71]

There is currently no way of predicting which infants will die because of SIDS. However, research has shown that sleeping on the back all the time rather than the stomach or side greatly decreases the risk of SIDS.[72] In response to this research, the federal government initiated a national Safe to Sleep campaign, which began in 1994 as the Back to Sleep campaign, to educate parents and health professionals that placing babies on their backs to sleep can reduce the risk of SIDS. Since the dissemination of the recommendation, more infants have been put to bed on their backs, and the rate of SIDS has fallen by more than 50%, demonstrating the power of a public health campaign (see **Figure 7.12**).[72]

Child Health

Good health during the childhood years (ages 1–9) is essential to each child's optimal development and this country's future. Children are less likely to become productive members of society if they grow up in poverty, live in a violent environment, have poor or mediocre childcare, or have no health insurance. Failure to provide timely and remedial care leads to unnecessary illness, disability, and death—events that are associated with much greater costs than the timely care itself. Vivid examples are the costs associated with late or no prenatal care given earlier in this chapter. For those who believe that access to basic care is a standard of justness and fairness in any socialized society, the United States sadly lingers behind many other nations in child health (see **Box 7.4**).[7]

> **Sudden infant death syndrome (SIDS)** sudden unanticipated death of an infant in whom, after examination, there is no recognized cause of death

---

BOX 7.4   How America Ranks Among 35 Industrialized Countries in Investing in and Protecting Children

First in gross domestic product
First in number of billionaires
30th in child poverty rates
32nd in income inequality

First in military spending
35th in protecting children against gun violence

20th in education spending
29th in preschool enrollment rates

30th in reading scores for 15 year olds
31st in math scores for 15 year olds

8th in health expenditures
30th in low birth weight rates
26th in immunization rates
31st in infant mortality rates
31st in teenage births (just ahead of Bulgaria)

Data from Children's Defense Fund. (2017). *The state of America's children.* Available at https://www.childrensdefense.org/reports/2017/the-state-of-americas-children-2017-report/

In an effort to improve care, the AAP promotes the concept of a "medical home," which is the provision of continuous, comprehensive, coordinated, family-oriented care. The physician not only addresses routine health issues and makes sure the child has all recommended immunizations, the physician also discusses growth and development, parenting, nutrition, safety, and psychosocial issues that may affect the child. Furthermore, the physician will coordinate with other providers to ensure the well-being of each child. When possible, having the same provider means continuity of care and a centralized location for a comprehensive record of the child's well-being. The provider should also work to ensure that care is culturally appropriate. The medical home can be in different types of locations, such as a physician's office or a health department, but this approach to care helps to provide effective and efficient care for children.[73]

Childhood Mortality

Childhood mortality rates are the most severe measure of health in children. The death of a child is an enormous tragedy for family and friends as well as a loss to the community. As mentioned in the introduction of this chapter, the mortality rates of children have generally declined over the past couple of decades.[6] Unintentional injuries are the leading cause of mortality in children (see **Figure 7.13**).[74] Many unintentional injury deaths among children are the result of motor vehicle crashes, which could be prevented with the appropriate use of child restraints, such as seat belts or car seats. In 2022, 43% of daytime and 57% of night-time fatalities in motor vehicle accidents were to unrestrained occupants.[75] Car seats reduce the likelihood of fatal injury in passenger cars by 71% for infants and by 54% for children 1 to 4 years of age. Education campaigns have had an impact on the number of children under 4 years of age as approximately 25% of those killed in 2022 were unrestrained. This is still too many deaths as it is preventable. Use of restraints when riding in a vehicle needs to be passed on to all passengers. In 2022, 43% of 8- to 12-year-olds and 58% of 13 to 14 year olds in fatal traffic crashes were unrestrained.[76] Although all 50 states have primary child restraint laws that allow law enforcement officers to stop a driver if a child is not restrained, the provisions of these laws vary from state to state.

Childhood Morbidity

Although childhood for many children represents a time of relatively good overall health, it is a time when far too many suffer from acute illness, chronic disease, and disabilities. Childhood morbidity includes unintentional injuries, child maltreatment, and infectious diseases.

Unintentional Injuries

Unintentional injuries are the leading cause of death among children (see **Figure 7.14**).[75] The leading causes of injuries among children are drowning, falls, suffocation, and injuries related to transportation (e.g., motor vehicle accidents) being struck/against, and bites (other than dog), including stings. While unintentional injuries are an important concern for all children, the

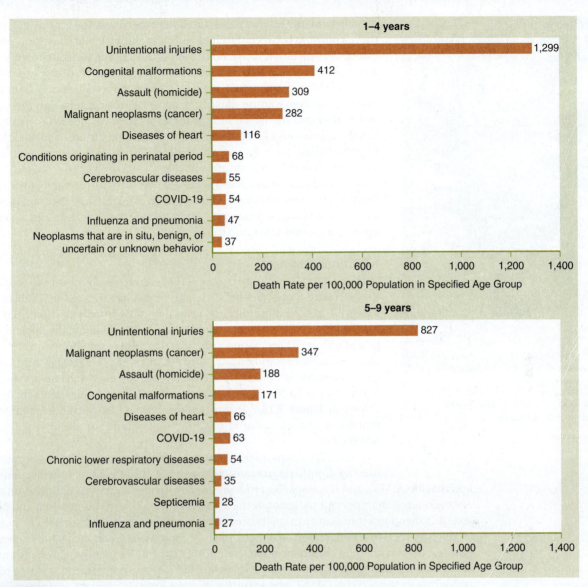

FIGURE 7.13   Leading causes of death in children aged 1 to 4 and 5 to 9; 2021.

Data from Curtin SC, Tejada-Vera B, Bastian BA. (2024) Deaths: Leading causes for 2021. *National Vital Statistics Reports; vol 73* no 4. Hyattsville, MD: National Center for Health Statistics. DOI: https://dx.doi.org/10.15620/cdc/147882. Available at https://www.cdc.gov/nchs/data/nvsr/nvsr73/nvsr73-04.pdf

type of accidents varies based on the child's age. For example, toddlers are at especially high risk of drowning, whereas older children are most at risk of transportation-related injuries.[77-79]

In addition to the physical and emotional effects on children and their families, these injuries have enormous financial costs. In fact, medical care and societal costs more than $78 billion per year for injuries to those 14 years of age and under.[77] Childhood injuries can deprive the country of the child's potential contributions. Looking at the causes of both fatal and nonfatal childhood injuries, it is evident that there are many opportunities for prevention.

Child Maltreatment

Child maltreatment is another source of injury to children. Child maltreatment includes physical abuse, neglect (physical, educational, emotional, and/or medical), sexual abuse, emotional abuse (psychological/verbal abuse and/or mental injury), and other types of maltreatment, such as abandonment, exploitation, and/or threats to harm the child. The causes of child maltreatment are not well understood. The impact of abuse depends on the age of the child and their stage of

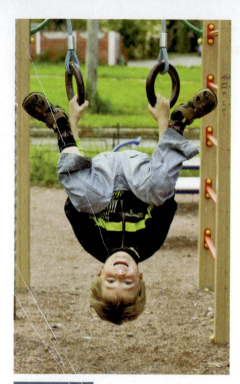

FIGURE 7.14 Unintentional injuries are the leading cause of childhood morbidity and mortality.

© Kitti/Shutterstock

development, the intensity and duration of the abuse, the type of abuse, and the relationship between the child and their abuser. Child abuse or neglect is associated with physical, psychological, behavioral, and societal consequences, which overlap and are intertwined. The consequences of adverse experiences during childhood can impact individuals throughout their entire lifetime. For example, children who are abused are more likely to engage in high-risk behaviors as they mature, which in turn increases their risk for long-term health consequences, such as sexually transmitted infections, cancer, and obesity. The impact of abuse can continue over multiple generations because individuals who were abused as children are more likely to victimize their own children.[80] The rate of children abused and neglected decreased to a 5-year low, with rates decreasing to a low of 8.1 per 1,000 children in 2021. Child maltreatment is a very complex societal issue with disparities seen by parent race, age, socioeconomic status, education, and substance use.[81]

Infectious Diseases

In the past, infectious diseases were the leading health concern for children in the United States, but public health action has resulted in a substantial reduction in both morbidity and mortality rates. Infectious disease control resulted from improvements in sanitation and hygiene and the implementation of universal vaccination programs. Because many vaccine-preventable diseases are more common and more deadly among infants and children, the CDC recommends vaccinating children against most vaccine-preventable diseases early in life. The 2024 recommended immunization schedule is shown in **Figure 7.15**.[82] Infectious diseases, which includes pneumonia, remains a leading cause of death among children under 5 years of age worldwide.[83]

The CDC keeps track of how many children receive key sets of vaccines like the diphtheria, tetanus, and pertussis (DTP); polio; measles, mumps, and rubella (MMR); and *Haemophilus influenzae* type b (Hib) vaccines. Immunization rates are considered an important indicator of the adequacy of health care for children and of the level of protection a community values related to preventable infectious diseases. The percent of children receiving vaccination coverage by age 24 months has remained similar over the past few years with 1% of children completely unvaccinated by 24 months. Coverage among children born during from 2019 to 2020 exceeded 90% for the recommended doses of the poliovirus vaccine, HepB, MMR, and varicella vaccine. Lowest coverage was observed for

Vaccine↓ Age→	Birth	1 month	2 months	4 months	6 months	12 months	15 months	18 months	19–23 months	2–3 years	4–6 years
Hepatitis B	HepB	HepB			HepB						
Rotavirus			RV	RV	RV						
Diphtheria, Tetanus, Pertussis			DTaP	DTaP	DTaP	DTaP					DTaP
Haemophilus influenzae type b			Hib	Hib	Hib	Hib					
Pneumococcal			PCV	PCV	PCV	PCV					
Inactivated Poliovirus			IPV	IPV	IPV						IPV
Influenza					Influenza (yearly)						
Measles, Mumps, Rubella						MMR					MMR
Varicella						Varicella					Varicella
Hepatitis A						HepA (2 doses)					

Range of recommended ages for all children except certain high-risk groups

FIGURE 7.15 Recommended immunization schedule for children aged 0 through 6 years—United States, 2024.

Data from Centers for Disease Control and Prevention. (2024). *Child and adolescent immunization schedule by age (addendum updated June 27, 2024)*, United States, 2024. Available at https://www.cdc.gov/vaccines/hcp/imz-schedules/child-adolescent-age.html?CDC_AAref_Val=https://www.cdc.gov/vaccines/schedules/hcp/imz/child-adolescent.html

influenza (61.3%) and the combined seven-vaccine series (69.1%) (DPT, polio, MMR, HepB, influenza type b, varicella, and pneumococcal infection).[84] A widening of the gap by poverty level was revealed for several vaccines in the 2022 data. Socioeconomic, demographic, and geographic disparities in vaccination coverage persist and are thus critical to address to ensure that all children are protected against vaccine-preventable diseases.[84]

All children should be immunized beginning at birth and according to schedules available from the CDC for birth through ages 6, 7 to 18 years of age, and adults 19 years of age and older.[82] By immunizing, the community safeguards its children against the potentially devastating effects of vaccine-preventable diseases as was recently experienced with the COVID-19 pandemic. No child should ever have to endure the effects of these diseases simply because they were not vaccinated on time.

In 1989, a measles epidemic occurred in the United States, leading to approximately 55,000 reported cases of measles and hundreds of deaths. Even though many of the infected children had seen a healthcare provider, investigation of the outbreak revealed that more than half of them had not been immunized. In response to that epidemic, the Vaccines for Children (VFC) program was created.[85] The VFC program provides vaccines to children whose families are not able to afford them, to ensure that all children have a better chance of getting their recommended vaccinations on schedule. Eligible children are those who are Medicaid-eligible, uninsured, underinsured, or an American Indian or Alaska Native. In 2022 alone, VFC distributed over 71.5 million doses of pediatric vaccines to participating provider locations.[86] With the goal of equitable access to vaccines for all U.S. children, VFC must continue in their effort as only 63.4% of VFC-eligible children were up to date with recommended vaccines, compared with 76.9% of non-VFC-eligible children. Recent years have seen a decrease in the VFC provider network; thus, there is a need for fresh strategies and innovative implementation of this important public health program.[86]

Despite improvements in vaccination rates historically and improved access to vaccines through the VFC program and the Affordable Care Act, fears about vaccine safety among parents continue to negatively impact vaccination. In March of 2024, an outbreak of measles originated in a temporary shelter for migrants in Chicago. Given the close gathering and the low vaccination coverage of shelter residents, as well as the high transmissibility of measles, there was the potential to spread rapidly among approximately 2,100 potentially exposed shelter residents. Within 6 days, there were a total of 57 associated confirmed measles cases, with 72% among persons who did not have documentation of measles vaccinations or were considered unvaccinated.[87] This outbreak, as well as others documented over the past 2 decades, demonstrate the need to ensure high vaccination rates among all people as well as timely public health interventions. The need for public health interventions and campaigns that are available where people reside and are culturally and linguistically accessible have never been more evident.[87]

Fears about the safety of vaccines were largely a response to the now-debunked work of British doctor Andrew Wakefield, whose now-retracted study claimed that vaccines were linked to the development of autism spectrum disorder. In the years since Dr. Wakefield's work was published, several large and rigorous studies by the IOM and the CDC have determined there is no link between autism and receipt of vaccines.[88] The COVID-19 pandemic reawakened the rise in concerns about vaccine safety and an increase in vaccine hesitancy. For many, this was the first time they recall that a population-wide vaccine was being recommended. Concerns centered around safety, including vaccine ingredients; skepticism about vaccine efficacy; risk vs. benefit with some suggesting the vaccine is riskier than the virus itself; limited trust in physicians, public health authorities, and the government; and concerns about health outcomes differing by race and ethnicity.[89] These concerns are consistent with documented MMR vaccine hesitancy.[90] The need to increase vaccine uptake continues and vaccine hesitancy is a public health threat. Addressing it is a collective responsibility. A multifaceted approach is required, including strategies to address individual concerns, and the benefit to communities is recommended.[89,90]

More stringent measures by the medical community are needed to ensure that all children are immunized. Opportunities to vaccinate are frequently missed by healthcare practitioners in primary care settings that do not routinely inquire about the immunization status of the child.

Parents and health practitioners need to work together to ensure that youth are protected from communicable diseases; some states have started immunization registries to facilitate timely vaccination by notifying providers when a vaccination is due.[91]

Community Programs for Women, Infants, and Children

In the preceding pages, many problems associated with maternal, infant, and child health have been identified. Solutions for many of these problems have been proposed, and in many cases, programs are already in place. Some of these programs are aimed at preventing or reducing the levels of maternal and infant morbidity and mortality, whereas others are aimed at the prevention or reduction of childhood morbidity and mortality.

The federal government has a multitude of health programs housed in a variety of agencies to serve the needs of our nation's children. The majority of these programs help meet the needs of many children. However, others are **categorical programs**, meaning they are only available to people who can be categorized into a specific group based on disease, age, geography, financial need, or other variables. This means that too many children fall through the cracks and are not served. Some children require services from multiple programs, which complicates the eligibility determination for each child. At times, this can lead to an inefficient system of child health care. Nonetheless, federal programs have contributed to a monumental improvement in maternal, infant, and child health. We discuss some of the more consequential government programs and their past successes and future objectives in the following sections.

Maternal and Child Health Bureau

In 1935, Congress enacted Title V of the Social Security Act. Title V is the only federal legislation dedicated to promoting and improving the health of our nation's mothers and children. Since its enactment, Title V-sponsored projects have been incorporated into the ongoing healthcare system for children and families. Although Title V has been modified over its history, the fundamental goal has remained constant—continued progress in the health, safety, and well-being of mothers and children. The most notable landmark achievements of Title V are projects that have produced "guidelines for child health supervision from infancy through adolescence; influenced the nature of nutritional care during pregnancy and lactation; recommended standards for prenatal care; identified successful strategies for the prevention of childhood injuries; and developed health safety standards for out-of-home child care facilities."[92]

In 1990, the Maternal and Child Health Bureau (MCHB) was established as part of the Health Resources and Services Administration (HRSA) in the U.S. Department of Health and Human Services to administer Title V funding. This means the MCHB is charged with the responsibility for promoting and improving the health of our nation's mothers, children, and their families.[93] To fulfill its mission, the MCHB has maternal and child health programs funded through block grants to[94]:

- Reduce infant deaths
- Provide better access to quality healthcare services for:
  - Women who need prenatal, delivery, and postnatal care
  - Women and children with low incomes who need preventive and primary care services
  - Women and children who have trouble finding care where they live
  - Children with special healthcare needs, including rehabilitative services
- Deliver family-centered, community-based, systems of coordinated care for children with special healthcare needs
- Set up toll-free hotlines so that pregnant women with infants and children who are eligible for Medicaid can apply for that help

The MCHB works on accomplishing its goals through the evidence-based strategies that improve access to quality health care and services, strengthen the health workforce, build healthy communities, improve health equity, and strengthen program operations.

Women, Infants, and Children Program

The Special Supplemental Nutrition Program for **Women, Infants, and Children (WIC)** is designed to provide a variety of nutritional and health-related goods and services to pregnant, postpartum, and breastfeeding women, infants up to 1 year of age, and children under the age of 5 years who are found to be at nutritional risk. The WIC program began as a pilot in 1972 and received permanent federal funding in 1974, in response to growing evidence linking nutritional inadequacies to mental and physical health defects. Congress intended that WIC, unlike other food programs, would serve as "an adjunct to good health care, during critical times of growth and development, to prevent the occurrence of health problems."[95]

The U.S. Department of Agriculture (USDA) administers WIC. The USDA administers grants to the states, where the WIC programs are most often offered through county health departments, hospitals, mobile clinics, community centers, schools, public housing sites, migrant health centers and camps, and Indian health service facilities (see **Figure 7.16**).[96] Pregnant, postpartum, or breastfeeding women, infants, and children up to age 5 years are eligible if they meet the following three criteria: (1) residency in the state in which they are applying, (2) income requirements (applicant must have a household income between 100% and 185% of the federal poverty income guidelines), (3) determination to be at "nutritional risk" by a health professional.[97]

Since WIC's inception as a national nutrition program, it has grown dramatically. In 1974, the average number of monthly WIC participants was 88,000; in 2023, that number was approximately 6.5 million women, infants, and children. Among WIC participants, children make up approximately one-half, infants one-quarter, and women one-quarter (see **Figure 7.17**).[98]

The WIC program has proven to be one of the most effective ways to improve the health of mothers, infants, and young children. Research indicates that participation in the WIC program during pregnancy provides women with a number of positive outcomes, some of which include birth to babies with higher birth weights, fewer fetal and infant deaths, and an increased rate of breastfeeding initiation.[99] In fact, rates of breastfeeding initiation among WIC participants has increased steadily with a rate of 41.5% in 1998 to a rate of 71.6% in 2020. However, rates continue to vary greatly across states (**Figure 7.18**).[99] The WIC program is also cost-effective. Historic USDA research has shown that for every dollar invested in WIC, taxpayers save on future Medicaid expenditures.[100] For this reason, the WIC program continues to receive strong bipartisan support in Congress.

Women, Infants, and Children (WIC) a special supplemental food program for women, infants, and children, sponsored by the USDA

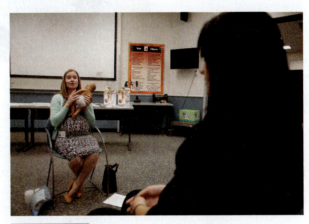

FIGURE 7.16 The WIC program has proven to be extremely effective in improving the health of woman, infants, and children in the United States.

© Jim Urquhart/Reuters

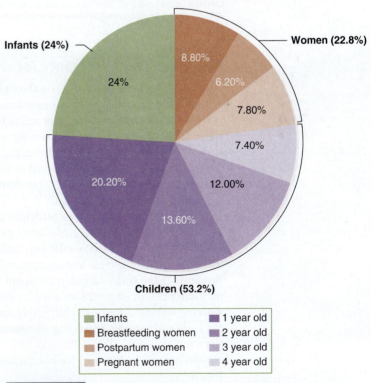

FIGURE 7.17 Distribution of individuals who participated in WIC.

Note: The percentage of children by age group is calculated from the total number of children by age group as a percentage of total WIC participation.

Data from U.S Department of Agriculture, Food and Nutrition Service. (2023). *WIC participant and program characteristics 2020 final report.* Available at https://www.fns.usda.gov/wic/participant-program-characteristics-2020

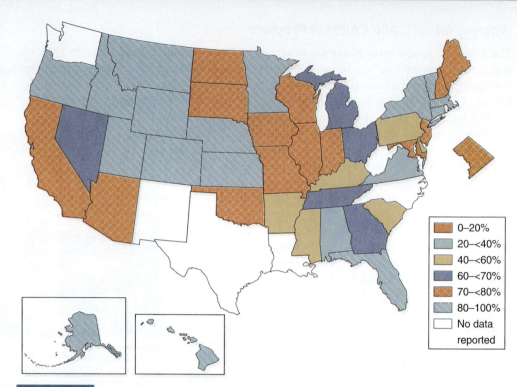

FIGURE 7.18 Breastfeeding initiation rates by state for WIC infant participants, ages 6 to 13 months; 2020.

Data from U.S Department of Agriculture, Food and Nutrition Service. (2023). *WIC participant and program characteristics 2020 final report.* Available at https://www.fns.usda.gov/wic/participant-program-characteristics-2020

Providing Health Insurance for Women, Infants, and Children

All children deserve to start life on the right track and to have access to comprehensive health services that provide preventive care when they are well and treatment when they are ill or injured. Health insurance provides access to critical preventive medical services as well as acute medical care in the case of illness or injury. When compared with children who are privately insured or have governmental insurance, children without health insurance are much more likely to have necessary care delayed or receive no care for health problems, putting them at greater risk for hospitalization.[100] Therefore, providing health insurance to low-income children is a critical healthcare safety net.

The government has two principal programs aimed at providing healthcare coverage to low-income children: the Medicaid program and the State Children's Health Insurance Program (formerly called SCHIP, now called CHIP). Medicaid, created in 1965, provides medical assistance for certain low-income individuals and families, mostly women and children. Medicaid is the single largest provider of health insurance for children in the United States, providing health coverage for over 37 million children.[101] A major reason that Medicaid is working well for American children is the multiphase program for preventive health called the Early and Periodic Screening, Diagnostic, and Treatment (EPSDT) for individuals younger than the age of 21. The Medicaid EPSDT provides children of low-income families with comprehensive and preventive healthcare screening and medically necessary diagnosis and treatment.[102]

Although the Medicaid program is a critical healthcare program for low-income children, being poor does not automatically qualify a child for Medicaid. Medicaid eligibility is determined by each state based on various age and income requirements. As a result, Medicaid coverage varies across the states and leaves a significant number of poor children uninsured. To broaden coverage to low-income children, Congress created CHIP under provisions in the

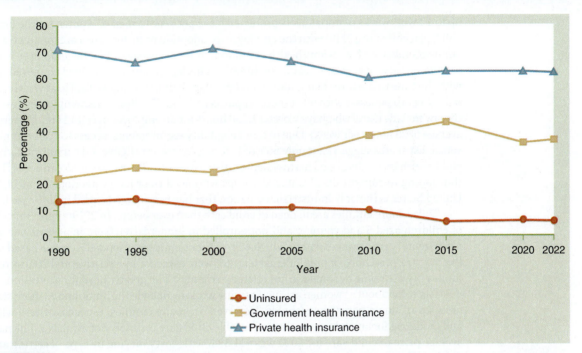

FIGURE 7.19   Percentage of children covered by health insurance, by type of insurance, select years 1990–2022.

Data from (1) Child Trends. (2017). *Health care coverage for children.* Available at https://www.childtrends.org/indicators/health-care-coverage; (2) Keisler-Starkey, K. & Bunch, L.N. (2021). *U.S. Census Bureau, Current Population Reports, P60-274, Health Insurance Coverage in the United States: 2020*, U.S. Government Publishing Office, Washington, DC; (3) Keisler-Starkey, K., Bunch, L.N., & Lindstrom, R.A. (2023). *U.S. Census Bureau, Current Population Reports, P60-281, Health Insurance Coverage in the United States: 2022*, U.S. Government Publishing Office, Washington, DC.

Balanced Budget Act of 1997. Coverage eligibility for CHIP is also determined by the state, as long as they meet the minimum guidelines set by the federal government.[101] In 2024, CHIP covered approximately 7.1 million children who were not covered by Medicaid.[101]

Government-funded health insurance is an important source of coverage for children, and its significance has been growing. Government health insurance coverage for children increased from 23.3% of all children in 1999 to 36.1% in 2022. During the same time period, the percentage of children with private health insurance coverage decreased from 70% in 1999 to 61.8% in 2022 (see **Figure 7.19**).[103,104] The success in increasing the number of children with coverage is attributable not just to Medicaid but also to the combined effects of Medicaid and CHIP. In 2022, approximately 5.4% of children younger than the age of 19 were uninsured,[104] a decrease that has been attributed to expansion of coverage under the Affordable Care Act.

Providing Child Care

Experiences during the first years of childhood significantly influence the health of a child. Research shows that early investments in the nurturing of children provide major advantages for families and society later. Whereas parents should accept the primary responsibility for raising their children, the government can assist families who need help making important investments. Two important investments into the health and welfare of America's children involve support for parenting during the first months of life and supporting the child's need for secure relationships with a small number of adults in safe settings as they develop during the first few years of life.

The **Family and Medical Leave Act (FMLA)** was signed into law in 1993 and provides job protection for individuals for medical- or family-related needs, including support for new parents. Evidence has shown that FMLA can be a valuable contributor to improving maternal and child health as it has been associated with improved child health, promoting breastfeeding, and improving a mother's physical and mental health, among other benefits.[105] The FMLA grants

Family and Medical Leave Act (FMLA) federal law that provides up to a 12-week unpaid leave to men and women after the birth of a child, an adoption, or an event of illness in the immediate family

up to 12 workweeks of unpaid, job-protected leave per year to men or women for the birth of a child, placement of a child with the employee for adoption or foster care, care for an immediate family member with a serious health condition, or medical leave when the employee is unable to work because of a serious health condition.[106] This legislation has provided employed parents with the time to nurture their children and develop their parenting skills. However, the FMLA only affects businesses with 50 or more employees within 75 miles. Those employees covered by the law include those who have worked 1,250 hours for an employer over a 12-month period (an average of 25 hours per week). Due to strict eligibility requirements, access to FMLA is not universal. Estimates suggest that only 56% of U.S. employees are eligible. Like many maternal and child health issues discussed in this chapter, disparities exist in terms of who can access FMLA, thus failing to support disadvantaged groups who need their job protection the most.[105] The United States is the only industrialized nation that has not enacted a paid infant-care leave.[107]

Today, more families are in need of child care than ever before. In 2019, approximately 59% of children aged 5 and younger and not enrolled in kindergarten were in at least one weekly nonparental care arrangement of which 62% of those children attended a center-based setting like daycare, preschool, or prekindergarten; 38% were cared for by a relative; and 20% were cared for in a private home by someone not related to them.[108] The greater need for professional child care has come about as women are increasingly working outside the home and as more children grow up in single-parent households. However, for many families, especially those with low and moderate incomes, high-quality, affordable child care is simply not available. The national average price of child care for 2023 was $11,582, with costs varying by type of setting and the state in which a family resides.[109] The costs decrease as children get older; however, parents often pay for childcare for more than one child at a time. These costs are beyond the reach of many working parents, as it is estimated to take 32% of a single parent with children's median household income to afford this national average. The lack of high-quality child care prevents children from entering school ready to learn, hinders their success in school, and limits the ability of their parents to be productive workers.[109]

In 1990, Congress passed the Child Care and Development Block Grant Act (CCDBG), which provides child care subsidies for low-income children and funding to improve the quality of child care services through the Child Care and Development Fund (CCDF). With the creation of the CCDF, states were able to provide additional assistance to many more low-income families.[110] However, in 2020, of the 10.9 million children eligible for child care subsidies under federal law, only 18% received subsidies. Due in part to restrictions on income eligibility set by individual states, only approximately one in five children who are eligible for child care assistance under federal law receive help. Children in deeper poverty, younger children ages 1 through 5 years, and Black, non-Hispanic children who were federally eligible for subsidies were most likely to receive subsidies.[111] This means that too many parents are unable to obtain necessary child care assistance.

Other Advocates for Children

Numerous groups advocate for children's health and welfare. Among them are the Children's Defense Fund, UNICEF, and the American Academy of Pediatrics.

Children's Defense Fund

Since 1973, the Children's Defense Fund (CDF; www.childrensdefense.org) has been working to create a nation in which the network of family, community, private-sector, and government supports for children is so tightly intertwined that no child can slip through the cracks. The CDF is a private, nonprofit organization headquartered in Washington, D.C., dedicated to providing a voice for the children of America. It has never accepted government funds and supports its programs through donations from foundations, corporate grants, and individuals. The CDF's work is rooted in the Civil Rights and Women's movements and is focused on overcoming systematic inequities for the nation's children and youth, working at the intersection of well-being and racial justice. The CDF engages in advocacy, community organizing, direct service, and public policy work.[112]

United Nations Children's Fund

Founded in 1946, UNICEF (www.unicefusa.org) is the only organization of the United Nations assigned exclusively to children. This organization works with other United Nations members, governments, and nongovernmental organizations to improve child conditions through community-based services in primary health care, basic education, and safe water and sanitation in more than 190 developing countries. UNICEF gathers data on the health of children throughout the world. UNICEF has assisted in mass vaccinations and has been involved in other international health efforts to protect children.[113]

American Academy of Pediatrics

The AAP (www.aap.org) was founded in 1930 by 35 pediatricians who saw the need for an independent pediatric forum to address children's needs. When the AAP was established, the idea that children have special developmental and health needs was a new one. Preventive health practices now associated with child care, including immunizations and regular health exams, were only just beginning to change the custom of treating children as "miniature adults." The AAP is committed to the attainment of optimal physical, mental, and social health and well-being for all infants, children, adolescents, and young adults. The activities and efforts of the AAP include research, advocacy for children and youth, philanthropy, and public and professional education.[114]

Chapter Summary

- Maternal, infant, and child health are important indicators of a community's overall health. Maternal health encompasses the health of women of childbearing age from prepregnancy through pregnancy, labor, and delivery, and in the postpartum period. Infant and child health refers to individuals through 9 years of age.

- Families are the primary unit in which infants and children are nurtured and supported regarding healthy development. Significant increases in births to unmarried women in the last 2 decades are among the many changes in American society that have affected family structure and the economic security of children. Teenage childbearing represents a significant social and financial burden on both the family and the community.

- The establishment of local family planning clinics with Title X funding has resulted in an improvement in maternal and child health indicators for the communities served.

- High-quality prenatal care is one of the fundamentals of a safe motherhood program. Ensuring early initiation of prenatal care during pregnancy greatly contributes to reductions in perinatal illness, disability, and death for the mother and the infant.

- Good health during the childhood years (ages 1 to 9) is essential for each child's optimal development and the United States' future. The United States cannot hope for every child to become a productive member of society if children in this country are allowed to grow up with poor or mediocre child care, without health insurance, living in poverty, or living in a violent environment.

- The federal government has many health programs within various agencies helping states to serve the needs of our nation's children. The majority of these programs are well respected and help to meet the needs of many children.

Scenario: Analysis and Response

We have learned that a lack of prenatal care increases the risk of premature delivery and possible health problems for the infant.

1. If Joan had received prenatal care, how could it have helped in the normal development of the infant? How could the doctor have counseled Joan?

2. How could Joan have found out about opportunities for affordable prenatal care?

3. The cost of treating Joan's infant could run into the hundreds of thousands of dollars, and there is no guarantee that the child will survive. Do you think it would be more cost-effective to ensure prenatal care to

all women or to continue under the system that is in place now? How would you suggest the United States approach this problem?

4. What programs mentioned in this chapter could have helped Joan?

5. Visit the USDA website (www.usda.gov) and read about WIC. After reading about WIC, do you think this is something that could help Joan with the raising of her child? Why or why not?

Review Questions

1. What has been the trend in infant mortality rates in the United States in the last 15 years? What is the current rate? How does this rate compare with that of other industrial countries?

2. Why are preconception and prenatal care so important for mothers and infants? What types of services are included?

3. What are the consequences of teen pregnancy to the mother? To the infant? To the community?

4. What is included in family planning? Why is family planning important?

5. Discuss the pro-life and pro-choice positions on abortion.

6. Why was the *Roe v. Wade* court decision so important? How has the overturning of this decision impacted women's access to abortion?

7. What are the leading causes of death in children ages 1 to 4 and ages 5 to 14 years?

8. Why are childhood immunizations so important?

9. What is the WIC program?

10. Why is health insurance important for women, infants, and children?

11. Name three groups that are advocates for the health of children and what they have done to show their support.

Activities

Write a two-page paper summarizing the results and/or information you gain from one of the following activities.

1. Survey 10 classmates and friends and ask them what leads to teen pregnancy. What prompts adolescents to risk pregnancy when they have adequate knowledge of contraception? Ask if they know anyone who became pregnant as an adolescent. Are the reasons given the same as your own? Divide your list into categories of personal beliefs, barriers to action, and social pressure. For example, a comment that might fit under beliefs is, "They don't think they can get pregnant the first time"; under barriers, "They are too embarrassed to buy contraception"; and under social pressure, "All the messages in society promoting sex." Which of the three categories had the most responses? Does this surprise you? What implications does this have for programs trying to reduce the incidence of teen pregnancy?

2. Call your local health department and ask for information about the local WIC program. Ask permission to visit and talk to a representative about the program and clientele.

3. Visit, call, or get on the website of your state health department and obtain information concerning the number of childhood communicable diseases reported in your state. What are your state laws concerning immunization of children? Does your state provide immunizations free of charge? What qualifications must a person meet to receive free immunizations?

4. Call a local obstetrician's office and ask if the office accepts Medicaid reimbursement. What is the normal fee for prenatal care and delivery? If the provider does not take Medicaid, ask to whom they would refer a pregnant woman with no private insurance.

5. Create a record of your own (or a family member's) immunizations. Find out when and where you were immunized for each of the immunizations listed in Figure 7.15. Are there any immunizations that are still needed? When are you scheduled to get your next tetanus toxoid immunization?

6. Explore your state's current laws regarding abortion. Investigate what services are available for women under 18 and for 18 and older. If your state does not permit abortion, what options are available to a woman who does not want to stay pregnant? How far would she need to travel to access services? What would this cost?

7. Examine child care options in your community. Does your campus offer child care for students? What does child care cost for a full-time student? What kind of planning ahead might a parent need to do in order to access quality child care?

8. Research birth to five programs/initiatives (often called school readiness) in your state. Examine how they use

public health programs and services to strengthen early childhood development and school readiness. What resources might you suggest the group use to strengthen their efforts? What can you apply from the community action efforts of the birth to five programs to what you learned in this chapter?

References

1. Pillitteri, A. (2013). *Maternal and child health nursing: Care of the childbearing and childrearing family* (7th ed.). J. B. Lippincott.

2. Ely, D. M., & Driscoll, A. K. (2023). Infant mortality in the United States: Provisional data from the 2022 period linked birth/infant death file. *National Vital Statistics Rapid Release, Report No. 33.* Available at https://www.cdc.gov/nchs/data/vsrr/vsrr033.pdf

3. Trost, S., Beauregard, J., Chandra, G., Njie, F., Berry, J., Harvey, A., & Goodman, D. A. (2022). *Pregnancy-Related Deaths: Data from Maternal Mortality Review Committees in 36 US States, 2017-2019.* Available at https://www.cdc.gov/maternal-mortality/media/pdfs/Pregnancy-Related-Deaths-Data-MMRCs-2017-2019-H.pdf

4. U.S. Department of Health and Human Services, Health Resources and Services Administration, Maternal and Child Health Bureau. (2015). *Child Health USA 2014.* Available at http://mchb.hrsa.gov/chusa14/dl/chusa14.pdf

5. United Health Foundation. (2019). *America's Health Rankings Annual Report 2019.* Available at https://assets.americashealthrankings.org/app/uploads/ahr_2019annualreport.pdf.

6. Kochanek, K. D., Murphy, S. L., Xu, J., & Arias, E. (2024). *Mortality in the United States, 2022.* NCHS Data Brief, No. 492, March 2024. Available at https://www.cdc.gov/nchs/data/databriefs/db492.pdf

7. Children's Defense Fund. (2023). *2023 State of America's Children Report.* Available at https://www.childrensdefense.org/tools-and-resources/the-state-of-americas-children/

8. United States Census Bureau. (2024). *Current population survey (CPS)—subject definitions.* https://www.census.gov/programs-surveys/cps/technical-documentation/subject-definitions.html

9. Friedman, M. (2003). *Family nursing: Research, theory and practice* (5th ed.). Appleton & Lange.

10. Osterman, M. J., Hamilton, B. E., Martin, J. A., Driscoll, A. K., & Valenzuela, C. P. (2024). Births: Final Data for 2022. *National Vital Statistics Reports, 73*(2). Available at https://www.cdc.gov/nchs/data/nvsr/nvsr73/nvsr73-02.pdf

11. Shah, P. S., Zao, J., Ali, S., & Knowledge Synthesis Group of Determinants of Preterm/LBW Births. (2011). Maternal marital status and birth outcomes: A systematic review and meta-analyses. *Maternal and Child Health Journal, 15*(7), 1097–1109.

12. Balayla, J., Azoulay, L., & Abenhaim, H. A. (2011). Maternal marital status and the risk of stillbirth and infant death: A population-based cohort study on 40 million births in the United States. *Women's Health Issues, 21*(5), 351–355.

13. Hans, S. L., & White, B. A. (2019). Teenage childbearing, reproductive justice, and infant mental health. *Infant Mental Health Journal, 40*(5), 690–709. Available at http://dx.doi.org/10.1002/imhj.21803

14. Merklinger-Gruchala, A. (2023). Marital status, father acknowledgement, and birth outcomes: Does the maternal education matter? *Int J Environ Res Public Health, 20*(6), 4868. Available at https://www.ncbi.nlm.nih.gov/pmc/articles/PMC10048939/

15. Sedge, G., Finer, L. B., Bankole, A., Eilers, M. A., & Singh, S. (2015). Adolescent pregnancy, birth, and abortion rates across countries: Levels and recent trends. *Journal of Adolescent Health, 56,* 223–230. Available at http://www.jahonline.org/article/S1054-139X(14)00387-5/pdf

16. Power to Decide. (2018). *Progress pays off.* Available at https://powertodecide.org/sites/default/files/media/savings-fact-sheet-national.pdf

17. Youth.gov. (2024). *The Adverse Effects of Teen Pregnancy.* Available at https://youth.gov/youth-topics/pregnancy-prevention/adverse-effects-teen-pregnancy

18. Jackson, S. (1993). Opening session comments: Laying the groundwork for working together for the future. *Journal of School Health, 63*(1), 11.

19. Rossen, L. M., Hamilton, B. E., Abma, J. C., Gregory, E.C., Beresovsky, V., Resendez, A. V., et al. (2023). Updated methodology to estimate overall and unintended pregnancy rates in the United States. *National Center for Health Statistics. Vital Health Stat 2*(201). Available at https://dx.doi.org/10.15620/cdc:124395. https://www.cdc.gov/nchs/data/series/sr_02/sr02-201.pdf

20. Centers for Disease Control and Prevention. (2024). *Reproductive health: Unintended pregnancy.* Available at https://www.cdc.gov/reproductive-health/hcp/unintended-pregnancy/index.html

21. Nelson, H. D., Darney, B. G., Ahrens, K., et al. (2022). Associations of unintended pregnancy with maternal and infant health outcomes: A systematic review and meta-analysis. *JAMA, 2022; 328*(17), 1714–1729. doi: 10.1001/jama.2022.19097

22. Guttmacher Institute. (2024). *Unintended pregnancy in the United States: Fact Sheet, January 2019.* Available at https://www.guttmacher.org/fact-sheet/unintended-pregnancy-united-states

23. Mosher, W. D., Jones, J., & Abma, J. C. (2012). Intended and unintended births in the United States: 1982–2010. *National Vital Statistics Reports, 55.* Available at http://www.cdc.gov/nchs/data/nhsr/nhsr055.pdf

24. U.S. Department of Health and Human Services. (2021). *2021 Title X Final Rule Summary.* Available at https://opa.hhs.gov/sites/default/files/2021-10/2021-Title-X-Final-Rule-One-Pager-October-2021.pdf

25. Clochard, A., Killewald, P., Larson, A., Leith, W., Paxton, N., Troxel, J., & Wong, M. (2023). *Family Planning Annual Report: 2022 National Summary.* Washington, DC: Office of Population Affairs, Office of the Assistant Secretary for Health, Department of Health and Human Services.

26. U.S. Department of Health and Human Services, Office of Population Affairs. (2024). *Title X statutes, regulations, and legislative mandates.* Available at https://opa.hhs.gov/grant-programs/title-x-service-grants/title-x-statutes-regulations-and-legislative-mandates

27. Frederiksen, B., Salganicoff, A., Gomez, I., & Salganicoff. (2023). *Rebuilding the Title X network under the Biden administration.* Kaiser Family Foundation. Available at https://www.kff.org/womens-health-policy/issue-brief/rebuilding-the-title-x-network-under-the-biden-administration

28. U.S. Department of Health and Human Services, Office of Population Affairs. (2000). *42 CFR Part 59, Standards of compliance for abortion-related services in family planning services projects.* Available at http://www.hhs.gov/opa/title-x-family-planning/title-x-policies/program-guidelines/final-rules-42-cfr-59.html

29. Planned Parenthood Federation of America. (2024). *Our History.* Available at https://www.plannedparenthood.org/about-us/who-we-are/our-history

30. Planned Parenthood Federation of America. (2024). *Mission.* Available at https://www.plannedparenthood.org/about-us/who-we-are/mission

31. Planned Parenthood Federation of America. (2023). *Annual report.* Available at https://www.plannedparenthood.org/about-us/facts-figures/annual-report

32. Guttmacher Institute. (2019). *Publicly supported family planning services in the United States: Likely need, availability and impact.* Available at https://www.guttmacher.org/fact-sheet/publicly-supported-FP-services-US

33. Guttmacher Institute. (September 1, 2023). *State laws and policies Insurance coverage of contraceptives.* Available at https://www.guttmacher.org/state-policy/explore/insurance-coverage-contraceptives

34. Long, M., Frederiksen, B., Ranji, U., Diep, K., & Salganicoff, A. (2019). *Many women use preventive services, but gaps in awareness of insurance coverage requirements persist: Findings from the 2022 KFF women's health survey.* Available at https://www.kff.org/womens-health-policy/issue-brief/many-women-use-preventive-services-but-gaps-awareness-insurance-coverage-requirements-persist-findings-from-2022-kff-womens-health-survey/

35. Ranji, U., Salganicoff, A., Sobel, L., & Gomez, I. (2019). *Financing family planning services for low-income women: The role of public programs.* Kaiser Family Foundation. Available at https://www.kff.org/womens-health-policy/issue-brief/financing-family-planning-services-for-low-income-women-the-role-of-public-programs/

36. Cornell University Law School, Legal Information Institute. (n.d.). *Roe v. Wade.* 410 U.S. 113 (1973). Available at http://www.law.cornell.edu/supct/html/historics/USSC_CR_0410_0113_ZS.html

37. Supreme Court of the United States. (2022). *Dobbs, state health officer of the Mississippi department of health, et al., v. Jackson women's health organization et al.* Available at https://www.supremecourt.gov/opinions/21pdf/19-1392_6j37.pdf

38. Kortsmit, K., Nguyen, A. T., Mandel, M. G., Hollier, L. M., Ramer, S., Rodenhizer, J., & Whiteman, M. K. (2023). Abortion surveillance—United States, 2021. *Morbidity and Mortality Weekly Report, 72(9),* 1-29. Available at https://www.cdc.gov/mmwr/volumes/72/ss/ss7209a1.htm

39. Guttmacher Institute. (2023). *The state abortion policy landscape one year post-Roe.* Available at https://www.guttmacher.org/2023/06/state-abortion-policy-landscape-one-year-post-roe

40. Alan Guttmacher Institute. (2024). *Global abortion* Available at https://www.guttmacher.org/global/abortion

41. Hoyert, D. L. (2024). Maternal mortality rates in the United States, 2022. *NCHS Health E-Stats.* doi: https://dx.doi.org/10.15620/cdc/152992. https://www.cdc.gov/nchs/data/hestat/maternal-mortality/2022/maternal-mortality-rates-2022.htm

42. Centers for Disease Control and Prevention. (2024). *Pregnancy mortality surveillance system.* Available at https://www.cdc.gov/reproductivehealth/maternal-mortality/pregnancy-mortality-surveillance-system.htm

43. Petersen, E. E., Davis, N. L., Goodman, D., Cox, S., Mayes, N., Johnston, E., Syverson, C., Seed, K., Shapiro-Mendoza, C. K., Callaghan, W. M., & Barfield, W. (2019). Vital signs: Pregnancy-related deaths, United States, 2011–2015, and strategies for prevention, 13 states, 2013–2017. *Morbidity and Mortality Weekly Report, 68*(18), 423–429. Available at https://www.cdc.gov/mmwr/volumes/68/wr/mm6818e1.htm?s_cid=mm6818e1_w#T1_down

44. World Health Organization. (2024). *Maternal mortality.* Available at https://www.who.int/news-room/fact-sheets/detail/maternal-mortality

45. American Academy of Family Physicians. (2015). *Preconception care* [Position paper]. Available at http://www.aafp.org/about/policies/all/preconception-care.html

46. Robbins, C., Boulet, S. L., Morgan, I., et al. (2018). Disparities in preconception health indicators—Behavioral Risk Factor Surveillance System, 2013–2015, and Pregnancy Risk Assessment Monitoring System, 2013–2014. *MMWR Surveill Summ;* 67(No. SS-01), 1–16. doi: http://dx.doi.org/10.15585/mmwr.ss6701a1

47. Centers for Disease Control and Prevention. (2024). *About planning for pregnancy.* Available at https://www.cdc.gov/pregnancy/about/index.html

48. Child Trends DataBank. (2015). *Late or no prenatal care: Indicators on children and youth.* Available at http://www.childtrends.org/wp-content/uploads/2014/07/25_Prenatal_Care.pdf

49. U.S. Department of Health and Human Services, Health Resources and Services Administration, Maternal and Child Health Bureau. (2014). *Child Health USA 2013.* Available at http://www.mchb.hrsa.gov/publications/pdfs/childhealth2013.pdf

50. Martin, J. A., & Osterman, M. J. (2023). Changes in prenatal care utilization: United States, 2019–2021. *National Vital Statistics Reports; vol 72* no 4. Hyattsville, MD: National Center for Health Statistics. doi: https://dx.doi.org/10.15620/cdc:12570651.

51. Osterman, M. J., & Martin, J. A. (2018). Timing and adequacy of prenatal care in the United States, 2016. *National Vital Statistics Reports, vol 67* no 3. Hyattsville, MD: National Center for Health Statistics.

52. Ely, D. M., & Driscoll, A. K. (2023). Infant mortality in the United States: Provisional data from the 2022 period linked birth/infant death file. *National Center for Health Statistics. Vital Statistics Rapid Release; no 33.* Hyattsville, MD: National Center for Health Statistics. doi: https://doi.org/10.15620/cdc:133699.

53. Curtin, S C., Tejada-Vera, B., & Bastian, B. A. (2024). Deaths: Leading causes for 2021. *National Vital Statistics Reports; 73*(4). Hyattsville, MD: National Center for Health Statistics. 2024. doi: https://dx.doi.org/10.15620/cdc:147882. https://www.cdc.gov/nchs/nvss/index.htm

54. Hill, L., Artiga, S., & Ranji, U. (2022). *Racial disparities in maternal and infant health: Current status of efforts to address them.* Kaiser Family Foundation. Available at https://www.kff.org/racial-equity-and-health-policy/issue-brief/racial-disparities-in-maternal-and-infant-health-current-status-and-efforts-to-address-them/

55. March of Dimes. (2024). *Prematurity profile.* Available at https://www.marchofdimes.org/peristats/reports/united-states/prematurity-profile

56. Behrman, R. E., & Stith Buter, A. (Eds.). (2006). *Preterm birth: Causes, consequences, and prevention.* National Academies Press.

57. March of Dimes. (2018). *Why at least 39 weeks is best for your baby.* Available at http://www.marchofdimes.com/pregnancy/why-at-least-39-weeks-is-best-for-your-baby.aspx

58. Main, E., Oshiro, B., Chagolla, B., Bingham, D., Dang-Kilduff, L., & Kowalewski, L. (2010). *Elimination of non-medically indicated (elective) deliveries before 39 weeks gestational age* [California Maternal Quality Care Collaborative Toolkit to Transform Maternity Care]. California Department of Public Health; Maternal, Child and Adolescent Health Division. (First edition published by March of Dimes. Contract #08-85012.) Available at http://www.cdph.ca.gov/programs/mcah/Documents/MCAH-EliminationOfNon-Medically-Indicated Deliveries.pdf

59. University of Michigan Medicine. (2018). *Physical growth in newborns.* Available at https://www.uofmhealth.org/health-library/te6295

60. March of Dimes. (2021). *Low birthweight.* Available at https://www.marchofdimes.org/find-support/topics/birth/low-birthweight

61. American Pregnancy Association. (2024). *Intrauterine growth restriction (IUGR): Small for gestational age (SGA).* Available at https://americanpregnancy.org/healthy-pregnancy/pregnancy-complications/intrauterine-growth-restriction/

62. Institute of Medicine. (n.d). *Healthy weight gain during pregnancy.* Available at https://webassets.nationalacademies.org/whattogain/

63. U.S. Department of Health and Human Services. (2024). *Healthy People 2030: Objectives and data.* Available at https://health.gov /healthypeople/objectives-and-data

64. March of Dimes. (2023). *Alcohol during pregnancy.* Available at https://www.marchofdimes.org/find-support/topics/pregnancy /alcohol-during-pregnancy

65. Gosdin, L. K., Deputy, N. P., Kim, S. Y., Dang, E.P., & Denny, C. H. (2022). Alcohol consumption and binge drinking during pregnancy among adults aged 18–49 years — United States, 2018–2020. *MMWR Morb Mortal Wkly Rep, 71,* 10–13. doi: http://dx.doi.org /10.15585/mmwr.mm7101a2. Available at https://www.cdc.gov /mmwr/volumes/71/wr/mm7101a2.htm

66. National Institute on Drug Abuse. (2020). *Substance use while pregnant and breastfeeding.* Available at https://nida.nih.gov /publications/research-reports/substance-use-in-women /substance-use-while-pregnant-breastfeeding

67. American Academy of Pediatrics. (2022). Policy statement: Breastfeeding and the use of human milk. *Pediatrics, 150(1),* e2022057988. Available at https://doi.org/10.1542/peds.2022 -057988. Available at https://publications.aap.org/pediatrics /article/150/1/e2022057988/188347/Policy-Statement-Breastfeeding -and-the-Use-of?autologincheck=redirected

68. Centers for Disease Control and Prevention. (2023). *Breastfeeding benefits both baby and mom.* Available at https://www.cdc.gov /breastfeeding/features/breastfeeding-benefits.html

69. Centers for Disease Control and Prevention. (2023). *Breastfeeding among U.S children born 2013-2020, CDC National Immunization Survey-Child.* Available at https://www.cdc.gov/breastfeeding/data /nis_data/results.html

70. Baby-Friendly USA. (2024). *10 steps to successful breastfeeding.* Available at https://www.babyfriendlyusa.org/for-facilities /practice-guidelines/10-steps-and-international-code/

71. Centers for Disease Control and Prevention. (2023). *Sudden unexpected infant death and sudden infant death syndrome.* Available at https://www.cdc.gov/sids/data.htm

72. National Institutes of Health, Eunice Kennedy Shriver National Institute of Child Health and Human Development (NICHD), Safe to Sleep. (2024). *About SIDS and safe infant sleep.* https://safetosleep .nichd.nih.gov/

73. American Academy of Pediatrics. (2024). *Medical home.* Available at https://www.aap.org/en/practice-management/medical-home/

74. Curtin S. C., Tejada-Vera B., & Bastian B. A. (2024). Deaths: Leading causes for 2021. National *Vital Statistics Reports, 73*(4) Hyattsville, MD: National Center for Health Statistics. doi: https://dx.doi .org/10.15620/cdc/147882. https://www.cdc.gov/nchs/data/nvsr /nvsr73/nvsr73-04.pdf

75. National Center for Statistics and Analysis. (2024, July). *Passenger vehicles: 2022 data* (Traffic Safety Facts. Report No. DOT HS 813 592). National Highway Traffic Safety Administration. Available at https://crashstats.nhtsa.dot.gov/Api/Public/View Publication/813592

76. National Center for Statistics and Analysis. (2024, June). *Children: 2022 data* (Traffic Safety Facts. Report No. DOT HS 813 575). National Highway Traffic Safety Administration.

77. Centers for Disease Control and Prevention. (2024). *WISQARS Fatal and Nonfatal Injury Reports.* Available at https://wisqars.cdc.gov /reports

78. Centers for Disease Control and Prevention. (2024). *Preventing drowning.* Available at https://www.cdc.gov/drowning/prevention /index.html

79. Centers for Disease Control and Prevention. (2024). *Child passenger safety.* Available at https://www.cdc.gov/child-passenger-safety /about/index.html

80. Child Welfare Information Gateway. (2019). *Long-term consequences of child abuse and neglect.* Washington, DC: U.S. Department of Health and Human Services, Administration for Children and Families, Children's Bureau. Available at https://www.child welfare.gov/resources/long-term-consequences-child-abuse-and -neglect/

81. U.S. Department of Health & Human Services, Administration for Children and Families, Administration on Children, Youth and Families, Children's Bureau. (2023). *Child Maltreatment 2021.* Available at https://www.acf.hhs.gov/cb/data-research/child -maltreatment.

82. Centers for Disease Control and Prevention. (2024). *Child and adolescent immunization schedule by age, United States, 2024.* Available at https://www.cdc.gov/vaccines/schedules/hcp/imz /child-adolescent.html

83. World Health Organization. (2020). *Children: Improving survival and well-being.* Available at https://www.who.int/news-room /fact-sheets/detail/children-reducing-mortality

84. Hill, H. A., Yankey, D., Elam-Evans, L. D., Chen, M., & Singleton, J. A. (2023). Vaccination coverage by age 24 months among children born in 2019 and 2020 — National Immunization Survey-Child, United States, 2020–2022. *MMWR Morb Mortal Wkly Rep, 72,* 1190–1196. doi: http://dx.doi.org/10.15585/mmwr.mm7244a3. Available at https://www.cdc.gov/mmwr/volumes/72/wr /mm7244a3.htm#

85. Centers for Disease Control and Prevention. (2023). *Vaccines for children (VFC) program.* Available at https://www.cdc.gov /vaccines/programs/vfc/index.html

86. Centers for Disease Control and Prevention (2023). *The vaccines for children (VFC) program: A retrospective of the program's first 30 years.* Available at https://storymaps.arcgis.com /stories/9284cdacff094798931c386bd64a897a

87. Gressick, K., Nham, A., Filardo, T. D., et al. (2024). Measles outbreak associated with a migrant shelter — Chicago, Illinois, February– May 2024. *MMWR Morb Mortal Wkly Rep, 73,* 424–429. doi: http:// dx.doi.org/10.15585/mmwr.mm7319a1. Available at https://www .cdc.gov/mmwr/volumes/73/wr/mm7319a1.htm

88. Centers for Disease Control and Prevention. (2024). *Autism and vaccines.* Available at https://www.cdc.gov/vaccinesafety/concerns /autism.html

89. Razai, M. S., Chaudhry, U.A., Doerholt, K., Bauld, L., & Majeed, A. (2021). COVID-19 vaccination hesitancy. *BMJ, 37,* n1138. (Published 20 May 2021) Available at https://doi.org/10.1136/bmj.n1138 Available at https://www.bmj.com/content/373/bmj.n1138

90. Novilla, M.L., Goates, M. C., Redelfs, A. H., Quenzer, M., Novilla, L.K., et al. (2023). Why parents say no to having their children vaccinated against measles: *A systematic review of the social determinants of parental perceptions on MMR vaccine hesitancy. Vaccines, 11(5),* 926. doi: 10.3390/vaccines11050926 Available at https://www.ncbi .nlm.nih.gov/pmc/articles/PMC10224336/

91. Centers for Disease Control and Prevention. (2023). *Immunization information systems (IIS).* Available at https://www.cdc.gov /vaccines/programs/iis/index.html

92. Association of Maternal and Child Health Programs. (2023). *Title V overview.* Available at https://amchp.org/title-v/

93. U.S. Department of Health and Human Services, Health Resources and Services Administration, Maternal and Child Health. (2020). *About us.* Available at https://mchb.hrsa.gov/about-us

94. U.S. Department of Health and Human Services, Health Resources and Services Administration, Maternal and Child Health. (2023). *Title V maternal and child health (MCH) services block grant.* Available at https://mchb.hrsa.gov/programs-impact /title-v-maternal-child-health-mch-services-block-grant

95. National Archives. (2024). *Code of Federal Regulations: Title 7BIIA Part 246: Special supplemental nutrition program for women, infants, and children.* Available at https://www.ecfr.gov/current /title-7/subtitle-B/chapter-II/subchapter-A/part-246

96. U.S. Department of Agriculture, Food and Nutrition Service. (2024). *Special supplemental nutrition program for women, infants, and children (WIC).* Available at https://www.fns.usda.gov/wic

97. U.S. Department of Agriculture, Food and Nutrition Service. (2024). *WIC eligibility requirements.* Available at https://www.fns.usda.gov /wic/wic-eligibility-requirements

98. U.S. Department of Agriculture, Food and Nutrition Service. (2024). *WIC data tables.* Available at https://www.fns.usda.gov/pd /wic-program

99. U.S. Department of Agriculture, Food and Nutrition Service. (2023). *WIC participant and program characteristics 2020 final data.* Available at https://www.fns.usda.gov/wic /participant-program-characteristics-2020

100. Institute of Medicine. (2002). *Health insurance is a family matter.* Available at https://nap.nationalacademies.org/read/10503 /chapter/1#ii\

101. Centers for Medicare and Medicaid Services. (2024). *March 2024 Medicaid & CHIP enrollment data highlights.* Available at https:// www.medicaid.gov/medicaid/program-information/medicaid -and-chip-enrollment-data/report-highlights/index.html

102. Centers for Medicare and Medicaid Services. (2024). *Early and periodic screening, diagnostic, and treatment.* Available at https://www .medicaid.gov/medicaid/benefits/early-and-periodic-screening -diagnostic-and-treatment/index.html

103. DeNavas-Walt, C., Proctor, B. D., & Smith, J. C. (2013). *Income, poverty, and health insurance coverage in the United States: 2012.* U.S. Census Bureau, Current Population Reports, P60-243. Available at http://www.census.gov/content/dam/Census/library /publications/2013 /demo/p60-245.pdf

104. Keisler-Starkey, K., Bunch, L. N., & Lindstrom, R. A. (2023). U.S. Census Bureau. *Current Population Reports, P60-281, Health Insurance Coverage in the United States: 2022,* U.S. Government Publishing Office, Washington, DC.

105. Jones, K., & Tasneem, F. (n.d.). *FMLA eligibility of underserved communities.* Prepared for U.S. Department of Labor. Available at https://www.dol.gov/sites/dolgov/files/OASP/evaluation/pdf /American%20University_Final_20220105_508.pdf

106. U.S. Department of Labor. (2024). *Family and medical leave (FMLA).* Available at https://www.dol.gov/general/topic/benefits-leave/fmla

107. Livingston, G., & Thomas, D. (2019). *Among 41 countries, only U.S. lacks paid parental leave.* Pew Research Center. Available at https://www.pewresearch.org/short-reads/2019/12 /16/u-s-lacks-mandated-paid-parental-leave/

108. National Center for Education Statistics. (2024). *Fast facts: Child care.* Available at https://nces.ed.gov/fastfacts/display.asp?id=4

109. Child Care Aware of America. (2024). *Child care at a standstill: Price and landscape analysis.* Available at https://www.childcareaware .org/thechildcarestandstill/#PriceofCare

110. Cohen, A. J. (1996). A brief history of federal financing for child care in the United States. *The Future of Children, 6*(2), 26–40.

111. U.S. Department of Health and Human Services, Office of the Assistant Secretary for Planning and Evaluation. (2024). *Estimates of child care eligibility and receipt for fiscal year 2020.* Available at https:// aspe.hhs.gov/reports/estimates-child-care-eligibility-receipt -fy-2020

112. Children's Defense Fund. (2024). *About us.* Available at https://www .childrensdefense.org/about-us/

113. UNICEF. (2024). *About UNICEF.* Available at https://www.unicef .org/about-unicef

114. American Academy of Pediatrics. (2024). *About the AAP.* Available at https://www.aap.org/

CHAPTER 8

Adolescents, Young Adults, and Adults

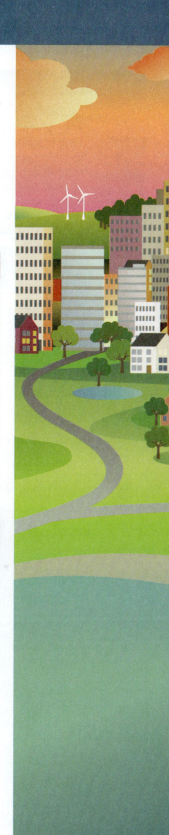

Chapter Outline

Chapter Objectives

After studying this chapter, you will be able to:

1. Explain why it is important for community health workers to be aware of the different health concerns of the various age groups in the United States.

2. Define the following groups by age: adolescents, young adults, and adults.

3. Briefly describe key demographic characteristics of adolescents and young adults.

4. Summarize what the Youth Risk Behavior Surveillance System (YRBSS) and the Behavioral Risk Factor Surveillance System (BRFSS) are and what type of data they generate.

5. Provide a brief behavioral risk profile for adolescents, young adults (including college students), and adults.

6. Outline the health profiles for the various age groups—adolescents, young adults, and adults—listing the major causes of mortality, morbidity, and risk factors for each group.

7. Give examples of community health strategies for improving the health status of adolescents, young adults, and adults.

Scenario

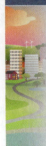

Annie and Connor are about halfway through their sophomore year at a local high school in an urban area. This year, as chance would have it, they have similar class schedules and have ended up eating lunch together in the school cafeteria every day.

One day during lunch, Annie mentioned to Connor that her friend, Dayna, who is also a high school student, recently went to the doctor and was diagnosed with type 2 diabetes. Dayna was told that more and more kids her age are being diagnosed with this disease. Connor replied that he thought that only adults had that type of diabetes. Annie stated that she is

concerned for Dayna because Dayna's doctor told her that she must start eating more fresh fruits and vegetables, drinking less sugary beverages, and exercising on a daily basis, or else she will be at risk of developing serious health problems from having diabetes. Apparently, Dayna doesn't know where to buy fruits and vegetables because the corner store she visits every day before and after school only sells candy, soda, and alcohol, and she does not want to exercise outside because there has been a lot of violence in her neighborhood lately. Connor said that he thought Dayna might just have to move away from the neighborhood to be healthy.

Introduction

In this chapter, we present a profile of the health of Americans in two different groups—adolescents and young adults (10–24 years of age) and adults (25–64 years of age). Please note that different organizations and agencies use various age ranges to categorize adolescents and young adults. The age range of 10–19 years is used for adolescents in this text because it is used by leading health organizations, such as the World Health Organization.[1] Just like the age groups of Americans presented elsewhere in the text, each of these groups has its own set of health risks, problems, and assets to contribute to the solution of their health problems. Viewing these age-group profiles enables public health workers to detect the causes of disease, injury, and death for specific priority populations and to propose interventions to reduce those causes. Effective interventions aimed at specific population age groups can reduce the risk factors that contribute to disease, injury, and death, and increase the protective factors that enhance the well-being for these groups as well as the entire population. We hope that you, the student, will become knowledgeable about the specific health problems and solutions to these problems of each age group and also become mindful of the subpopulations within these groups that are at special risk.

The years of life between the ages of 10 and 64 are some of the most productive, if not the most productive, of people's lives. Consider all that takes place during these years. Many people will complete their formal education, meet and commit to their lifelong partners, become parents and raise a family, find and develop their vocation, earn their greatest amount of wealth, actively engage in the development of their community, travel more than during any other time in their lives, become aunts or uncles and grandparents, become valued employees, serve as role models and mentors, and plan and save for retirement.[2] However, recent research shows that, for a variety of reasons, an increasing number of adolescents and young adults are delaying some of these life choices and taking longer to become independent. It is also during this time that individuals typically enjoy some of the best health of their lives as well as have their current and future health and health behaviors shaped by their environment and life circumstances.

Adolescents and Young Adults

Adolescents and young adults are considered to be those people who fall into the 10- to 24-year-old age range. The individuals in this age group are considered important by our society because they represent the future of our nation. This period of development of adolescence and young adulthood, often combined when reporting data about young people, can be further

Adolescents and young adults people who fall into the 10- to 24-year-old age range

split into two subgroups. "Adolescence is generally regarded as the period of life from puberty to maturity."[3] This may not be an easy stage of life for individuals because it is a period of transition from childhood to adulthood. Adolescence "is a time when children psychologically move from areas of relative comfort and emotional security to places and situations that are far more complex and often much more challenging."[4] In addition to the psychological changes, this population of teenagers is also experiencing "hormonal changes, physical maturation, and frequently, opportunities to engage in risky behaviors."[3]

Young adults also face many physical, emotional, and educational changes. For example, many young adults complete their physical growth and maturity, and experience those situations and opportunities previously mentioned. Couple the demands of these personal changes with the demands of a fast-paced, ever-changing society and it is easy to see why this stage in life is considered one of the most difficult.[5] However, this stage of life can also be fulfilling. The combined period of adolescence and young adulthood is a critical one in terms of health. It is during this period in one's life that many health-related beliefs, attitudes, and behaviors are adopted and challenged.[3,4,6] During this stage of life, young people have increased freedom and access to health-compromising substances and experiences—such as alcohol, tobacco, other drugs, and sexual risk taking—as well as opportunities for health-enhancing experiences, such as regularly scheduled exercise, healthful diets, and opportunities to engage in behaviors and experiences that benefit their communities.[3,4,6] It is also during this stage that lifestyles are often established and shaped, resulting in long-term influences on health in later years of life. The concept that health status and environmental exposures in the early part of one's life will impact their adult health status is called the *life course approach* to understanding health and disease.[7] This is an important concept because it helps explain how every stage of a person's life impacts the individual's long-term health. Thus, those risk behaviors as well as protective factors in the adolescent and young adult years will have an influence on that person's well-being throughout their lifetime.

Demography

Several demographic variables affect the health of this age group, but the four variables that are most important to community health are the number of young people, their living arrangements, their employment status, and their access to health care. Please note that for some of the adolescent data in this chapter, especially for young adolescents (ages 10–14), information for children will also be included due to how the data were collected and reported. Mortality and morbidity information for young adolescents is discussed elsewhere in the text.

Number of Adolescents and Young Adults

According to the 2020 U.S. Census, 10- to 24-year-olds made up approximately one-fifth of the U.S. population.[8] As we look to the future, the proportion of adolescents and young adults in the overall population will decrease as a result of the older population living longer (12.8% in 2019 to 11.1% in 2060). Yet, the total number of adolescents will continue to grow.[9] The racial and ethnic makeup of adolescents will become increasingly diverse (see **Figure 8.1**). In 2019, nearly half of adolescents identified as a racial or ethnic minority. While approximately 51% of adolescents identified as non-Hispanic White, it is estimated that by 2050, this percentage will drop to 40.8%. with a significant increase among those who identify as Hispanic.[9]

Living Arrangements

The percentage of children younger than 18 years old living in a single-parent family has been on the rise ever since 1965. In fact, the percentage increased sharply in the 1970s and continued to rise slowly through the 1990s. The sharp rise in the 1970s can be attributed to the great increase in the divorce rate.[5] In 2023, 27.5% of 12- to 17-year-olds lived in single-parent families.[10] For children under 18 years old, Black children (55.0%) and Hispanic children (32.7%) were more likely to live in a single-parent home than White children (23.9%).[11] Regardless of race and ethnicity, children in a single-parent family are more likely to be living with their

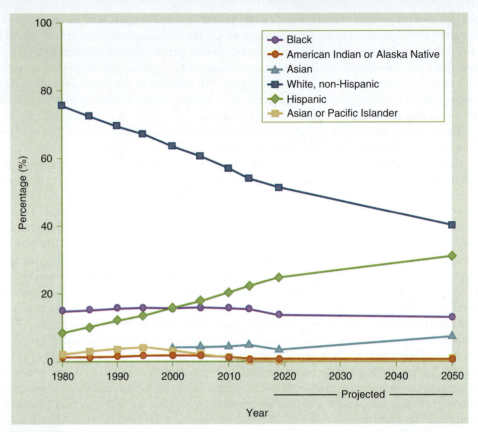

FIGURE 8.1 Race and Hispanic origin of adolescents 10–19 years of age: United States 1980–2050.

Data from (1) MacKay, A. P., and Duran, C. (2007). *Adolescent Health in the United States*. Hyattsville, MD: National Center for Health Statistics, 9; (2) U.S. Department of Health and Human Services. (2017). The Changing Face of America's Adolescent. Available at https://www.hhs.gov/ash/oah/facts-and-stats/changing-face-of-americas-adolescents/index.html. (3) U.S. Census Bureau. (2020). Annual Estimates of the Resident Population by Sex, Age, Race, and Hispanic Origin for the United States: April 1, 2010 to July 1, 2019 (NC-EST2019-ASR6H). Retrieved from https://www.census.gov/newsroom/press-kits/2020/population-estimates-detailed.html

mother than their father (22.6% with mother, 4.9% with father).[10] Family household statistics on single-parent families are only a snapshot of children's living status during a single year. It is widely believed that children from single-parent households have more adverse health outcomes.[12] There are many factors for this, and causes differ greatly among families. Income is one such factor, with children in single-parent households being two times more likely to live in poverty in a male household family and nearly four times more likely in a female household family than their peers in two-parent households.[13] It is also important to note that the number of children in households with same-sex parents is growing. While same-sex parent families have different social factors to navigate, the protective factors of two parents also extend to their children.[14,15]

Employment Status and Healthcare Access

From 1960 to the early 1980s, when there were significant increases in the participation of young women in the labor force, the proportion of adolescents and young adults in the labor force remained relatively constant. As we moved into the early 2000s, the employment: population ratios for teens and young adults dipped, likely as a result of the two recessions. Participation in the labor force remained relatively low, particularly for high school-age students, due to the encouragement of high schoolers to seek unpaid internship experiences to meet high school graduation requirements and improve prospects for attending college. Furthermore, the

BOX 8.1   The ACA, Adolescents, and Young Adults

Some of the ways the ACA is affecting adolescents and young adults are as follows:

- Increasing insurance coverage by allowing young adults to remain on their parents' plan through age 26 and other mechanisms.
- Prohibiting plans from imposing pre-existing condition exclusions (starting in 2010 for children and adolescents and in 2014 for adults).
- Establishing insurance marketplaces (exchanges) where consumers can shop for, compare, and purchase insurance.

- Reducing premiums and cost-sharing in plans purchased in the marketplace through subsidies and tax credits for many low-income individuals.
- Expanding Medicaid (required for children and adolescents; a state option for adults).
- Requiring coverage of certain preventive services without cost-sharing.

Data from National Adolescent and Young Adult Health Information Center. Available at http://nahic.ucsf.edu/resources/aca/

lengthened transition into adulthood due to the growing need for higher levels of educational attainment to secure employment has had an impact on the labor force for 16- to 24-year-olds.[16] In 2023, the youth labor force made up 32.8% of the overall labor force for 16- to 19-year-olds and 66.6% for 20- to 24-year-olds.[17] Like with many of the characteristics discussed already, when the unemployment rates of this age group are separated by race and ethnicity, differences appear. For example, regardless of sex, Black adolescents and young adults are more likely to be unemployed than Whites, thus exemplifying the disparities.[17]

Engagement in the labor force is important to community and public health because most health insurance, and thus access to health care, is connected to employment status. In 2022, 86% of young adults aged 19 to 25 had health insurance coverage, compared with 94.6% of children aged from birth to 18 years.[18] Prior to the passage of the Patient Protection and Affordable Care Act (ACA), only 75% of young adults had health insurance.[19] The ACA, as discussed elsewhere in the text, gave Americans, especially young adults aged 19 to 26 years, increased access to health insurance and health care. Prior to the ACA, studies showed that young adults had less access to health care and tended to use emergency departments for care more than adolescents.[20] After the ACA, studies showed a small yet significant decrease in young adult usage of the emergency department.[21] Since the implementation of the ACA, it is clear that gains have been made to improve access to health care for young adults. More research is still needed to truly understand the full impact. **Box 8.1** highlights ways the ACA impacts adolescents and young adults.

A Health Profile

With regard to the health profile of this age group, four major areas stand out—mortality, morbidity from specific infectious diseases, health behavior and lifestyle, and protective factors. The following information will be presented with the recognition that it is known and emphasized throughout this chapter that an individual's behavior and overall lifestyle are heavily impacted by factors both within and outside of their control.[22] This is increasingly recognized by the community health workforce, and strategies to improve the health and well-being of the adolescent and young adult population are, including approaches that will modify the environment to support healthy lifestyles.

Mortality

Although, on average, adolescents and young adults are a healthy segment of the U.S. population, adolescents and young adults suffer their share of life-threatening problems.[5] As it has been with most other age groups, the death rate for adolescents and young adults has significantly declined. Between 1950 and 2013, the death rate of adolescents and young adults aged 15 to 24 years declined by nearly 50%, from 128.1 to 64.8 per 100,000.[19] Mortality data for early adolescents

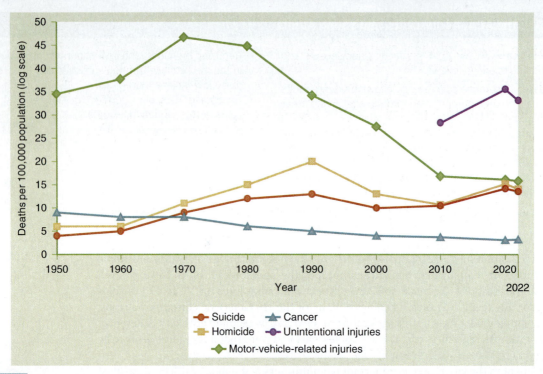

FIGURE 8.2   Death rates for leading causes of death for ages 15 to 24, 1950–2022.

Data from National Center for Health Statistics. (2018). Health, United States, 2017: With Special Feature on Mortality. Hyattsville, MD; National Safety Council. (2024). Historical fatality trends: deaths by age group. https://injuryfacts.nsc.org/motor-vehicle/historical-fatality-trends/deaths-by-age-group; Centers for Disease Control and Prevention, National Center for Health Statistics. National Vital Statistics System, Provisional Mortality on CDC WONDER Online Database. (2024) Provisional leading causes of death rates by age for 2022. https://wonder.cdc.gov/; Centers for Disease Control and Prevention, National Center for Health Statistics. (2024). Drug overdose deaths in the United States, 2002-2022. https://www.cdc.gov/nchs/products/databriefs/db491.htm; Centers for Disease Control and Prevention, National Center for Health Statistics. (2022). Drug overdose deaths in the United States, 2001–2021. https://www.cdc.gov/nchs/products/databriefs/db457.htm

(10–13 years of age) showed a similar decline. This decline in death rates for adolescents and young adults, like that for children, can be attributed to advances in medicine and injury and disease prevention as well as behavior change among this age group.[9,19] Nearly 10 years later, and postpandemic, the death rate for 15- to 24-year-olds was 79.5 in 2022, which is down from 88.9 in 2021.[23] The death rate increase between 2013 and 2022 demonstrates the continued need for targeted public health initiatives.

Regardless of race or ethnicity, adolescent and young adult males have much higher mortality rates than adolescent and young adult females.[21] Mortality rates for males and females were highest among Black adolescents and young adults.[24] Much of the physical threat to those ages10 to 24 stems from their behavior and their environment rather than from disease.[1,24] For young people overall, nearly three-fourths of all mortality can be attributed to three causes—unintentional injuries (39.9%; mainly motor vehicle crashes: 25.5%), suicide (17.0%), and homicide (16.6%).[25] Mortality from unintentional injuries in this age group declined during the last half of the twentieth century. For example, since 1990, the mortality rates for deaths from motor vehicle–related injuries for 15- to 24-year-old people has declined by almost 55%[19] (see **Figure 8.2**).

When we examine the mortality data among 15- to 24-year-old people by gender and race, distinct differences exist. Males are approximately three times more likely than females to be involved in a fatal motor vehicle crash. American Indian or Alaska Native individuals are two times more likely than Black or Hispanic people to be killed in a motor vehicle crash and nearly three times more likely than White individuals 15 to 24 years of age.[25] Similarly, homicide rates are nearly six times higher and suicide rates are more than four times higher for 15- to 24-year-old males than females. Homicide rates are concerningly high for

Black males at a rate of 114.8, which is more than four times the rate for American Indian or Alaska Native males (28.2), the next closest group. Suicide rates are two times higher among American Indian or Alaska Natives and Native Hawaiian or Other Pacific Islanders than Black and White people, which are the next closest groups.[24] Race and gender are not the risk factors for violent death, per se, but rather socioeconomic status and environment. Differences in homicide rates between races are significantly reduced when socioeconomic factors are taken into consideration. When such disproportionate race and gender disparities are identified, as are seen in this age group, the need to continue to address structural and economic disparities is vital.

Morbidity

Although a higher proportion of adolescents and young adults survive to age 24 than ever before, this group still experiences a number of different communicable diseases. Due to medical advances and knowledge regarding immunizations, certain communicable diseases, such as measles, have been nearly eradicated.[26] Changes to the immunization schedule (number and frequency of vaccinations) has significantly reduced the number of measles cases.

The other diseases that cause considerable morbidity in adolescents and young adults are sexually transmitted diseases (STDs), also known as sexually transmitted infections (STIs; see **Table 8.1**), with young people 15 to 24 years of age acquiring half (49.8%) of all reported cases of STIs in 2022 (chlamydia, gonorrhea, and syphilis). This population is at higher risk of acquiring STIs for a combination of behavioral, biological, and cultural reasons.[27] Whereas many STIs are completely curable with antibiotics, some viral infections, such as human immunodeficiency virus (HIV) or human papillomavirus (HPV), can be treated but never cured.[27] The effects of some STIs can last a lifetime. For example, some forms of HPV are the precursor to cervical cancer, and the effects of chlamydia, if untreated, can lead to infertility. As in the case of HIV, the precursor to acquired immunodeficiency syndrome (AIDS), the result may even be death,

TABLE 8.1 Number of Reported Cases (and Incidence Rates) of Selected Communicable Diseases Among 15- to 24-Year-Old People, 1981 to 2022

Disease	1981#	1990#	2000	2010	2020	2022
AIDS	—	1,715	1,567 (4.16)	7,217 (16.75) (reported as HIV)	22 (0.05)	26 (0.06)
Chlamydia	—	—	508,736 (1,349.42)	930,338 (2,159.69)	10,119 (24.69)	9,937 (24.69)
Gonorrhea*	617,994	384,490	212,679 (564.13)	193,869 (450.05)	3,065 (7.48)	3,073 (7.64)
Measles	94	5,646	17 (0.05)	7 (0.02)	—	4 (0.01)
Syphilis*	12,965	16,408	1,338 (3.55)	10,629 (24.67)	81 (0.20)	97 (0.24)
Tuberculosis	2,198	1,867	1,623 (4.31)	1,220 (2.79)	152 (0.37)	157 (0.38)

Notes: # = rates not available; — = data not collected; * = civilian cases only, primary and secondary. Incidence rates per 100,000 population.

Data from Centers for Disease Control. Morbidity and Mortality Weekly Report: Annual Summaries, various years; Summary of Notifiable Diseases—United States, 2000. Morbidity and Mortality Weekly Report, 49(53): 23; and Summary of Notifiable Diseases—United States, 2008. Morbidity and Mortality Weekly Report, 57(54): 32–33. Summary of Notifiable Diseases—United States, 2010. Morbidity and Mortality Weekly Report, 59(53): 39–40. Centers for Disease Control and Prevention. (2019) National Notifiable Diseases Surveillance System, 2018 Annual Tables of Infectious Disease Data. Available at https://www.cdc.gov/nndss/infectious-tables.html

2020 Data Source: Centers for Disease Control and Prevention. (2023). Nationally Notifiable Infectious Diseases and Conditions, United States: Annual Tables. https://wonder.cdc.gov/nndss/static/2020/annual/2020-table4-H.pdf

2022 Data Source: Centers for Disease Control and Prevention. (2024). Nationally Notifiable Infectious Diseases and Conditions, United States: Annual Tables. https://wonder.cdc.gov/nndss/static/2021/annual/2021-table4-H.pdf

although people with HIV are living long healthy lives when they are diagnosed and treated soon after infection.[28] Chlamydia is the most common curable STI among this age group with 57.7% of all cases of chlamydia reported among persons aged 15 to 24 years in 2022. Disparities continue to exist among rates of reported STIs. For example, in 2022, Black people made up 12.6% of the U.S. population, but accounted for 31.1% of all cases of chlamydia, gonorrhea, and syphilis cases.[27]

Timely medical care is important in managing STIs—treatment of the person infected as well as reducing the likelihood of infecting a sexual partner. The COVID-19 pandemic resulted in significant disruptions in STI-related prevention and care activities. Thus, surveillance data must be cautiously interpreted. While the number of cases of STIs reported in 2022 was higher than the number reported in 2020, the 2022 numbers are lower than cases reported prior to the COVID-19 pandemic. Nonetheless, STIs continue to be a significant public health concern, particularly for this age group. Prevention and control efforts remain important.[29]

In terms of HIV, 20% of all new HIV infections in the United States in 2022 were found in youth ages 13 to 24.[28] The rate of new infections is declining. Unfortunately, like with other STIs, certain groups are disproportionately affected. Specifically, Black and Hispanic people made up 70% of estimated new HIV infections in 2022,[30] affirming the need for population-specific public health campaigns.

Health Behaviors of High School Students

Whereas many behavioral patterns begin during the childhood years, others begin in adolescence and young adulthood. During this period of experimentation, young people are susceptible to developing harmful behaviors, such as the abuse of tobacco and other drugs, driving under the influence, and carrying a weapon.

In 1990, the Centers for Disease Control and Prevention (CDC) initiated the YRBSS to better track selected health behaviors among young people. The YRBSS includes a national school-based survey, as well as state, territorial, tribal, and district surveys. In the spring of 1991, CDC conducted for the first time the national school-based Youth Risk Behavior Survey (YRBS). This survey continues to be conducted biennially during odd-numbered years among national probability samples of 9th- through 12th-grade students from private and public schools. In 1990, the CDC began offering to each state and to selected local education departments the YRBSS questionnaire and fiscal and technical assistance to conduct the YRBS. Data are gathered from a representative sample of youth from most states and several large urban school districts.[31] During the time the YRBSS has been in operation, it has proved to be helpful at both the state and local levels. A number of states and local communities have put programs and policies into place to reduce risk behaviors in youth. Continued support of YRBSS will help monitor and ensure the success of many public health and school health programs. Results of the 2021 survey, which was conducted during the COVID-19 pandemic, are included in the following sections. The 2021 findings reflect shifts in youth demographics, with increased percentages of racial and ethnic minority youth and LGBQ+ youths compared with previous YRBSS cycles providing guidance in developing health equity strategies to address long-term disparities.[31]

Behaviors That Contribute to Unintentional Injuries

Four different behaviors of high school students that relate to unintentional injuries are regularly monitored as part of the YRBSS: seat belt use, riding with a driver who has been drinking alcohol, driving after drinking alcohol, and texting or e-mailing while driving a vehicle. During the years studied, the numbers of students engaging in these risky behaviors have declined. Yet concerns remain as 14.1% of students nationwide had, in the 30 days preceding the survey, ridden with a driver who had been drinking alcohol in 2021. Of those same students, 36.1% of students had texted or e-mailed while driving a vehicle on at least 1 day in the 30 days before the survey, demonstrating that nearly one in seven high school students engaged in risky behaviors while in a motor vehicle.[32]

Behaviors That Contribute to Violence

Behaviors that contribute to violence-related injuries of high school students include engaging in a physical fight, engaging in dating violence, having been forced to have sexual intercourse, engaging in school-related violence, including bullying, suicide ideation, and suicide attempts. Nationwide, nearly one in seven students (15%) had been bullied on school property in the past 12 months before the survey and 15.9% of students reported being electronically bullied within the 12 months before the survey.[32] Females and students who identify as gay, lesbian, bisexual, or questioning are more likely to experience bullying behaviors than males or students who identify as heterosexual. Males are more likely than females to get into a fight. The percentage of students who are forced to have sexual intercourse is higher for females (13.5%) and students who identify as gay, lesbian, bisexual, or questioning (21.9%) than males (3.3%) and heterosexual students (5%). Also, the percentage of students who seriously consider suicide is higher for those who identify as gay, lesbian, bisexual, or questioning (48.1%) and females (30%) than males (14.3%) and heterosexual students (15%). The percentage of students who attempt suicide is also higher for students who identify as gay, lesbian, bisexual, or questioning (24.1%) and females (13.3%) than males (663%) and heterosexual students (6.3%).[32]

Tobacco Use

The use of tobacco products represents one of the most widespread, high-risk health behaviors for this group. In 2023, less than 2% of high school students nationwide were current smokers—that is, smoked on at least 1 day in the past 30 days. While this is a significant decrease from 1995, when 34.8% of students were current smokers, it does not fully capture student smoking behavior of high school students as youth use e-cigarettes, or vapes, more than any other tobacco product.[33] In 2023, one of every 10 high school students reported they had used e-cigarettes in the past 30 days, with more females than males reporting current e-cigarette use.[34] With one in two U.S. youth who have tried e-cigarettes reporting current use, the concern is great. Of additional worry is that e-cigarettes can be used to deliver other substances, such as cannabis. Nearly one in three middle and high school students who had ever used an e-cigarette reported using marijuana in the device.[34] The vast majority of people who become dependent on nicotine develop that dependency before the age of 18 (see **Figure 8.3**).[33]

Because use of tobacco that begins during adolescence can lead to a lifetime of nicotine dependence and a variety of negative health consequences, the federal government has exerted considerable effort to keep tobacco out of the hands of adolescents. Many believed, and data from the YRBSS verified, that most adolescents have had easy access to tobacco products. E-cigarettes have presented new challenges in our national tobacco prevention efforts. Most middle and high school students who vape first start with flavored products, such as fruit, candy, mint, or menthol flavors. The availability of flavored vapes is reported as one of the top 10 reasons youth try e-cigarettes.[35]

The most sweeping changes related to the sale of cigarettes came in 1998 when 46 state attorneys general agreed to a settlement with tobacco companies. (Florida, Minnesota, Mississippi, and Texas were not included in the settlement because they had already settled individually with the tobacco companies.) The settlement called for the companies to make payments of $206 billion to the states over 25 years, beginning in 2000, and to finance antismoking programs in exchange for the states dropping their healthcare lawsuits for smokers who were treated with Medicaid funds. In addition to paying the states, the tobacco companies agreed to spend $1.7 billion to

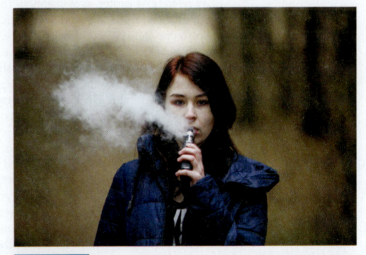

FIGURE 8.3 Electronic cigarettes are the most commonly used tobacco product among youth with one out of 10 high school students reporting they had used e-cigarettes in the past 30 days.[33]

© Aleksandr Yu/Shutterstock

study youth smoking and to finance antismoking advertising and accept restrictions on marketing practices that appeal to children, such as the use of cartoon characters (e.g., "Joe Camel").[36] Although policy and prevention efforts have continued to positively affect the number of children who begin smoking, as can be observed by the 2009 passing of the Family Smoking Prevention and Tobacco Control Act, which, for the first time, granted the U.S. Food and Drug Administration (FDA) the authority to regulate the manufacturing, marketing, and distribution,[36] states are spending only $1 in tobacco revenue to fight tobacco use, while tobacco companies are outspending prevention efforts 12 to 1 in the marketing of their products.[37]

The invention of e-cigarettes has once again changed the challenges in prevention and cessation of tobacco use. While states and other localities have worked to address tobacco-related issues through advocacy efforts and the establishment of policies, enormous challenges remain. Most recently, in December of 2019, the federal government increased the minimum legal sale age for tobacco to 21.[38] However, many public health professionals would like to see stronger policies and laws, such as banning flavored e-cigarettes to help curb the skyrocketing numbers of youth who use these products.[39]

Alcohol and Other Drugs

Although, for some, the first use of alcohol or other drugs begins during the childhood years, for most, experimentation with these substances occurs during the adolescent and young adult years. For example, 15% of students surveyed for the YRBSS in 2021 indicated that they drank alcohol (more than a few sips) for the first time prior to 13 years of age.[32] Of all high school students, 22.7% reported drinking during the previous month and 10.5% engaged in binge drinking (five or more drinks of alcohol in a row).[32] Furthermore, 27.8% of high school students have tried marijuana with nearly one-sixth (15.8%) reporting use within the past 30 days.[32]

Although 15.8% of all high school students have used marijuana during the preceding month, alcohol use and abuse continue to be major problems for adolescents. In addition to the use of marijuana, 13.3% of high school students are reporting the use of other illicit drugs (cocaine, inhalants, heroin, methamphetamines, ecstasy, or hallucinogens) one or more times during their life.[32] Additionally, the 2021 YRBSS data indicated a rising concern for adolescents and young adults reporting misuse and abuse of prescription drugs as 12.2% of students surveyed had taken prescription pain medication (e.g., OxyContin, Percocet, Vicodin, codeine, or hydrocodone) without a doctor's prescription or differently from how a doctor told them to use it at least once.[32]

Sexual Behaviors That Contribute to Unintended Pregnancy and Sexually Transmitted Infections

As referenced earlier, adolescents in the United States continue to experience high rates of unintended pregnancies and STIs, including HIV infection. YRBSS data from 2021 show that nearly one-third (30.0%) of all high school students have engaged in sexual intercourse sometime in their lifetime. The prevalence of sexual intercourse ranged between 15.9% for 9th-graders to 48.4% for 12th-graders. While data show differences as students get older, data do not show large differences by gender and race. Reported differences exist based on sexual identity—more students identifying as bisexual (39.9%) and gay, lesbian, and bisexual (38.2%) than heterosexual (29.2%) report having had sexual intercourse. **Table 8.2** shows the trends of selected sexual risk behaviors for high school students since 1995. These findings have important implications for the need for comprehensive sexual education prior to high school.

The teenage birth rate has declined more than 70% since its peak in 1991 to 13.6 births per 1,000 in 2022. Although these are positive changes, teenage pregnancy remains a significant concern with more than 143,700 teen girls in the United States between the ages of 15 and 19 becoming pregnant each year.[40] Children born to teen mothers are more likely to have a higher risk for low birth weight or infant mortality, rely more heavily on funded health care, have higher rates of foster placement, have lower school achievement, and give birth as a teen.[41] In addition to the health risks associated with teenage pregnancies for both mother and child, there are educational, economic, and psychosocial risks to the mother and father as well.[41] Consequently, due to these negative health and psychosocial outcomes, the public health community must take steps to prevent pregnancy in the adolescent population.

TABLE 8.2 Percentage of High School Students Who Reported Selected Sexual Risk Behaviors, by Selected Year—Youth Risk Behavior Survey, United States

Behavior	1995	2005	2015	2021
Ever had sexual intercourse	53.1	46.8	41.2	30.0
Ever had sexual intercourse with four or more partners	17.8	14.3	11.5	6.0
Had sexual intercourse at least once during the 3 months preceding the survey	37.9	33.9	30.1	20.7
Used alcohol or drugs before last sexual intercourse	24.8	23.3	20.6	20.6
Did not use any method to prevent pregnancy (among students who were currently sexually active)	15.8	12.7	13.8	13.7
Used or partner used condom at last sexual intercourse	54.4	62.8	56.9	51.8

Data from Centers for Disease Control and Prevention. (2024). *YRBS Explorer: Explore youth risk behavior survey questions – United States, 2021.* https://yrbs -explorer.services.cdc.gov/#/

Physical Activity and Sedentary Behaviors

Lack of physical activity by young people is an ongoing concern. In 2021, 45.3% of students had not been physically active for at least 60 minutes per day on 5 or more days during the 7 days prior to the YRBSS survey. Males (54.7%) were more likely than females (35.9%) to engage in sufficient physical activity. Nationally, 15.8% of students had not participated in 60 minutes of any kind of physical activity that increased their heart rate or made them breathe hard some of the time on at least 1 day during the 7 days preceding the survey.[32] In contrast, approximately three-quarters (75.9%) of students had spent 3 or more hours per day on screen time (TV, computer, smart phone, or other electronic device, not counting time spent doing schoolwork).[32]

Overweight and Weight Control

Much like the concern for insufficient physical activity, the concern regarding students becoming overweight has been a public health priority due to the negative health consequences associated with being overweight and obese, such as the potential to develop type 2 diabetes, as well as a variety of other health issues.[42] In 2021, 16.3% of high school students had obesity, and 16.0% were overweight, while 32.3% described themselves as slightly or very overweight. Almost one-half of students were trying to lose weight (45.7%).[32] While many policies and practices have been implemented over the past 2 decades, adequate physical activity and healthy eating practices among young people remain a public health priority.

Mental Health

While there have always been concerns about adolescent mental health, the isolation experienced during the COVID-19 pandemic brought national attention to the challenges young people experience. In 2021, nearly one in three (42%) high school students reported having felt so sad or hopeless for at least 2 weeks in the past year they could not engage in regular activities, and more than one in five (22%) students reported they had seriously considered suicide.[32] Female students, lesbian, gay, bisexual, queer, or questioning students are even more likely to experience poor mental health.[32] Like many of the other risk behaviors, poor mental health increases students' risk of engaging in harmful sexual behaviors and substance use.[43] Much work is needed to ensure students are receiving the services needed to build resilience and mental health skills as the consequences of poor mental health impacts not only the individual but their family and community.

Health Behaviors of College Students

Two currently available data sources regarding the health behaviors of college students are the National College Health Assessment III (NCHA-III)[44] and Monitoring the Future.[45] The NCHA-IIIb, first implemented in the spring of 2000, is a national, nonprofit research effort organized by the American College Health Association.[44] Monitoring the Future is conducted at the University of Michigan's Institute for Social Research and, since its inception in 1975, has been funded by the National Institute on Drug Abuse. Monitoring the Future specifically examines drug behaviors and related attitudes of a broad participant age range: 8th, 10th, and 12th graders to adults through age 60,[45] whereas the NCHA-III examines a wide range of health behaviors in college students. These data sources, among others, can be helpful to those responsible for delivering health promotion education and services to many of the 15.4 million students enrolled in the nation's colleges and universities.[46]

Behaviors That Contribute to Unintentional Injuries

As mentioned throughout this chapter, the use of alcohol, both by the injured individual or a person whom the individual is with at the time of injury, is a common cause of unintentional injuries among adolescents and young adults, especially college-age students.[9,19] These injuries are often associated with the use of a motor vehicle at the time of the incident,[9] but this is not always the case. Unintentional injuries have been the leading cause of death for young adults throughout the past 50 years.[19]

Tobacco and Marijuana Use

Historically, a significant difference in cigarette use had been observed between noncollege and college young adults. The most recent data no longer show that difference.[44] Concern has now shifted to vaping nicotine (see **Figure 8.4**). Monitoring the Future began collecting data on vaping among young adults in 2017. Since 2017, past-30-day prevalence has more than tripled

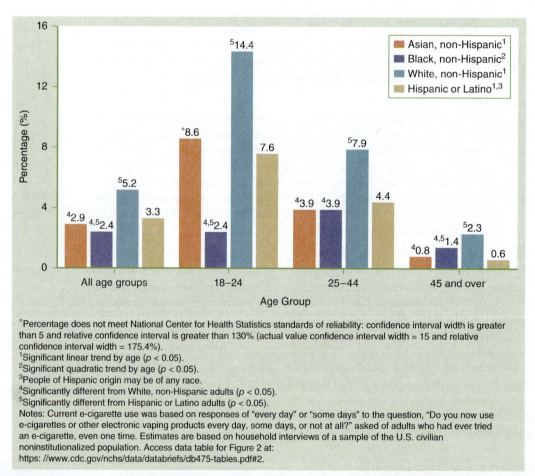

*Percentage does not meet National Center for Health Statistics standards of reliability: confidence interval width is greater than 5 and relative confidence interval is greater than 130% (actual value confidence interval width = 15 and relative confidence interval width = 175.4%).
[1]Significant linear trend by age ($p < 0.05$).
[2]Significant quadratic trend by age ($p < 0.05$).
[3]People of Hispanic origin may be of any race.
[4]Significantly different from White, non-Hispanic adults ($p < 0.05$).
[5]Significantly different from Hispanic or Latino adults ($p < 0.05$).
Notes: Current e-cigarette use was based on responses of "every day" or "some days" to the question, "Do you now use e-cigarettes or other electronic vaping products every day, some days, or not at all?" asked of adults who had ever tried an e-cigarette, even one time. Estimates are based on household interviews of a sample of the U.S. civilian noninstitutionalized population. Access data table for Figure 2 at: https://www.cdc.gov/nchs/data/databriefs/db475-tables.pdf#2.

FIGURE 8.4   Percentage of adults aged 18 and over who currently use e-cigarettes by age group and race and Hispanic origin, 2021.

Reproduced from Centers for Disease Control and Prevention, National Center for Health Statistics. (2023). Current Electronic Cigarette Use Among Adults Aged 18 and Over: United States, 2021. https://www.cdc.gov/nchs/data/databriefs/db475.pdf

among college young adults (from 5.4% in 2017 to 18.9% in 2022) and among noncollege young adults (from 7.0% in 2017 to 23.2% in 2022).[44] Similar to the vaping nicotine data, prevalence of vaping marijuana was also higher for noncollege than college young adults, with 18.9% of noncollege young adults reporting vaping marijuana in the past 30 days compared with 11.2% of college young adults.[44] Additionally, daily use of marijuana is also significantly different for these two groups with 14.5% of noncollege students compared with 4.7% of college young adults reporting daily marijuana use in 2022.[44]

Alcohol and Other Drug Use

College and university campuses have long been thought of as places where alcohol and other drugs have been abused. **Table 8.3** shows that alcohol was the drug of choice on college campuses in 2022, with 62.5% of the students reporting that they had consumed alcohol in the previous 30 days.[45] Table 8.3 also shows that illicit drug use has significantly decreased since 1980.[45] **Figure 8.5A** presents the more than 40-year trend for alcohol use on college campuses. The figure shows that the number of individuals consuming one or more drinks over the past 30-day period has remained fairly stable for the past 25 years, with approximately 62.5% of college students having consumed alcohol.[45] **Figure 8.5B** demonstrates a decrease in the number of college students participating in binge drinking, which is commonly defined as consuming five or more drinks in a row, which is encouraging.[45] According to the National College Health Association, 22% of males and females binge drank on at least one occasion during the 2 weeks prior to survey administration.[44] Excessive alcohol intake is associated with a number of adverse consequences, including motor vehicle crashes, alcohol poisoning, STIs and unintended pregnancy, and various forms of violence.[47]

Sexual Behaviors That Contribute to Unintended Pregnancy and Sexually Transmitted Diseases

Like adolescents, many college students are at risk for unintended pregnancies and STIs through the practice of unprotected sexual activity. Approximately 41% of all gonorrhea cases and 58% of all chlamydia cases occur among persons under 25 years of age.[27] In addition, 48.5% of college students used a condom or another protective barrier the last time they had vaginal intercourse in the 30 days prior to being surveyed, and 18.5% relied on the withdrawal method for pregnancy prevention.[44]

Mental Health

Like high school students, young adults in college experienced significant mental health challenges during the COVID-19 pandemic. Anxiety (31.5%) and depression (24.1%) are reported by a significant number of college students. Women (36.4%; 26.4%) and transgender/gender

TABLE 8.3 Trends in 30-Day Prevalence of Various Types of Drugs Among Full-Time College Students

	Percentage Who Used in Past 30 Days					
	1980	1990	2000	2010	2020	2022
Any illicit drug other than marijuana	20.7	4.4	6.9	8.1	6.0	2.9
Marijuana	34.0	14.0	20.0	17.5	24.5	22.1
Vaping Marijuana	NA	NA	NA	NA	12.4	11.2
Alcohol	81.8	74.5	67.4	65.0	55.7	62.5
Cigarettes	25.8	21.5	28.2	16.4	4.1	6.4
Vaping Nicotine	NA	NA	NA	NA	18.6	18.9

Notes: NA = data not available.

Data from Schulenberg, J. E., Patrick, M. E., Johnston, L. D., O'Malley, P. M., Bachman, J. G., & Miech, R. A., (2021). *Monitoring the Future national survey results on drug use, 1975–2020: Volume II, College students and adults ages 19–60.* Ann Arbor: Institute for Social Research, The University of Michigan. Available at https://monitoringthefuture.org/results/

Patrick, M. E., Miech, R. A., Johnston, L. D., & O'Malley, P. M. (2023). *Monitoring the Future panel study annual report: National data on substance abuse among adults ages 19 to 60, 1976–2022.* Monitoring the Future Monograph Serices. Ann Arbor: Institute for Social Research, The University of Michigan. Available at https://monitoringthefuture.org/results/

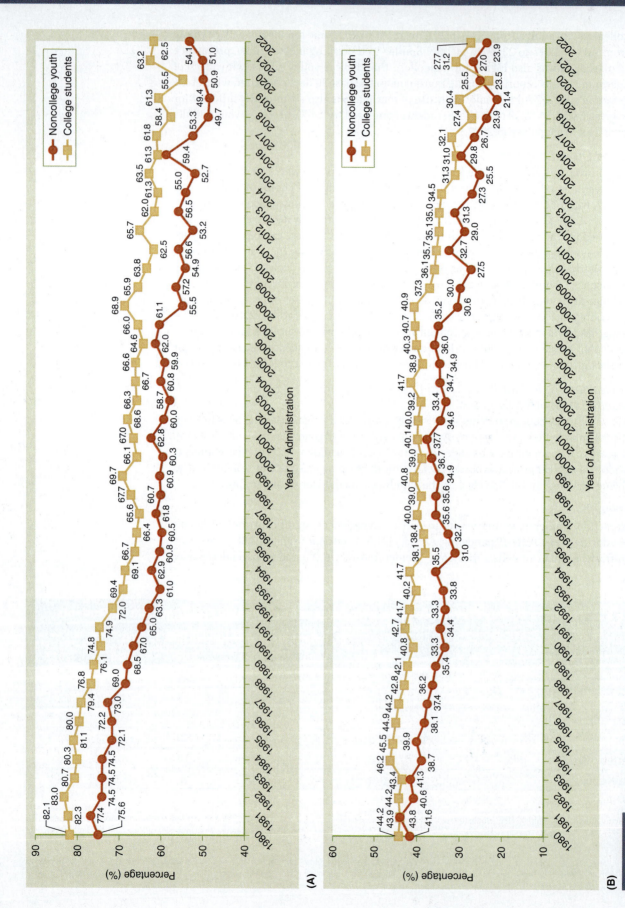

FIGURE 8.5 **A.** Alcohol: trends in 30-day prevalence among college students vs. others 1 to 4 years beyond high school. **B.** Alcohol: trends in 2-week prevalence of five or more drinks in a row among college students vs. others 1 to 4 years beyond high school.

nonconforming (60.9%; 56.4%) college students report experiencing anxiety and depression at much higher rates than males (15.1%; 12.3%).[44] Additionally, college students report high levels of loneliness and stress.[44] When the mental health challenges young adults are experiencing are combined with other risky behaviors discussed earlier, the health of young adults becomes significantly concerning. Early and ongoing health education and public health campaigns geared toward their most high-risk behaviors and the most at-risk populations will help ensure that young people make healthy choices now and throughout their lifetime.

> **Protective factors** factors that increase an individual's ability to avoid risks or hazards, and promote social and emotional competence to thrive in all aspects of life

Protective Factors

So far in this chapter, the health problems of the adolescent and young adult age groups have been highlighted. However, protective factors must also be considered in the equation of the overall health of these populations. **Protective factors** are "individual or environmental characteristics and conditions that promote the health and emotional well-being of children and adolescents."[47] An example of a protective factor is school connectedness or engagement, which is defined as, "the belief by students that adults and peers in the school support, value, and care about their individual well-being as well as their academic progress."[48] Students who feel more connected to school are[48]:

- Less likely to engage in risky behaviors (violence, sexual health, and harmful substance use).
- More likely to engage in positive health behaviors (physical activity and healthy eating).
- More likely to have higher grades and test scores, have better school attendance, and graduate from high school.
- Less likely to have emotional distress and thoughts of suicide among adolescents.

Another example of a protective factor for adolescents and young adults is community service. It has been shown that adolescents who volunteer in their community engage in fewer risk behaviors, have a stronger connection to their community, do better in school, and are more likely to volunteer as adults.[49,50] Thus, it may be more efficient and effective to focus limited public health resources on increasing the protective factors, rather than exclusively focusing on decreasing the health problems.

Community and Public Health Strategies for Improving the Health of Adolescents and Young Adults

There are no easy, simple, or immediate solutions to reducing or eliminating the health problems of adolescents and young adults. Community health is affected by four major factors—physical factors, community organizing, individual behavior, and social and cultural factors. Of these four factors, two need special attention when dealing with the health problems of adolescents and young adults—social and cultural factors and community organizing. Many health problems originate from the social and cultural environments in which people have been raised and live, and the cultural and social norms that have been with us, in some cases, for many years.

Take, for example, the use of alcohol. It is safe to say that one of the biggest health problems facing adolescents and young adults in the United States today is the use of alcohol. Alcohol contributes to all of the leading causes of mortality and morbidity in these age groups. If the norm of a community is to turn its back on adolescents consuming alcohol or young adults (of legal age) abusing alcohol, efforts need to be made to change the culture. However, in most communities, cultural and social norms do not change quickly. Efforts to turn these health problems around will need to be community-wide in nature and sustained over a long period of time. By "community-wide," we mean the involvement of all the stakeholders in a community, not just those who are associated with health-related professions—in other words, a community organizing effort is needed. By "sustained over a long period," we mean institutionalizing the change in the culture. For examples of programs that have been effective in preventing or reducing substance use and other related high-risk behaviors in communities and schools, including college campus communities, visit the SAMHSA (Substance Abuse and Mental Health Services Administration) Evidence-Based Practices Resource Center website at https://www.samhsa.gov

/resource-search/ebp, which includes a searchable online registry of mental health and substance use interventions that have been reviewed and rated by independent reviewers.[51]

To change the culture as it relates to adolescents' use of alcohol, research has shown that alcohol prevention efforts need to be a part of a comprehensive school health education effort and should include components outside of the classroom. Thus, prevention programs need to include components that focus on changing norms, interaction among peers, social skills training, and developmental and cultural appropriateness.[52-54] Although the adolescent and young adult age group encounters many health issues that are described in this chapter, these individuals are typically the healthiest segments of the U.S. population. The health challenges experienced by this age group need to be addressed at every level, especially the community level. The members of this age group also need to be involved in creating and implementing the solutions to these health challenges for these strategies to be effective.[55] These strategies should not only focus on decreasing the health problem but also on increasing the protective factors associated with that health problem.

Adults

The adult age group (those 25 to 64 years old) represents slightly more than half of the U.S. population.[8] The size of this segment of the overall population is expected to remain stable over the next several decades, but in proportion to the rest of the population, this segment will become smaller. Therefore, provisions to deal with the health concerns of this age group will need to be maintained.

A Health Profile

The health profile of this age group of adults is characterized primarily by mortality from chronic diseases stemming from poor health behaviors impacted by health-detracting environments, and as previously mentioned, the health behaviors, events, and exposures experienced during the earlier years of life.[7]

Mortality

With life expectancy at birth between 75 and 80 years,[19] most Americans can expect to live beyond their 65th birthday. However, many do not. During the 1950s and 1960s, many of the leading causes of death in this age group resulted from preventable conditions associated with unhealthy behaviors and lifestyles. Since that time, the public health and medical communities have recognized how the environment, social, and cultural factors shape an individual's behavior.[56] As such, many adults have quit smoking, and more Americans than ever before are exercising regularly and eating healthier diets. These lifestyle improvements, along with successes in public health, such as an increased focus on the built environment (i.e., advocating for the need for more sidewalks vs. more roads) and advances in medicine, have resulted in a significant decline in the death rate for adults.

In the past, the leading causes of death for adults were reported only for the 25- to 64-year-old age group. More recently, the adult years have been subdivided into two groups: 25 to 44 years and 45 to 64 years, with some data being reported in 5- or 10-year age spans. In 2022, the death rate for all adults aged 25 to 34 years was 163.4 and 35 to 44 years 255.4.[23] The leading causes of death for adults aged 25 to 34 in 2022 were unintentional injuries, suicide, homicide, heart disease, and cancer. For 35- to 44-year-olds, the leading causes of death were unintentional injuries, heart disease, cancer, suicide, and chronic liver disease and cirrhosis.[24] In 2021, COVID-19 was the second leading cause of death for 25- to 44-year-olds, but by 2022, it had fallen to the seventh leading cause.[24] When these mortality data were broken down in 2021 (the most current data available) by age, sex, and race, some differences appear. For both age groups, the five leading causes of death were the same but differ in rank order by race and ethnicity, except for liver disease among Hispanic 35- to 44-year-olds, which ranked in their

TABLE 8.4   2021 Death Rates for Adults Ages 25–34 and 35–44 (rate per 100,000 population)

Cause	White, Non-Hispanic		Black, Non-Hispanic		Hispanic	
	25–34 (173.7)	35–44 (287)	25–34 (296.8)	35–44 (465.3)	25–34 (155.7)	35–44 (236.3)
Unintentional injuries	84.2	96.9	92.0	104.4	62.3	58.6
COVID-19	9.6	27.4	21.4	59.3	19.7	55.1
Cancer	7.7	26.7	9.7	34.6	8.1	20.9
Heart disease	8.1	27.8	20.2	65.8	6.1	17.3
Suicide	23.0	23.6	16.7	11.9	14.4	10.1
Homicide	5.3	5.2	71.2	45.5	14.0	9.6
Chronic liver disease and cirrhosis	4.0	14.6	—	8.2	4.3	13.2
Diabetes mellitus	2.4	5.7	6.8	16.3	1.7	5.3
Stroke	1.2	3.8	2.4	11.3	1.3	4.9
HIV	—	—	4.9	6.7	—	1.9
Pregnancy, childbirth and peurperium	1.4	—	1.2	—	1.7	—

Data from Curtin SC, Tejada-Vera B, Bastian BA. (2024). Deaths: Leading causes for 2021. National Vital Statistics Reports; vol 73 no 4. Hyattsville, MD: National Center for Health Statistics. DOI: https://dx.doi.org/10.15620/cdc/147882. https://www.cdc.gov/nchs/data/nvsr/nvsr73/nvsr73-04.pdf

top five. In addition, HIV was a leading cause of death for Black and 35- to 44-year-old Hispanic people but not for White people (see **Table 8.4**).[26]

In 2022, the death rate for 45- to 54-year-olds was 453.3 per 100,000, and for 55- to 64-year-olds, it was 992.1 per 100,000.[24] The majority of these deaths were the result of noncommunicable health problems, including cancer, heart disease, unintentional injuries, COVID-19, liver disease, suicide, diabetes, and stroke. In 2021, (the most recent available data presented by race and ethnicity) the disparities among Black, Hispanic, and White people are apparent when the leading causes of death are examined in **Table 8.5**.

Cancer

Since 1983, the number one cause of death in the adult age group for people ages 45 to 54 and 55 to 64 has been cancer (malignant neoplasms). Cancer death rates for both age groups have decreased since 1950 (175.1 and 390.7 per 100,000 in 1950 compared with 82.5 and 249.8 per 100,000 in 2022).[24] Four types of cancers account for these large numbers—prostate, lung, and colorectal for men; and breast, lung, and colorectal for women.[57] The leading cause of cancer deaths and the most preventable type of cancer for both men and women is lung cancer.[57] This trend is expected to continue as large numbers of smokers continue to age. Of all lung cancer deaths, upward of 80% can be attributed to smoking.[58] Another leading cause of death resulting from cancer is colorectal cancer. Risk factors for this type of cancer include being overweight or obese, a diet high in red or processed meats, smoking, and moderate to heavy alcohol consumption.[58]

Breast cancer is the other cancer of much concern. Although it is less deadly than lung cancer, the number of cases of breast cancer is more than twice that of lung cancer in women.[57] Because of increased community awareness and the availability of diagnostic screening for breast cancer, survival rates are much higher than for lung cancer. It is important for women 40 years of age and older to comply with the screening recommendations for early detection.[59]

Cardiovascular Diseases

Some of the greatest changes in cause-specific mortality rates in adults are those for the cardiovascular diseases. Age-adjusted mortality rates from heart disease dropped from 588.8 per 100,000 in 1950 to 79.9 per 100,000 for 45- to 54-year-olds and 203.7 per 100,000 for 55- to 64-year-olds in 2022, whereas deaths from strokes dropped from 180.7 per 100,000 to 13.8 and 33.7 per 100,000, respectively, during the same period of time.[24] While the age ranges reported

TABLE 8.5   2021 Death Rates for Adults Ages 45-54 and 55-64 (rate per 100,000 population)

Cause	White, Non-Hispanic		Black, Non-Hispanic		Hispanic	
	45–54 (529.9)	55–64 (1097.8)	45–54 (827.8)	55–64 (1681.3)	45–54 (433.1)	55–64 (932.7)
Heart disease	85.1	205.3	168.3	366.2	48.0	131.5
Cancer	87.6	264.7	103.4	322.7	60.8	170.0
COVID-19	75.3	146.2	132.4	242.0	128.6	272.0
Unintentional injuries	83.2	76.1	110.4	133.4	54.2	58.1
Chronic liver disease and cirrhosis	28.2	43.4	17.9	32.6	25.5	45.4
Chronic lower respiratory disease	9.9	49.8	—	41.1	—	10.8
Diabetes mellitus	16.4	37.7	36.7	81.5	16.0	44.9
Stroke	11.8	29.4	28.7	70.8	12.9	29.1
Suicide	24.6	21.8	—	—	8.3	—
Septicemia	5.7	14.2	—	—	—	10.8
Homicide	—	—	24.0	—	6.1	—
Nephritis, nephrotic syndrome, and nephrosis	—	—	15.6	35.1	5.7	15.2
Hypertension and hypertensive renal disease	—	—	13.1	30.1	—	—

Data from Curtin SC, Tejada-Vera B, Bastian BA. (2024). Deaths: Leading causes for 2021. National Vital Statistics Reports; vol 73 no 4. Hyattsville, MD: National Center for Health Statistics. DOI: https://dx.doi.org/10.15620/cdc/147882. https://www.cdc.gov/nchs/data/nvsr/nvsr73/nvsr73-04.pdf

have changed over the years, a significant decrease in mortality rates is evident. These changes are primarily the result of public health efforts, including changes to the environment, which have encouraged people to stop smoking, increase their physical activity, and eat more nutritiously. The reduction or postponement of deaths from heart disease has resulted in cancer becoming the leading cause of deaths in adults aged 45 to 64.[24]

Health Behaviors

Many of the risk factors associated with the leading causes of morbidity and mortality in American adults are associated with health behaviors that are influenced by an individual's environment and other social determinants of health, such as income, access to food, and education.[60] Adults are in a position to take action, by modifying their health behaviors, to improve their health status. However, environmental support systems need to be in place to encourage these health behaviors or else it becomes increasingly difficult for these individuals to live a healthy lifestyle. We know that today, more than ever before, adults are watching what they eat, wearing their seat belts, controlling their blood pressure, and exercising with regularity. The prevalence of smoking among adults has declined, as has the incidence of drinking and driving. Although these are encouraging signs, much more can be done.

As with the other age groups discussed in this chapter, the National Center for Health Statistics (NCHS) collects self-reported behavior risk data on adults. These data are collected via the Behavioral Risk Factor Surveillance System (BRFSS). One limitation of the data from this system is that they are collected, and usually reported, on all adults older than 18 years of age; the data are not broken down by the specific age groups (18–24, 25–44, and 45–64) discussed in this chapter. More detailed information about the health behaviors of adults in the United States is presented next.

Risk Factors for Chronic Disease

The best single behavioral change Americans can make to reduce morbidity and mortality is to stop smoking. Cigarette smoking causes nearly one of five deaths in the United States each year.[61] Smoking tobacco, no matter the form (cigarettes or vape) is a significant risk factor for cancer, heart disease, and stroke. In 2021, 11.5% of those aged 18 years and older smoked.

This is a decline from 20.9 in 2005. This amounts to about 28.3 million Americans.[61] The proportion of Americans who smoke has dropped considerably since 1965, when 40% of all Americans smoked, but the consequences on individual health remain.[19] In general, smoking rates are higher among males, people with fewer years of education, and those with lower incomes.[61] The use of e-cigarettes is likely to have an impact on the demographics impacted by smoking behaviors as younger people report much more use (see Figure 8.4).

Three other interrelated risk factors that contribute to disease and death in this age group are lack of exercise, poor nutrition, and drinking too much alcohol. Although American adults are exercising more than ever before, few are exercising on a regular basis. In 2020, only 24.2% U.S. adults met the recommendations for aerobic and muscle-strengthening activity.[62] Although it was once thought that **intensity** had to be high for cardiovascular benefits from exercise to accrue, best practice recommendations encourage adults to engage in 150 minutes per week of moderate-intensity aerobic physical activity as well as engaging in muscle-strengthening activities 2 or more days per week.[63]

Poor dietary habits are associated with an increased risk for type 2 diabetes, hypertension, heart disease, certain cancers, and micronutrient deficiencies. While two-thirds (67.3%) of adults reported eating fruit on a given day and nearly all (95%) ate vegetables,[64] more than 80% of Americans have dietary patterns that are low in vegetables and fruits.[65]

The consequence of poor dietary habits and physical inactivity is obesity, in addition to the other chronic diseases mentioned previously. More than two in five (41.9%) U.S. adults have obesity, which is a significant increase from 30.5% in 1999–2000.[66] Like the leading causes of death, obesity affects some groups more than others (see **Figure 8.6**).

> **Intensity** cardiovascular workload measured by heart rate

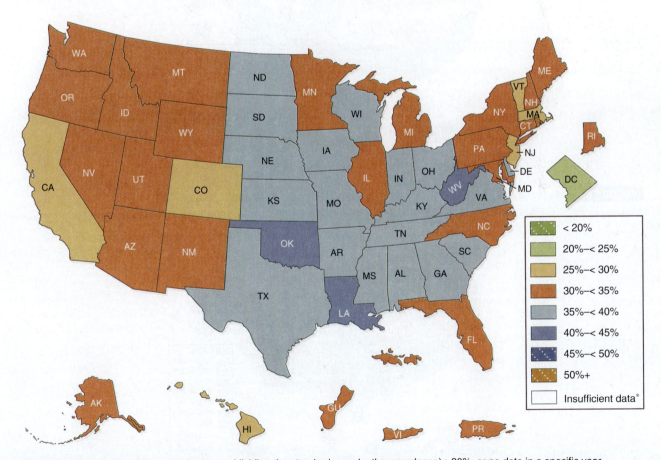

*Sample size <50, the relative standard error (dividing the standard error by the prevalance) ≥30%, or no data in a specific year.

FIGURE 8.6   **A.** Prevalence of obesity among U.S. adults by State, 2022.

Note: Obesity is defined as a BMI >30, or about 30 pounds overweight for a 5-foot, 4-inch person.

Reproduced from Centers for Disease Control and Prevention. *Obesity: Adult obesity prevalence maps.* https://www.cdc.gov/obesity/php/yata-research/adult-obesity-prevalence-maps.html

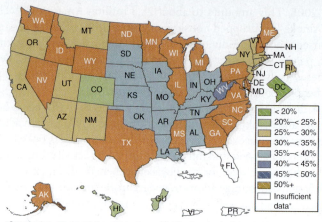

FIGURE 8.6 **B.** Prevalence of obesity among Non-Hispanic White adults, by State, 2020-2022.

Reproduced from Centers for Disease Control and Prevention. *Obesity: Adult obesity prevalence maps.* https://www.cdc.gov/obesity/php/data-research/adult-obesity-prevalence-maps.html

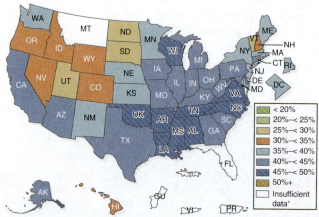

FIGURE 8.6 **C.** Prevalence of obesity among Non-Hispanic Black adults, by State, 2020-2022.

Reproduced from Centers for Disease Control and Prevention. *Obesity: Adult obesity prevalence maps.* https://www.cdc.gov/obesity/php/data-research/adult-obesity-prevalence-maps.html

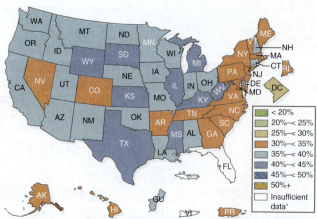

FIGURE 8.6 **D.** Prevalence of obesity among Hispanic adults, by State, 2020-2022.

Reproduced from Centers for Disease Control and Prevention. *Obesity: Adult obesity prevalence maps.* https://www.cdc.gov/obesity/php/data-research/adult-obesity-prevalence-maps.html

Obesity in the United States is truly an epidemic. **Body mass index (BMI)** is the primary way obesity is measured in the U.S. population, and in the adult population, a BMI of 30 or greater indicates that an individual is obese.[67] The key to maintaining an appropriate weight throughout life is a combination of healthy eating and exercise. It is widely recognized that a person's environment, including society and other life circumstances, impacts their ability to engage in these behaviors. Thus, increasingly, public health practitioners are implementing strategies to change policies, systems, and the environment to support healthier living for all individuals.[68]

As with other age groups, alcohol consumption often places adults at greater health risk. In 2022, about 52.9% of adult Americans reported consuming alcohol in the previous month, while just over one-quarter (23.5%) of people aged 18 and older reported binge drinking in the past month.[69] Those who engage in binge drinking and heavy alcohol use are at the greatest risk for developing a dependence on alcohol and for developing such alcohol-related health problems as liver and heart disease, mental health problems, dementia, and family problems.[47]

One does not have to become dependent on alcohol to have a drinking problem. Alcohol contributes to society's problems in many other ways. As noted elsewhere in this text, alcohol increases the rates of homicide, suicide, family violence, and unintentional injuries, such as those from motor vehicle crashes, boating incidents, and falls. The use of alcohol by pregnant women can cause fetal alcohol spectrum disorder, which can lead to several types of birth defects and disability.[70] Clearly, alcohol consumption adversely affects the health and well-being of Americans.

Awareness and Screening of Certain Medical Conditions

A number of regular, noninvasive or minimally invasive health screenings are recommended for adults, such as screenings for hypertension, diabetes, high blood cholesterol, and cancer.

Blood pressure is the force of blood pushing against the walls of the blood vessels. There is no "ideal" blood pressure. Instead, the acceptable blood pressure falls within a range considered healthy, and an adult's (age 20 and over) blood pressure should be less than 120/80 mm Hg. High blood pressure, or **hypertension stage one**, exists when systolic pressure is equal to or greater than 130 mm of mercury (Hg) and/or diastolic pressure is equal to or greater than 80 mm Hg for extended periods of time (more than one blood pressure reading). Hypertension stage two exists when systolic pressure is equal to or greater than 140 mm of mercury and/or diastolic pressure is equal to or greater than 90 mm of mercury. A hypertensive crisis exists when a person's systolic pressure is equal to or greater than 180 mm of mercury and/or diastolic pressure is equal to or greater than 120 mm of mercury.[71] Statistics show that hypertension is found in about one-half of adults in the United States, and only one-quarter of those individuals have their condition under control, making it a significant risk factor for cardiovascular disease in the United States.[72] Fortunately, once detected, hypertension is a risk factor that is highly modifiable (see **Figure 8.7**). The most desirable means of controlling hypertension is through a combination of diet modification, appropriate physical exercise, and weight management. In cases in which these measures prove ineffective, hypertension can usually still be controlled with medication. The keys to reducing morbidity and mortality resulting from hypertension are mass screenings that result in early detection of previously unidentified cases and their appropriate treatment.[71]

Diabetes results from failure of the pancreas to make or use a sufficient amount of insulin. Without insulin, food cannot be properly used by the body. Diabetes cannot be cured, but it can be controlled through a combination of diet, exercise, medications, and insulin injections. As reported earlier in the chapter, diabetes is one of the leading causes of death for adults, especially adults aged 45 to 64.[23] Disparities exist by race and ethnicity, education level, and socioeconomic status.[73] Many deaths resulting from diabetes could be postponed if diabetes was detected and treated appropriately. Approximately

Body mass index (BMI)
the ratio of weight (in kilograms) to height (in meters squared)

Hypertension stage one
a systolic pressure equal to or greater than 130 mm Hg and/or diastolic pressure equal to or greater than 80 mm Hg for extended periods of time

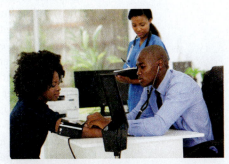

FIGURE 8.7 Hypertension is a highly modifiable risk factor.
© Michaeljung/Shutterstock

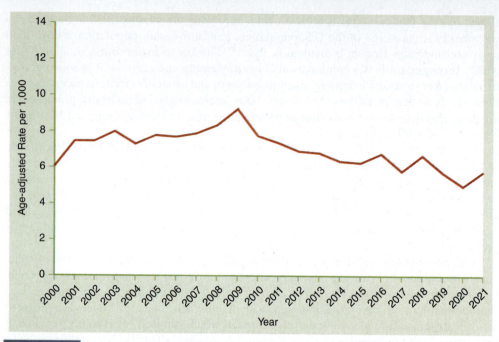

FIGURE 8.8 Trends in age-adjusted incidence of diagnosed diabetes among adults aged 18 years or older, United States, 2000-2021.

Reproduced from Centers for Disease Control and Prevention. (2024). National diabetes statistics report. Available at https://www.cdc.gov /diabetes/php/data-research/index.html

38.4 million Americans, or 11.6% of the U.S. population, are estimated to have diagnosed or undiagnosed diabetes with nearly 1.2 million new cases diagnosed each year.[73] An additional 38.0% of adults are estimated to have prediabetes. The percentage of adults with diagnosed diabetes has begun to see a slight reduction in recent years, but the number of individuals with diabetes or at risk of diabetes remains a public health concern. (see **Figure 8.8**).[73]

Cholesterol is a soft, fatlike substance that is necessary to build cell membranes. The cholesterol needed for healthy body function is produced by the liver and other cells in the body, with the remainder coming from the foods we eat, specifically animal products. Elevated cholesterol levels in blood can put people at greater risk for heart disease and stroke. The higher the cholesterol level, the greater the risk.[74] A person's cholesterol level is affected by certain health conditions, such as diabetes, lifestyle, age, and family history.[74] Although we cannot modify our age and family history, we can reduce our risk by engaging in healthy lifestyle behaviors.

Dietary factors are associated with four of the 10 leading causes of death in this age group. Many dietary components are involved in the diet–health relationship, but chief among them is the disproportionate consumption of foods high in fat and added sugars, often at the expense of foods high in complex carbohydrates and dietary fiber. Limiting sugars, saturated fats, and sodium to the recommended dietary levels will go a long way in reducing a person's risk for diabetes, hypertension, heart disease, and stroke.[66] Approximately 10% of adults over age 20 years has high cholesterol, which puts them at a substantially greater risk for developing heart disease. Like diabetes, the key to controlling high cholesterol is screening and treatment.[75]

The other prevalent medical condition in this age group that should be screened for on a regular basis is cancer. As noted earlier, malignant neoplasms (cancer) are the leading cause of death in 45- to 64-year-old people.[23] The American Cancer Society recommends a number of screenings for various age groups (see **Table 8.6**). However, many more adults in the United States could be getting screened. The earlier that cancer is detected, the greater the chance for successful treatment.

TABLE 8.6 Summary of American Cancer Society Guidelines for the Early Detection of Cancer

Cancer Site	Population	Test or Procedure	Frequency
Breast	Women, age 40+	Mammography	Women ages 40–44 should have a choice to start annual breast cancer screenings. Women age 45 to 54, annual screenings. Women 55 and older, mammograms every 2 years.
Cervix	People, ages 25–65	Pap test Pap test plus HPV test	Cervical cancer screening should begin at age 25. People ages 25-65, HPV test every 5 years; Pap test every 3 years. People aged 65+ who have had regular cervical testing in the past 10 years with normal results should not be tested for cervical cancer. Those with a history of a serious cervical precancer should continue to be tested for at least 25 years after that diagnosis, even if testing goes past age 65.
Colorectal	Men and women, starting at age 45	Stool-based test or visual exam based on healthcare provider recommendation and insurance coverage.	Regular intervals dependent on type of testing starting at age 45. If an individual is in good health, they continue screening until 75. Individuals between 76 and 85 should consult their doctor.
Endometrial	Women, at menopause	At the time of menopause, women at average risk should be informed about risks and symptoms of endometrial cancer and strongly encouraged to report any unexpected bleeding or spotting to their physicians.	
Lung	Individuals ages 50 to 80 who smoke or used to smoke AND have at least a 20 pack-per-year history of smoking	Low-dose helical computed tomography (LDCT) scan of the chest	
Prostate	Men, ages 50+ in consultation with a healthcare provider. African American men or men whose father or brother had prostate cancer before age 65 should discuss screening starting at age 45.	Prostate-specific antigen blood test (PSA) with or without a rectal exam	

Data from American Cancer Society. (2024). American Cancer Society guidelines for early detection of cancer. Available at http://www.cancer.org/healthy /find-cancer-early/cancer-screening-guidelines/american-cancer-society-guidelines-for-the-early-detection-of-cancer

Community and Public Health Strategies for Improving the Health of Adults

As noted in the previous pages, adults in the United States face a number of health issues. Even so, for most individuals, the years between 25 and 64 are some of the healthiest of their lifetimes. A key for keeping these people healthy is to understand that the health status of adults is often impacted by their current and previous health behaviors, as well as factors, such as socioeconomic status—especially poverty and education level—along with previous influences on their health throughout their lives (i.e., exposure to violence as a child, childhood health status, etc.). Health behaviors are complex and heavily influenced by societal factors and an individual's local community. Consequently, it is important that community health workers understand that it is not enough to provide health education to adults about how to change behaviors that they have often exhibited for a significant part of their lifetime. Policy, systems, and environmental change strategies must also accompany health education strategies. For example, in order to reverse the obesity epidemic, we must change our physical and food environments. Specific federal guidelines have been developed to guide local communities in the effort to improve access to healthy foods and physical activity.[76,77] Learning from tobacco prevention and control efforts, we can guide communities in addressing other major health challenges. Tobacco control has required personal and community-level interventions—from screening and cessation efforts to smoking restrictions, media campaigns, and increasing the cost to purchase tobacco.[78] Thus, community health workers must recognize that the health of one person is not just an individual responsibility but also a community responsibility.

Chapter Summary

- Adolescence and young adulthood (10 to 24 years old) and adulthood (25 to 64 years old) are the most productive periods of people's lives. Although most people enjoy good health during these years, there is substantial room for improvement.

- The overall health status of these age groups could be improved by reducing the prevalence of high-risk behaviors (e.g., cigarette smoking/vaping, excessive alcohol consumption, and physical inactivity), increasing participation in health screenings, institutionalizing preventive health care, and making environments more health enhancing in our society.

- Nearly 75% of adolescent and young adult mortality can be attributed to motor vehicle crashes, other unintentional injuries, homicide, and suicide.

- Adolescents and young adults remain at considerable risk for STIs.

- College students are at considerable risk for STIs due to unprotected sexual activity and the use of alcohol and other drugs.

- Mortality rates for older adults (45 to 64 years old) have declined in recent years, but cancer is still the overall leading cause of death, followed by cardiovascular disease.

- Reductions in deaths from cardiovascular diseases in adults have been substantial, but health problems resulting from unhealthy behaviors—such as smoking, poor diet, and physical inactivity—can be reduced further if environments are created to help support healthy behaviors (e.g., increased access to fruits and vegetables, the creation of more walkable communities, etc.).

- No matter how the health of adolescents and young adults and adults in the United States is broken down and described, it can be summarized by saying that the health of Americans in these age groups has come a long way in the past 50 years, but there is still room for improvement.

Scenario: Analysis and Response

1. What are the primary reasons that Annie stated that might have caused Dayna to develop diabetes?

2. Comment on the attitudes of Annie and Connor about Dayna's recent diabetes diagnosis. Do you agree with

Connor that the only way for Dayna to be healthy is to move away from the neighborhood where she lives? Why or why not?

3. If you were a community health worker in this urban community that has limited places where residents can purchase healthy food and safely exercise outside, what could you do to help young people like Dayna?

4. Do high schools have an obligation to develop prevention programs, including offering physical activity opportunities at school, to keep students healthy? Why or why not?

5. Say you were friends with Annie. She got so concerned with Dayna's health problem that she wanted to take action, especially to figure out how to help the local corner store that Dayna visits every day offer healthy foods for her. She thought that maybe she would do an online search to see if there are any corner stores that offer healthy foods and how they do it. You told her that you would help her see if there is anything on the Internet. Go online and use a search engine (e.g., Google, Bing) and enter "healthy corner stores." What did you find that might be of help to Annie?

Review Questions

1. Why is it important for community and public health workers to be aware of the significant health problems of the various age groups in the United States?

2. Why are the number of adolescents and young adults, living arrangements, and employment status such key demographic characteristics of young people with regard to community health? Briefly summarize the data available on these characteristics.

3. What are the leading causes of death for adolescents and young adults, and for adults?

4. What are the Youth Risk Behavior Surveillance System (YRBSS) and the Behavioral Risk Factor Surveillance System (BRFSS), and what type of data do they generate?

5. What are the behaviors that put each of these cohorts—adolescents, college students, and adults—at greatest risk, and how does a person's environment impact these behaviors?

6. How would you summarize the health profile of the two cohorts (adolescents and young adults and adults) presented in this chapter?

Activities

1. Assess the most recent results of the Youth Risk Behavior Surveillance System (YRBSS) and the Behavioral Risk Factor Surveillance System (BRFSS) for your state. Review the data presented, and then prepare a two-page summary on the "Health Behavior Profile of the Adolescents, Young Adults, and Adults" of your state.

2. Obtain data presenting the 10 leading causes of death according to age and race for the age groups presented in this chapter. Review the data and prepare a summary paper discussing conclusions that can be drawn about race, the leading causes of death, and age.

3. Interview a small group (about 10) of adults (aged 45–64) about their present health status. Ask them questions about their health behavior and health problems. Then summarize the data you collect in writing, and compare it with the information in this chapter on this age group. How are the data similar? How do they differ?

4. Pick either adolescents and young adults or adults, and write a two-page paper that presents ideas on how the health profile of that age group can be improved in your state.

5. Access the American College Health Association data. Do a walking tour of your college campus and notice the types of communication that is being shared (e.g., bulletin boards, bathroom stalls, digital signs, student health center, etc.) and programs being offered. Based on the current ACHA data and what you observe on your campus, what conclusions can you draw about the health education messaging and programming occurring on your campus and the health of the students on campus. Make recommendations for additional content or strategies for ensuring the target audience is being reached.

6. Access one of the CDC's online databases (YRBS Explorer, CDC WONDER, WISQARS). Select an age group and a leading cause of death. Do a deep dive to see what you can learn related to this population and health behavior. Use your findings to engage in a discussion board or group chat. Be prepared to share the following: a few key facts, things that surprised you, things that concern you, and recommendations for improving the health of this population and this health condition.

References

1. World Health Organization. (2024). *Adolescent health.* Available at https://www.who.int/health-topics/adolescent-health/#tab=tab_1

2. Berlin, G., Furstenberg, F. F., & Waters, M. C. (2010). Introducing the issue: Transition to adulthood. *The Future of Children, 20*(1), 3–18.

3. MacKay, A. P., Fingerhut, L. A., & Duran, C. R. (2000). *Health, United States, 2000 with adolescent health chartbook.* National Center for Health Statistics.

4. Seffrin, J. R. (1990). The comprehensive school health curriculum: Closing the gap between state-of-the-art and state-of-the-practice. *Journal of School Health, 60*(4), 151–156.

5. Snyder, T., & Shafer, L. (1996). *Youth indicators, 1996* (NCES 96-027). U.S. Department of Education, National Center for Education Statistics.

6. Valois, R. F., Thatcher, W. G., Drane, J. W., & Reininger, B. M. (1997). Comparison of selected health risk behaviors between adolescents in public and private high schools in South Carolina. *Journal of School Health, 67*(10), 434–440.

7. Power, C., Kuh, D., & Morton, S. (2013). From developmental origins of adult disease to life course research on adult disease and aging: Insights from birth cohort studies. *Annual Review of Public Health, 34*, 7–28.

8. U.S. Census Bureau. (2023). *Age and sex composition 2020: 2020 census briefs.* Available at https://www2.census.gov/library/publications/decennial/2020/census-briefs/c2020br-06.pdf

9. U.S. Department of Health and Human Services. (2024). *Adolescent health data: America's diverse adolescents.* Available at https://opa.hhs.gov/adolescent-health/adolescent-health-data/americas-diverse-adolescents

10. U.S. Census Bureau. (2023). *Children's living arrangements.* Available at https://www.census.gov/library/visualizations/interactive/childrens-living-arrangements.html

11. U.S. Census Bureau. (2023). Parent/child family groups with children under 18. Available at https://www.census.gov/library/visualizations/interactive/parent-child-family-groups.html

12. Amato, P. R. (2005). The impact of family formation change on the cognitive, social, and emotional well-being of the next generation. *The Future of Children, 15*(2), 75–96.

13. Shrider, E. A., & Creamer, J. (2023). *Poverty in the United States: 2022* (Current Population Reports, P60-280). U.S. Census Bureau, U.S. Government Publishing Office. Available at https://www.census.gov/content/dam/Census/library/publications/2023/demo/p60-280.pdf

14. Potter, D. (2012). Same-sex parent families and children's academic achievement. *Journal of Marriage and Family, 74*(3), 556–571. doi.org/10.1111/j.1741-3737.2012.00966.x

15. Bos, H. M., Gelderen, L. R., & Gatrell, N. K. (2016). Same-sex and different-sex parent households and child health outcomes: Findings from the National Survey of Children's Health. *Journal of Developmental and Behavioral Pediatrics, 37*(3), 179–187. Available at http://dx.doi.org/10.1097/DBP.0000000000000288

16. Congressional Research Service. (2018). *Youth and the labor force: Background and trends.* Available at https://crsreports.congress.gov/product/pdf/R/R42519

17. U.S. Bureau of Labor Statistics. (2024). *Labor force statistics from the current population survey.* Available at https://www.bls.gov/cps/cpsaat03.htm

18. Keisler-Starkey, K., Bunch, L. N., & Lindstrom, R. A. (2023). *Health Insurance Coverage in the United States: 2022.* Available at https://www.census.gov/library/publications/2023/demo/p60-281.html

19. National Center for Health Statistics. (2015). *Health, United States, 2014: With special feature on adults age 55–64.* NCHS.

20. Chua, K. P., Schuster, M. A., & McWilliams, J. M. (2013). Differences in health care access and utilization between adolescents and young adults with asthma. *Pediatrics, 131*(5). Available at http://dx.doi.org/10.1542/peds.2012-2881

21. Akosa Antwi, Y., Moriya, A. S., Simon, K., & Sommer, B. D. (2015). Changes in emergency department use among young adults after the Patient Protection and Affordable Care Act's dependent coverage provision. *Annals of Emergency Medicine, 65*(6), 664–672. Available at http://dx.doi.org/10.1016/j.annemergmed.2015.01.010

22. First International Conference on Health Promotion. (1986). *The Ottawa Charter for Health Promotion.* World Health Organization. Available at http://www.who.int/healthpromotion/conferences/previous/ottawa/en/

23. Kochanek, K. D., Murphy, S. L., Xu, J. Q., & Arias, E. (2024). *Mortality in the United States, 2022. NCHS Data Brief, no 492.* Hyattsville, MD: National Center for Health Statistics. doi: https://dx.doi.org/10.15620/cdc:135850 https://www.cdc.gov/nchs/data/databriefs/db492.pdf

24. Centers for Disease Control and Prevention, National Center for Health Statistics. National Vital Statistics System, Provisional Mortality on CDC WONDER Online Database (2024). *Provisional death rates by age, gender and race for 2024.* Available at https://wonder.cdc.gov/

25. National Safety Council. (2024). *Historical fatality trends: Deaths by age group, 2021.* Available at https://injuryfacts.nsc.org/motor-vehicle/historical-fatality-trends/deaths-by-age-group/

26. Curtin, S. C., Tejada-Vera, B., & Bastian, B. A. (2024). *Deaths: Leading causes for 2021.* National Vital Statistics Reports, 73(4). National Center for Health Statistics. doi: https://dx.doi.org/10.15620/cdc:147882. Available at https://www.cdc.gov/nchs/data/nvsr/nvsr73/nvsr73-04.pdf

27. Centers for Disease Control and Prevention. (2024). *Sexually transmitted infection surveillance, 2022.* Available at https://www.cdc.gov/std/statistics/2022/default.htm

28. Centers for Disease Control and Prevention. (2024). *Fast facts: HIV in the US by age.* Available at https://www.cdc.gov/hiv/data-research/facts-stats/age.html

29. Centers for Disease Control and Prevention. (2024). *Sexually transmitted infections surveillance, 2022: Impact of COVID-19 on STIs.* Available at https://www.cdc.gov/std/statistics/2022/impact.htm

30. Centers for Disease Control and Prevention. (2024). *HIV: Fast facts: HIV in the US by race and ethnicity.* Available at https://www.cdc.gov/hiv/data-research/facts-stats/race-ethnicity.html

31. Centers for Disease Control and Prevention. (2023). Youth risk behavior surveillance—United States, 2021. *Morbidity and Mortality Weekly Report*, Supplement, 72(1), 1–102. Available at https://www.cdc.gov/healthyyouth/data/yrbs/index.htm

32. Centers for Disease Control and Prevention. (2024). *YRBS Explorer: Explore youth risk behavior survey questions – United States, 2021.* Available at https://yrbs-explorer.services.cdc.gov/#/

33. Centers for Disease Control and Prevention. (2023). *Youth and tobacco use.* Available at https://www.cdc.gov/tobacco/data_statistics/fact_sheets/youth_data/tobacco_use/

34. Centers for Disease Control and Prevention. (2024). *Smoking and tobacco use: E-cigarette use among youth.* Available at https://www.cdc.gov/tobacco/e-cigarettes/youth.html

35. Centers for Disease Control and Prevention. (2024). *Smoking and tobacco use: Why youth vape.* Available at https://www.cdc.gov/tobacco/e-cigarettes/why-youth-vape.html

36. American Heart Association, American Cancer Society, Campaign for Tobacco-Free Kids, and American Lung Association. (2024).

Broken promises to our children: A state-by-state look at the 1998 state tobacco settlement 25 years later. Available at https://www.tobaccofreekids.org/what-we-do/us/statereport

37. Campaign for Tobacco-Free Kids. (2023). *FDA authority over tobacco.* Available at https://www.tobaccofreekids.org/what-we-do/us/fda

38. U.S. Food & Drug Administration. (2024). *Tobacco 21.* Available at https://www.fda.gov/tobacco-products/retail-sales-tobacco-products/tobacco-21

39. American Cancer Society Cancer Action Network. (2024). *Effective policies known to prevent tobacco use and address tobacco-related disparities.* Available at https://www.fightcancer.org/policy-resources/effective-policies-known-prevent-tobacco-use-and-address-tobacco-related

40. Centers for Disease Control and Prevention, National Center for Health Statistics. (2024). *Teen births.* Available at https://www.cdc.gov/nchs/fastats/teen-births.htm

41. Youth.gov. (2024.). *Adverse effect.* Available at https://youth.gov/youth-topics/pregnancy-prevention/adverse-effects-teen-pregnancy

42. Centers for Disease Control and Prevention. (2022). *Overweight & obesity: Consequences of obesity.* Available at https://www.cdc.gov/obesity/basics/consequences.html

43. Centers for Disease Control and Prevention. (2023). *Promoting mental health and well-being in schools: An action guide for school and district leaders.* Available at https://www.cdc.gov/healthyyouth/mental-health-action-guide/index.html Available at https://www.cdc.gov/healthyyouth/mental-health-action-guide/pdf/DASH_MH_Action_Guide_508.pdf

44. American College Health Association. (2024). *ACHA National College Health Assessment III: Reference group executive summary fall 2023.* ACHA. Available at https://www.acha.org/NCHA/ACHA-NCHA_Data/Publications_and_Reports/NCHA/Data/Reports_ACHA-NCHAIIIb.aspx

45. Patrick, M. E., Miech, R. A., Johnston, L. D., & O'Malley, P. M. (2023). *Monitoring the future panel study annual report: National data on substance use among adults ages 19 to 60, 1972-2022.* Institute for Social Research, The University of Michigan. Available at https://monitoringthefuture.org/results/annual-reports/

46. U.S. Department of Education. (2024). *Fast facts.* National Center for Education Statistics. Available at https://nces.ed.gov/fastfacts/display.asp?id=98

47. Centers for Disease Control and Prevention. (2024). *Drink less, be your best: What is excessive drinking?* Available at https://www.cdc.gov/drinklessbeyourbest/excessivedrinking.html

48. Centers for Disease Control and Prevention. (2023). *School connectedness.* Available at https://www.cdc.gov/healthyschools/school_connectedness.htm

49. University of Nevada, Reno Extension. (2024). *Young volunteers: The benefits of community service.* Available at https://extension.unr.edu/publication.aspx?PubID=4307

50. Opportunity Nation. (2014). *Connecting youth and strengthening communities: The data behind civic engagement and economic opportunity.* Available at http://opportunitynation.org/app/uploads/2014/09/Opportunity-Nation-Civic-Engagement-Report-2014.pdf

51. Substance Abuse and Mental Health Services Administration. (2024). *Evidence-based practices resource center.* Available at https://www.samhsa.gov/resource-search/ebp

52. Dusenbury, L., & Falco, M. (1995). Eleven components of effective drug abuse prevention curricula. *Journal of School Health, 65,* 420–425.

53. National Consensus for School Health Education. (2022). *National Health Education Standards: Model Guidance for Curriculum and Instruction (3rd Edition).* Available at www.schoolhealtheducation.org

54. Centers for Disease Control and Prevention. (2022). *Health education curriculum analysis tool (HECAT).* CDC. Available at https://www.cdc.gov/healthyyouth/hecat/index.htm

55. Minkler, M., & Wallerstein, N. (Eds.). (2003). *Community-based participatory research for health.* Jossey-Bass Publishers.

56. Centers for Disease Control and Prevention. (2019). *Social determinants of health (SDOH).* Available at https://www.cdc.gov/about/priorities/why-is-addressing-sdoh-important.html

57. National Cancer Institute. (2024). *Cancer stat facts: Common cancer sites.* Available at https://seer.cancer.gov/statfacts/html/common.html

58. American Cancer Society. (2017). *More than 4 in 10 cancers and cancer deaths linked to modifiable risk factors.* Available at https://www.cancer.org/research/acs-research-news/more-than-4-in-10-cancers-and-cancer-deaths-linked-to-modifiable-risk-factors.html

59. American Cancer Society. (2024). American Cancer Society guidelines for early detection of cancer. Available at http://www.cancer.org/healthy/find-cancer-early/cancer-screening-guidelines/american-cancer-society-guidelines-for-the-early-detection-of-cancer

60. Centers for Disease Control and Prevention. (2024). *Social determinants of health (SDOH).* Available at https://www.cdc.gov/about/priorities/why-is-addressing-sdoh-important.html

61. Centers for Disease Control and Prevention. (2023). *Current cigarette smoking among adults in the United States.* Available at http://www.cdc.gov/tobacco/data_statistics/fact_sheets/adult_data/cig_smoking/index.htm

62. Elgaddal, N., Kramarow, E. A. & Reuben, C. (2022). Physical activity among adults aged 18 and over: United States, 2020. *NCHS Data Brief No. 443, August 2022.* https://www.cdc.gov/nchs/data/databriefs/db443.pdf

63. Office of Disease Prevention and Health Promotion. (2018). *Physical activity guidelines* (2nd ed.). Available at https://health.gov/our-work/nutrition-physical-activity/physical-activity-guidelines/current-guidelines

64. Ansai, N., & Wambogo, E. A. (2021). Fruit and vegetable consumption among adults in the United States, 2015-2018. *NCHS Data Brief No. 397, February 2021.* Available at https://www.cdc.gov/nchs/data/databriefs/db397-H.pdf

65. U.S. Department of Agriculture and U.S. Department of Health and Human Services. (2020). Dietary Guidelines for Americans, 2020-2025. 9th Edition. Available at DietaryGuidelines.gov

66. Centers for Disease Control and Prevention. (2024). *Obesity: Adult obesity facts.* Available at https://www.cdc.gov/obesity/php/data-research/adult-obesity-facts.html

67. Centers for Disease Control and Prevention. (2024). *BMI: Adult BMI categories.* https://www.cdc.gov/bmi/adult-calculator/bmi-categories.html

68. Galuska, D. A., Fulton, J. E., & O'Neal, L. J. (2024). Data for decision makers: Finding policy, systems, and environmental solutions for public health problems. *Preventing Chronic Disease 2024; 21:240165.* DOI: http://dx.doi.org/10.5888/pcd21.240165. Available at https://www.cdc.gov/pcd/issues/2024/24_0165.htm

69. National Institute on Alcohol Abuse and Alcoholism. (2024). *Alcohol facts and statistics.* Available at https://www.niaaa.nih.gov/alcohols-effects-health/alcohol-topics/alcohol-facts-and-statistics

70. March of Dimes. (2024). *Alcohol during pregnancy.* Available at https://www.marchofdimes.org/find-support/topics/pregnancy/alcohol-during-pregnancy

71. American Heart Association. (2024). *Facts about high blood pressure.* Available at https://www.heart.org/en/health-topics/high-blood-pressure/the-facts-about-high-blood-pressure

72. Centers for Disease Control and Prevention. (2024). *High blood pressure facts*. Available at https://www.cdc.gov/high-blood-pressure/data-research/facts-stats/index.html

73. Centers for Disease Control and Prevention. (2024). *National diabetes statistics report*. Available at https://www.cdc.gov/diabetes/php/data-research/index.html

74. American Heart Association. (2024). *Control your cholesterol*. Available at https://www.heart.org/en/health-topics/cholesterol/about-cholesterol

75. Centers for Disease Control and Prevention. (2024). *High cholesterol facts*. Available at https://www.cdc.gov/cholesterol/data-research/facts-stats/

76. Centers for Disease Control and Prevention. (2024). *Physical activity: Guidelines and recommended strategies*. Available at https://www.cdc.gov/physical-activity/php/guidelines-recommendations/index.html

77. Centers for Disease Control and Prevention. (2024). *Obesity: Obesity strategies: What can be done*. https://www.cdc.gov/obesity/php/about/obesity-strategies-what-can-be-done.html

78. Ockene, J. K., Edgerton, E. A., Teutsch, S. M., Marion, L. N., Miller, T., Genevro, J. L., Loveland-Cherry, C. J., Fielding, J. E., & Briss, P. A. (2007). Integrating evidence-based clinical and community strategies to improve health. *American Journal of Preventive Medicine, 32*, 244–252.

CHAPTER 9

Older Adults

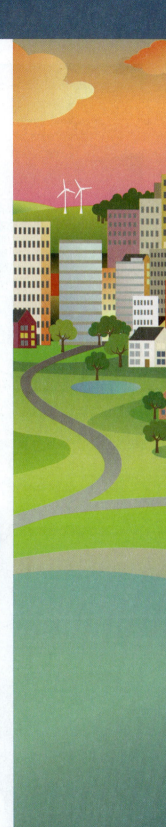

Chapter Outline

Chapter Objectives

After studying this chapter, you will be able to:

1. Identify the characteristics of an aging population.
2. Define the following groups—*old, young old, middle old,* and *old old.*
3. Refute several commonly held myths about the older adult population.
4. Describe the factors that affect the size and age of a population.
5. Define fertility and mortality rates and explain how they affect life expectancy.
6. Explain the difference between dependency and labor-force ratios.
7. Describe older adults with regard to marital status, living arrangements, racial and ethnic background, education, economic status, and geographic location.

8. Discuss the effects of chronic conditions and physical impairments on older adults.
9. Explain how health behaviors can improve the quality of later life.
10. Briefly outline elder abuse and neglect in the United States.
11. Illustrate the six instrumental needs of older adults.
12. Explain the role of caregivers with older adults in the United States.
13. Describe different housing options available to older adults.
14. Briefly summarize the Older Americans Act of 1965.
15. List the commonly provided services for older adults in most communities.
16. Explain the difference between respite care and adult day care.

Scenario

John and Glenda have been looking forward to retirement since both of their children moved out of the area. John, who worked in healthcare finance for nearly 40 years, recently had both of his knees replaced in anticipation of the traveling he was planning to do once the sale of their home went through. Glenda, who had retired years earlier from teaching school, kept her days busy volunteering at the local hospital and caring for her grandchildren. Up until recently, both were in good health and spent many weekends working in their large yard in North Carolina. Upon retirement, they worked to pare down their belongings to fit in a much smaller home that they had recently purchased in Florida. Although they now lived on a fixed income, the profit from the sale of their home and the small investments that they had made over the years allowed them the income they needed to live out the retirement they had dreamed about.

However, with a cruise planned to set sail in April of 2020, life was getting ready to take a drastic change. Within a week, their upcoming cruise was canceled, all volunteers of the hospital were let go, restaurants were closing, and no toilet paper was anywhere to be found. The cause of this was a worldwide pandemic known as COVID-19 (or Coronavirus) and it stopped the world in its tracks.

Now, instead of traveling and going out with friends, days were spent inside, isolated, and in panic that at any time, one of them could get sick. Although the effects of the pandemic did slowly subside, and life returned to a new normal, many of their friends were gone as they either succumbed to COVID-19, moved away to live with family, or overlooked routine health care in fear of going out, resulting in advancing stages of illnesses. Glenda even developed a mild case of COVID-19, and despite a quick recovery, she is still dealing with the effects of limited lung capacity.

John and Glenda now look to the future with a mix of optimism and anxiety. They are optimistic that they will be able to travel again and visit with their children and grandchildren but anxious that they will not be able to live out their years being as active as they were just a few years before. Not only did Glenda's illness affect her ability to breathe, but the costs associated with treating COVID-19 tapped into some of their retirement funds. Nevertheless, John and Glenda feel that they are up to the challenge and adventure of aging into the future and take satisfaction in looking back at lives well lived.

Introduction

The U.S. population is growing older and living longer. The number of older adults in America and their proportion of the total population increased dramatically during the twentieth and early twenty-first centuries. To put this into perspective, this means that as of 2020, one in six people in the country was age 65 or older.[1] And, of this population, those aged 85 and older are taking up a larger share of this group.[2] For the first time in U.S. history, a significant number of Americans will achieve older adult status. We need only look around us to see the change that is taking place (see **Figure 9.1**). With better health care, improved communication, and increased longevity, the volume of older adults remaining active within the community continues to increase. Senior centers, retirement villages, and assisted-living facilities are being built in record numbers. And today, more than ever before, many people belong to multigenerational families, where there are opportunities to develop long-lasting relationships with parents, grandparents, and great-grandparents. There are now families in which members of three successive generations receive monthly Social Security checks. In the twenty-first century, the economic, social, and health issues associated with the growing proportion of people older than age 65 in the United States have become major political concerns. In this chapter, we will look to create a better understanding of terminology related to this population, assess relevant demographics, and look at what special needs and services are associated with this growing community of older adults.

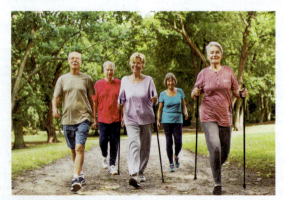

FIGURE 9.1 The number of older adults in the United States is on the rise, and they are more energetic than previous cohorts.

© alvarez/E+/Getty Images

Definitions

How old is old? The ageless baseball pitcher Satchel Paige once said, "How old would you be if you didn't know how old you was [sic]?" Although his English might be found wanting, Paige's point is important (see **Figure 9.2**). A person's age might depend on who measures it and how they define it. Children might see their 35-year-old teacher as old, whereas the 35-year-old teacher might regard her 61-year-old principal as old. Age is and always will be a relative concept.

In the United States and other developed countries, people are considered *old* once they reach the age of 65. But because there are a number of people who are very active and healthy at age 65 and will live a number of productive years after 65, researchers have subdivided old into the *young old* (65–74), the *middle old* (75–84), and the *old old* (85 and over). These distinctions can be important for community health programming. Not only does the government use this information to determine funding for programs, such as public transportation and healthcare servicing centers, but the private sector will use this information to help determine where best to place goods and services. We can assume there are likely to be significant differences between a 65-year-old and a 95-year-old person, for example, just as there are between a 15-year-old and a 45-year-old person. But with the latter group growing proportionally faster, the need for alternative goods and services is in a state of flux.

Many terms have been used to describe individuals who are 65 years of age and older, including "seniors, senior citizens, golden agers, retired persons, mature adults, elderly, aged, and old people. There is no clear preference among older people for any of these terms."[3] We can also assume preferences will change with various generations.

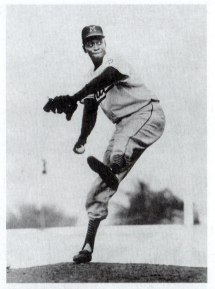

FIGURE 9.2 Some would say you are only as old as you think you are. (Satchel Paige remained active in professional baseball long after reaching the age at which others retired.)

© AP/Shutterstock

Myths Surrounding Aging

Like other forms of prejudice and discrimination, **ageism** is the result of ignorance, misconceptions, and half-truths about aging and older adults. Because many people do not interact with older people on a daily basis, it is easy to create a stereotypical image of older adults based on the atypical actions of a few or negative images in the media.

When you think of older people, who comes to mind? Do you immediately think of a lonely man with a disheveled appearance sitting on a park bench or an older person lying in a nursing home bed making incomprehensible noises? Or do you think of Harrison Ford or Morgan Freeman (who turned 81 and 86 years old, respectively, in 2023) in action packed or high suspense movies and shows?

Both Ferrini and Ferrini as well as Dychtwald and Flower have identified a number of commonly held myths about older adults.[3,4] They are presented here to remind us that older adults are not depressed, lonely and disengaged, but rather are independent, capable, and valuable resources for our communities. Do not forget that several U.S. presidents have been eligible for Social Security and Medicare while in office.

Here are some of the myths, followed by the reasons why they are only myths:

1. Myth: "Old people are lonely and ignored by their families."

    Truth: Older adults are the least likely to be lonely of any age group; those who live alone are likely to be in close contact, either in person, by email, or by telephone, with close friends and/or their family.

2. Myth: "Old people are senile."

    Truth: Cognitive impairments are the result of disease and are not a guaranteed part of older adulthood.

> **Ageism** a form of prejudice and discrimination resulting from ignorance, misconceptions, and half-truths about aging and older adults

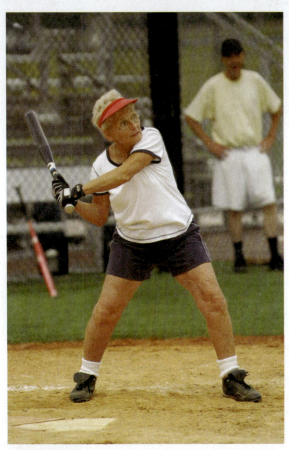

FIGURE 9.3   Many older adults are remaining active well after retirement age.
© Glenda/Shutterstock

3. Myth: "Most old people are sickly."

Truth: Most older people do have at least one chronic health problem, but the majority of older adults live active lifestyles.

4. Myth: "Old people no longer have any sexual interest or ability."

Truth: Sexual interest may or may not diminish with age, but there is an alteration in sexual response. Nonetheless, many older adults in reasonably good health have active and satisfying sex lives.

5. Myth: "Older people are unproductive."

Truth: Older adults are more likely to be retired, but they are very likely to be productively engaged at home and in the community. The number of older adults engaged in professional employment is at an all-time high.

Although a number of issues and concerns facing older adults are presented later in this chapter, the majority of older adults in the United States today are active and well (see **Figure 9.3**).

Demography of Aging

The demography of aging is typically defined as a study of those who are 65 years and older and of the variables that bring about change in their lives. In the following paragraphs, some of the demographic features of the elder population, including size, growth rate, and the factors that contribute to this growth are revealed. We also discuss other demographic characteristics of this population, such as living arrangements, racial and ethnic composition, geographic distribution, economic status, and housing.

Size and Growth of the Older Adult Population in the United States

The number of older adults and the proportion of the total population made up of older adults grew significantly during the twentieth and early twenty-first centuries. Demographers' projections suggest that populations will continue to age, not only in this country, but in most other countries as well. In 2011, members of the baby boomer generation (1946-1964) began to turn 65. It is estimated that by 2060, approximately 23% of the population, or 94.7 million people, will be 65 or older.[5] The population aged 85 and older is currently the fastest-growing segment of the older population. During this same time, it is expected that the percentage of people aged 18 and younger will decline and for the first time in U.S history, the older adult population will outnumber the population of children.[5] **Figure 9.4** shows the difference in the population pyramid of 1960 and the projections for 2060.

As one might guess, the projected growth of the older adult population is expected to raise the **median age** of the U.S. population. As of 2021, the median age for the U.S. population was 38.8 years.[6] Projections put the median age at 39 years by 2035 where it will remain until 2050.[7]

Median age the age at which half of the population is older and half is younger

Factors That Affect Population Size and Age

It is a common misconception that all populations will age with time; that is not necessarily true. Fertility rates and mortality rates both play a significant role in the "age" of any population.

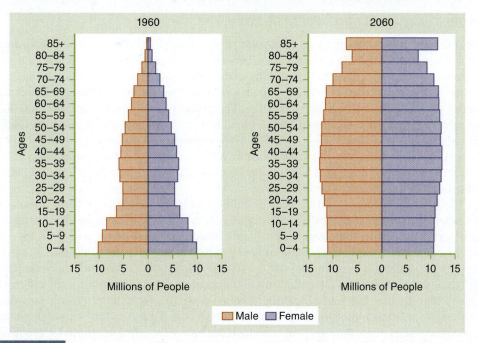

FIGURE 9.4   **A.** Population of the United States in 1960. **B.** Projected resident population of the United States in 2060.

Reproduced from U.S. Census Bureau. National population projections, 2017: From pyramid to pillar: A century of change, population of the U.S. Available at https://census.gov/library/visualizations/2018/comm/century-of-change.html

Fertility Rates

The *fertility rate* is an expression of the number of births per 1,000 women of childbearing age (15–44) in the population during a specific time period. Fertility rates in the United States were at their highest at the beginning of the twentieth century. Those rates dipped during the Depression years (1929-1939) but rebounded after World War II (1965). The period of consistently high fertility rates immediately following World War II has become known as the "baby boom years," hence the name *baby boomers* for those born between 1946 and 1964. During those years, 76 million babies were born. As the baby boomers continue to age, a "human tidal wave" (bulge) progressively moves up the U.S. age pyramid. While our society has attempted to adjust to the size and needs of the baby boomer generation, it has had a dramatic impact on society and politics, family dynamics, social security, health care, and retirement age. This generation, however, has grown up with improved healthcare, economic and educational systems, as well as a decreased risk of nutritional deficiency and improved immunology.[8]

Mortality Rates

The *mortality*, or *death rate* (usually expressed in deaths per 100,000 population) also has an impact on the aging population. The annual crude mortality rate in the United States in 1900 was 1,720 per 100,000. Recent data from 2021 shows that this figure has dropped by nearly half, or 879.7 per 100,000.[9]

The decrease in the annual mortality rate achieved over the twentieth century was the result of triumphs in medical science and public health practice.

Another demographic variable that interacts with the mortality rate is life expectancy. Although the mortality rate in the United States has been fairly constant for over 20 years, life expectancy has continued to increase. In 1900, life expectancy at birth was 47.3 years. This has increased to 76.4 as of 2021.[9] Whereas the increase in life expectancy in the first half of the twentieth century could be attributed to the decrease in infant and early childhood deaths, the increase in life expectancy since 1970 can be traced to the postponement of death among the middle-aged and older adult population.

Dependency ratio a ratio that compares the number of individuals whom society considers economically unproductive to the number it considers economically productive

Total dependency ratio the dependency ratio that includes both youth and old

Youth dependency ratio the dependency ratio that includes only youth

Old-age dependency ratio the dependency ratio that includes only the old

Labor-force ratio a ratio of the total number of those individuals who are not working to the number of those who are

Dependency and Labor-Force Ratios

Other demographic signs of an aging population are changes in dependency and labor-force ratios. The **dependency ratio** is a comparison between those individuals whom society considers economically unproductive (the nonworking or dependent population) and those it considers economically productive (the working population). Traditionally, the productive and nonproductive populations have been defined by age. The productive population includes those who are aged 15 to 64 years. The unproductive population includes both youth (under the age of 15) and the older population (65+ years). When the dependency ratio includes both youth and old, it is referred to as a **total dependency ratio**. When only the youth are compared with the productive group, the term used is **youth dependency ratio**; when only the old are compared, it is called **old-age dependency ratio**.

Changes in dependency ratios "provide an indirect broad indication of periods when we can expect the particular age distribution of the country to affect the need for distinct types of social services, housing, and consumer products."[10] Communities can refer to dependency ratio data as a guide for making the best social policy decisions and as a way to allocate resources. For example, leaders in a community with a relatively high youth dependency ratio compared with the old-age dependency ratio may want to concentrate community resources on programs, such as education for the young, health promotion programs for children, special programs for working parents, and other youth-associated concerns. Communities with high old-age dependency ratios might increase programs for older adults, including programs for caregivers and flexible employment opportunities.

The total dependency ratio is then calculated by adding together the number of youth and the old, then dividing this by the number of those in the labor force, times 100. Over the years, this dependency ratio is progressively climbing. For example, in 2010, in the United States, this ratio was 49.0; however, this number climbed to 53.7 in 2019. This is primarily driven by the growth of the 65 and older population and thus will guide future social policy.[11]

Such an increase in the old-age dependency ratio provides an interesting political scenario because the costs to support youth and the old are not the same. Parents pay directly for most of the expenditures to support their children, with the primary exception being public education, which is paid for by taxes. In contrast, much of the support for elders comes from tax-supported programs, such as Social Security, Medicare, and Medicaid. To meet the impending burden of expenditures for the older adults, taxes will most certainly need to be raised or benefits reduced. Therefore, the two questions for the future are: (1) Will the productive population be willing to pay increased taxes to support older adults? and (2) Will services to older adults be drastically reduced?

Although dependency ratio data clearly show one trend, they are merely an estimate and should not be the only accepted estimate. In truth, the dependency ratios are based on the assumption that everyone of productive age supports all members of the nonproductive age group. Obviously, this is not the case. Many of those in the productive age group (for instance, homemakers, those who are unemployed, and those who are disabled) do not participate in the paid labor force. Conversely, many teenagers and older adults do. Thus, dependency ratios, in some situations, could provide misleading figures for decision makers.

Other experts believe that labor-force ratios also need to be considered. **Labor-force ratios** differ from dependency ratios in that they are based on the number of people who are actually working and those who are not, independent of their ages. When labor-force participation rates are used to calculate the labor-force ratios, it is projected that the burden of support for the labor force in the future will be somewhat lighter than that projected through dependency ratios. This is because of the fact that baby boomers plan to work longer than members of the previous generations.[12] Nonetheless, under either method of calculation, the ratio of workers to dependents will be lower in the future than it is today.

Other Demographic Variables Affecting Older Adults

Other demographic variables that affect the community and public health programs of older Americans include marital status, living arrangements, racial and ethnic composition, geographic distribution, economic status, and housing.

Marital Status

As of the 2018 American Community Survey, 49.3% of the male population was married whereas only 46% of the female population was married. Of these, 8.7% of the female population was widowed and only 2.6% of the male population was widowed.[13] There are three primary reasons for these differences. First, men have shorter average life expectancies (73.2 years in 2021) than women (79.1 years in 2021) and, therefore, are shown to predecease their wives.[14] Second, men tend to marry women who are younger than themselves. Finally, men who lose a spouse through death or divorce are more likely to remarry than women in the same situation. These statistics reveal that most older men have a spouse for assistance, especially when health fails, whereas most women do not. Widowed women tend to have a closer and wider network of social support but generally suffer from a lowered financial status upon widowhood[3] (see **Figure 9.5**).

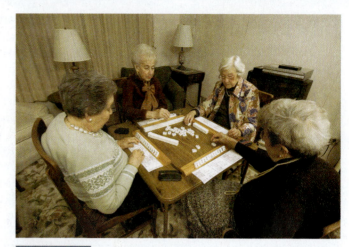

FIGURE 9.5 Older women are three times more likely to be widowed than older men.

© rj lerich/Shutterstock

In 2021, the number of divorced or separated elders rose slightly from 15% to 16% of the older U.S. population.[15] As more baby boomers move into their older years, the number of divorced older adults will grow substantially. These divorced older adults represent a new type of need group—those who lack the retirement benefits, insurance, and net worth assets associated with being married.

Living Arrangements

"The living arrangements of America's older population are linked to income, health status, and the availability of caregivers."[16] In 2021, 60% of noninstitutionalized older adults lived with their spouses, and 27% lived alone.[15] Older women are more likely to live alone than older men. The proportion of those living alone is projected to remain about the same, but the numbers are expected to increase dramatically over the next 20 years.[4,5] Reasons for these increased numbers revolve around the aging of the baby boomers and the improved economic status of older adults, coupled with their strong desire to live as independently as possible.

Only a small percentage of the older adult population in the United States resides in nursing homes. In line with previous statistics, in 2019, approximately 1.2 million of those aged 65 years and older were living in nursing homes, with the proportion of these residents increasing by age.[15] This percentage is down from previous years, in part as a result of the increase in other housing options and community services discussed later in this chapter. Of those who do live in nursing homes, older women at all ages have higher usage rates than men do. Approximately three-fourths of nursing home residents are women, and more than half of all nursing home residents are older than 85 years.

Racial and Ethnic Composition

As the older adult population grows larger, it will also grow more diverse, reflecting the demographic changes in the U.S. population as a whole. As with previous surveys, the largest percentage of the United States population remains white (non-Hispanic). However, the breakdown of minorities is as follows as of 2020: 12% non-Hispanic African American, 13% Asian, 10% Native Hawaiian/Pacific Islander, 12% American Indian/Alaskan, 8% Hispanic, and 6% classified as multiracial.[15] It is expected that in the coming decades, the percentage of older whites will decline and older Americans of Hispanic origin will become the largest older racial or ethnic minority group in the United States.[3]

A number of health disparities exist among racial and ethnic minority groups in the United States. Health professionals will have to work to achieve cultural competence in the services they provide to older adults of diverse backgrounds.[3]

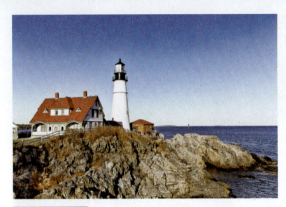

FIGURE 9.6   Recent trends have shown an increase in older adults in the state of Maine.

© imageBROKER/Angela to Roxel/imageBROKER/Getty Images

Geographic Distribution

The distribution of older adults across the United States varies greatly. Fifty-one percent of older adults lived in just 9 states in 2020. California, Florida, and Texas had the largest population numbers. The state with the highest percentage of older adults aged 65 years and older in 2020 was Maine at 22%, followed closely by Florida, West Virginia and Vermont each at 21%.[15] **(Figure 9.6)**.[15]

Economic Status

Significant improvements have occurred with regard to the income and economic position of older adults in recent decades. In 1970, approximately 25% of elders lived at or below poverty level; however, this statistic dramatically dropped to 9% by the year 2020. However, another 4.6% are considered "near poor" for this same year.[15]

Following a 5-year survey from 2018–2022, the primary source of income for older householders was Social Security, which accounted for just above one-half of their income. The remaining sources of income were from earnings income (19.3%) and pension/retirement (17.2%).[5] Because slightly more than a quarter of older adult income comes from the earnings income and retirement/pensions, they are economically more vulnerable to circumstances beyond their control, such as the loss of a spouse; deteriorating health and self-sufficiency; changes in Social Security, Medicare, and Medicaid legislation; and inflation.

Education

Older adults in the United States have completed fewer years of formal education than their younger counterparts. However, the education level has increased dramatically in recent decades. The percentage of older adults who completed high school rose drastically from 28% in 1970 to 89% in 2021.[15] In addition to this, approximately one-third of this same population went on to complete at least one higher educational degree.[15] Baby boomers are the most educated cohort in the history of the United States, so it is expected that future older adults will have achieved higher educational attainment than today's older adults.[3]

Housing

In general, the majority of older Americans live in adequate, affordable housing.[8] Of the 14.1 million households headed by persons aged 75 and older in 2019, 77% (10.8 million) owned their homes and 23% (3.3 million) rented.[15] Older adults' homes tend to be older, of lower value, and in greater need of repairs than the homes of their younger counterparts.[17]

But it is not just the general upkeep of these homes that can be problematic, but rather a question of whether or not these homes are adapted for their aging needs.[18] In addition, for others within a lower tax bracket, housing can become a burden. The cost of utilities, real estate taxes, insurance, repairs, and maintenance have forced many to sell their property or live in a less-desirable residence.

A Health Profile of Older Adults

The health status of older adults has improved over the years, both in terms of living longer and remaining functional. The percentage of older persons who are chronically disabled—those with impairments for 3 months or longer that impede daily activities—has been slowly falling. However, the most consistent risk factor of illness and death across the total population is age; in general, the health status of older adults is not as good as their younger counterparts. In this section of the chapter, we examine some of the health concerns of aging, including mortality, morbidity, and health behaviors and lifestyle choices.

Mortality

When looking at the overall mortality and reasons that people die, many consistent trends can be noted in the causes of death. However, these trends can vary considerably by age group. According to the National Vital Statistics Report for 2020, the top three leading causes of death were heart disease, cancers, and COVID-19, accounting for just over half of all deaths in the older population.[19] When broken down even farther, for those aged 85 and older, COVID-19 was the second-leading cause of death over cancers.[19] What is interesting to note here is that COVID-19 was only added as a cause of death as of the year 2020. Nevertheless, the overall age-adjusted mortality rate for older adults has continued to fall. The primary reason for this has been the declining death rates for heart disease and stroke. Despite such drops, heart disease remains the leading cause of death in this age group and is responsible for nearly one-fourth of all deaths—many of them being preventable.[19] Diseases highly impacted by behaviors and modifiable risk factors continue to be a focus of community health efforts (see **Box 9.1**).

Morbidity

Morbidity, or the condition of suffering from a specific illness or condition, may or may not affect the overall quality of life of an individual. Many morbidities, however, do affect one's ability to perform specific activities and can be classified as either chronic conditions or impairments. Of all of the chronic conditions that limit, arthritis ranks high on the list at 47%.[15] Other conditions, while just as important to manage, may not have the same immediate disabling effect. These include illnesses, such as heart disease (14%) and diabetes (21%).[15] Most of these chronic conditions will lead to an eventual loss in functioning with 39% of this population reporting difficulty with walking and climbing stairs and 8% reporting difficulty with self-care.[15] However, with the advent of medications and surgical treatment options available now, older adults are benefiting from restorative treatments and reducing the need for assistance with many activities of daily living, such as personal hygiene, simple transfers, and ambulation.[8]

Chronic Conditions

As stated before, chronic conditions are systemic health problems that are designated as chronic if they persist for longer than 3 months. Many of these conditions, such as arthritis, hypertension, diabetes, heart disease, and emphysema may or may not be life-threatening

---

BOX 9.1   *Healthy People 2030:* Objectives

Diabetes

Goal: Reduce the burden of diabetes and improve quality of life for all people who have, or are at risk for, diabetes.

Objective D-09: Reduce the rate of all-cause mortality among adults diagnosed with diabetes.

Target: 13.7 deaths per 1,000 person years

Baseline: 15.2 deaths per 1,000 person years among adults aged 18 years and over with diagnosed diabetes in 2010–2015 (age adjusted to the year 2000 standard population)

Target-setting method: Percent improvement

Data source: National Health Interview Survey (NHIS), Centers for Disease Control and Prevention (CDC)/National Center for Health Statistics (NCHS); National Death Index (NDI), CDC/NCHS

Objective D-07: Increase the proportion of adults with diabetes using insulin who monitor their blood sugar daily.

Target: 94.4%

Baseline: 89.0% of adults aged 18 years and over diagnosed with diabetes using insulin performed self-monitoring of blood glucose at least once daily in 2017 (age adjusted to the year 2000 standard population)

Target-setting method: Percentage point improvement

Data source: Behavioral Risk Factor Surveillance System (BRFSS), CDC/National Center for Chronic Disease Prevention and Health Promotion (NCCDPHP)

For Further Thought

If you were given the responsibility of getting people with diabetes using insulin to monitor their blood sugar daily, what community health activities would you use?

Data from U.S. Department of Health and Human Services, Office of Disease Prevention and Health Promotion. (2020). *Healthy People 2030*. Available at https://health.gov/healthypeople/objectives-and-data/browse-objectives/diabetes

and most older adults suffer from at least one, if not more, of these conditions.[15] Chronic conditions of older adults vary by gender and race. The most common chronic conditions reported by those aged 65 and older in the United States are hypertension, arthritis, heart disease, cancer, and diabetes.[16] The actual number of chronic conditions increases with age; therefore, limitations from activities become increasingly prevalent with age. Furthermore, many chronic conditions can result in impairments, such as the loss of sight from diabetes. They create a burden on health and economic status, impede ability to engage with family and friends, and increase the demand for caregivers. What is of public policy concern is the need for, and potential lack of, resources to care for this aging population. Improved management of chronic conditions can and will lead to reduced disability with a dramatic impact on healthcare costs.[8]

Impairments

Impairments are deficits in the functioning of one's sense organs or limitations in one's mobility or range of motion. Like chronic conditions, impairments are far more prevalent in older adults. The primary impairments that affect older adults are sensory impairments (i.e., vision, hearing, postural balance, or loss of feeling in the feet), physical limitations, and memory impairments.[20] Oral health problems and the absence of natural teeth not only create verbal and communication difficulties but also can affect general health and nutrition (see **Figure 9.7**). Unfortunately, the majority of older adults (65 years or older) are covered primarily by Medicare services. Therefore, these impairments are not likely to be addressed as traditional Medicare does not cover most dental care. In addition, Medicare does not cover prescription glasses, dentures, or hearing aids and exams for fittings.[20]

Sensory impairments increase with age, and their prevalence will increase as life expectancy increases. In 2020, 21% of older adults reported having vision difficulties.[15] "Age is the strongest predictor of hearing loss among adults aged 20 to 69, with the greatest amount of hearing loss in the 60 to 69 age group."[21] However, it is important to note that of those aged 70 and older who would benefit from the use of a hearing aid, only 30% have even used them.[21]

Falls are of great concern with older adults, particularly those with balance impairments. One in four older adults falls each year, and one in five falls causes serious injury, with over

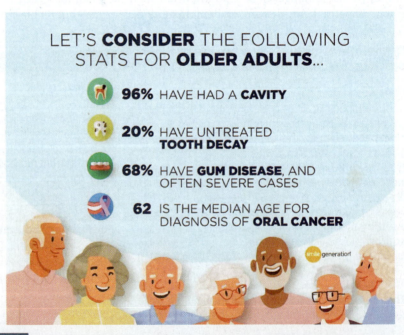

FIGURE 9.7   Oral health for older adults can affect overall health in later years.

https://www.smilegeneration.com/blog/ask-a-dentist/the-connection-between-aging-and-oral-health/. Courtesy of SmileGeneration.com.

95% of hip fractures in older adults caused by falls.[22] The death rate from falls has been growing steadily in the United States over the past decade.[22] Balance impairment may be in part why so many older adults have physical limitations. *Physical limitations* refer to older adults having difficulty performing any of these eight physical activities: (1) walking a quarter of a mile—about three city blocks; (2) walking up 10 steps without resting; (3) standing or being on their feet for about 2 hours; (4) sitting for about 2 hours; (5) stooping, bending, or kneeling; (6) reaching over their head; (7) using their fingers to grasp or handle small objects; or (8) lifting or carrying something as heavy as 10 pounds, such as a full bag of groceries.[23] Like sensory impairments, physical limitations increase with age. Memory impairments are not a natural part of aging, but connected to diseases, illnesses, or conditions more commonly affecting older adults. Currently, Alzheimer's disease is the leading cause of memory loss in older adults. Like rates for chronic conditions, rates for impairments in older adults differ by gender and race.

Health Behaviors and Lifestyle Choices

As of 2020, only 20% of the population from age 65 to 74 rated their health as fair or poor, with a slight increase to 27% for those over the age of 75.[15] There is no question that health behavior and social factors play significant roles in helping older adults maintain health in later life. Some older adults believe that they are too old to gain any benefit from changing their health behaviors. This, of course, is not true; it is never too late to make a change for the better.

In interviews, older adults generally report more favorable health behaviors than their younger counterparts. Most older Americans are less likely to consume large amounts of alcohol, smoke cigarettes (only 9% are current smokers), or be overweight or obese (30% were considered obese).[15] However, it should be noted that abusing alcoholic beverages, smoking cigarettes, and being overweight or obese decreases life expectancy, so the number of those over age 65 years reporting these factors is likely to be decreased.

Even though older adults generally report better health behaviors than their younger counterparts, there is still room for improvement. The health behaviors that can most affect the health of older adults are healthy eating, exercise, and immunizations. These issues play a major role in preventing or delaying the onset of chronic diseases.

Physical Activity

Helping to promote a healthier lifestyle is the responsibility of every healthcare practitioner. Many of the costly ailments associated with aging and inactivity can be managed with regular physical activity.[24] Although the population in this age group is increasing, the amount of activity they engage in is declining, with most being sedentary in nature. While all adults will experience some loss of physical functioning due to the aging process, even small increases in physical activity have been shown to help slow or mitigate many of these chronic conditions, such as diabetes, arthritis, cardiovascular disease, and even dementia.[24] In a recent report from the Department of Health and Human Services, the recommendation for most older adults is to participate in at least 150 minutes of moderate-intensity aerobic activity and at least 2 days of muscle strengthening each week.[24] Currently, less than 15% of this population in the United States gets this recommended amount of physical activity.[15] Of most concern is that longevity, quality of life, fall risk, and direct healthcare costs can be greatly impacted by this inactivity. Regular exercise can help to benefit anyone at any age and these benefits go far in promoting healthy aging.

Nutrition

"The foods and beverages that people consume have a profound impact on their health. The scientific connection between food and health has been well documented for many decades, with substantial evidence showing that healthy dietary patterns can help people achieve and maintain good health and reduce the risk of chronic diseases throughout all stages of the lifespan".[25] Dietary quality and requirements for older adults vary greatly, depending on life circumstances. Both obesity and malnutrition can pose challenges with the older adult population in the United States. Although the types of nutrients needed are the same for people of all age groups, the amount of each nutrient needed can vary as people age. Some dietary concerns for older adults include reduced sodium intake, reduced caloric needs from added sugars and fats, increased vegetable consumption, and increased water consumption.[25]

Obesity

As with all age groups, the number of obese people aged 65 and over in the United States has increased in recent decades. In 2020, adults in the age range of 60 and up had a recorded obesity rate of 41.5% compared with only 35% in 2014.[16,26] Many of the leading causes of premature and preventable death are a result of obesity-related conditions, including type 2 diabetes, stroke, and heart disease.[26]

Cigarette Smoking

According to the most recent data from the Centers for Disease Control and Prevention, 8.3% of all adults aged 65 and older are current cigarette smokers, with a larger percentage of male smokers compared with their female counterparts.[27] Of special concern are the number of older adults who are former smokers. Chronic lower respiratory diseases are the third-leading cause of death among older adults, which indicates the cumulative effect of cigarette smoking over many years of life.[16]

Vaccinations

Immune systems tend to weaken over time, which increases the risk of infectious diseases. The use of vaccines, however, can be some of the safest ways to help prevent communicable illnesses. According to the Centers for Disease Control and Prevention, adults who are 65 and older are recommended to stay up-to-date on vaccines to address COVID-19, influenza, pneumonia, shingles, as well as a recent rise in RSV (respiratory syncytial virus).[28] As of 2020, 75% of this population reported having received the influenza vaccine in the last year, but this number has been steadily declining.[28,29] And, of this population, 68% had received at least one pneumococcal vaccine.[15] In contrast, 95% had received at least one dose of the COVID-19 vaccine.[15] Age-associated illness places this age group at the greatest risk for complications, increased hospitalizations, and death from COVID-19.[30]

Although vaccination rates have improved over time, significant racial disparities occur. Vaccine coverage continues to be lowest for the Black and Hispanic adults compared with White and Asians.[31]

Mistreatment of Older Adults

Reports of elder abuse and neglect have increased greatly in recent years. Perhaps a substantial part of the increase in these numbers was the result of all 50 states having passed some form of elder abuse prevention laws. Although the laws and definitions of terms vary from state to state, all states have reporting systems. Prior to the reporting systems, many incidences of abuse were never recorded. Even with reporting systems in place, it is difficult to determine the actual number of older adults experiencing some form of mistreatment.

Generally, the first line of contact in the reporting of elder abuse is with Adult Protective Services.

"Adult Protective Services (APS) are those services provided to ensure the safety and well-being of elders and adults with disabilities who are in danger of being mistreated or neglected, are unable to take care of themselves or protect themselves from harm, and have no one to assist them. Interventions provided by Adult Protective Services include, but are not limited to, receiving reports of adult abuse, exploitation, or neglect, investigating these reports, case planning, monitoring, and evaluation. In addition to casework services, Adult Protection may provide or arrange for the provision of medical, social, economic, legal, housing, law enforcement, or other protective, emergency or supportive services."[32]

According to the first-ever National Elder Abuse Incidence Study, released in 1998, an estimated total of 551,000 persons older than 60 years had experienced abuse (physical, emotional/psychological), neglect, or self-neglect in a domestic setting during the year of the study.[33] This study also revealed the following:

- Female elders are abused at a higher rate than elder men.
- Elders 80 years and older are abused or neglected at two to three times the rate of their proportion of the elderly population.
- In almost 90% of all elder abuse and neglect incidents where a perpetrator is identified, the perpetrator is a family member, and two-thirds of the perpetrators are adult children or spouses.
- Victims of self-neglect are usually depressed, confused, or extremely frail.

Instrumental Needs of Older Adults

Six instrumental needs that determine lifestyles for people of all ages have been identified as income, housing, personal care, health care, transportation, and community facilities and services.[34] However, the aging process can alter these needs in unpredictable ways. Whereas those older adults in the young old group (age 65–74 years) usually do not experience appreciable changes in their lifestyles relative to these six needs, older adults in the middle old group (age 75–84 years) and the old old group (age 85 and older) eventually do. The rest of this chapter explores these six needs, discusses their implications, and describes community services for older adults.

Income

Although the need for income continues throughout one's life, achieving older adult status often reduces the income needs. Perhaps the major reduction occurs with one's retirement. Retirees do not need to purchase job-related items, such as special clothing or tools, pay union dues, or join professional associations. Expenses are further reduced because retirees no longer commute every day, buy as many meals away from home, or spend money on business travel. Reaching older adult status also usually means that children are grown and no longer dependent, and, as noted earlier, the home mortgage has often been retired. Taxes are usually lower because income is lower. In addition, many community services are offered at reduced prices for older adults.

However, aging usually means increased expenses for health care and for home maintenance and repairs that aging homeowners can no longer do themselves. Despite these increased costs, the overall need for income seems to decrease slightly for people after retirement.

As noted earlier in this chapter, the main sources of income for older adults are Social Security, pensions (e.g., government employee pensions, private pensions, or annuities), earnings from jobs, income from assets (e.g., savings accounts, stocks, bonds, real estate), and other miscellaneous sources (e.g., public assistance for poor older adults). Social Security income can account for anywhere between 50% to 90% of a retiree's income with the average monthly income of $1,782 monthly, or $21,384 annually.[35] Approximately 97% of older adults from the ages of 60 to 89 years are currently receiving Social Security benefits or will receive them in their lifetime.[35] In recent years, the income of older adults has improved. When income and other assets are combined, the economic status of older adults and those younger than 65 years is not that far apart. However, the fact remains that 10.2% of the older population lives at or below poverty level, a number that has increased from pre-pandemic levels.[36] Certain subgroups of older adults have higher rates. Unmarried women and minorities have the highest poverty rates. Married persons have the lowest poverty rates.[15,36]

Housing

Housing, a basic necessity for all, is a central concern for older adults in terms of needs and costs. It is an important source of continuity for older adults. A home is more than just a place to live. It is a symbol of independence; a place for family gatherings; a source of pleasant memories; and a link to friends, the neighborhood, and the community.[34]

When housing for older adults is examined, the major needs are appropriateness, accessibility, adequacy, and affordability. These needs are not independent of each other; in fact, they are closely intertwined. Older adults may live in affordable housing, but the housing may not be appropriate for their special needs. Or, certain housing may be accessible, but it may not be affordable, or there may not be an adequate number of units available to meet demand.

Housing requirements may change more rapidly than housing consumption during the course of retirement years as a result of changes in household composition, decreasing mobility, and/or increasing morbidity. Thus, the single biggest change in the housing needs of older adults is the need for special modifications because of physical limitations. Such modifications can be very simple—such as handrails for support in bathrooms—or more complex—such as chair lifts for stairs. Sometimes, there is need for live-in help, whereas at other times, disabilities may force older adults to leave their homes and seek specialized housing.

The decision to remove older adults from their long-term residences is not made easily. Because of the psychological and social value of the home, changing an older adult's place of residence has negative effects for both the older adult and the family members who help make the arrangements for the move. Recognizing the importance of a home and independence, families often feel tremendous conflict and guilt in deciding to move an older relative. Although moving an older adult is very difficult, it is often best for all involved. For example, moving a frail person from a 2-story to a 1-story home makes good sense, and moving an older adult from a very large home to a smaller home or an apartment is logical. A variety of housing options is available for older adults based on their needs and personal preferences. The following are general categories of housing options for older adults and their family members to explore.

Independent Living

Many older adults continue to live independently in their own home, condominium, or apartment. A variety of community services (discussed later in this chapter) are available in the home to assist older adults in maintaining their independence. Some independent older adults choose to move from a long-term private residence into a group setting, often referred to as independent living apartments, **retirement communities**, or senior housing (see **Figure 9.8**). Independent living settings are for older adults who require little to no assistance with daily activities.

Assisted Living

Assisted living facilities offer housing options for individuals who need a wide range of support services to help them with activities of daily living, such as medication management, bathing, dressing, and meals. Assisted living residents do not require the level of care that nursing home residents need. The level of care is assessed upon moving into the facility and reassessed whenever their condition changes, such as after a hospitalization.[37]

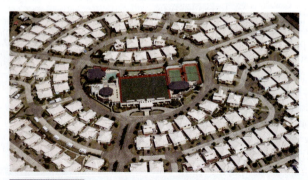

FIGURE 9.8   The number of planned retirement communities in the United States continues to rise.

Assisted living residences can vary greatly from high-rise buildings, to multibuilding campuses, to mansion-style homes. Most of them offer standard services, including the following[37]:

- Meals served in a common dining area
- Housekeeping services
- Transportation
- Laundry services
- Social and recreational activities
- 24-hour staff available to respond to both scheduled and unscheduled needs
- Assistance with eating, bathing, dressing, toileting, and other activities of daily living
- Medication management

Costs for assisted living can vary dramatically according to the facility, location, and services needed. As the cost of living for the average American continues to increase, so does the cost of care for the older adult. According to the National Council on Aging, the costs associated with living in an assisted living facility in 2023 were $4,500 per month.[38] Often, this care is funded through a combination of personal savings and assets, since Medicare and Medicaid will only cover the costs of health care received and not room and board costs.[38]

Continuing Care Retirement Communities

Continuing care retirement communities (CCRCs) offer a variety of levels of assistance in the same building, campus, or community. Moving from facility to facility can be costly and time consuming. CCRC facilities help to mitigate this by offering housing options that can manage a variety of conditions and stages of life. For example, there may be independent apartments or homes that can progress the resident to an assisted living facility should the need arise. And, if health conditions continue to deteriorate, the resident can transfer to the skilled nursing facility for more full-time care. "Residents can move from one level to another based on their individual needs, but usually stay within the CCRC."[39]

The focus of CCRCs is guaranteed lifelong residence and health care. They are typically paid for through long-term contracts/leases, large entry fees, and monthly fees. Additional services may require extra fees. Unfortunately, CCRCs are financially beyond the reach of many older adults.

Nursing Homes (Skilled Nursing Facilities) and Home Health Care

Nursing homes, otherwise known as skilled nursing facilities, offer a more comprehensive care program for people who suffer from chronic, debilitating conditions that affect their ability to self-care. Residents in these facilities are monitored 24 hours a day by registered nursing staff as well as staff that care for basic needs.[40] Nursing homes may provide short-term care for those needing rehabilitation or who are convalescing from a hospitalization. They also provide long-term care for those who are not able to return to an independent state of living. In addition to full-time care for the chronically ill, some nursing homes will also have a designated area for residents who are suffering from Alzheimer's and other forms of dementia. As of 2023, 58% of all long-term care residents were Alzheimer's patients.[40]

The costs associated with these more involved living arrangements can be quite cost prohibitive and are a major concern for individuals, families, and the government. The costs associated with living in a nursing home continue to rise with the average monthly cost of $7,908 for a semiprivate room and $9,034 for a private room.[40] Payment responsibility is dependent on many factors, including type of care needed, type of insurance coverage one has, and financial status. Options for payment include private payments, long-term care insurance, Medicare, and Medicaid. Although there are many government funding options to help cover the extensive costs associated with living in a nursing home, most individuals will have to pay privately. However, Medicare will cover a short-term nursing home stay, also known as rehabilitation, which generally follows a qualifying inpatient stay at a hospital.[40] If an individual has a long-term care insurance policy, nursing home stays are generally a covered part of the policy.

Continuing care retirement communities (CCRCs) planned communities for older adults that guarantee a lifelong residence and health care

Home health care healthcare services provided in the patient's place of residence

Activities of daily living (ADLs) tasks, such as eating, toileting, dressing, bathing, walking, getting in and out of a bed or chair, and getting outside

Functional limitation difficulty in performing personal care and home management tasks

Instrumental activities of daily living (IADLs) more complex tasks, such as handling personal finances, preparing meals, shopping, doing housework, traveling, using the telephone, and taking medications

Informal caregiver one who provides unpaid assistance to one who has some physical, mental, emotional, or financial need limiting their independence

As an alternative to these institutional services, many patients may receive medical treatment, therapy services and homemaker services in their residence for a lower cost than many inpatient settings. This home health care is often provided by nurses, home health aides, and personal care workers. Some of these services are covered by Medicare; however, a significant portion may need to be paid out of pocket.

Affordable Housing

Of all of the housing problems that confront older adults, the availability of affordable housing is the biggest. Unfortunately, the older adults who are most in need of such housing are often frail and disabled, have low incomes, and live in rural areas. The U.S. Department of Housing and Urban Development (HUD) works to provide safe, decent, affordable housing for older adults and other groups. HUD housing, also known as Section 8 Housing, does assist with finding seniors a place to reside; however, the wait list can be quite lengthy. These communities, "typically do not offer services like housekeeping and personal care services, but some do offer services, such as care coordination and wellness programs."[40] Eligibility and types of housing options are based on income and other criteria. Individuals can work with a HUD-approved housing counselor to determine qualifications.[41]

Personal Care

Although most older adults are able to care for themselves, there is a significant minority who require personal assistance for an optimal or even adequate existence. The size of this minority increases as the older adults attain middle old and old old status.

The following four different levels of tasks have been identified with which older adults may need assistance:

1. *Instrumental tasks.* Tasks, such as housekeeping, transportation, maintenance on the automobile or yard, and assistance with business affairs
2. *Expressive tasks.* Those that include emotional support, socializing and inclusion in social gatherings, and trying to prevent feelings of loneliness and isolation
3. *Cognitive tasks.* Assistance that involves scheduling appointments, monitoring health conditions, reminding elders of the need to take medications, and in general, acting as a backup memory
4. *Tasks of daily living.* Tasks, such as eating, bathing, dressing, toileting, walking, getting in and out of bed or a chair, and getting outside

Note that this last group of tasks, in addition to being a part of this listing, has special significance. These specific items have been used to develop a scale called **activities of daily living (ADLs)** and provide healthcare providers with an objective criterion on which to measure functional limitations. A **functional limitation** refers to the difficulty in performing personal care and home management tasks. However, ADLs do not cover all aspects of disability and are not sufficient by themselves to estimate the need for long-term care. Many times, these activities of daily living can be modified to allow the person to independently perform a task, such as using an assistive device to improve safety with walking, or bathroom modifications to allow for independent toileting or bathing. Some older adults have cognitive impairments that are not measured by ADLs. An additional, commonly used measure called **instrumental activities of daily living (IADLs)** measures more complex tasks, such as handling personal finances, preparing meals, shopping, doing housework, traveling, using the telephone, and taking medications.[41]

Caregivers

When older adults begin to need help with one or more ADLs or IADLs, it is usually a spouse, adult children, or other family members who first provide the help, thus assuming the role of informal caregivers. An **informal caregiver** has been defined as one who provides unpaid care or assistance to one who has some physical, mental, emotional, or financial need that limits their independence. According to a study run by the Behavioral Risk Factor Surveillance System (BRFSS), 22.3% of adults reported providing informal care within the past 30 days for a family member who is experiencing a health problem or disability.[43] This position of informal caregiver can take on many roles. For example, someone can be a **care provider**, or one that helps to identify the needs of an individual as well as personally perform the service. Or, a provider can be a **care manager**, who helps to identify specific needs for an individual, but does not provide the service. The arrangements made by a care manager can be either through volunteers or paid assistance for services.

With the aging of the population, it is now highly probable that many, if not most, adults can expect to have some responsibility as caregivers for their parents (see **Figure 9.9**). "Caregiving can affect the caregiver's life in a myriad of ways, including his/her ability to work, engage in social interactions and relationships, and maintain good physical and mental health."[43] Providing care for a loved one can be both rewarding and mentally and physically draining. Many caregivers report that they have experienced or are currently experiencing some type of decline in their health because of these demands.[43] In addition to compromised health, caregivers also often experience less personal freedom and privacy, and are economically impacted due to their caregiving responsibilities. Even though caregiving can provide many challenges, caregivers may also experience positive feelings about their role. Caring for a loved one can provide fulfillment and feelings of "giving back." Additionally, caregivers may extend their personal networks to include others with similar experiences and feel a sense of purpose and meaning in life.

The need for personal care and paying for long-term care services for older adults is projected to increase in the coming years. As noted elsewhere in this chapter, long-term care services can be very expensive for many Americans. Because of the financial burden, many opt to purchase long-term care insurance policies. These policies can be expensive if purchased late in life when the need for long-term care services are the greatest. However, they often provide older adults with sufficient income protection against the depletion of assets. The high premiums and copayment costs of long-term care policies mean that many Americans cannot afford them unless they are willing to purchase them when they are younger and the costs are lower.[44,45]

To assist caregivers, federal legislation was passed called the Older Americans Act Amendments of 2000 (Public Law 106-501). This law established the National Family Caregiver Support Program (NFCSP), which has been administered by the Administration on Aging (AoA) of the U.S. Department of Health and Human Services. The program provides grants to states based on the percentage of their population aged 70 and over. The funding is used to support services that assist families and informal caregivers to keep loved ones at home for as long as possible. The NFCSP grantees help to provide the following five types of services[46]:

- Information to caregivers about available services
- Assistance to caregivers in gaining access to the services
- Individual counseling, organization of support groups, and caregiver training
- Respite care
- Supplemental services, on a limited basis

Eldercare support for working caregivers is a growing concern in the United States as more women are in the workplace and the percentage of the age 85+ population, those with the greatest needs, grows. In fact, it is estimated that one of every six employees is performing the dual tasks of work and caregiving responsibilities.[47] As such, many employers are implementing programs to support these caregivers. In turn, employers are reaping the benefits of being able to retain quality employees, enhance employee loyalty, and reduce unexcused absences.

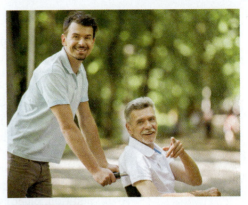

FIGURE 9.9 Adult children are gaining greater responsibility as caregivers.

© VGstockstudio/Shutterstock

Care provider one who helps identify the health care needs of an individual and also personally performs the caregiving service

Care manager one who helps identify the health care needs of an individual but does not actually provide the healthcare services

Health Care

Health care is a major issue for all segments of society, particularly for older adults. Although significant progress has been made in extending life expectancy, a longer life does not necessarily mean a healthier life. Health problems naturally increase with age. With these problems comes a need for increased healthcare services.

Older adults are the heaviest users of healthcare services. In 2022, 95.1% of adults 65 years and older reported having visited a physician in the last 12 months compared with 81.2% for those between the ages of 35 and 49.[48] They are also hospitalized more often and for longer stays. Although persons 65 years of age and older only represented 18% of the total population in 2021, they accounted for 36% of total health spending,[49] and they spent over twice as much per person on prescription drugs as those younger than 65 years. In addition, older adults have higher usage rates for professional dental care, vision aids, and medical equipment and supplies than people younger than 65 years. Usage of healthcare services increases with age, and much of the money spent on health care is spent in the last years of life.

Whereas private sources, such as employer-paid insurance, are the major sources of healthcare payment for people younger than 65 years old, public funds are used to pay for the majority of the healthcare expenses for older adults. Medicare, which was enacted in 1965 and became effective July 1, 1966, provides almost universal health insurance coverage for older adults. Medicare coverage, however, is biased toward hospital care, whereas chronic care health needs, such as eyeglasses, hearing aids, and most long-term services are not covered (see **Figure 9.10**).

In 2020, the Medicare program had approximately 63 million enrollees and as of 2022, had expenditures totaling $744 billion.[50] In addition to the increased volume of Medicare participants, the average per-person spending has also increased from $5,800 in 2000 to $15,700 in

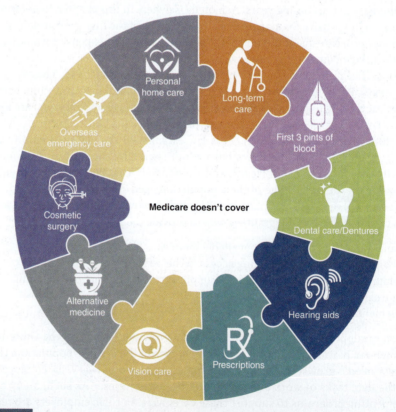

FIGURE 9.10   Many services are not covered by traditional Medicare Services.

2022.[50] Based on current trends, the net Medicare output is projected to be nearly $1.7 trillion by 2033.[50] In addition, Medicaid, a federal-state program that was also approved in 1965, helps to cover the healthcare costs of poor older adults, primarily for nursing home care (continuing care), home health care, and prescription drugs. The most recent survey calculated that 7.2 million older adults are currently covered by their state's Medicaid program, with many of them being dual enrolled in both Medicare and Medicaid.[51] Numerous changes have occurred to Medicare over the years, but the need for ongoing change remains inevitable as the first of the baby boomers turned 65 years old, and thus became eligible for Medicare in 2011. Therefore, future legislators will be forced to choose from among the following alternatives: (1) raising taxes to pay for the care, (2) reallocating tax dollars from other programs to pay for care, (3) cutting back on coverage presently offered, (4) offering care to only those who truly cannot afford it otherwise (also known as *means testing*), or (5) completely revamping the present system under which the care is funded.

In the meantime, the importance of instilling in Americans the value of preventing the onset of chronic diseases through healthy living cannot be overstated. Although it is not possible to prevent all chronic health problems, encouraging healthy behaviors is a step in the right direction.

Transportation

As of 2020, there were about 48 million Americans 65 years of age and older who were licensed drivers—a 68% increase from 2000.[52] The ability to drive provides a sense of independence in all older adults, and losing this privilege can lead to a sense of loneliness and depression. However, due to both ailing health and general costs associated with maintaining an automobile, many older adults find they are unable to continue with this task.

To help prepare our healthcare professionals, family members, and concerned community members to have effective conversations about driver safety and community transportation issues with older adults, including alternatives to driving, the National Highway Traffic Safety Administration (NHTSA) has a variety of resources available.[53] For information, visit www.nhtsa.gov.

Community Facilities and Services

As has been mentioned previously, one of the most common occurrences of the aging process is loss of independence. Even some of the most basic activities of adults become major tasks for older adults because of low income, ill health, and lack of transportation. Because of the limitations of older adults and the barriers they must face, they have special needs with regard to community facilities and services. If these needs are met, the lifestyles of older adults are greatly enhanced. If not, they are confronted with anything from a slight inconvenience to a poor quality of life.

With a view toward improving the lives of older adults, Congress enacted the **Older Americans Act of 1965 (OAA)** and has amended it several times. Among the programs created by key amendments are the national nutrition program for older adults, the state and area agencies on aging, and other programs (e.g., the caregiver program discussed earlier) to increase the services and protect the rights of older Americans.

Although the initial act was important, the services and facilities available to older adults were greatly improved after the passage of the 1973 amendments, which established the state departments on aging and area agencies on aging. These systems inform, guide, and link older persons to available, appropriate, and acceptable services to meet their needs. The amendments were written to provide the state and area agencies with the flexibility to develop plans that allow for local variations.

Although it has been mentioned many times previously, it is important to note that one of the most challenging problems facing many older adults is their loss of independence. Simple

Older Americans Act of 1965 (OAA) federal legislation to improve the lives of older adults

Meals on Wheels a community-supported nutrition program in which prepared meals are delivered to individuals in their homes, usually by volunteers

Homebound a person unable to leave their home for normal activities

Congregate meal programs community-sponsored nutrition programs that provide meals at a central site, such as a senior center

activities can become major tasks for the older adults as a result of low income, ill health, and lack of transportation. Because of these barriers, many older adults have special needs when it comes to community facilities and services. As a result of these needs, congress enacted the Older Americans Act of 1965 (OAA). Additionally, although many of the programs were designed to increase the services and protect the rights of older Americans, it wasn't until 1973 that amendments to this act greatly enhanced the programs and services. These services include, but are not limited to, nutritional supportive services, family caregiver support services, long-term care ombudsman services, and services to prevent abuse, neglect, and the exploitation of older adults.[54]

The specific needs of each community can vary greatly, depending on the population within that region. Even the names of the local agencies (few of which are called area agencies on aging) can vary a great deal. Individuals can find their local area agency on aging by visiting www.eldercare.acl.gov.

It is important to keep in mind, however, that the growth in our nation's older adult population, combined with this population's financial ability to pay for service, has created an entrepreneurial atmosphere surrounding adult care services. In some larger communities, or in those communities with a large number of older residents, the range of services can be astonishing. All of these services vary greatly in costs. In the following sections, we provide brief descriptions of facilities and services available in many communities.

Meal Service

The 1972 amendments to the OAA outlined a national nutrition program for older adults and provided funds for communities to establish meal services. Today's meal services are provided through home-delivered meal and congregate meal programs. The concept of the home-delivered meal programs (often known as **Meals on Wheels**) is the regular delivery of meals—usually once a day, 5 days per week—to **homebound** individuals. These meals are prepared in a central location, sometimes in a hospital, school, or senior center, and are delivered by community volunteers.

Congregate meal programs are provided for individuals who can travel to a central site, often within senior centers or publicly funded housing units. Usually, it is the noon meal that is provided. Generally, these meals are funded by federal and state monies and make use of commodity food services (see **Figure 9.11**)[1]. Congregate meal programs were gaining in popularity until the COVID-19 pandemic dramatically altered the landscape for gathering programs yet heightened the need for these programs at the same time. "As a result, communities, families, and providers quickly adopted new, creative ways to continue providing nutritious meals, and found ways to keep connected with clients and community members."[55]

Both types of meal programs are strictly regulated by federal and state guidelines to ensure that the meals meet standard nutritional requirements. The cost of the meals varies by site and client income level. Older adults may pay full price, pay a portion of the cost, or just make a voluntary contribution.

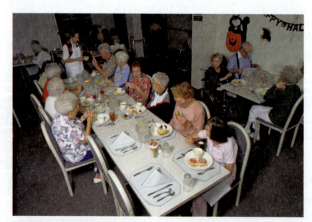

FIGURE 9.11 Congregate meal programs are not only valuable because of the enhanced nutrition but also because of the social interaction.

© Ken Hammond/USDA

Homemaker Service

For a number of older adults, periodic homemaker services can be the critical factor enabling them to remain in their own homes. For these individuals, physical impairment restricts their ability to carry out normal housekeeping activities, such as house cleaning, laundry, and meal preparation. The availability of these services allows many older adults to live semi-independently and delays their moving in with relatives or into group housing.

Adult Day Care

Adult daycare programs provide care during the daytime hours for older adults who are unable to be left alone. These services are modeled after child daycare. Most programs offer meals, snacks, and social activities for the clients. Some either provide or make arrangements for the clients to receive therapy, counseling, health education, or other health services. Other daycare programs are designed for older adults with special needs, such as clients with Alzheimer's disease, those who are blind, or veterans. Adult daycare programs allow families to continue with daytime activities while still providing the primary care for a family member.

Respite Care

Respite care is planned, short-term care. Such care allows families who provide primary care for an older family member to leave them at home or alone in a supervised care setting for anywhere from a day to a few weeks. Respite services can provide full care, including sleeping quarters, meals, bathing facilities, social activities, and the monitoring of medications. This is the service most frequently requested by informal caregivers. Such a program allows primary caregivers to take a vacation, visit other relatives, or be otherwise relieved from their constant caregiving responsibilities.

Senior Centers

With the enactment of the OAA, funds were provided to develop multipurpose senior centers to provide services, such as: fellowship, meals, recreation, legal assistance, income counseling, tax return assistance, program referrals, employment services, and other types of aid. In the last few years, a number of communities have built or upgraded senior centers with the goal of improving the lives of 40 million people by the year 2030.[56]

Other Services

There are many other services available to older adults in some communities. Usually, larger communities and those with more older adults provide a greater variety of services. The types of services provided in any one community are limited only by the creativity of those providing the service. In some communities, **visitor services** have been implemented to ensure some form of social interaction and social contact with homebound older adults. This service is typically performed on a voluntary basis, often through churches and other social organizations.

Adult day care programs daytime care provided to older adults who are unable to be left alone

Respite care planned short-term care, usually for the purpose of relieving a full-time informal caregiver

Visitor services one individual taking time to visit with another who is unable to leave their residence

Chapter Summary

- The median age of the U.S. population is at an all-time high and will continue to increase through the first third of this century.
- There are many myths about the older adult population.
- The increasing median age is affected by decreasing fertility rates and declining mortality rates.
- We are now at a point in history when a significant portion of Americans will assume some responsibility for the care of their aging parents.
- One of the most common occurrences of the aging process is the reduction in independence.
- An aging population presents the community with several concerns, which means legislators and tax-payers will be faced with decisions about how best to afford the costs (Social Security, government employee pensions, Medicare, etc.) of an ever-increasing old-age dependency ratio.
- Communities will need to deal with the special needs of income, housing, personal care, health care, transportation, and community facilities and services for older adults.
- All projections indicate that the incomes of older adults will remain lower than those of the general population, that the need for affordable and accessible housing will increase, that there will be increased needs for personal services and care, that health care needs and costs will increase, and that the demand for barrier-free transportation will increase for older adults.

Chapter Objectives   (continued)

7. Discuss selected sociodemographic characteristics across populations that experience health disparities in the United States.

8. List the six priority areas of the *Race and Health Initiative*.

9. Define concepts within multicultural competence and the importance of each related to minority community and public health.

Scenario 1

Isabel is an international student in a graduate program at your local university and just became a close contact for someone who tested positive for COVID-19. She is to quarantine for the required 14 days at her apartment. Isabel's English language skills are limited, and the county health department uses an automated system for contact tracing.

Introduction

The United States is a country rife with diversity and rich heritage, a cultural profile that has evolved from centuries of cultural exchange between both indigenous peoples and immigrants that each carry traditions, languages, culinary preferences, and myriad other customs. Within the nation's complex history, the role of race and ethnicity have evolved due to ever-shifting dynamics of power, privilege, and oppression in society. In order to meet the health needs of diverse populations and advance the goal of achieving health equity for all, one must first understand the underlying causes for many of today's health disparities between racial and ethnic populations throughout the United States.

As defined by the National Institute on Minority Health and Health Disparities, **minority health** refers to the distinctive health characteristics and attributes of racial and/or ethnic populations who are socially disadvantaged due in part to being subject to racist or discriminatory acts and are underserved in health care. Racial and ethnic minority populations include American Indian or Alaska Native, Asian, Black or African American, Hispanic or Latino American, and Native Hawaiian and Pacific Islander peoples.[1] The research literature suggests racial and ethnic minorities experience poorer health status, lower levels of insurance coverage, and inadequate access to healthcare services. Given current and estimated demographic shifts in the U.S. population, decreasing health disparities is imperative to ensure the future health of all Americans.[2]

Health disparities are health differences with adverse effects on a disadvantaged population compared with a reference population, based on one or more health outcomes. Populations with health disparities are socially disadvantaged, due in part, to being subject to racist and discriminatory acts, or continually underserved in health care.[1] In addition to most racial and ethnic populations, other populations that experience notable health disparities include people with lower socioeconomic status, underserved rural communities, sexual and gender minority groups, and people with disabilities.[1] One example of health disparities can be seen in current life expectancies across racial and ethnic populations. Between 2019 and 2021, all groups at birth experienced a decline in life expectancy; however, life expectancy for American Indian and Alaskan Native people was only 65.2 years, compared with 76.4 years for White people[3] (see **Figure 10.1**).

Although progress has been made in advancing the health status of racial and ethnic minorities, more work will need to be done before these disparities are entirely eliminated.

Minority health refers to the distinctive health characteristics and attributes of racial and/or ethnic minority populations who are socially disadvantaged due in part to being subject to racist or discriminatory acts and are underserved in health care

Health disparities refers to health differences with adverse effects on a disadvantaged population compared with a reference population, based on one or more health outcomes

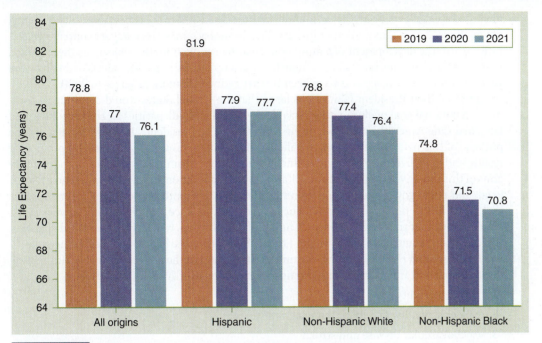

FIGURE 10.1 Life expectancy in years by race/ethnicity, 2019–2021.

Data from Arias E, Tejada-Vera B, Kochanek KD, Ahmad FB. Provisional life expectancy estimates for 2021. Vital Statistics Rapid Release; no 23. Hyattsville, MD: National Center for Health Statistics. August 2022. DOI: https://dx.doi.org/

The U.S. government, along with professional and community-based health organizations, has devoted significant resources to the elimination of health disparities, and these are now incorporated as a goal of the Healthy People Initiative (*Healthy People 2030*). Concurrently, efforts to document and address health disparities in this country are being made and have been strengthened through provisions of the Patient Protection and Affordable Care Act of 2010 (ACA).

One of the most comprehensive reports dealing with racial and ethnic health disparities in the United States is the Institute of Medicine's report titled, *Unequal Treatment: Confronting Racial and Ethnic Disparities in Health Care*. In addition to identifying health disparities, the report proposed a blueprint for addressing them as a nation.

Other noteworthy reports include the annual National Health Care Quality and Disparities Reports produced by the Agency for Healthcare Research and Quality, which seek to quantify disparities and propose strategies to eliminate them. An advantage of these annual reports over similar efforts lies in the fact that they can track changes over a period of time.[4,5]

Other government efforts include the Centers for Disease Control and Prevention's (CDC's) Racial and Ethnic Approaches to Community Health (REACH), which is designed to educate and empower people to seek and obtain needed health services; the Communities Putting Prevention to Work (2010–2012); the U.S. Department of Health and Human Services (HHS) Strategic Action Plan to End the Tobacco Epidemic (2010); and Efforts to Reduce Disparities in Influenza Vaccination. All of these programs have the overarching goal of equalizing the health status of all population groups in the United States. HHS has also developed an Action Plan to Reduce Racial and Ethnic Health Disparities,[5] and in 2013, released its second Health Disparities and Inequalities Report, which sought to "identify and address the factors that lead to health disparities among racial, ethnic, geographical, socioeconomic, and other groups so that barriers to health equity can be removed." An overall tool utilized by the federal government to achieve these goals is reflected in *Healthy People 2030* and in funding priorities for research and healthcare services.

The genesis of these national efforts can be traced to the landmark 1985 *Secretary's Task Force Report on Black and Minority Health* report, which first documented the health status disparities of minority groups in the United States.[6] This report provided documentation about health disparities experienced by members of under-represented groups. Specifically, the report identified six causes of death that accounted for more than 80% of the excess mortality observed among Black Americans and other groups. The *Secretary's Task Force Report* contributed significantly to the development of a number of Healthy People Initiative objectives that resulted in some measurable decreases in age-adjusted death rates for six specific causes of death by the year 2020, and these objectives have been further refined for more progress in 2030.[7]

In 1997, then-President Clinton declared that the United States would continue to commit to a national goal of eliminating racial and ethnic health disparities by the year 2010, and launched One America in the twenty-first Century: The President's Initiative on Race.[8] The purpose of this national effort was to enhance efforts in (1) preventing disease, (2) promoting health, and (3) delivering care to racial and ethnic minority communities.[8] One of the primary aims of this initiative consisted of consultation and collaboration among federal agencies; state, local, and tribal governments; and community professionals to research and address issues that affect health outcomes.[8] It is not surprising that this Race and Health Initiative is still a key component of the *Healthy People 2030*'s broad health goal to "eliminate health disparities, achieve health equity, and attain health literacy to improve the health and well-being of all."[7]

The Race and Health Initiative committed the nation to the ambitious goal of eliminating health disparities among racial and ethnic groups in six priority areas, including:

1. infant mortality

2. cancer screening and management

3. cardiovascular disease and stroke

4. diabetes

5. HIV/AIDS

6. adult and child immunization

The Race and Health Initiative reaffirmed the government's extensive focus on minority health issues by emphasizing the six health issues that account for a substantial burden of disease that is highly modifiable if appropriate interventions are applied. Thus, the Race and Health Initiative was intertwined with the Healthy People Initiative and the goals of the nation for the next decade and beyond.

For each of the six health disparities just mentioned, it is important to ask why each of these disparities exists. How are these related to the social determinants of health? How does power and privilege contribute to these health problems? For example, the infant mortality rate among Black Americans is consistently higher than White Americans. When looking carefully at infant mortality, many contributing factors exist for Black women that White women may not experience. The concept of "weathering" among young Black women (the age of a woman's body being significantly older than its years due to sociological disadvantage), for example, may be a factor not considered in prior interpretations of infant mortality data.[9]

Social Determinants of Health and Disparities in Health

The World Health Organization describes the social determinants of health as "the non-medical factors that influence health outcomes."[10] These factors include the conditions that people are born, grow, work, live, and age. Beyond the individual, there are also forces and systems shaped by economic policies, social norms, development agendas, and political systems.[9] In the United States, *Healthy People 2030* addresses the social determinants of health through its goal of creating social, physical, and economic environments that promote attaining the full potential for health and well-being for all.[7] Given the critical role played by social determinants of health, it is important to examine at least two key social determinants of health among racial and ethnic groups in the United States—education and income—because the literature suggests that they predict the greatest proportion of health status variance among individuals worldwide. According to the United States Census Bureau, educational attainment and median income vary by race and ethnicity with lower educational attainment associated with lower median income[11] (see **Table 10.1**).

TABLE 10.1 Educational Attainment and Household Median Income by Race and Ethnic Origin in the United States

Race or Ethnicity	High School Degree or Higher [1]	Bachelor's Degree or Higher [1]	Median Income [2]
Black	88.30%	25.40%	$52,860
American Indian/Alaska Native	78.10%	16.80%	$52,810
Asian	88.20%	57.40%	$108,700
Hispanic or Latino Origin	73.10%	20.40%	$62,800
Native Hawaiian and Other Pacific Islander	87.60%	19.80%	$72,411
White, not Hispanic or Latino	94.20%	39.50%	$81,060
Total population	87.30%	30.90%	$74,755

Data from [1] U.S. Census Bureau. (2022). *"Educational Attainment."* American Community Survey, ACS 5-Year Estimates Subject Tables [Table S1501]. Retrieved from https://data.census.gov/table/ACSST1Y2022.S1501 [2] Kollar, M., & Guzman, G. (2023, September 12). *Income in the United States: 2022.* Census.gov. https://www.census.gov/library/publications/2023/demo/p60-279.html#:-:text=Real%20median%20household%20income%20was,and%20Table%20A%2D1)

Furthermore, these social determinants of health are not always direct in nature—they are what are referred to as indirect causal associations or intermediary factors. For example, poverty by itself may not cause disease and death; however, by precluding adequate nutrition, preventive medical care, and housing, it leads to increased morbidity and premature mortality.

Race is a social construct, rather than a biologic category, reinforced by a population's social context. More than 90% of the differences in genetic makeup occur within racial and ethnic groups rather than between the groups.[12] Despite being a social construct, ignoring and minimizing race or being "colorblind" has real public health consequences. Race by itself is not the driver of health inequities. Instead, inequities often stem from **structural racism** or the historic disenfranchisement and discrimination of particular marginalized groups, including communities of color. These groups have historically been prevented from obtaining resources needed to be healthy and are disproportionately exposed to a combination of health risks, such as poverty, violence, poor neighborhood conditions, and environmental health hazards. The impact of racism on public health cannot be understated; racism shapes access to health resources and contributes to growing health disparities between and across communities.[13]

Public health research has long studied social determinants of health and explored their impact on the well-being of individuals. Many of these studies have shown that better health is associated with more years of education and having more income, a more prestigious job, and living in superior neighborhoods. Similarly, elevated levels of morbidity, disability, and mortality are associated with less education, lower income, poverty, unemployment, and poor housing. An extensive amount of research documents that social determinants of health play a significant role in the association of race and ethnicity with health and life expectancy. Furthermore, research in the last few decades indicates that the relationship between socioeconomic status (SES) and health occurs at every socioeconomic level and for a broad range of SES indicators, including life expectancy.[10]

This relationship between SES and health can be described as a gradient.[15] For example, research has documented that the more family income increases above the poverty threshold, the more health improves, and that the greater the gap in income, the greater the gap in health. Similarly, the percentage of individuals reporting good to excellent health increases with higher income levels.

This gradient effect between SES and health has important implications that are related to the gap between the privileged and underprivileged, or the "haves and have nots." In the United States, many disparities still exist between all racial and ethnic groups related to level of education and income (see Table 10.1). In the United States, communities of color often intersect with low socioeconomic rankings. These low rankings become a significant community health concern when one recognizes that progress toward the *Healthy People 2020* objectives

Structural racism refers to the totality of ways in which societies foster racial discrimination through mutually reinforcing systems of housing, education, employment, earnings, benefits, credit, media, health care, and criminal justice. These patterns and practices in turn reinforce discriminatory beliefs, values, and distribution of resources[14]

was found to be greatest among higher SES groups and least among the lower SES groups. In essence, progress toward improved health outcomes is broadly reduced for communities of color and especially reduced for those with the lowest SES. It is yet to be determined what, if any, improvements will be made with the development and implementation of the *Healthy People 2030* objectives.

Diversity and Health Equity

Although the term **diversity** has different meanings for different people, its importance is central to every public health professional's practice. According to Dicent Taillepierre (2016), diversity is an appreciation and respect for differences and similarities in the workplace (and beyond), including the varied perspectives, approaches, and competencies of coworkers and populations served.[16] Within diversity, issues, such as representation, sociodemographic (lived experience), linguistic and other characteristics, practice, technical expertise, and applied approaches must be taken into account in the community health workplace and with the many communities served in order to achieve health equity.[16] Diversity is dynamic; a single person cannot be an expert of all identities. However, everyone can take the opportunity to reflect on their own identities, learn about the identities of others, and celebrate the similarities and differences people share. For many, diversity is synonymous with race and ethnicity, and although the focus of this chapter is, in fact, on the major racial and ethnic groups in the United States, it is important to remember that diversity is much more extensive and intersects with other similarities and differences among people.

According to the U.S. Census Bureau, the population is projected to be over 338 million in 2025.[17] In the same year, projections estimate that 57.8%% of Americans, the **majority**, self-identify as "White, non-Hispanic."[18] The remaining 42.2% of the U.S. population are members of what are traditionally viewed as racial or ethnic **minority groups**.[17] In 2024, the updated OMB Directive 15 guidance states that going forward, "majority" and "minority" terminology should be removed and limited in use, except when statistically accurate and used for statistical descriptions or when legal requirements call for, use of the terms.[19]

Since the 1970s, the United States has been becoming more racially and ethnically pluralistic. Estimates suggest that by 2045, a majority of the total U.S. population will comprise racial minorities.[20] Increases in population by racial and ethnic minorities will be accomplished by corresponding decreases in the non-Hispanic White population, which is projected to represent 44.9% of the U.S. population by 2060.[17]

People of Hispanic or Latino origin—people of Cuban, Mexican, Puerto Rican, South or Central American, or other Spanish culture or origin, regardless of race—were considered the fastest growing ethnic group for most of the last 2 decades.[21] The U.S. Asian population has the fastest growth rate of any major racial or ethnic group, and has been considered the fastest growing ethnic group since the 2010 Census.[22] Between 2000 and 2019, the Asian population grew by 81% (from 10.5 million to 18.9 million) with expected growth to pass 35 million by 2060.[23] Additionally, the rising number of people who self-report as "two or more races" is expected to significantly affect the pluralistic growth in the United States.[20] As seen in **Table 10.2**, the "two or more races" population is projected to double from 3.02% of the population in 2022 to 6.08% of the population by 2060.[18]

One of the primary aims of the Race and Health Initiative consisted of consultation and collaboration among federal agencies; state, local, and tribal governments; and community professionals to research and address issues of education, income, environment, and other socioeconomic factors that affect health outcomes, and ultimately, health equity. Potential health outcomes are inseparable from a variety of other social problems, making simple solutions unlikely. It is also known that multiple resources are required to resolve these social and economic problems, and that solutions to these problems for one group may not work for another.

Whether a public health practitioner is working with a community that shares their identities or not, the experiences of one person or group are not a monolithic representation of

TABLE 10.2   Projected Population Distribution by Race and Ethnic Origin: Projections for the United States: 2022–2060 (in thousands)

Characteristics	Population						Change from 2022 to 2060	
	2022		2030		2060			
	Number	Percent	Number	Percent	Number	Percent	Number	Percent
Total Population	**333,288**	**100.00**	**345,074**	**100.00**	**364,287**	**100.00**	**30,999**	**9.30**
One race	323,217	96.98	332,809	96.45	342,122	93.92	18,905	−3.06
White	251,602	75.49	255,570	74.06	247,459	67.93	−4,143	−7.56
Non-Hispanic White	196,226	58.88	193,347	56.03	163,630	44.92	−32,596	−13.96
Black or African American	45,400	13.62	47,622	13.80	53,997	14.82	8,597	1.20
American Indian and Alaska Native	4,382	1.31	4,593	1.33	5,046	1.39	664	0.08
Asian	20,954	6.29	24,051	6.97	34,357	9.43	13,403	3.14
Native Hawaiian and Other Pacific Islander	879	0.26	973	0.28	1,263	0.35	384	0.09
Two or More Races	10,071	3.02	12,264	3.55	22,165	6.08	12,094	3.06
Hispanic or Latino	63,664	19.10	71,677	20.77	97,994	26.90	34,330	7.80

Note: 2022 is the base population estimate for the projections. Race and Hispanic origin data in the 2023 National Population Projections do not currently reflect the results of the 2020 Census. Hispanic origin is considered an ethnicity, not a race. Hispanics may be of any race. Responses of "Some Other Race" from the decennial census are modified to be consistent with the race categories that appear in our input data. To learn more about the "Modified Race" process, go tô http://www.census.gov/programs-surveys/popest/technical-documentation/research/modified-race-data.html

Note: Percentages will not add to 100 because Hispanic or Latino may be any race.

Modified from U.S. Census Bureau. (2023, October). 2023 National Population Projections Tables: Main Series. Retrieved from census.gov: https://www.census.gov/data/tables/2023/demo/popproj/2023-summary-tables.html

that population's culture, assets, needs, or health challenges in every context. Using a public health lens can help identify trends and gaps in health services to create targeted solutions to common health problems. However, in order for solutions to be meaningful, sustainable, and implemented with fidelity, the work of a public health practitioner must acknowledge and celebrate the unique perspectives of the populations they work with. Having an identity that is systemically discriminated against is traumatic; individuals from a minority groups face additional barriers to safely navigating American society and health care in particular.

For many individuals, the exposure to a new or different culture can present some unforeseen challenges where the person experiences some level of trauma. Exposure to the healthcare system in itself can be a traumatic experience, especially within systems that are not designed to be intuitive and accessible.

It could be as simple as going to a clinic visit for the first time and understanding the check-in procedures or being diagnosed with a terminal illness and the intensive medical procedures entailed or receiving a bill and filing a claim. Understanding where a community member is on the continuum of their exposure to U.S. health care and related resources can aid in providing the best quality healthcare experience that will meet their needs, wherever they may be in the process. Similarly, a community health education specialist should build rapport with community members and educate themselves on the communities with which they work. Understanding the spaces that exist and naming one's own positionality will significantly shape how to best engage and treat a community.

Community health education specialists should understand how their own culture is internalized. When one individual's culture is compared with another culture, is it just considered different, or is it considered to be better or lesser than that of another culture? For example,

Ethnocentrism when an individual believes the customs and practices of one's own culture are superior to those of others

Race the socially constructed categorization of parts of a population based on physical appearance due to particular historic social and political forces

Ethnicity refers to a subcultural group within a multicultural society. Membership in an ethnic group is usually based on a common national or tribal heritage

Operationalize to define a concept so that it can be measured

there are many homes where shoes are expected to be removed because they may have light colored carpet or the household observes a religious teaching. In other homes, there is no such requirement. Is there a right or wrong way with regard to the shoe requirement? In this context, preferences are neither right nor wrong—just different. However, there are times when an individual believes that the customs and practices of one's own culture are superior to those of others, which is termed **ethnocentrism**. Ethnocentrism occurs along a continuum, on one end of which a person thinks their culture is superior but is still respectful of someone else's culture, while on the other end, a person displays a great deal of prejudice and intolerance toward someone from a different culture. Ethnocentric practices can impede the ability of a community health education specialist in delivering the most relevant and appropriate education due to their personal conviction about their own culture, and this could adversely affect health outcomes.

Racial and Ethnic Classifications

It is standard practice for medical practitioners and public health professionals to describe participants and populations in terms of "race" or "ethnicity." Unfortunately, these terms are often used interchangeably when in fact they are not. The term **race** refers to, "the categorization of parts of a population based on physical appearance due to particular historical social and political forces.[24]" Despite this widely used classification, it should be noted that there are no scientifically established genotypes to delineate race, which leads to a subjective categorization into racial categories through social construction.

Ethnicity refers to a subcultural group within a multicultural society. Membership in an ethnic group is usually based on a common national or tribal heritage. Hutchinson and Smith have proposed that the definition of an ethnic group includes six main features, including the following[25]:

1. A common proper name, to identify and express the "essence" of the community

2. A myth of common ancestry that includes the idea of common origin in time and place and that gives an ethnie a sense of fictive kinship

3. Shared historic memories, or better, shared memories of a common past or pasts, including heroes, events, and their commemoration

4. One or more elements of common culture, which need not be specified but normally include religion, customs, and language

5. A link with a homeland, not necessarily its physical occupation by the ethnie, only its symbolic attachment to the ancestral land, as with diaspora peoples

6. A sense of solidarity on the part of at least some sections of the ethnie's population

In the United States, racial and ethnic categories are used in statistical activities and program administration reporting, including the monitoring and enforcement of civil rights (see **Table 10.3**). In the 1980s, the regulations used for the statistical classification of racial and ethnic groups by federal agencies were based on the 1978 publication by the Office of Management and Budget (OMB) of Directive 15, titled, *Race and Ethnic Standards for Federal Statistics and Administrative Reporting.*[26] This directive presented brief rules for classifying persons into four racial categories (American Indian or Alaska Native, Asian or Pacific Islander, Black, and White) and two ethnic categories (of Hispanic origin or not of Hispanic origin). Directive 15 was not intended to be scientific or anthropologic in nature, but rather, a way to **operationalize** race and ethnicity, and its guidelines provided the standards by which federal government agencies collected and classified racial and ethnic data in the 1980s and 1990s.

In 1997, classification standards expanded race from four to five categories by separating the "Asian or Pacific Islander" category into two categories: "Asian" and "Native Hawaiian or Other Pacific Islander." Other additions included acceptable substitutions when referring to an individual, such as using "Latino" instead of "Hispanic.[27]" The 1997 version of the standards were used in developing and measuring the *Healthy People 2030* objectives.

TABLE 10.3 Definitions for Racial and Ethnic Populations

Race and/or Ethnicity	Definition
American Indian or Alaska Native	A person having origins in any of the original peoples of North, South and, Central America.
Asian	A person having origins in any of the original peoples of Central or East Asia, Southeast Asia, or South Asia
Black or African American	A person having origins in any of the Black racial groups of Africa
Native Hawaiian and Pacific Islander	A person having origins in any of the original peoples of Hawaii, Guam, Samoa, or other Pacific Islands
White	A person having origins in any of the original peoples of Europe.
Middle Eastern or North African	A person having origins in any of the original peoples of the Middle East or North Africa
Hispanic or Latino	Includes individuals of Mexican, Puerto Rican, Salvadoran, Cuban, Dominican, Guatemalan, and other Central or South American or Spanish culture or origin.

Data from Office of Management and Budget. (2024, March 29). *Revisions to OMB's Statistical Policy Directive No. 15: Standards for Maintaining, Collecting, and Presenting Federal Data on Race and Ethnicity.* Retrieved from Federal Register: https://www.federalregister.gov/documents/2024/03/29/2024-06469/revisions-to-ombs-statistical-policy-directive-no-15-standards-for-maintaining-collecting-and

As of March of 2024, the OMB released updated guidelines and key revisions used to collect information on race and ethnicity, including[19]:

- Combined question for race and ethnicity
- Adding Middle Eastern or North African as a new minimum category
- Collecting additional detail to ensure further disaggregation in the collection, tabulation, and presentation of data when useful and appropriate.

Table 10.3 features the updated definitions of the race and/or ethnicity categories, as well as the inclusion of the new Middle Eastern and North African category.

Of particular interest to community health professionals are the requirements to collect data for diverse populations at federally funded programs and the need to develop culturally and linguistically appropriate materials for providers and consumers.[24] In practice; however, it should be noted that when referring to race and ethnicity, it is important to use the terminology preferred by the individual or community.

Health Data Sources and Their Limitations

The reporting of accurate and complete race and ethnicity data provides essential information to focus and evaluate public health interventions aimed at under-represented populations. However, because of the diversity in race and ethnicity in the U.S. population, community health practitioners and researchers have long recognized many crucial issues in the way that racial and ethnic variables are assessed in the collection, analysis, and dissemination of health information.

Self-reported data regarding race and ethnicity may be unreliable because individuals of varied cultures and heritage and multiple races may have difficulty selecting their racial or ethnic identity on standardized forms. Whenever person-level demographic data are needed, it is important to use best practices and standards.[28] Nonfederal health data systems may operationalize race and ethnicity differently, making data comparisons difficult and susceptible to inaccuracies.

Bias in data continues to be a priority for public health professionals. Healthcare providers are increasingly using healthcare algorithms (a computation, often based on statistical or mathematical models, that helps medical practitioners make diagnoses and decisions for treatments) and artificial intelligence (AI), to diagnose illnesses, write treatment plans, predict

Acculturation one cultural group learns and adopts elements of another cultural group, integrating them into their original culture

Assimilation the complete adoption of the ways of life of the new cultural group, resulting in the assimilated group losing nearly all of its original or native culture. A potential outcome of acculturation

health risks, and more. With the expansion of artificial intelligence to assist in patient assessment and treatment within contemporary medicine, awareness of bias in data is critical in preventing the perpetuation of discrimination. Algorithms and AI are tools built on existing data; if those data are not from a representative sample or the operations are not informed by feedback from the populations in question, the groups excluded can potentially have their health needs eclipsed by overgeneralized operations, receive poorly curated health services, and eventually worsen health outcomes.[29] Race is often used as a factor for capturing genetic differences, despite evidence suggesting race is not a reliable proxy.[30] By embedding race into healthcare data and decision making, the use of such algorithms can unintentionally perpetuate racial disparities in health.

One component of the ACA is the continued upgrading of data collection on race and ethnicity in public health surveys; therefore, the HHS continues to work with health data systems that do not collect self-reported race or ethnicity on individuals to do so. Increasing both the reliability and amount of data will assist in monitoring and assessing the outcomes related to meeting the proposed goal of *Healthy People 2030* to "eliminate health disparities, achieve health equity, and attain health literacy to improve the health and well-being of all."[7]

The next section provides a broad overview of selected characteristics of public health trends, health behaviors, and practices among the larger racial, ethnic, and other populations with health disparities in the United States. However, caution is needed to avoid stereotyping because there is a considerable amount of heterogeneity within and between groups. Making summary statements regarding cultural beliefs can cause harm if a public health practitioner relies too heavily on summaries, rather than centering the lived experiences of the populations with whom they are working. Additionally, some members of a racial or ethnic group may experience varying degrees of **acculturation** within mainstream U.S. society, including **assimilation** into American culture.[31] Therefore, health behaviors cannot be predicted with race or ethnicity alone.

Populations of Hispanic or Latino Origin Overview

The Hispanic or Latino population is one of the most rapidly growing ethnic groups in the United States. In 2022, Americans of Hispanic or Latino origin constituted 19.1% of the total U.S. population, making them the largest racial or ethnic minority group in the nation.[17] Based on the OMB Directive 15 revisions in 1997, the only ethnic distinction that the U.S. government makes is "Hispanic" or "non-Hispanic" and; therefore, many Americans of Hispanic or Latino origin are racially classified as White.[27]

More people of Hispanic or Latino origin live in the United States than in any other place in the world outside of Mexico. A decreasing number of immigrants from this population group, however, has led the U.S. Census Bureau to scale back their population growth estimate for the next few decades.[17] Current U.S. policies regarding documentation and citizenship of Hispanic or Latino individuals may also play a factor in exacting a count of immigration from Hispanic and Latino countries. Based on the 2021 American Community Survey, California, Texas, and Florida are home to the largest populations of Hispanic or Latino people, followed by New York and Arizona (see **Figure 10.2**).[32]

People of Hispanic or Latino origin are a heterogeneous group representing people living in vast geographic regions extending from Mexico to South America. People of Mexican origin are the largest Hispanic and Latino origin group in the United States, followed by Puerto Ricans. **Table 10.4** shows the distribution of Hispanic populations by country of origin.[31]

Education is a common social determinant of health considered in understanding a population's public health picture. According to the U.S. Census Bureau, 74.2% of people of Hispanic or Latino origin age 25 and older obtained at least a high school diploma in 2021, an increase from 64.3% in 2011. Additionally, 20.6% of the Hispanic or Latino population age 25 or older received a bachelor's degree or higher, an increase from 14.1% in 2011.[33] The high school completion rate increased for all racial and Hispanic or Latino origin groups, which can be seen in **Figure 10.3**.[34]

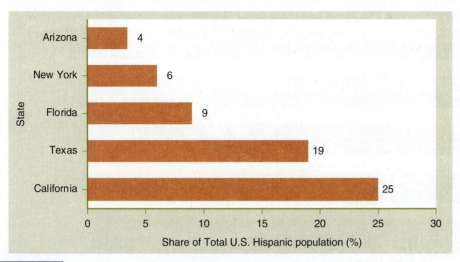

FIGURE 10.2 Top five states by share of U.S. Hispanic population—2021.

Reproduced from Moslimani, M., & Noe-Bustamante, L. (2023, August 16). Facts on Latinos in the U.S. Retrieved from Pew Research Center: https://www.pewresearch.org/hispanic/fact-sheet/latinos-in-the-us-fact-sheet/

TABLE 10.4 Hispanic Origin Profiles—2021	
	Number
Mexican	36,634,000
Puerto Rican	5,800,000
Salvadoran	2,500,000
Dominican	2,400,000
Cuban	2,400,000
Guatemalan	1,800,000
Colombian	1,400,000
Honduran	1,100,000
Spaniard	990,000
Ecuadorian	830,000
Peruvian	710,000
Venezuelan	640,000
Nicaraguan	450,000
Argentinean	290,000
Panamanian	240,000
Chilean	190,000
Costa Rican	180,000
Total	58,838,000

Note: The 17 largest U.S. Hispanic groups by origin (based on self-described race or ethnicity)

Data from Moslimani, M., Lopez, M. H., & Noe-Bustamante, L. (2023, August 16). 11 facts about Hispanic origin groups in the U.S. Retrieved from Pew Research Center: https://www.pewresearch.org/short-reads/2023/08/16/11-facts-about-hispanic-origin-groups-in-the-us

Linked with education is earning power. As described in Table 10.1, the median income of Hispanic or Latino households was $62,800 in 2022, higher than the median income of Black households ($52,860) and American Indian/Alaska Native households ($52,810);

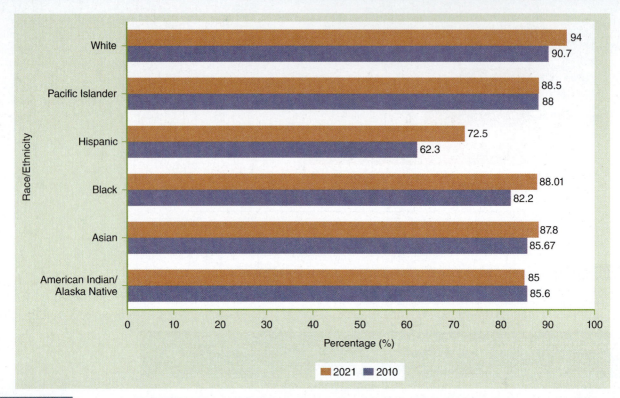

FIGURE 10.3   High school completion age 25 years and older by race/ethnicity. Educational attainment of a high school diploma or higher among individuals 25 years and older, compared between 2010 and 2021.

Note: Includes completion of high school through equivalency programs, such as a GED program.

Data from the National Center for Education Statistics. (2023, February). *Table 104.40. Percentage of persons 18 to 24 years old and 25 years old and over, by educational attainment, race/ethnicity, and selected racial/ethnic subgroups: 2010 and 2021.* Retrieved from ncese.ed.gov: https://nces.ed.gov/programs/digest/d22/tables/dt22_104.40.asp

however, their median was significantly lower than Asian households ($108,700) and White households ($81,060).[35] The poverty rate for people of Hispanic or Latino origin was 16.7% in 2022, a little under twice the rate for non-Hispanic White Americans (9.5%).[36]

Hispanic or Latino origin adults experience decreased access to health services and utilization of health care, a disparity compared with non-Hispanic White populations. Access to health services is limited among Hispanic/Latino adults, as 19.1% among the nonelderly do not have health insurance coverage.[37] Additionally, 34% denied having a doctor or healthcare provider.[38] Utilization of health care is limited among Hispanic/Latino adults as 36% reported they did not receive a routine medical checkup in the past 12 months[38] and 44% did not visit a dentist in the past 12 months.[37] When reviewing mental health utilization, only 36% of adults of Hispanic or Latino origin with any mental illness received mental health services and 14% reported to have 2 weeks or more of mentally unhealthy days in the past month[38] (see **Table 10.5** and **Table 10.6**).

Through a combination of Spanish traditions, indigenous practices throughout Latin America, and religion, there are some cultural practices that a public health professional might observe among people of Hispanic or Latino Origin. These practices should not be generalized to the entire population, but might be a consideration in certain community health contexts. Some health behaviors and beliefs one might observe include the perception of good physical health as a matter of fortune or divine determination, prioritizing collective and family care over self, and showing respect to others with a higher perceived authority.[39] Again, these behaviors and attitudes should not be assumed of someone simply because they identify as Hispanic or Latino but are provided to encourage openness to how others conceptualize or respond to health messages.

TABLE 10.5 Health Coverage, Access, and Utilization by Race and Ethnicity

Racial or Ethnic Group	Adults Reporting Fair or Poor Health Status, 2021 (%) [1]	Uninsured Among Nonelderly (Age 0–64), 2022 (%) [1]	No Doctor or Health Care Provider, 2021 [2]	No Routine Medical Checkup in the Past 12 Months, 2021 [2]	Did Not Seek Care due to Cost [2]	Did Not Visit Dentist or Dental Clinic in Past 12 Months [2]
American Indian/ Alaska Native	25%	19.1%	24%	30%	15%	45%
Asian	9%	6.0%	19%	33%	7%	36%
Black	20%	10.0%	18%	21%	14%	38%
Hispanic or Latino	21%	18.0%	34%	36%	18%	44%
Native Hawaiian/ Pacific Islander	12%	12.7%	21%	29%	14%	40%
White	14%	6.6%	16%	30%	9%	32%

Data from Hill, L., Ndugga, N., & Artiga, S. (2023, March 15). Key Data on Health and Health Care by Race and Ethnicity. Retrieved from kff.org: https://www .kff.org/racial-equity-and-health-policy/report/key-data-on-health-and-health-care-by-race-and-ethnicity/#HealthCoverage; Hill, L., Artiga, S., & Damico, A. (2024, January 11). Health Coverage by Race and Ethnicity, 2010–2022. Retrieved from kff.com: https://www.kff.org/racial-equity-and-health-policy/issue-brief /health-coverage-by-race-and-ethnicity

The leading causes of death for Americans of Hispanic or Latino origin can be seen in **Table 10.7**. When considering these larger national trends, a community health education specialist can reflect on how their programs engage people of Hispanic or Latino origin, as well as the opportunities and barriers to address and prevent the most common causes of death.

TABLE 10.6 Mental Health Status, Services, Mental Illness and Substance Use Disorder, and Suicide Rates by Race and Ethnicity

Racial or Ethnic Group	Adults with 14 or More Mentally Unhealthy Days in Past 30 Days, 2021 (%) [1]	Adults with Any Mental Illness Who Received Mental Health Services, 2021 [1]	Adults with Mental Illness and Substance Use Disorder, 2020 [1]	Suicide Death Rates (per 100,000), 2020 [2]	Age-Adjusted Drug Overdose Deaths (per 100,000), 2021 [3]
American Indian/ Alaska Native	21	N/A	N/A	23.9	56.6
Asian	11	25%	N/A	6.8*	4.7
Black	16	39%	28%	7.7	44.2
Hispanic or Latino	14	36%	27%	7.5	21.1
Native Hawaiian/ Pacific Islander	12	N/A	N/A	N/A	20.1
White	15	52%	36%	16.8	36.8

*Aggregate of Asian and Pacific Islander data.

Note: [1] Persons of more than one race are not included in the data. Insufficient data that did not allow analysis were excluded. Includes individuals ages 18 years and older.

Data from [1] Hill, L., Ndugga, N., & Artiga, S. (2023, March 15). Key Data on Health and Health Care by Race and Ethnicity. Retrieved from kff.org: https://www .kff.org/racial-equity-and-health-policy/report/key-data-on-health-and-health-care-by-race-and-ethnicity/#HealthCoverage; [2] Centers for Disease Control and Prevention. (2020). Fatal Injury Reports, National, Regional and State, 1981–2020. Retrieved from WISQARS: wisqars.cdc.gov/fata-reports; [3] Spencer, M. R., Miniño, A. M., & Warner, M. (2022, December). Drug Overdose Deaths in the United States, 2001–2021. Retrieved from National Center for Health Statistics: https:// www.cdc.gov/nchs/products/databriefs/db457.htm

TABLE 10.7   Leading Causes of Death Among Hispanic or Latino Population, 2021

1. COVID-19
2. Diseases of the heart
3. Malignant neoplasms
4. Accidents (unintentional injuries)
5. Cerebrovascular diseases
6. Diabetes mellitus
7. Alzheimer's disease
8. Chronic liver disease and cirrhosis
9. Chronic lower respiratory disease
10. Nephritis, nephrotic syndrome, and nephrosis
11. Intentional self-harm (suicide)
12. Assault (homicide)
13. Essential hypertension and hypertensive renal disease
14. Influenza and pneumonia
15. Septicemia

Black or African American Population Overview

Black or African American people have origins in any of the Black racial groups from Africa. Note that not all Black Americans trace their roots to the African continent, so allowing a person to self-identify is key to meeting their cultural needs. In 2022, Black Americans constituted 13.6% of the population, making them the second largest racial minority group in the nation.[17] The Black American population has grown by more than 10 million since 2000, when 36.2 million of the U.S. population identified as Black, marking a 32% increase over roughly two decades.[40] Black Americans live in all regions of the United States; notably, more than half (56%) live in southern states[40] (see **Figure 10.4**).

Educational attainment for Black Americans is on the rise. From 2010 to 2021, completion of high school or higher by age 25 increased from 82.2% to 88.1%, comparable to the completion rates of Asian (87.8%) and NHPI (88.5%) racial groups.[34] In 2022, approximately one in four of all Black adults aged 25 and older have a bachelor's degree or more education.[40]

Despite growths in educational attainment, earnings for Black people remain low compared with other racial groups. In 2022, the median income of Black Americans was $52,860, barely second lowest to the median income of American Indian/Alaska Native households ($52,810).[35] With earnings remaining low comparatively in a time of increasing costs of living, the poverty rate reveals similar trends: in 2022, the poverty rate among Black Americans was 21.4%, a stark contrast to the national poverty rate of 12.6%.[36] Additionally, in the same year, the non-Hispanic White population had a poverty rate of 9.5%, indicating that Black Americans were 2.25 times more likely to live in poverty than White Americans.[41] The states with the highest rates of poverty among Black people include Iowa (37.5%), Wyoming (37.0%), and West Virginia (32.6%).[36]

The United States has a long history of discrimination and harm against Black Americans, which continues to shape and influence the health of this population to this day. The transgenerational trauma deeply rooted in historic injustices, especially for Black Americans, poses a significant barrier to healthy, holistic relationships with U.S. health systems.[42] No matter the time period, there are continual examples of medical mistreatment against Black people. Black people have been subject to inferior treatment since the inception of slavery in the American colonies, these systems of harm persisting throughout the history of the country.[42] Historic laws forbade enslaved people from providing health care to each other, under the threat of

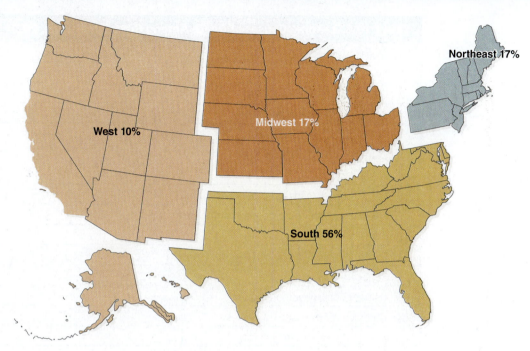

Note: Figures may not add to 100% due to rounding. "Black" refers to people who self-identify as Black, including single-race Black, multiracial Black and Black Hispanic people.

FIGURE 10.4   Majority of the U.S. Black population lives in the South, 2022.

Reproduced from Moslimani, M., Tamir, C., Budiman, A., Noe-Bustamante, L., & Mora, L. (2024, January 18). *Facts About the US Black* Population. Retrieved from Pew Research Center: https://www.pewresearch.org/social-trends/fact-sheet/facts-about-the-us-black-population/#:-:text=An%20estimated%2047.9%20million%20people%20in%20the%20U.S.%20identified%20as,increase%20over%20roughly%20two%20decades

death, consequentially driving the growth of an underground system of health care. Even if health services were offered by untrained providers, underground services were preferable to the health care available through White enslavers that were typically inadequate or dehumanizing, if available at all.

Issues did not resolve following emancipation. After the Civil War, poverty, discrimination, and poor living conditions led to a high prevalence of disease, disability, and death among Black Americans, the long-term effects continuing to this day.[43] Lacking access to more formalized health care, first by enslavement and then by segregation and discrimination, many Black Americans had to depend on traditional health methods.[44] These traditional methods include curing illnesses with roots, herbs, barks, and teas by an individual knowledgeable about their use. Many Black Americans continue to use traditional health methods today because they are acceptable, available, and affordable.

Mistrust in the healthcare system persists, a combination of historic wrongs and ongoing negative experiences. In a survey conducted by Pew Research Center, 55% of Black adults reported having a negative experience with healthcare providers in the past and younger Black women were more likely to have had a wider range of negative healthcare experiences.[45] Among survey participants, 75% of Black respondents have heard or read about the government-sponsored Tuskegee study that led to the unethical treatment of Black men diagnosed with syphilis.[45] With this context in mind, public health practitioners must remember to not interpret someone's hesitance as noncompliance or difficult behavior; these behaviors are rooted in generations of medical trauma. Many Black Americans remain skeptical about medical research, with 61% believing that medical research misconduct is just as likely today as it has been in the past.[45]

Black adults experience disparities in access to health services and utilization of health care compared with White populations.[13] Access to health services is limited among African American/Black adults with 10% of the nonelderly going uninsured and 18% reporting they do not have a doctor or healthcare provider, compared with White Americans at 6.6% and 16%,

TABLE 10.8 Leading Causes of Death Among Black Americans, 2021

| 1. Diseases of heart |
| 2. Malignant neoplasms |
| 3. COVID-19 |
| 4. Accidents (unintentional injuries) |
| 5. Cerebrovascular diseases |
| 6. Diabetes mellitus |
| 7. Assault (homicide) |
| 8. Chronic lower respiratory diseases |
| 9. Nephritis, nephrotic syndrome, and nephrosis |
| 10. Alzheimer's disease |
| 11. Essential hypertension and hypertensive renal disease |
| 12. Septicemia |
| 13. Influenza and pneumonia |
| 14. Chronic liver disease and cirrhosis |
| 15. Intentional self-harm (suicide) |

Note: Data excludes respondents of Hispanic or Latino origin.

Data from Centers for Disease Control and Prevention, National Center for Health Statistics. National Vital Statistics System, Mortality 2018-2021 on CDC WONDER Online Database, released in 2021. Data are from the Multiple Cause of Death Files, 2018-2021, as compiled from data provided by the 57 vital statistics jurisdictions through the Vital Statistics Cooperative Program. Accessed at https://wonder.cdc.gov/controller/saved/D158/D385F400

respectively.[38] Utilization of health care is limited among Black adults with 14% reporting they did not seek care due to cost and 21% did not receive a routine medical checkup in the past 12 months.[37] They were also less likely to receive treatment for mental illness than White adults and had the second highest rate of drug overdose deaths across all race and ethnicity groups.[46] (refer to Table 10.5 and Table 10.6).

The health status of Black Americans is influenced by all of these factors. See **Table 10.8** for the leading causes of death.

Asian American, Native Hawaiian, and Pacific Islander Population Overview

The term *Asian American* refers to over 20 million people who trace their roots to more than 20 countries in East Asia, Central Asia, Southeast Asia, and South Asia, each with unique histories, cultures, languages, and other characteristics.[22] The term *Native Hawaiian and Pacific Islander* (NHPI) refers to the over 879,000 people who have origins from the Pacific Islanders, including Hawaii, Samoa, Chamorro, Tonga, Marshall Islands, and Fiji.[47] In 2022, Asian Americans accounted for 6.3% of the U.S. population and NHPI people accounted for 0.26%.[17] Between 2000 and 2019, the Asian American population has increased in every state and the District of Columbia, demonstrating some of the fastest growth of a racial group.[23] Among the total Asian American population, 57% were born in another country, including 71% of Asian American adults—a stark contrast compared with 14% of all Americans and 17% of all adults.[22] Asian American populations are generally concentrated in the western states (45%), the Northeast (19%), and parts of the South (24%).[22]

Native Hawaiian alone or in any combination was one of the three largest detailed NHPI groups reported in all 10 counties with the largest NHPI alone or in combination populations in the country; less than half (46.7%) of this population live in Hawaii, down from 55% in

2010.[48] Isolated populations, chronic workforce limitations, weak governance arrangements, aging and inadequate health facilities, and supply chain difficulties interact to challenge primary healthcare delivery across the Pacific Islands.[49] Additionally, the proportions of several detailed NHPI groups living in California and Hawaii declined while the shares of these populations increased in other states across the country.[48] In June of 1999, President Clinton signed Executive Order (EO) 13125 to improve the quality of life of Asian Americans and Pacific Islanders through increased participation in federal programs where they may be underserved and by collecting separate data on each group to decrease the concealment of substantial socioeconomic and health differences between the two groups.[44] This EO attempted to address a significant concern regarding the reporting of data for these two different groups; however, even throughout the early 2000s, most federal agencies were still collecting and reporting aggregate data for Asians and Pacific Islanders, citing methodologic and funding constraints.[50] It would not be until the 2010 decennial census when data for these groups would be disaggregated.

The experiences of Asian American, Native Hawaiian, and Pacific Islander peoples are not interchangeable, but limitations in data collection and analysis can obscure underlying disparities. Often, the data—and therefore, experiences—of smaller Asian and NHPI groups are dismissed as insignificant or lumped in with another group during analysis for the sake of reliability, validity, and reproducibility of data.[47] As public health practitioners, collecting disaggregated data reduces bias against Asian American and NHPI groups. These data can also point to growing disparities and prevent the exacerbation of health inequities. Producing accurate data supports community narratives and drives action toward enduring solutions for Asian American, Native Hawaiian, and Pacific Islander constraints.[51]

In 2021, disaggregated health coverage data reveals the disparities among Asian American and NHPI populations. NHPI nonelderly adults were twice as likely to be uninsured as Asian adults.[37] They were also twice as likely to not seek care due to cost barriers than Asian Americans.[38] Twenty-one percent of NHPI people also reported they did not have a doctor or healthcare provider. There was little disaggregated data at the federal level about disparities in mental health measures. These data highlight the importance of disaggregating this population to have a better understanding of their health needs.

Immigration is an integral part of Asian American community growth, as many are seeking better economic and employment opportunities, and/or are reuniting with family members. Even among those who have come from the same country, immigration to the United States weaves a rich tapestry of narratives and timelines, resulting in a racial group with highly variant generations with equally variant motivations and lived experiences. For example, some families may have immigrated well over 100 years ago as laborers, some families send one family member overseas to pave the way for their relatives over many years, and some enter the country with a freshly minted professional degree in search of a career. In contrast to Asian populations, there is no large-scale immigration of NHPI people into the continental United States. These differences contribute to substantial diversity in acculturation, socioeconomic status, and health behaviors.

Approximately 87.8% of Asian Americans and 88.5% of Pacific Islanders aged 25 years and older had a high school diploma in 2021, but the rates for educational attainment within this group have wide ranges between subgroups.[34] Among the 56.7% of Asian Americans aged 25 years and older who received a bachelor's degree, they were more likely a South Asian person (72.8%) than a Southeast Asian person (31.9%). Even among the same subgroup, significant variation exists: while both Indian and Bhutanese people are categorized as South Asian, 77.2% of Indian Americans have a bachelor's degree vs. 19% of Bhutanese Americans.[34] Unfortunately, aggregated data masks the large variation within this population (see **Figure 10.5**).

With the sheer breadth of the Asian American and NHPI population, a summary of health beliefs, attitudes, and behaviors of all Asian Americans would be inaccurate and likely perpetuate harmful stereotypes. Again, given the multiple generations and national origins, there may be significant heterogeneity even within the same family. Medicine and health practices originating from Asia have influenced Western medicine. **Integrative medicine** combines evidence-based

Integrative Medicine combines evidence-based conventional medicine and evidence-based complementary therapies to achieve appropriate care

54% of U.S. Asians have a bachelor's degree or more education

% of those ages 25 and older with a bachelor's degree or more, by origin group, 2019

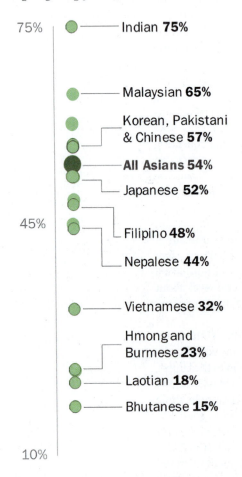

- Indian **75%**
- Malaysian **65%**
- Korean, Pakistani & Chinese **57%**
- All Asians **54%**
- Japanese **52%**
- Filipino **48%**
- Nepalese **44%**
- Vietnamese **32%**
- Hmong and Burmese **23%**
- Laotian **18%**
- Bhutanese **15%**

Note: Data not available for all Asian origin groups. "Chinese" includes those identifying as Taiwanese. See methodology for more. Source: Pew Research Center analysis of 2017-2019 American Community Survey (IPUMS).

PEW RESEARCH CENTER

FIGURE 10.5 Asian American Populations with Bachelor's Degree or Higher

conventional medicine and evidence-based complementary therapies to achieve appropriate care.[52] As a result of this cultural exchange, a public health practitioner may encounter these health beliefs and practices among various populations and not limited to Asian American groups, such as practices based in Traditional Chinese Medicine (TCM) and Ayurveda, which share some themes around holistic well-being. For example, the ultimate goal of TCM treatment is to balance one's life force, or qi, by modifying environmental factors, internal emotions, and lifestyle to optimize health.[53]

If Asian Americans had an aversion to health care available in the United States, this would be expected in the data. However, Asian Americans were the least likely racial group to avoid care due to cost, 81% had at least one doctor, and nonelderly Asian Americans were more likely to be insured than any other racial group.[37] Their access and utilization rates were comparable to the rates of White Americans. In short, just as with any population, public health practitioners should center the experience and health needs communicated directly by the group over personal assumptions.

Due to the aforementioned social determinants of health and disparities that exist for subgroups within the Asian American, Native Hawaiian, and Pacific Islander populations, there are higher risks for particular illnesses and conditions. The leading causes of death are found in **Table 10.9**.

American Indian and Alaska Native Population Overview

The American Indian and Alaska Native (AI/AN) population accounted for 1.31% of the total U.S. population in 2022.[17] American Indian and Alaska Native describe persons belonging to the Tribal nations of the continental United States (American Indians) and the Tribal nations and villages of Alaska (Alaska Natives), not to be used interchangeably with *Native American*. This term includes all Native people of the United States and its trust territories (including American Indians, Alaska Natives, Native Hawaiians, Chamorros, and American Samoans), as well as persons from Canadian First Nations and Indigenous communities in Mexico, Central America, and South America who are U.S. residents.[54] Of note, AI/AN people are the only racial or ethnic group that must submit blood quantum results and Tribal affiliation documentation (Certificate Degree of Indian Blood) in order to receive health benefits set up through the many treaties signed between the U.S. government and Tribal nations. American Indians and Alaska Natives are members of the original Indigenous peoples of North America, the original stewards of the land that now comprise the United States; this history and ancestry is reflected in over 574 federally recognized Indian Tribes.[55] This number does not include AI/AN Tribes that have not received federal recognition.[56]

Land is of great spiritual and cultural significance to Tribal nations, many Tribes relying on the land for subsistence and their local economies.[54] Between 1887 and 1934, approximately 90 million acres were taken by the U.S. government and nearly ⅔ of reservation lands were taken from Tribal nations and given to settlers as a result of the General Allotment Act of 1887.[54] In 2020, 56 million acres of the United States was held in trust by the federal government for Tribal nations, the largest reservation of which covers similar acreage as West Virginia. Some

TABLE 10.9   Leading Causes of Death Among Asian American, Native Hawaiian, and Pacific Islander People, 2021

Rank	Asian American [1]	NHPI [2]
1	Malignant neoplasms	COVID-19
2	Diseases of heart	Diseases of heart
3	COVID-19	Malignant neoplasms
4	Cerebrovascular diseases	Accidents (unintentional injuries)
5	Accidents (unintentional injuries)	Diabetes mellitus
6	Diabetes mellitus	Cerebrovascular diseases
7	Alzheimer disease	Nephritis, nephrotic syndrome, and nephrosis
8	Essential hypertension and hypertensive renal disease	Chronic lower respiratory diseases
9	Chronic lower respiratory diseases	Alzheimer's disease
10	Nephritis, nephrotic syndrome, and nephrosis	Intentional self-harm (suicide)
11	Influence and pneumonia	Essential hypertension and hypertensive renal disease
12	Intentional self-harm (suicide)	Septicemia
13	Parkinson's disease	Influenza and pneumonia
14	Septicemia	Chronic liver disease and cirrhosis
15	Chronic liver disease and cirrhosis	Assault (homicide)

Note: Data excludes respondents of Hispanic or Latino origin.

Data from [1] Centers for Disease Control and Prevention, National Center for Health Statistics. National Vital Statistics System, Mortality 2018-2021 on CDC WONDER Online Database, released in 2021. Data are from the Multiple Cause of Death Files, 2018-2021, as compiled from data provided by the 57 vital statistics jurisdictions through the Vital Statistics Cooperative Program. Accessed at https://wonder.cdc.gov/controller/saved/D158/D385F402 [2] Centers for Disease Control and Prevention, National Center for Health Statistics. National Vital Statistics System, Mortality 2018–2021 on CDC WONDER Online Database, released in 2021. Data are from the Multiple Cause of Death Files, 2018–2021, as compiled from data provided by the 57 vital statistics jurisdictions through the Vital Statistics Cooperative Program. Accessed at https://wonder.cdc.gov/controller/saved/D158/D385F457

nations hold a few acres or no land at all.[57] The experience of one AI/AN community is not equivalent to another's distinct customs, language, and beliefs, but all share a common history of colonial disruption.

It has been estimated that prior to European colonization, 12 million AI/AN people lived and flourished throughout what is now the United States. Exposure to diseases and ecological changes introduced by colonists decimated the AI/AN population. Despite the destruction and oppression of the AI/AN people and their sovereignty throughout US history, AI/AN people persist and continue to build up thriving communities, reclaiming their narratives from a violent past.[56] This transgenerational trauma and cultural assimilation has contributed to significant systemic social and economic inequities, ultimately reflecting in the health status of AI/AN people today. In 2022, the median income for AI/AN households was $52,810, the lowest of all racial and ethnic groups.[35] Their poverty rate for that same year was 24.5%, the highest poverty rate among all racial and ethnic groups.[36] AI/AN people aged 25 and older had the second lowest high school or higher completion rate.[34] The disparities seen in educational attainment for AI/AN people is even more evident for those aged 25 years and over with at least a bachelor's degree (14.2%), compared with 31.4% of the non-Hispanic White population.[34]

Racial and ethnic groups, including the AI/AN population, have a higher prevalence of chronic health conditions, which in turn suggests a need for a higher frequency of healthcare visits and interactions with their physicians and providers; insufficient cultural competency can hinder communication and thereby elevate the risk of misdiagnosis and undermining trust.[58] With over 574 Tribes, including urban Native populations, the health practices of AI/AN cannot be summarized in one paragraph. Every individual presents a unique set of backgrounds and circumstances, necessitating the creation of personalized solutions. As a community health education specialist, this might look like using an integrative approach and being open to health practices prioritized by the target population.

U.S. Government, Tribal Sovereignty, and the Provision of Health Care

Although classified by definition and for statistical purposes as a minority group, AI/AN peoples are unlike any other ethnic or racial group in the United States. Tribal members are citizens of three sovereigns: their Tribe, the United States, and the state in which they reside.[54] At the heart of nearly every issue, public health included, is the government status of a Tribe: self-government is essential if AI/AN communities are to continue protecting their unique culture and identities.

AI/AN adults experience disparities in health status, access to health services, and utilization of health care compared with White populations. One in four (25%) of AI/AN adults reported fair or poor health status, compared with 14% of White adults.[38] AI/AN adults were also 1.5 times more likely to not have a doctor or healthcare provider and nearly three times more likely to be uninsured than White nonelderly adults.[38] Mental health outcomes had some of the most striking disparities, with 21% of AI/AN adults reporting 14 or more poor mental health days in the past month[38] and the highest rate of deaths by suicide across all racial and ethnic groups.[59] Utilization of health care is limited among American Indian/Alaska Native adults, as 70% of adults reported having a routine medical checkup in the past 12 months and 55% visited a dentist in the past 12 months[37] (refer to Table 10.5 and Table 10.6). Contributing factors to this could be the distance needed to travel for covered services, a lack of culturally competent providers, and generations of oppressions.

The health services provided for Native Americans after the signing of the early treaties were limited. It was not until 1921, when the Snyder Act created the Bureau of Indian Affairs (BIA) Health Division, that more emphasis was given to providing health services to Native Americans. In 1954, with the passage of Public Law 83-568, known as the Transfer Act, the responsibility of health care for Native Americans was transferred from the Department of Interior's BIA to the U.S. Public Health Service (PHS), which created the Indian Health Service (IHS) to carry out these responsibilities.

In keeping with the concept of Tribal sovereignty, the Indian Self-Determination and Education Assistance Act (PL 93-63) of 1975 authorized the IHS to involve Tribes in the administration and operation of all or certain programs under a special contract. It authorized the IHS to provide grants to Tribal nations, on request, for planning, development, and operation of health programs.[57] Today, a number of programs are managed and operated under contract by AI/AN nations.[54]

Indian Health Service

The IHS is responsible for providing federal health services to the 574 federally recognized Native American and Alaska Native Tribes.[54] This agency operates hospitals, clinics, and health stations, and a variety of other programs. The IHS website (www.ihs.gov) offers a wealth of information for both patients and the general public.

Due to the social determinants of health and issues with accessing health care, there are many health concerns leading to morbidity and mortality in the Native American/Alaska Native population. The leading causes of death among this population group are listed in **Table 10.10**.

Middle Eastern and North African American Population Preview

Contrary to other populations, Middle Eastern and North African (MENA) Americans are not considered a unique racial group according to the U.S. government. This creates a challenge for these individuals, as some are currently classified as White in the system, whereas others

TABLE 10.10 Leading Causes of Death Among American Indians/Alaska Native Population, 2021

1. COVID-19
2. Diseases of heart
3. Malignant neoplasms
4. Accidents (unintentional injuries)
5. Chronic liver disease and cirrhosis
6. Diabetes mellitus
7. Chronic lower respiratory diseases
8. Cerebrovascular diseases
9. Intentional self-harm (suicide)
10. Nephritis, nephrotic syndrome, and nephrosis
11. Alzheimer's disease
12. Influenza and pneumonia
13. Assault (homicide)
14. Septicemia
15. Essential hypertension and hypertensive renal disease

Note: Data exclude respondents of Hispanic or Latino origin.

Data from Centers for Disease Control and Prevention, National Center for Health Statistics. National Vital Statistics System, Mortality 2018-2021 on CDC WONDER Online Database, released in 2021. Data are from the Multiple Cause of Death Files, 2018-2021, as compiled from data provided by the 57 vital statistics jurisdictions through the Vital Statistics Cooperative Program. Accessed at https://wonder.cdc.gov/controller/saved/D158/D385F551

fall into other racial categories. There was a chance that at least Middle Eastern Americans would be counted separately on the 2020 U.S. Census, but the government failed to add this category in time. Instead, a write-in section was included under the race selection box. This means that this population, with specific needs, cultures, and customs, remained counted as White or other racial groups. Without data to identify health disparities, MENA Americans would potentially be overlooked and underserved at a systems level, a significant barrier to health equity. However, with the March of 2024 revisions to OMB'S Statistical Policy Directive No. 15, Middle Eastern or North African will be added as a minimum reporting category that is separate and distinct from the White category.[19]

As a result of these data biases, providing accurate and quality data about MENA Americans remains difficult until the statistical revisions are fully accepted and implemented. Using responses to ancestry and birthplace questions as a proxy for respondents likely to self-identify as MENA, there is an estimate of 3.8 million people with either Middle Eastern or North African ancestry.[60] MENA immigrants were 4.9% of the total foreign-born population in 2021, totaling 2.2 million MENA immigrants, and nearly 70% were naturalized citizens.[60]

Over 26 different countries are represented within the MENA category. The three largest MENA groups were Lebanese, Iranian, and Egyptian.[61] California, Michigan, and New York had the largest MENA populations, but they are spread throughout the country (see **Figure 10.6**). There are some common misconceptions about the MENA population. MENA is not interchangeable with someone identifying as Arab or Muslim. *Arab* refers to people who speak Arabic as a native language and identify themselves as Arabs; *Muslims* are those who practice the religion of Islam.[62] While religion and language can be a significant part of someone's identity, these facets cannot be assumed from racial identity alone. As a public health professional, one must be aware of the stereotypes they have been exposed to and be open to learning about the true experiences of the populations supported.

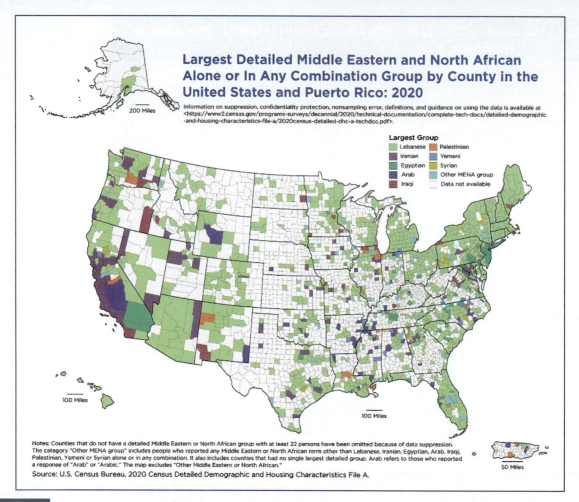

FIGURE 10.6   Largest Detailed Map of Middle Eastern and North African alone or in any combination group by count, 2020.

Reproduced from Marks, R., Jacobs, P., & Coritz, A. (2023, September 21). Lebanese, Iranian and Egyptian Populations Represented Nearly Half of the MENA Population in 2020 Census. Retrieved from census.gov: https://www.census.gov/library/stories/2023/09/2020-census-dhc-a-mena-population.html

Intersectionality in Community and Public Health

Although this chapter focuses on the public health context around race and ethnicity in the United States, addressing the needs of a community go beyond recognizing the racial and ethnic identities of a group. **Intersectionality**, a term constructed by Kimberlé Crenshaw in 1989 to talk about the complexity of Black women and how they are perceived in society; the term describes how race, class, gender, and other individual characteristics "intersect" with one another and overlap.[63] The concept of intersectionality is important to community health education specialists because all components of an individual matter when assessing, planning, implementing, and evaluating both individual and community programming and policy efforts in order to achieve health equity for all underrepresented people. Inequities often stem from historic disenfranchisement and discrimination, including communities of color, low-income populations, people with disabilities, and members of the LGBTQ community.[13]

Intersections with Race and Ethnicity Throughout the COVID-19 Pandemic

The intersections of a person's identity are especially important to understand the disparities in health outcomes following the onset of the COVID-19 pandemic. While all groups experienced an increase in premature mortality, the rate rose more for people of color than for White people.

Intersectionality describes how race, class, gender, and other individual characteristics "intersect" with one another and overlap

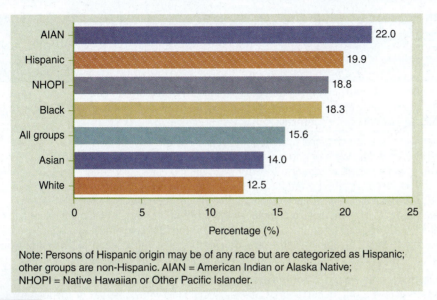

FIGURE 10.7 Average years of life lost per premature excess death under age 75 during the COVID-19 pandemic, by race/ethnicity, March 28, 2020, to December 31, 2022.

Reproduced from McGough, M., Lo, J., Amin, K., Artiga, S., Hill, L., & Cox, C. (2023, April 24). Racial disparities in premature deaths during the COVID-19 pandemic. Retrieved from Health Systems Tracker: https://www.healthsystemtracker.org/brief/racial-disparities-in-premature-deaths-during-the-covid-19-pandemic

Between 2019 and 2022, the all-cause mortality rate among people under age 75 increased by 33% for Hispanic and AIAN people, 28% for Native Hawaiian or Pacific Islander people, 22% for Asian people, and 21% for Black people, in contrast to a 14% increase for White people.[64] Black and Hispanic or Latino people also had a higher risk of COVID-19 infection compared with White individuals.[65] During the pandemic, premature deaths among people of color resulted in more years of life lost than among White people (see **Figure 10.7**).

The root causes of these disparities lie in the intersecting identities combined with race and ethnicity. Possible factors contributing to the racial disparities include family structures and household type, occupations, and access to services and supplies. Racial and ethnic minority groups are more likely to live in multi-generational households or shared accommodations, making isolation more difficult and increasing the risk of transmission.[65] Additionally, people of color are more likely to have essential worker occupations, increasing their risk of exposure to COVID-19; while Black Americans make up 15% of the workforce, they made up 30% of bus drivers, 23% of personal care aides, and 20% of food service workers in 2020.[66] Additionally, 4% of nurses nationwide are Filipino American, but accounted for about 25% of registered nurses who died of COVID-19, labor statistics suggesting Filipino nurses are more likely than White nurses to work in intensive care units.[67] On top of all of this, nationwide shortages of personal protective equipment meant that many essential workers had to recycle single-use materials or forego PPE altogether.[65] The COVID-19 pandemic continues to highlight gaps in health equity and demonstrates the consequences of trying to ameliorate a public health crisis without an intersectional lens.

Using an intersectional lens, one can recognize that racial and ethnic groups do not exist in a vacuum, and individuals will likely have some overlap with other communities that experience similar, but distinct, health challenges. According to the NIH, health disparities are identified using one or more of the following health outcomes[1] (see **Table 10.11** for Populations with Health Disparities):

- Higher incidence and/or prevalence and earlier onset of disease
- Higher prevalence of risk factors, unhealthy behaviors, or clinical measures in the causal pathway of a disease outcome
- Higher rates of condition-specific symptoms, reduced global daily functioning, or self-reported health-related quality of life using standardized measures

TABLE 10.11   NIH Populations with Health Disparities

NIH Populations with Health Disparities

Population	Description
Racial and ethnic minority groups[1]	The minority race and/or ethnicity categories defined by OMB are American Indian or Alaska Native, Asian, Native Hawaiian and Pacific Islander, Black or African American, Hispanic or Latino, and Middle Eastern or North African.
People with lower socioeconomic status (SES)[1]	Individuals from disadvantaged backgrounds, defined as those who meet two or more of the following criteria: Were or currently are homeless; were or currently are in the foster care system, as defined by the Administration for Children and Families; were eligible for the Federal Free and Reduced Lunch Program for 2 or more years; have/had no parents or legal guardians who completed a bachelor's degree; were or currently are eligible for Federal Pell grants; received support from the Special Supplemental Nutrition Program for Women, Infants, and Children (WIC) as a parent or child; grew up in one of the following areas: a) a U.S. rural area, as designated by the Health Resources and Services Administration, or b) a Centers for Medicare and Medicaid Services-designated Low-Income and Health Professional Shortage Areas.
Sexual and gender minority (SGM) groups[2]	Include, but are not limited to, individuals who identify as lesbian, gay, bisexual, asexual, transgender, Two-Spirit, queer, and/or intersex. Individuals with same-sex or -gender attractions or behaviors and those with variations in sex characteristics are also included. These populations also encompass those who do not self-identify with one of these terms but whose sexual orientation, gender identity or expression, or reproductive development is characterized by nonbinary constructs of sexual orientation, gender, and/or sex.
People with disabilities[1]	Individuals with disabilities, who are defined as those with a physical or mental impairment that substantially limits one or more major life activities, as described in the Americans with Disabilities Act of 1990, as amended.

Note: OMB Directive 15 updated in March 2024 with the newest addition of Middle Eastern and North African as a race and/or ethnicity category.

Data from NIH. (2019, November 22). Notice of NIH's Interest in Diversity. Retrieved from https://grants.nih.gov/grants/guide/notice-files/NOT-OD-20-031.html; NIH. (2024, January 17). Sex, Gender, and Sexuality. Retrieved from nih.gov: https://www.nih.gov/nih-style-guide/sex-gender-sexuality

- Premature and/or excessive mortality from diseases where population rates differ
- Greater global burden of disease using a standardized metric

Individuals practicing in community health education and related fields must be aware of the diversity within and among populations to best meet their needs through program and policy development and related advocacy efforts.

Using consistent and affirming language is a key part of building trust as a community health education specialist. With the expansion of language when discussing gender and sexuality, it would be remiss to not build a baseline knowledge of common terms to explore this facet of a person's or group's identity. **Gender** is a multidimensional social and cultural construct that includes gender roles, expressions, behaviors, activities, power dynamics, and/or attributes that a given society associates with being a woman, man, girl, or boy, as well as relationships with each other. As a social construct, gender varies from society to society and can change over time.[68] **Gender identity** refers to an individual's innermost concept of self as male, female, a blend of both, or neither; this identity is not necessarily visible to others.[68] **Sexual Orientation** describes a person's emotional, romantic, or sexual feelings toward other people or no people.[69] **Gender expression** is how one chooses to convey one's gender identity through behavior, clothing, and other external characteristics. An outsider cannot accurately glean someone's gender identity and sexual orientation from gender expression alone.

Sexuality can be both fluid and complex, and individuals may be less likely to discuss issues regarding sexual orientation, gender identity, and gender expression, especially if stigma exists within their community context. Therefore, it is important to let the people or groups describe their sexuality without bias or judgment. For example, a community health education specialist cannot assume a man is at higher risk for HIV because he was seen holding hands with another man. Holding hands is not a reliable indicator of sexual activity, but the specialist assumed

Gender a multidimensional social and cultural construct that includes gender roles, expressions, behaviors, activities, power dynamics, and/or attributes that a given society associates with being a woman, man, girl, or boy, as well as relationships with each other

Gender identity refers to an individual's innermost concept of self as male, female, a blend of both, or neither; this identity is not necessarily visible to others

Sexual orientation a person's emotional, romantic, or sexual feelings toward other people or no people

Gender expression how one chooses to convey one's gender identity through behavior, clothing, and other external characteristics

someone's sexual orientation and their behaviors. This bias could have inadvertently prevented the individual from accessing the appropriate care, therapy, or programming.

Diverse populations and the communities within them can and will vary in their values, beliefs, and structure. A person's identities beyond those already discussed, such as religion, physical appearance, veteran status, and weight add additional layers to navigating a healthy life. Making an effort to understand these nuances will better equip a public health professional to address a population's needs in a meaningful way, bringing everyone closer to true health equity.

Scenario 2

At a maternal and child health fair, you table for your university's health clinic. You excitedly share resources with new and expecting parents. At the event, a young Black person wearing a loose sweater and overalls covered with paint approaches you and introduces themself as Rhian. Before they have a chance to say more, you share your resources for new fathers and sessions for couples. You give him a brochure and encourage him to give it to his wife. Rhian frowns and says, "Actually, I'm the one expecting."

Immigrant and Refugee Population Health

As of May of 2023, more than 110 million individuals were forcibly displaced worldwide. This marks the largest ever single-year increase in forced displacement.[70] Forty-one percent of all displaced people are children, but they only make up 30% of the world's population.[71] A **refugee** likely cannot return home because of war, violence, or fear of persecution for reasons of race, religion, nationality, political opinion, or membership in a particular social group. War and ethnic, tribal, and religious violence are leading causes of refugee populations fleeing their home countries. Refugees arriving in the United States may be seeking political asylum, refuge from war, or escape from famine or other environmental disaster. The United States admitted only 11,411 refugees in the fiscal year of 2021, the lowest number since Congress passed the 1980 Refugee Act for those fleeing persecution in their home countries; in 2022, President Joseph Biden Jr. increased the refugee cap to 125,000.[72]

The term **immigrant** refers to a person living in a country other than that of their birth.[73] It describes individuals who migrate from another country for the purpose of seeking permanent residence and hopefully a better life. The United States has a checkered past in welcoming people from other countries that often is reflected in its immigration policies. These policies have provided the foundation for distinct waves of legal immigration to the United States from different countries.

Approximately 46.2 million immigrants resided in the United States by the end of 2022, more than three-quarters of whom reside lawfully.[74] Immigrant populations contribute to the expansion of the U.S. population and during the last decade, more than 7.7 million immigrants became naturalized citizens.[75] Mexican, Indian, and Filipino immigrants had the most approved naturalizations in 2023 (See **Table 10.12**).

Although all refugees and immigrants who enter the United States can be classified into one of the existing racial and ethnic categories used by our government, their immigration status adds a significant intersection of race and/or ethnicity and citizenship, resulting in a lived experienced distinct from those born in the United States. A majority of refugee populations are young and many are poor, have lower levels of formal education, and limited transferrable work skills. Contrasting this, recent immigrants have much higher rates of education attainment compared with U.S. natives. In 2022, among immigrants who arrived since 2010, 45.2% had a bachelor's degree or higher, compared with 38.0% of U.S. natives.[76]

The difficulties facing immigrants and refugees in the United States—including finding employment, obtaining access to education, and utilizing appropriate physical health and mental health services—represent significant barriers to the social integration of refugees into American society. Immigrant and refugee populations face some of the harshest circumstances

Refugee someone who has been forced to flee their country because of persecution, war, or violence

Immigrant individual who migrates from one country to another for the purpose of seeking permanent residence. Other terms for immigrant include "migrant," "foreign born," and "international migrant."[73] Immigrants can be classified as naturalized citizens, permanent residents, refugee/asylee, twilight status, or unauthorized.[73]

TABLE 10.12 Top 10 Countries of Birth with Approved Naturalizations in the United States, 2023

Country of birth	Number of Approved Naturalizations
Mexico	111,500
India	59,100
Philippines	44,800
Dominican Republic	35,200
Cuba	33,200
Vietnam	32,800
China	25,800
El Salvador	21,100
Jamaica	20,200
Colombia	17,100
All Others	477,800
Total	878,500

Reproduced from US Citizenship and Immigration Services. (2024, January 12). *Naturalization Statistics.* Retrieved from uscis. gov: https://www.uscis.gov/citizenship-resource-center/naturalization-statistics

and enter other countries in search of a better life, but are often met with unkind institutional barriers and discrimination. Despite these struggles, immigrant and refugee populations continue to enrich the communities they find themselves in and create opportunities for cultural exchange and appreciation. The role of the community health education specialist is to lift some of the burdens off their shoulders through advocacy, connecting these populations to relevant resources, and amplifying their stories.

Addressing Bias to Become Multiculturally Competent

With shifting U.S. demographics and greater research, knowledge, and cultural exchange throughout the country, health systems must be responsive to diversity and create inclusive environments where everyone thrives. This increased interest is not only being found among healthcare providers but also among patients, policymakers, educators, and accreditation and credentialing agencies.

At least a portion of the unequal treatment of disparate groups, such as racial and ethnic minority groups, is attributed to *bias*. **Bias** refers to a prejudice in favor of or against one thing, person, or group compared to another, usually in a way that is considered unfair. These biases may be held by a person, group, or institution and can yield negative or positive results. Everyone has bias. Having bias does not mean that someone is immediately a harmful person. However, when bias is not identified and actions are taken based on those biases, bias-based harm can occur. When someone holds a bias, but is not aware of its existence, it is termed **unconscious (implicit) bias**. People discern patterns based on information gathered from their lived experiences and social contexts, and they develop subconscious neural connections that influence their actions. For example, if an individual is walking down the street and all of a sudden, pedestrians on both sides of the street begin to run, most individuals will run with the crowd because their subconscious mind has determined that there is danger, despite not having a direct encounter with the reason why the others are running.

While breaking into a jog is a neutral outcome of bias, there are examples where actions informed by bias lead to inequities. For example, if a community health education specialist read a demographic report that stated almost 100% of Black households in their city speak English, they might develop a bias that Black communities do not need materials in another

Bias a prejudice in favor of or against one thing, person, or group compared with another usually in a way that is considered to be unfair

Unconscious (implicit) bias when someone holds a bias but is not aware of its existence

language. They plan several events for predominately Black communities and only prepare English materials. When the programs start, most events go without complaint. However, at one event, community members ask for Spanish materials because they have a multilingual family and another person asks where the ASL interpreter will be positioned; these families are told only English is available and that there are no interpretation services, thus creating an inequity in health literacy access.

The good news is that biases, even implicit biases, are manageable. According to the National Institute for Children's Health Quality (2019), there are seven steps that may be used to help manage implicit bias[77]:

1. *Acknowledge your bias.* As stated earlier, everyone experiences biases. However, not everyone is aware of the biases they may possess. A helpful resource to identify your unknown biases is called an Implicit Association Test (IAT). The IAT measures the attitudes or stereotypes subconsciously associated with different concepts like age or race. Take a test at https://implicit.harvard.edu/implicit/takeatest.html.

2. *Challenge your current negative biases.* Monitor how you treat someone who is different from you. Explore why you may treat them differently. Reflect on whether or not you hold assumptions about this person. Try to establish shared similarities. Afterward, seek out materials that counter that false or negative assumption you may hold, such as podcasts, articles, books, and other media by creators with identities that are different from your own.

3. *Be empathetic.* Be intentional about becoming personally connected with communities that have similar and different identities as you. Find opportunities to learn more about populations with whom you do not regularly engage and proactively learn about other communities.

4. *See differences.* Embrace the experiences of others by not being "colorblind." The ability to see color is not the issue; it is the response to or the adverse treatment of the color we see that poses the issue.

5. *Be an ally.* When you see someone who is experiencing bias, become an advocate on their behalf. One can use bystander intervention techniques to prevent or stop bias-based harm. Step up and be a voice to address the bias even if it may be difficult or frightening.

6. *Recognize that this is stressful and painful.* Becoming aware of your own biases often means facing uncomfortable truths about the ways you might have perpetuated bias-based harm in the past and the privileges you hold. Be intentional about remaining present, deeply breathe, and inquire. Collectively, these will help to overcome your biases.

7. *Engage in dialogue.* Since biases are based in prejudice, being open and curious counters preconceived notions. Many individuals appreciate that you ask and don't assume and are more than willing to share their preferences with you, but also accept if someone declines to educate you about their identity.

Becoming aware of and managing bias is part of becoming a multiculturally competent professional. The HHS and the Office of Minority Health and Health Disparities published revised standards for culturally and linguistically appropriate services (CLAS) in health care[78] (see **Box 10.1**). These criteria are the first comprehensive and nationally recognized standards of cultural and linguistic competence in healthcare service delivery that have been developed. In the past, national organizations and federal agencies independently developed their own standards and policies; the result was a wide spectrum of ideas about what constitutes culturally appropriate health services. The CLAS report went further and defined **cultural and linguistic competence** as

> a set of congruent behaviors, attitudes, and policies that come together in a system, agency, or among professionals that enables effective work in cross-cultural situations. Culture refers to integrated patterns of human behavior that include language, thoughts, communications, actions, customs, beliefs, values, and institutions of racial, ethnic, religious, or social groups. Competence implies having the capacity to function effectively as an individual and an organization within the context of the cultural beliefs, behaviors, and needs presented by consumers and their communities.[73]

Cultural and linguistic competence a set of congruent behaviors, attitudes, and policies that come together in a system, agency, or among professionals, that enables effective work in cross-cultural situations

BOX 10.1   Standards for Culturally and Linguistically Appropriate Services in Health Care

Standard	Standard Description	Practical Application Examples
Principal standard	Provide effective, equitable, understandable, and respectful quality care and services that are responsive to diverse cultural health beliefs and practices, preferred languages, health literacy, and other communication needs.	
Governance, Leadership, and Workforce		
Standard #2	Advance and sustain organizational governance and leadership that promotes CLAS and health equity through policy, practices, and allocated resources.	Identify CLAS as a priority within agency's strategic plan. (Note: Include SMART objectives or benchmark.) Review and appropriately amend agency bylaws, personnel policies, and any other operational procedures (i.e., grant review process) to ensure cultural appropriateness. Ensure that CLAS-related activities are part of the annual budget.
Standard #3	Recruit, promote, and support a culturally and linguistically diverse governance, leadership, and workforce that are responsive to the population in the service area.	Intentionally recruit individuals from diverse backgrounds (i.e., ethnic minorities) on the agency's board of directors, staff executives and management, and staff frontline workers.
Standard #4	Educate and train governance, leadership, and workforce in culturally and linguistically appropriate policies and practices on an ongoing basis.	Mandate or provide an annual cultural humility and/or CLAS training for all board of directors, executive leadership, middle managers, and frontline staff and volunteers.
Communication and Language Assistance		
Standard #5	Offer language assistance to individuals who have limited English proficiency and/or other communication needs, at no cost to them, to facilitate timely access to all health care and services.	Identify an agency process for determining language assistance services and other communication needs. Train staff on the new process for language assistance services and communication. Periodically report language assistance services data to all staff and modify and reiterate the process. Ensure that language assistance services are in the annual budget.
Standard #6	Inform all individuals of the availability of language assistance services clearly and in their preferred language, verbally, and in writing.	Ask about language assistance services experience from clients regularly.
Standard #7	Ensure the competence of individuals providing language assistance, recognizing that the use of untrained individuals and/or minors as interpreters should be avoided.	Ensure that individuals providing language assistance are certified or licensed to do so. Check on the authenticity and credibility of the certifying body. Ask clients to identify and rate their satisfaction with the person(s) providing interpretation services as part of the evaluation.

BOX 10.1   Standards for Culturally and Linguistically Appropriate Services in Health Care

Standard #8	Provide easy-to-understand print and multimedia materials and signage in the languages commonly used by the populations in the service area.	Member check all print, multimedia, and signage—meaning conduct focus groups, interviews, or surveys with clients about user-friendliness of print, multimedia, and signage materials.
Engagement, Continuous Improvement, and Accountability		
Standard #9	Establish culturally and linguistically appropriate goals, policies, and management accountability, and infuse them throughout the organizations' planning and operations.	Integrate CLAS practices in the agency's standard operating procedures for every service line.
Standard #10	Conduct ongoing assessments of the organization's CLAS-related activities and integrate CLAS-related measures into assessment measurement and continuous quality improvement activities.	Ensure that CLAS-related goals are integrated in the annual performance measures of staff at all levels. Incorporate CLAS objectives in all departmental management plans. Ensure that CLAS is part of the client and staff satisfaction, and at a minimum report annually on the findings.
Standard #11	Collect and maintain accurate and reliable demographic data to monitor and evaluate the impact of CLAS on health equity and outcomes and to inform service delivery.	Mandate the self-reporting of demographic information by client.
Standard #12	Conduct regular assessments of community health assets and needs, and use the results to plan and implement services that respond to the cultural and linguistic diversity of populations in the service area.	Conduct an agency-wide implicit association test (IAT), and develop and implement an organizational response. Create an advisory board or council comprising clients to provide ongoing feedback about CLAS-related issues and resolutions for your agency.
Standard #13	Partner with the community to design, implement, and evaluate policies, practices, and services to ensure cultural and linguistic appropriateness.	Establish a Diversity or Equity Committee that is comprised of someone from the board, staff at management level, and staff at frontline level that can recommend the crafting of CLAS-related goals, policies, and practices for the organization. Obtain input from external partners about observed CLAS practices of your organization by personnel via survey, interview, or focus group.
Standard #14	Create conflict and grievance resolution processes that are culturally and linguistically appropriate to identify, prevent, and resolve conflicts or complaints.	Host employee listening sessions conducted by an independent third party to obtain culturally appropriate grievance and conflict resolution procedures for your agency.
Standard #15	Communicate the organization's progress in implementing and sustaining CLAS to all stakeholders, constituents, and the general public.	Use your agency's social media, newsletters, and other mass communications to promote CLAS, and highlight success of CLAS implemented by the board, staff, and/or volunteers.

Cultural communication
a process that helps to serve as a sense-making function to better understand the meaning people ascribe to the verbal and nonverbal messages and behaviors of others

Intracultural communication communication with members of the same culture or subculture

Intercultural communication communication with members of different cultures or subcultures

Cross-cultural communication communication with members across cultures from different nations

Microaggressions the everyday slights, insults, putdowns, invalidations, and offensive behaviors that people experience in daily interactions with generally well-intentioned individuals who may be unaware that they have engaged in demeaning ways

Based on this definition, culture is a vital factor in both how community health professionals deliver services and how community members respond to community health programs and preventive interventions. In a society as culturally diverse as the United States, community health education specialists need to be able to communicate with different communities and understand how culture influences health behaviors.[79] It is important that community health promotion/disease prevention programs be understandable and acceptable within the cultural framework of the focus population.

Intercultural Communication

Communication is the most important way that community health education specialists form trusting relationships with members of the community. Trust is a major factor in determining whether recommended health behaviors will be adopted. Each time there is an exchange between community health education specialists and community members, cultural communication is taking place whereby trust is fostered or compromised. **Cultural communication** is a process that helps to serve as a sense-making function to better understand the meaning people ascribe to the verbal and nonverbal messages and behaviors of others. This sense-making endeavor helps both community health education specialists and community members create meaning to the exchange.

There are three primary contexts for cultural communication experienced by community health education specialists. Many will experience communication with members of the same culture or subculture, which is **intracultural communication**. Conversely, many will experience communication with members of different cultures or subcultures, which is **intercultural communication**. Similarly, many will experience communication with members across cultures from different nations, which is **cross-cultural communication**. All three contexts provide an opportunity for community health education specialists to build trusting relationships.

Educating oneself, such as through reading a community health textbook, can help prevent miscommunications, but sometimes learning through mistakes happens. In conversations with community members, a common form of bias-based harm are microaggressions.

Microaggressions are the everyday slights, insults, putdowns, invalidations, and offensive behaviors that people experience in daily interactions with generally well-intentioned individuals who may be unaware that they have engaged in demeaning ways.[80]. If a community member calls out the microaggression, be sure to use that as a learning opportunity and correct the language or behavior to prevent future harm.

For community health professionals whose role is to educate groups and communities of diverse cultural backgrounds, multicultural competence is critical.[79] Additionally, successful community health intervention and educational activities should be firmly grounded in an understanding and appreciation of the cultural characteristics of the group of interest. *Healthy People 2030* is firmly devoted to its principles that lead toward a United States in which health equity is achieved.

Empowering the Self and the Community

A principle deeply etched in the Healthy People Initiative with respect to achieving equity is the ideal that the greatest opportunities for reducing health disparities are in empowering individuals to make informed healthcare decisions and in promoting communitywide safety, education, and access to health care.[20] Given its importance in decreasing health disparities, it is not surprising that this principle is also found in the United Nations Sustainable Development Goals, which went into effect in 2015.[81]

A strategy to achieve the goals set forth in *Healthy People 2030* and the Sustainable Development Goals is to promote empowerment of historically disempowered communities, such as populations with health disparities. Community empowerment refers to the process of enabling communities to increase control over the factors and decisions that shape their lives.[82] People are their own assets, and the role of the external agent (such as a community health educator) is to catalyze, facilitate, or "accompany" the community in acquiring power. People are more cooperative, productive, and more likely to make positive changes when those in positions of authority do things *with* them, rather than *to* them or *for* them.[83] Community empowerment addresses the social, cultural, political and economic determinants that underpin health, and seeks to build partnerships in finding solutions.[82] Since empowerment hinges on the redistribution of power, naming how harm has historically disempowered a community and repairing that harm can create the foundations for healthier, sustainable communities.

Originally used as an approach in criminal justice that focuses on repairing harm rather than punishment, using a *restorative justice framework* can aid in addressing systemic harm and empower communities. A restorative strategy focuses on working with a community to resolve public health issues where the public health practitioner and community work together to understand what are the barriers to meeting expectations and how those barriers can be addressed.[84] Key to this approach is that the public health professional does not enter a community assuming they have the best approach with an already formed solution, but instead, requires cultural humility and centers collaboration to get to the core of an issue.

A final strategy to improve the health status of diverse populations includes a focus on health literacy, which is defined as "the degree to which individuals have the capacity to obtain, process, and understand basic health information and services needed to make appropriate health decisions.[85]" In order to achieve the health literacy goals embedded in *Healthy People 2030*, health education specialists must determine the language and health knowledge of their target community to best meet their needs.

By reflecting on the health disparities experienced across racial and ethnic populations, one can see the great progress and great challenges in achieving health equity for all people. Creating a country that prioritizes health equity for all people does not mean that every population and their solutions look the same. Rather, through multicultural collaboration and celebration of the diverse communities that make up the nation, every community can grow and achieve health equity.

Chapter Summary

- One of the great strengths of the United States has been, and remains, the diversity of its people.
- The social determinants of health impact the health status of all people, as these are part of their social, emotional, and physical environments.
- Health disparities persist among racial and ethnic minority populations due in part to being subject to structural racism and are underserved in health care.
- Socioeconomic status (SES) has been considered the most influential single contributor to premature morbidity and mortality by many public health researchers. Research in the last few decades indicates that the relationship between SES and health occurs at every socioeconomic level and for a broad range of SES indicators. This relationship between SES and health can be described as a gradient.
- The federal government has historically categorized the U.S. population into five racial groups (American Indian or Alaska Native, Asian, Black or African American, Native Hawaiian or Other Pacific Islander, and White) and two ethnic groups (Hispanic or Latino and non-Hispanic or non-Latino), but terminology changes over time.
- The reporting of accurate and complete race and ethnicity data provide essential information to implement and evaluate public health interventions aimed at minority populations.
- All cultural and ethnic groups hold concepts related to health and illness and associated practices for maintaining well-being or providing treatment when it is indicated.
- Significant strides in the improvement of health among racial and ethnic populations can be achieved if community and public health professionals become more multiculturally competent.
- Populations with health disparities must be empowered to solve their own problems, which will require amending the social, cultural, political, and economic determinants that underpin health.

Scenario 1: Analysis and Response

1. How should you approach this situation with regard to contact tracing?

2. What follow-up questions should you ask Isabel before assuming she does or does not understand contact tracing?

3. How could the protocol be equitably changed to help Isabel with understanding her quarantine situation?

4. What forms of cultural communication might assist the health education specialist in this situation?

5. What parts of Isabel's identity might play into this situation?

Scenario 2: Analysis and Response

1. What were some of the biases, or assumptions, about Rhian?

2. What questions should have been asked before assuming what materials and needs Rhian would have?

3. If you were tabling with someone else and saw this happen, what are some ways you could intervene and make amends in the situation?

4. Based on what was shared in the scenario, what are some identities you share with Rhian? What are some differences? From the differences, where and how did you learn about those identities?

5. What are some potential intersecting identities that Rhian has that would prompt considering additional resources and supports? What are some follow-up questions you have?

Review Questions

1. Why is it said that the United States was built on diversity?

2. Discuss how the social determinants of health impact the health status of AI/AN, Asian, Black, Hispanic or Latino, NHPI, and White people. What are some similarities? What are some key differences? How do these drive public health action?

3. What is the Office of Management and Budget's Directive 15?

4. Why is it important for community health education specialists to be aware of the significant health disparities affecting specific racial or ethnic groups across the United States?

5. What changes have taken place since the 1985 landmark report, *The Secretary's Task Force Report on Black and Minority Health*?

6. How did the intersection of socioeconomic status and race and/or ethnicity play a role in health outcomes during the COVID-19 pandemic?

7. Why is it important for community health professionals to be multiculturally competent?

8. How does a community health education specialist reduce their own implicit bias?

9. Discuss the three types of communication presented in this chapter and how they are utilized when working with different populations.

10. What is the role of a community health specialist in community empowerment? How can a community health specialist empower a community to create a solution for a specific health issue?

Activities

1. Using the most recent U.S. Census report (available on the Internet), create a demographic profile of the state and county in which you live. Locate the following information—population; racial/ethnic composition; percentage of people represented by the different age groups, gender breakdown, and marital status; and percentage of people living in poverty.

2. Visit the U. S. Department of Health and Human Services Office of Minority Health website https://minorityhealth.hhs.gov/ and go to the Healthy People 2020 Health Disparities Data Widget. Explore a disparity not explained in the chapter and, using health indicators, develop charts to illustrate health statuses of these groups.

3. In a two- to three-page paper, present the proposal you would recommend to the President of the United States for eliminating health disparities between groups of people.

4. Identify a specific racial/ethnic minority group, and select a health problem. Study the topic and present in a three-page paper the present status of the problem, the future outlook for the problem, and what could be done to reduce or eliminate the problem.

5. Write a two-page position paper on "What are the main drivers of health disparities among racial and ethnic populations?"

References

1. National Institute on Minority Health and Health Disparities. (2023, October 3). *Minority health and health disparities definitions.* Retrieved February 19, 2024, from https://www.nimhd.nih.gov/about/strategic-plan/nih-strategic-plan-definitions-and-parameters.html

2. U.S. Census Bureau. (2019). *American fact finder.* Retrieved from Census.gov: https://factfinder .census.gov/faces/nav/jsf/pages /index.xhtml

3. Hill, L., & Artiga, S. (2023). *What is driving widening racial disparities in life expectancy?* Retrieved from KFF: https://www.kff.org/racial-equity-and-health-policy/issue-brief/what-is-driving-widening-racial-disparities-in-life-expectancy

4. U.S. Department of Health and Human Services. (2018). *National Health Care Quality and Disparities Report 2018.* Agency for Healthcare Research and Quality.

5. U.S. Department of Health and Human Services. (2015). HHS Action Plan to Reduce Disparities. Retrieved from aspe.hhs.gov: https://aspe.hhs.gov/sites/default/files/private/pdf/206166/Disparities ActionPlan.pdf

6. U.S. Department of Health and Human Services. (1988). *Report of the Secretary's Task Force on Black and Minority Health.* HHS.

7. U.S. Department of Health and Human Services Office of Disease Prevention and Health Promotion. (2020). *Healthy People 2030.* Retrieved from Healthy People: https://health.gov/healthy people /about/healthy-people-2030-framework.2020/default .aspx

8. The President's Initiative on Race. (1998). *One American in the 21st Century.* Retrieved from https://www.ncjrs.gov/pdffiles/173431.pdf

9. Geronimus, A. (1992). *The weathering hypothesis and the health of African-American women and infants: Evidence and speculations.* Ethnicity and Disease. Retrieved from https://www.ncbi.nlm .nih.gov/pubmed/1467758

10. World Health Organization. (2024). *Social determinants of health.* Retrieved from who.int: https://www.who.int/health-topics/social -determinants-of-health

11. U.S. Census Bureau. (2022). *Educational attainment. American Community Survey, ACS 5-Year Estimates Subject Tables [Table S1501].* Retrieved from data.census.gov: https://data.census.gov /table/ACSST1Y2022.S1501

12. Witherspoon, D. J., Wooding, S., Rogers, A. R., Marchani, E. E., Watkins, W. S., Batzer, M. A., & Jorde, L. B. (2007). Genetic similarities within and between human populations. *Genetics, 176*(1), 351–359. Retrieved from https://doi.org/10.1534/genetics.106.067355

13. American Public Health Association. (2023). *Racial equity & public health.* Retrieved from apha.org: https://www.apha.org/-/media/Files /PDF/advocacy/SPEAK/210825_Racial_Equity_Fact_Sheet.ashx

14. American Medical Association. (2021). What is structural racism? Retrieved from AMA-ASSN.org: https://www.ama-assn.org /delivering-care/health-equity/what-structural-racism

15. Donkin, A. J. (2014). *Social gradient.* The Wiley Blackwell Encyclopedia of Health, Illness, Behavior, and Society, 2172–2178.

16. Taillepierre, D. (2016). *Why diversity and inclusion matters in public health.* Retrieved from cdc.gov: https://www.cdc.gov /minorityhealth/internships

17. U.S. Census Bureau. (2023). *2023 National Population Projections Tables: Main Series.* Retrieved from census.gov: https://www .census.gov/data/tables/2023/demo/popproj/2023-summary-tables .html

18. U.S. Census Bureau, Population Division. (2023). *2023 National Population Projections Tables: Main series.* Retrieved from census. gov: https://www.census.gov/data/tables/2023/demo/popproj/2023 -summary-tables.html

19. Office of Management and Budget. (2024, March 29). *Revisions to OMB's Statistical Policy Directive No. 15: Standards for Maintaining, Collecting, and Presenting Federal Data on Race and Ethnicity.* Retrieved from Federal Register: https://www.federalregister.gov /documents/2024/03/29/2024-06469/revisions-to-ombs-statistical -policy-directive-no-15-standards-for-maintaining-collecting-and

20. Vespa, J. M. (2020). *Demographic turning points for the United States: Population projections for 2020 to 2060.* Retrieved from census.gov: https://www.census.gov/content/dam/Census/library /publications/2020/demo/p25-1144.pdf

21. Moslimani, M., Lopez, M. H., & Noe-Bustamante, L. (2023). *11 facts about Hispanic origin groups in the U.S.* Retrieved from Pew Research Center: https://www.pewresearch.org/short-reads/2023/08/16 /11-facts-about-hispanic-origin-groups-in-the-us/

22. Budiman, A., & Ruiz, N. G. (2021). *Key facts about Asian Americans, a diverse and growing population.* Retrieved from Pew Research Center: https://www.pewresearch.org/short-reads/2021/04/29 /key-facts-about-asian-americans/

23. Budiman, A., & Ruiz, N. (2021). *Asian Americans are the fastest-growing racial or ethnic group in the U.S.* Retrieved from pewresearch.org: https://www.pewresearch.org/short-reads /2021/04/09/asian-americans-are-the-fastest-growing-racial-or -ethnic-group-in-the-u-s/

24. Heurtin-Roberts, S. (2004). *Race and ethnicity in health and vital statistics.* Retrieved from hhs.gov: https://ncvhs.hhs.gov/wp-content /uploads/2014/05 /040902p1.pdf

25. Hutchinson, J., & Smith, A. (1996). *Introduction.* Ethnicity, 1–14.

26. U.S Office of Management and Budget. (1978). *Directive 15: Race and ethnic standards for federal statistics and administrative reporting.* U.S. Department of Commerce, Office of Federal Statistical Policy and Standards Statistical Policy Handbook, 37–38.

27. U.S. Office of Management and Budget. (1997). *Revisions to the standards for the classification of federal data on race and ethnicity.* OMB.

28. U.S. Department of Health and Human Services Office of Minority Health. (2018). *Data collection standards for race, ethnicity, primary language, sex and disability status.* Retrieved from hhs.gov: https:// minorityhealth.hhs.gov /omh/browse.aspx?lvl=2&lvlid=23

29. Colón-Rodríguez, C. J. (2023). Shedding light on healthcare algorithmic and artificial intelligence bias. Retrieved from minority-health.hhs.gov: https://minorityhealth.hhs.gov/news/shedding -light-healthcare-algorithmic-and-artificial-intelligence-bias

30. Jones, D. S., & Payton, F. C. (2021). *Racial bias in health care artificial intelligence.* Retrieved from NIHCM Foundation: https://nihcm.org /publications/artificial-intelligences-racial-bias-in-health-care

31. SAMHSA. (2015). Tip 59: Improving cultural competence. Retrieved from SAMHSA.gov: https://store.samhsa.gov/sites/default/files/sma14-4849.pdf

32. Moslimani, M., & Noe-Bustamante, L. (2023). *Facts on Latinos in the U.S.* Retrieved from Pew Research Center: https://www.pewresearch.org/hispanic/fact-sheet/latinos-in-the-us-fact-sheet/

33. U.S. Census Bureau. (2022). Census Bureau releases new educational attainment data. Retrieved from census.gov: https://www.census.gov/newsroom/press-releases/2022/educational-attainment.html

34. National Center for Education Statistics. (2023). *Table 104.40. Percentage of persons 18 to 24 years old and 25 years old and over, by educational attainment, race/ethnicity, and selected racial/ethnic subgroups: 2010 and 2021.* Retrieved from ncese.ed.gov: https://nces.ed.gov/programs/digest/d22/tables/dt22_104.40.asp

35. Guzman, G., & Kollar, M. (2023). Income in the United States: 2022. Retrieved from Census.gov: https://www.census.gov/library/publications/2023/demo/p60-279.html#:~:text=Real%20median%20household%20income%20was,and%20Table%20A%2D1

36. KFF. (2022). *Poverty rate by race/ethnicity.* Retrieved from kff.org: https://www.kff.org/other/state-indicator/poverty-rate-by-raceethnicity/?currentTimeframe=0&sortModel=%7B%22colId%22:%22Location%22,%22sort%22:%22asc%22%7D

37. Hill, L., Artiga, S., & Damico, A. (2024). *Health coverage by race and ethnicity, 2010-2022.* Retrieved from kff.com: https://www.kff.org/racial-equity-and-health-policy/issue-brief/health-coverage-by-race-and-ethnicity

38. Hill, L., Ndugga, N., & Artiga, S. (2023). *Key data on health and health care by race and ethnicity.* Retrieved from kff.org: https://www.kff.org/racial-equity-and-health-policy/report/key-data-on-health-and-health-care-by-race-and-ethnicity/#HealthCoverage

39. Rivera, G. M. (2016). *The Hispanic patient.* Retrieved from Coa.org: https://coa.org/2016/presentations/qme/7HispanicPatient101kkk.pdf

40. Moslimani, M., Tamir, C., Budiman, A., Noe-Bustamante, L., & Mora, L. (2024). Facts about the US Black population. Retrieved from Pew Research Center: https://www.pewresearch.org/social-trends/fact-sheet/facts-about-the-us-black-population

41. KFF. (2022). *Poverty rate by race/ethnicity.* Retrieved from kff.org: https://www.kff.org/other/state-indicator/poverty-rate-by-raceethnicity/

42. Miller, F., & Miller, P. (2021). Transgenerational trauma and trust restoration. *AMA Journal of Ethics,* 480–486.

43. Satcher, D. & Thomas, D. J. (1990). Dimensions of minority aging: Implications for curriculum development for selected health professions. In M. S. Harper (Ed.), Minority aging: Essential curricula content for selected health and allied health profession. In M. Harper, Minority aging: Essential curricula content for selected health and allied health profession (pp. 23-32). U.S Government Printing Office: HHS.

44. Airhihenbuwa, C. O., & Harrison, I. E. (1993). *Traditional medicine in Africa: Past, present and future.* In P. Conrad, & E. Gallagher, Healing and health care in developing countries. . Philadelphia, PA: Temple University Press.

45. Funk, C. (2022). *Black Americans' views of and engagement with science.* Retrieved from Pew Research Center: https://www.pewresearch.org/science/2022/04/07/black-americans-views-of-and-engagement-with-science/

46. Spencer, M. R., Miniño, A. M., & Warner, M. (2022). *Drug Overdose Deaths in the United States, 2001–2021.* Retrieved from National Center for Health Statistics: https://www.cdc.gov/nchs/products/databriefs/db457.htm

47. Pillai, D., Ndugga, N., & Artiga, S. (2023). *Health care disparities among Asian, Native Hawaiian, and other Pacific Islander (NHOPI) People.* Retrieved from KFF.org: https://www.kff.org/racial-equity-and-health-policy/issue-brief/health-care-disparities-among-asian-native-hawaiian-and-other-pacific-islander-nhopi-people/

48. Rico, B., Hahn, J. K., & Jacobs, P. (2023). *Chuukese and Papua New Guinean populations fastest growing pacific islander groups in 2020.* Retrieved from census.gov: https://www.census.gov/library/stories/2023/09/2020-census-dhc-a-nhpi-population.html

49. Craig, A. T., Beek, K., Gilbert, K., Soakai, T. S., Liaw, S.-T., & Hall, J. J. (2022). Universal health coverage and the Pacific Islands: An overview of senior leaders' discussions, challenges, priorities and solutions, 2015–2020. *International Journal of Environmental Research and Public Health.*

50. Ghosh, C. (2003). Healthy People 2010 and Asian Americans/Pacific Islanders: Defining a baseline of information. *American Journal of Public Health,* 2093–2098.

51. AAPI Data. (2024). *AAPI Data celebrates historic update to federal standards on the collection of race & ethnicity data.* Retrieved from aapidata.com: https://aapidata.com/blog/spd-15-statement-mar2024

52. Mayo Clinic. (2022). *Integrative medicine.* Retrieved from mayoclinic.org: https://www.mayoclinic.org/tests-procedures/complementary-alternative-medicine/about/pac-20393581

53. Mount Sinai. (n.d.). *Traditional Chinese medicine.* Retrieved from MountSinai.org: https://www.mountsinai.org/health-library/treatment/traditional-chinese-medicine#:~:text=What%20is%20the%20history%20of,stayed%20in%20Asia%20for%20centuries

54. National Congress of American Indians. (2020). *Tribal Nations and the United States: An introduction.* Washington, DC: Embassy of Tribal Nations.

55. USAGov. (n.d.). *Federally recognized American Indian tribes and Alaska Native entities.* Retrieved from usa.gov: https://www.usa.gov/indian-tribes-alaska-native53–55

56. Wilbur, M. (2018). I'm dreaming about a modern world that doesn't erase its indigenous intelligence. Retrieved from project562.com: 2018

57. Bureau of Indian Affairs. (n.d.). *Frequently asked questions - what is a federal Indian reservation?* Retrieved from bia.gov: http://www.bia.gov/FAQs/

58. Nahian, A., & Jouk, N. (2023). *Cultural competence in caring for American Indians and Alaska Natives.* Retrieved from National Library of Medicine: https://www.ncbi.nlm.nih.gov/books/NBK570619/

59. Centers for Disease Control and Prevention. (2020). *Fatal injury reports, national, regional and state, 1981 - 2020.* Retrieved from WISQARS: wisqars.cdc.gov/fata-reports

60. Forrester, A. (2023*). Middle Eastern or North African in U.S. government surveys: A preview of MENA demographics.* Retrieved from cato.org: https://www.cato.org/briefing-paper/middle-eastern-or-north-african-us-government-surveys-preview-mena-demographics

61. Marks, R., Jacobs, P., & Coritz, A. (2023). Lebanese, Iranian and Egyptian Populations represented nearly half of the MENA population in 2020 Census. Retrieved from census.gov: https://www.census.gov/library/stories/2023/09/2020-census-dhc-a-mena-population.html

62. PBS. (2002). *Global connections: The Middle East.* Retrieved from PBS: https://www.pbs.org/wgbh/globalconnections/mideast/questions/types/index.html

63. Crenshaw, K. (1989). *Demarginalizing the intersection of race and sex: A Black feminist critique of antidiscrimination doctrine, feminist theory and antiracist politics.* University of Chicago Legal Forum, 139–167.

64. McGough, M., Lo, J., Amin, K., Artiga, S., Hill, L., & Cox, C. (2023). *Racial disparities in premature deaths during the COVID-19 pandemic.* Retrieved from Health Systems Tracker: https://www

.healthsystemtracker.org/brief/racial-disparities-in-premature-deaths-during-the-covid-19-pandemic

65. Duong, K. N., Le, L. M., Veettil, S. K., Saidoung, P., Wannaadisai, W., Nelson, R. E., . . . Chaiyakunapruk, N. (2023). Disparities in COVID-19 related outcomes in the United States by race and ethnicity pre-vaccination era: An umbrella review of meta-analyses. *Frontiers in Public Health*.

66. Brown, J. L. (2022). Addressing racial capitalism's impact on Black essential workers during the COVID-19 pandemic: policy recommendations. *Journal of Racial and Ethnic Health Disparities*, 1597–1604.

67. Nazareno, J., Yoshioka, E., Adia, A. C., Restar, A., Operario, D., & Choy, C. C. (2021). From imperialism to inpatient care: Work differences of Filipino and White registered nurses in the United States and implications for COVID-19 through an intersectional lens. *Gender, Work & Organization*, 1426–1446.

68. NIH. (2024). *Sex, Gender, and Sexuality*. Retrieved from nih.gov: https://www.nih.gov/nih-style-guide/sex-gender-sexuality

69. NIH. (n.d.). *LGBTI-SafeZone Terminology*. Retrieved from NIH Office of Equity, Diversity, and Inclusion: https://www.edi.nih.gov/people/sep/lgbti/safezone/terminology

70. UNHCR. (n.d.). *Refugee statistics*. Retrieved from UNRefugees.org: https://www.unrefugees.org/refugee-facts/statistics/

71. UNHCR. (2023). *Five takeaways from the 2022 UNHCR Global Trends Report*. Retrieved from UNRefugees.org: https://www.unrefugees.org/news/five-takeaways-from-the-2022-unhcr-global-trends-report/

72. Krogstad, J. M., & Gonzalez-Barrera, A. (2022, January 11). *Key facts about U.S. immigration policies and Biden's proposed changes*. Retrieved from PewResearch.org: https://www.pewresearch.org/short-reads/2022/01/11/key-facts-about-u-s-immigration-policies-and-bidens-proposed-changes/

73. National Center for Cultural Competence. (2004). *Definitions of Cultural Competence*. NCCC Curricula Enhancement Series. https://nccc.georgetown.edu/curricula/culturalcompetence.html

74. Batalova, J. (2024). *Frequently requested statistics on immigrants and immigration in the United States*. Retrieved from MigrationPolicy.org: https://www.migrationpolicy.org/article/frequently-requested-statistics-immigrants-and-immigration-united-states

75. U.S. Citizenship and Immigration Services. (2024). *Naturalization statistics*. Retrieved from uscis.gov: https://www.uscis.gov/citizenship-resource-center/naturalization-statistics

76. U.S. Census Bureau. (2023). *Census Bureau releases new educational attainment data*. Retrieved from census.gov: https://www.census.gov/newsroom/press-releases/2023/educational-attainment-data

77. National Institute for Children's Health Quality. (2019). Implicit bias resource guide: A resource to increase health equity and address implicit bias. NICHQ.

78. U.S. Department of Health and Human Services Office of Minority Health. (2013). *The national CLAS standards*. Retrieved from HHS.gov: https://thinkculturalhealth.hhs.gov/clas/standards

79. SAMHSA. (2015). Tip 59: Improving cultural competence. Retrieved from SAMHSA.gov: https://store.samhsa.gov/sites/default/files/sma14-4849.pdf

80. Office of Inclusive Excellence and Community Engagement. (2020). *Microaggressions/microaffirmations*. Retrieved from UNC School of Medicine: https://www.med.unc.edu/inclusion/justice-equity-diversity-and-inclusion-j-e-d-i-toolkit/microaggressions-microaffirmations/

81. United Nations. (n.d.). *Sustainable development goals: 17 goals to transform our world*. Retrieved from UN.org: http://www.un.org/sustainabledevelopment/sustainable-development-goals/

82. World Health Organization. (2009). *Track 1: Community empowerment*. Retrieved from who.int: https://www.who.int/teams/health-promotion/enhanced-wellbeing/seventh-global-conference/community-empowerment

83. McCold, P., & Wachtel, T. (2003). *In Pursuit of Paradigm: A theory of restorative justice*. Retrieved from ResearchGate: https://www.researchgate.net/publication/237314664_In_Pursuit_of_Paradigm_A_Theory_of_Restorative_Justice#pf2

84. Pointer, L. (2018). *Learning to work "with" (the social discipline window)*. Retrieved from Linsdsey Pointer, PhD : https://lindseypointer.com/2018/02/18/learning-to-work-with-the-social-discipline-window/comment-page-1/

85. U.S. Department of Health and Human Services. (n.d.). *Quick guide to health literacy*. Retrieved from http://health.gov/communication/literacy/quickguide/factsbasic.htm

CHAPTER 11

Community Mental Health

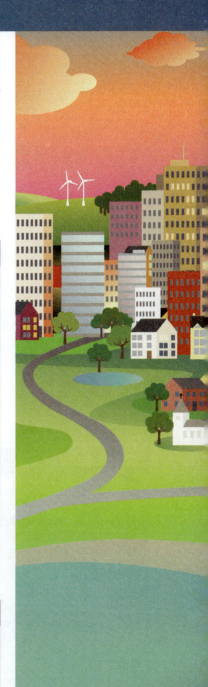

Chapter Objectives

After studying this chapter, you will be able to:

1. Define mental health and mental disorders, and explain the prevalence of mental disorders in the United States.

2. Explain what the *DSM-5-TR* is, and give examples of its limitations.

3. Give an example of how cultural differences can impact the diagnosis of mental disorder.

4. Cite specific examples of the causes of mental disorders.

5. Define stress, and explain its relationship to physical and mental health.

6. Briefly trace the history of mental health care in the United States, highlighting the major changes both before and after World War II.

7. Define the term *deinstitutionalization*, and list and discuss the forces that brought it about.

8. Describe community mental health centers as alternatives to state psychiatric hospitals.

9. Identify the major problems faced by people with mental illness who are homeless.

10. Illustrate some legal and practical issues affecting how society should deal with the problem of mental illness and violence.

11. Explain the difference between domestic violence and intimate partner violence and the mental health consequences of being a victim.

Chapter Objectives *(continued)*

12. Describe the mental health effects of the COVID-19 pandemic.

13. Describe mental health courts, assisted outpatient treatment, and the use of "legal leverage" to compel treatment.

14. Discuss the challenges facing law enforcement personnel when dealing with community residents who are struggling with acute symptoms of severe mental illness.

15. Define primary, secondary, and tertiary prevention as they relate to mental disorders, and give an example of each.

16. List and briefly describe the basic approaches to treating mental disorders and other ways to support people managing these problems.

17. Define self-help groups, give examples, and explain how they are helpful to their members.

18. Describe what "recovery" means for people with mental illness in the United States, and for those in less-developed countries, such as India or Tanzania.

19. Discuss what is meant by psychiatric rehabilitation, and list the kinds of services provided by effective programs.

20. Identify key clinical, multicultural, practical, and political challenges faced by the community mental health care system today.

21. Explain the federal government's role in supporting healthcare services to people with mental illness with respect to parity in insurance coverage, the Affordable Care Act, and integrative care.

Scenario

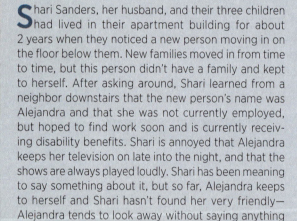

Shari Sanders, her husband, and their three children had lived in their apartment building for about 2 years when they noticed a new person moving in on the floor below them. New families moved in from time to time, but this person didn't have a family and kept to herself. After asking around, Shari learned from a neighbor downstairs that the new person's name was Alejandra and that she was not currently employed, but hoped to find work soon and is currently receiving disability benefits. Shari is annoyed that Alejandra keeps her television on late into the night, and that the shows are always played loudly. Shari has been meaning to say something about it, but so far, Alejandra keeps to herself and Shari hasn't found her very friendly—Alejandra tends to look away without saying anything when Shari passes her in the hallway. Shari also learned that Alejandra has recently returned from a tour in Afghanistan and she is recovering from a recent bout of mental illness, and that she is anxious about the demands of living as a civilian once again.

Shari noticed that every few days, a regular visitor arrived at the building in a van from the VA mental health services to spend an hour or so with Alejandra in her apartment. Shari wonders about the cost of all these services and thinks about the money she and her husband have to pay out of pocket for taxes and health care. She also worries if Alejandra has PTSD and may become a safety concern to herself or Shari's family if she is triggered. She knows that people with mental illness and veterans need to live somewhere, but why does it have to be in her building? Will Shari's children be safe?

Introduction

Mental illness is one of the major health issues facing every community. Approximately one in eight individuals worldwide lives with a mental disorder.[1] Mental disorders are associated with smoking, reduced activity, poor diet, obesity, and hypertension, and also contribute to unintentional and intentional injury. Mental disorders reduce average life expectancy, in some cases (involving substance use disorders, anorexia nervosa, schizophrenia, and bipolar disorder) by the same amount as does smoking more than 20 cigarettes a day.[2] Clearly, there is "no health without mental health."[3]

Approximately 23% of American adults (about 59 million people) have diagnosable mental disorders during a given year, and about 6% of adults in the United States have serious mental illness, that is, illness that interferes with some aspect of daily functioning. Only 50% of those diagnosed with a mental disorder received treatment in the last year.[4] Some of these people require only minimal counseling, followed by regular attendance at supportive self-help group meetings to remain in recovery, while others suffer repeated episodes of disabling mental illness. These individuals require more frequent medical and mental health treatment and more significant community support. Finally, there are the most severely disturbed individuals, who require repeated hospitalization.

Mental disorders typically begin early in life, with symptoms appearing by age 14 in half of the cases.[5] The tragic shootings at Virginia Tech and Northern Illinois University brought the issue of mental disorders in college students to national attention, and needs have increased in scope and complexity because many students now come to college with pre-existing disorders. In 2022, approximately 76% of college students reported moderate to severe levels of psychological distress. Thirty-six percent of college students utilized some form of mental health services, while more than 40% of the overall student population sought help at campus counseling centers.[6] The most common disorders reported by college students are anxiety and depression, (see **Table 11.1**).[6,7]

Because the needs of people with mental illness are many and diverse, the services required to meet these needs are likewise diverse; they not only include therapeutic services but also social services requiring significant community resources. As we explain, mental disorders and mental health care occur in a diverse social, cultural, and economic context that strongly influences how people cope with adversity, manifest emotional distress, and seek help, and have important ethical implications for proper diagnosis, treatment, and recovery.

Mental health emotional and social well-being, including one's psychological resources for dealing with day-to-day problems of life

Definitions

Mental health is the "state of successful performance of mental function, resulting in productive activities, fulfilling relationships with other people, and the ability to adapt to change and to cope with adversity."[8] Characteristics of people with good mental health include possessing a good self-image, having positive feelings about other people, and being able to meet the demands of everyday life.

Good mental health can be expressed as emotional maturity. In this regard, adults who have good mental health are able to do the following:

1. Function under adversity.
2. Change or adapt to changes around them.

TABLE 11.1 Most Common Mental Health Diagnoses in College Students, Mean age 21.3 Years

Diagnostic Characteristic	In College (%)
Any anxiety disorder	36.1
Any depressive disorder	28.4
Attention-Deficit Hyperactivity Disorder (ADHD)	14.2
Trauma and Stressor-Related disorders (including PTSD)	8.4
Eating disorders	7.3
Insomnia	7.3
Obsessive-Compulsive and related disorders (OCD)	7.0
Bipolar disorders	2.9
Autism Spectrum disorder	2.8
Alcohol or other drug-related abuse or addiction	1.5

Data from American College Health Association. American College Health Association-National College Health Assessment III: Undergraduate Student Reference Group Data Report Spring 2023. Updated April 2024. https://www.acha.org/wp-content/uploads/2024/07/NCHA-III_SPRING_2023_UNDERGRAD_REFERENCE_GROUP_DATA_REPORT.pdf

Mental illness collective term for all diagnosable mental disorders

Mental disorders health conditions characterized by alterations in thinking, mood, or behavior (or some combination thereof) associated with distress and/or impaired functioning

Major Depressive Disorder an affective disorder characterized by a dysphoric mood and/or loss of interest or pleasure in almost all usual activities or pastimes

Cultural competence service provider's degree of awareness with the specific culture of the population served, for example, proficiency in language(s) other than English, familiarity with cultural idioms of distress or body language, folk beliefs, and expectations or apprehensions regarding treatment procedures (such as medication or psychotherapy) and likely outcomes

3. Manage their tension and anxiety.

4. Find more satisfaction in giving than receiving.

5. Show consideration for others.

6. Curb hate and guilt.

7. Love others.

"**Mental illness** is a term that refers collectively to all diagnosable mental disorders. **Mental disorders** are health conditions that are characterized by alterations in thinking, mood, or behavior (or some combination thereof) associated with distress and/or impaired functioning."[8] People with mental illness have neurobiological disorders that prevent them from functioning effectively and happily in society. Many people with mental illness can be treated with medications and psychotherapy and are thus able to adapt successfully to community life.

Classification of Mental Disorders

The single most influential book in mental health is the *Diagnostic and Statistical Manual of Mental Disorders, Fifth Edition Text Revision* (*DSM-5-TR*), published by the American Psychiatric Association.[9] It identifies the various mental disorders, provides descriptive information and diagnostic instructions for each, and has significant implications for who merits a diagnosis, whether a treatment should be reimbursed by insurance, what school and social services a person is entitled to, the top priorities for mental health research, and what kinds of new therapeutic medications should be developed. This text can be considered a "living document" as it is being updated frequently, with experts in the field continuously working on making changes with the input of other colleagues and by information they gather in their own work with clients.

Disorders classified in *DSM-5-TR* are listed in **Table 11.2**.

Like preceding editions, *DSM-5-TR* places disorders in discrete categories on the basis of behavioral signs and symptoms rather than definitive tests or measurements of the brain or another body system. Given this lack of connection between diagnoses and unique biological pathologies, patients within each diagnostic category are heterogeneous in symptoms and responses to various treatments, including medications.[10]

Not surprisingly, given the multiple purposes it serves, *DSM-5-TR* has met with controversy. For example, one challenge in using a categorical system is to differentiate between cultural normative behaviors (e.g., speaking to one's ancestors) and a diagnosable disorder (e.g., Schizophrenia).[11] In addition, research shows that certain diagnoses have a tendency to occur alongside another diagnosis, the lifetime prevalence of being diagnosed with two or three disorders was found to be 27.7% overall but could be much higher, depending on the specific primary diagnosis (e.g., **Major Depressive Disorder**, Generalized Anxiety Disorder). When substance use is included as one of the co-occurring disorders, the statistic jumps to half of the people who experience a mental illness who will also be diagnosed with a substance use disorder or vice versa.

Differentiating people who are ill from those who are well based only on behavior inevitably ties diagnosis to culture rather than to precisely what is wrong with their brains, risking diagnostic error, inadequate treatment, patient disengagement, and poor clinical outcomes. Given the same symptoms, for example, Hispanics are more likely to be diagnosed with major depression than Whites or African Americans,[12] while African Americans are more likely than other groups to be diagnosed with schizophrenia.[13] Lack of **cultural competence**[14] (language proficiency, familiarity with cultural idioms of distress or body language) may lead a diagnostician to misinterpret a lack of direct eye contact, or colloquial speech that relies heavily on metaphors or describes contact with deceased relatives, as detachment from reality. The social context also affects diagnosis. Worldwide, for example, women are diagnosed with mood disorders more often than are men, but this difference is smaller in countries that have less traditional gender-role differences in employment opportunities, educational attainment, and

TABLE 11.2 Major Diagnostic Categories of Mental Disorders

Category	Examples
Neurodevelopmental disorders	Autism Spectrum disorder, Attention-Deficit/ Hyperactivity disorder, Tic disorders, Intellectual Development disorders
Schizophrenia Spectrum and Other Psychotic disorders	Schizophrenia, Delusional disorder, Brief Psychotic disorder, Schizophreniform disorder, Schizoaffective disorder
Bipolar and Related disorders	Bipolar I disorder, Bipolar II disorder, Cyclothymic disorder
Depressive disorders	Major Depressive disorder, Premenstrual Dysphoric disorder, Persistent Depressive disorder
Anxiety disorders	Specific Phobia, Panic disorder, Agoraphobia, Separation Anxiety disorder, Selective Mutism, Social Anxiety disorder, Generalized Anxiety disorder
Obsessive-Compulsive and Related disorders	Obsessive-Compulsive disorder, Body Dysmorphic disorder, Hoarding disorder, Trichotillomnia, Excoriation
Trauma- and Stressor-Related disorders	Posttraumatic Stress disorder, Acute Stress disorder, Reactive Attachment disorder, Disinhibited Social Engagement disorder, Adjustment disorders, Prolonged Grief disorder
Dissociative disorders	Dissociative I dentity disorder, Dissociative Amnesia, Depersonalization/Derealization disorder
Somatic Symptom and Related disorders	Somatic Symptom disorder, Illness Anxiety disorder, Functional Neurological Symptom disorder (Conversion disorder), Factitious disorder
Feeding and Eating disorders	Anorexia Nervosa, Bulimia Nervosa, Binge-Eating disorder, Pica, Rumination disorder, Avoidant/Restrictive Food Intake disorder,
Elimination disorders	Enuresis, Encopresis
Sleep-Wake disorders	Insomnia disorder, Hypersomnolence disorder, Narcolepsy
Sexual Dysfunctions	Erectile disorder, Female Sexual Interest/Arousal disorder, Female Orgasmic disorder, Genito-Pelvic Pain/Penetration disorder, Male Hypoactive Sexual Desire disorder
Gender Dysphoria	Gender Dysphoria
Disruptive, Impulse-Control, and Conduct disorders	Oppositional Defiant disorder, Intermittent Explosive disorder, Conduct disorder, Pyromania, Kleptomania
Substance-Related and Addictive disorders	Alcohol Use disorder, Cannabis Use disorder, Phencyclidine Use disorder, Hallucinogen Persisting Perception disorder, Inhalant Use disorder, Opioid Use disorder, Stimulant Use disorder, Tobacco Use disorder, Gambling disorder
Neurocognitive disorders	Delirium, Neurocognitive disorders; Frontotemporal, Vascular, Due to Alzheimer's Disease, Due to Traumatic Brain Injury, Due to HIV Infection, Due to Prion Disease, Due to Huntington's Disease, Due to Parkinson's Disease
Personality disorders	Personality disorders; Antisocial, Paranoid, Borderline, Histrionic Narcissistic, Avoidant, Obsessive-Compulsive,
Paraphilic disorders	Voyeuristic disorder, Exhibitionistic disorder, Frotteuristic disorder, Sexual Masochism disorder, Sexual Sadism disorder, Pedophilic disorder, Fetishistic disorder, Transvestic disorder

control of fertility.[15] A final concern is that diagnosis with a mental disorder can stigmatize a person by imposing negative stereotypes, prejudice, and discrimination that lead to mental distress, shame, avoidance of treatment, and fewer opportunities related to work and independent living. As a result, stigma may be the most debilitating aspect of a mental illness.[16] Despite these various problems, a reliable system for diagnosing mental disorders is essential for assessment, treatment, and research, and to guide the funding of all of these activities. *DSM-5-TR* remains the preferred tool for this purpose in the United States.

Causes of Mental Disorders

Symptoms of mental illness can arise from many causes, and the comorbidity that exists among disorders suggests they are not discrete conditions, each with a unique cause. Instead, a variety of mental disorders can result from genetic influences on complex brain functions that control a person's thoughts and emotions[17]; intrauterine infections[18]; preterm birth[19]; postnatal exposure to physical, chemical, and biological agents, including secondhand cigarette smoke[20]; head injury[21]; and diseases, such as syphilis, cancer, or stroke.

The brain is very sensitive to stress and other environmental influences as it develops during childhood and adolescence. In any given year, up to one in five children experiences a mental disorder,[22] yet less than half of children and adolescents who need mental health services receive them.[23] In adolescence, physical and hormonal changes intensify emotional reactivity, sensitivity to peer influence, impulsivity, and novelty-seeking, which undermines the self-control and regulation needed for effective participation in society.[24]

Mental disorders not only reflect biological vulnerability but also stress, social support, coping, and motivation to recover, making social experience a direct determinant of who gets a mental illness and how the illness unfolds. Some children face considerable adversity, including poverty, abuse, loss, neglect, trauma, and parental psychiatric disorder.[25] Every year, about 10% of children are physically or sexually abused. Early and cumulative adversity and maltreatment are believed to harm the development of the brain and affect later depression, post-traumatic stress disorder (PTSD), suicide attempts, drug and alcohol misuse, and criminal behavior.[26] Bullying in childhood (as a victim, perpetrator, or both) is associated with anxiety and mood disorders in adolescence and young adulthood,[27] as is excessive use of social media.[28] Social determinants of mental health, sometimes referred to as the "causes of the causes" of mental disorder, include inequality, discrimination and social exclusion, poor education, unemployment, poverty, housing instability, and poor access to care and to other resources.[29]

Clearly, stress is a significant cause of mental illness (see **Box 11.1**). For example, people who survive disasters and soldiers returning from combat face increased risk. Twenty percent of Manhattan residents living near the World Trade Center at the time of the attacks of September 11, 2001, had symptoms consistent with PTSD five to eight weeks after the attack, and nearly 10% suffered from depression, which occurred most often in those who had suffered losses as a result of the attack.[30] Ten years after Hurricane Katrina, many survivors continued to experience mental health problems related to the storm.[31] Military service increases one's risk of experiencing PTSD, depression, or other mental health problems[32] (see **Figure 11.1**). Disease pandemics, such as COVID-19, can provoke anxiety, depression, substance-use problems, and suicidal ideation, especially in younger adults, racial/ethnic minorities, essential workers like nurses, and unpaid adult caregivers. These mental health problems result from both morbidity and mortality caused by the disease and also the impact of physical distancing and stay-at-home orders.[33]

Immigrants and children of immigrants represent 24% of the U.S. population, and human migration may increase in response to climate change and other global events. Immigrants face significant stress, including separation from family, cultural and linguistic barriers, and new, sometimes unwelcoming environments; however, they access mental health services at lower rates than nonimmigrants.[40] Finally, among middle-aged White Americans (especially those with a high school education or less), suicides and substance use led to an unexpected rise in death rates between 1999 and 2014.[41] Suicide rates are rising in the United States, especially in younger adults, even as they decline in many other countries because of new restrictions on access to lethal means and improved mental health care.[42]

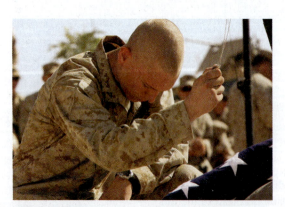

FIGURE 11.1 Military troops returning from duty in combat zones are heavy users of mental health services when these services are accessible.

Courtesy of Cpl. Brian Reimers/U.S. Marines.

BOX 11.1   Stress: A Contemporary Mental Health Problem

A stressful situation, whether caused by something in our environment like an upcoming work deadline, or a psychological cause like persistent worry about layoffs at work. Both of these can trigger stress hormones that produce physiologic changes, such as the heart pounding, breath quickening, muscles tensing, and sweat appearing. Stress is defined as one's psychological and physiologic response to stressors—Even Americans who believe they have good mental health carry out their everyday activities under considerable stress. Stressors can be subtle—such as having to wait in line, getting stuck in traffic, or having to keep an appointment[34]—or they can be major life events, such as getting married or divorced or losing a loved one. Although some exposure to stressors can be good, researchers have found that chronic stress can have long-term effects on a person's physical and mental health. Research suggests that chronic stress contributes to high blood pressure, promotes the formation of artery-clogging deposits, and causes brain changes that may contribute to anxiety, depression, and addiction. Preliminary research suggests that chronic stress may also contribute to obesity, both directly (causing people to eat more) and indirectly (decreasing sleep and exercise).[35] Relevant stressful events individuals may experience in their lifetime may include adverse childhood experiences (such as physical, emotional, and sexual abuse; neglect; parental separation or divorce; mental illness; substance use disorder; incarceration of a household member; or domestic violence), poor and unequal education, food insecurity, poor housing quality and housing instability, unemployment and underemployment, limited access to health care, poverty, and discrimination.[36]

The Fight or Flight Response is the body's natural physiologic response to a stressful, frightening, or dangerous situation. This response is activated by the perception of a threat, which then activates the sympathetic nervous system and releases hormones, preparing the body to either face a threat or run from it. The term was coined by Walter Cannon, an American physiologist who discovered that a subconscious and automatic series of fast-acting reactions occurred in the body to help manage threatening circumstances. Cannon also called this response the acute stress response. In recent years, physiologists and psychologists have refined Cannon's work and developed a better understanding of how people react to threats, and updating the fight or flight response to fight, flight, freeze, and fawn. The goal of jumping into fight, flight, freeze, or fawn is to decrease, end, or evade the danger and to return to a state of calm and control.

Fight Response: When you feel you are in danger but believe you can overpower the threat, your brain will send signals throughout your body to prepare for a physical fight.[37]

Signs to indicate you are in a fight response:

- Tight jaw or grinding of teeth
- Urge to punch something or someone
- Feeling intense anger or killing someone, even yourself
- Desire to stomp or kick
- Crying

- Glaring at people, conserving angrily
- Upset stomach, feels like knots or burning
- Attacking the source of the danger

Flight Response: When you believe the only way to overcome the danger is by running away, which, depending on the situation, could be the best decision.

Signs to indicate you are in a flight response:

- Exercising excessively
- Feeling fidgety or tense or trapped
- Constantly moving legs, feet, and arms
- Restless body that will not stop moving
- Sensation of numbness in extremities
- Dilated eyes, darting eyes

Freeze Response: When you don't feel like fighting or running away, you may freeze. Freeze is an inability to move or act against a threat.

Signs to indicate you are in a freeze response:

- Pale skin
- Sense of dread
- Feeling stiff, heavy, cold, numb
- Loud, pounding heart
- Decreasing heart rate
- Sensing tolerated stress

Fawn Response: May be used after the fight, flight, or freeze responses were unsuccessful. It is immediately trying to please to avoid conflict. Very common response in people who grew up in abusive families or situations, where the only chance of survival may be agreeableness and helpfulness.

Sign to indicate you are in a fawn response:

- Regardless of how poorly a person treats you, you are more concerned with making them happy than taking care of yourself.

Understanding the fight, flight, freeze, and fawn responses can help individuals identify their triggers and gain self-awareness, which can be used to slow down, assess the situation, recognize if it is a real threat, and gain control. [37]

Relationships and other social resources can mediate the effects of stress. People lacking support (in the form of marriage, church membership, social organization membership, and contacts with friends and relatives) face a greater risk than others of experiencing mental illness, alcohol and substance use, suicide, illness, and mortality, independent of their overall health, socioeconomic status, smoking, drinking, obesity, and utilization of health care.[38] Effective time management, goal setting, and prioritizing tasks help reduce stress, as does being realistic about one's abilities and expectations. Experts recommend a combination of physical, social, environmental, and psychological approaches to managing stress.[39] Physical approaches to stress reduction include good nutrition and adequate sleep and aerobic exercise. Healthy social interaction and optimizing environmental factors, such as noise, lighting, and living space can also reduce one's stress (see the American Institute of Stress website at www.stress.org).

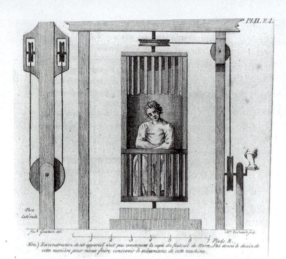

FIGURE 11.2 Treatment for mental illness in the eighteenth and nineteenth centuries was often inhumane and unsuccessful.

© National Library of Medicine

History of Mental Health Care in the United States

The response to mental illness in America has a history older than the country itself, and it is marked by enthusiastic reform movements followed by periods of widespread ambivalence toward people with mental disorders. Cyclical periods of reform often began when existing approaches to caring for those with mental illness became intolerable for society and ended when their economic burden became unbearable.

Mental Health Care Before World War II

In Colonial America, when communities were sparsely populated, "distracted" persons or "lunatics," as they were called, were generally cared for by their families or private caretakers, and only as a last resort became the responsibility of the local community. Institutionalization did not begin until the eighteenth century when people with mental disorders were placed in undifferentiated poorhouses or almshouses alongside people with intellectual disabilities, physical disabilities, and the otherwise deviant.[43]

By the early nineteenth century, the situation in the poorhouses and almshouses worsened and the first efforts were made to separate people by their type of disability. In 1751, Thomas Bond opened Pennsylvania Hospital, the first institution in America specifically designed to care for those with mental illness.[44] Conditions in the hospital were harsh (see **Figure 11.2**), and treatments, which consisted of "bloodletting, blistering, emetics, and warm and cold baths," were unpleasant.[45]

The Moral Treatment Era

Philippe Pinel of France developed a more humane approach that he called *traitement moral*, or in English, **moral treatment**, based on the assumption that environmental changes could affect an individual's mind and thus alter behavior.[43] In the United States, William Tuke put moral treatment into practice beginning in 1792.

People with mental illness were removed from the everyday life stressors of their home environments and given "asylum" in a quiet country environment, where they received a regimen of rest, light food, exercise, fresh air, and amusements. Moral treatment was initially deemed successful and soon spread,[46] but with rising immigration and urbanization, these asylums became overcrowded and indigent patients again ended up in poor houses. At this point, noted reformer Dorothea Lynde Dix (1802–1897; see **Figure 11.3**) began a tireless campaign to establish public hospitals to provide decent care to indigents with mental illness. When her lobbying for a federal law failed, Dix lobbied on a state-by-state basis. Her efforts were in most cases successful; all in all, Dix was personally involved in the founding of 32 public mental hospitals funded by individual states.[47]

The State Hospitals

The state mental hospitals were supposed to supply an environment in which therapeutic care was based on close personal relationships between patients and well-trained staff members, as prescribed in the methods of moral treatment (see **Figure 11.4**). Unfortunately, the chronic nature of mental illness made long-term or even lifetime hospital stays increasingly the norm.[47] "Maximum capacities" were quickly reached, exceeded, and repeatedly revised upward. Personalized care became impractical, and physical restraints provided the most efficient way to manage patients on large wards.[44] States repeatedly cut funding for these institutions until all that remained was custodial care by an overworked staff that turned over frequently.

By 1940, the population in state mental institutions had grown to nearly one-half million, and staff caseloads became so large that only subsistence care was possible.

Moral treatment a nineteenth century treatment in which people with mental illness were removed from the everyday life stressors of their home environments and given "asylum" in a rural setting, including rest, exercise, fresh air, and amusements

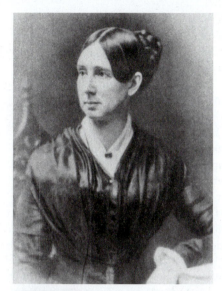

FIGURE 11.3 Dorothea Dix helped to establish public mental hospitals in many states.

© National Library of Medicine

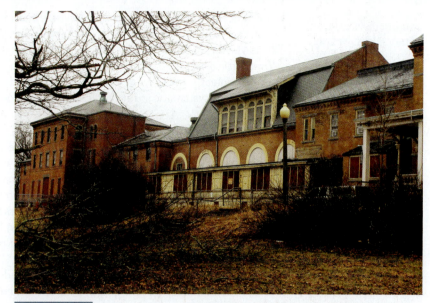

FIGURE 11.4 The state mental hospital was at one time viewed as the appropriate public response to the needs of those with mental illness.

© Aswphotos134/Shutterstock

In response to this situation, dramatic new approaches to treatment were developed, including **electroconvulsive therapy (ECT)** and **lobotomy**. ECT (**Figure 11.5**) uses electric current to produce convulsions in patients with severe depression who have not responded to medication or who are at imminent risk of suicide or other acute clinical condition.[48]

The lobotomy, in which nerve fibers of the brain are severed by surgical incision, was popularized by Portuguese neuropsychiatrist Antônio Egas Moniz, and by U.S. neurologist Walter Freeman. Freeman streamlined the procedure with his invention of the so-called ice-pick lobotomy, enabling him and other physicians to perform tens of thousands of lobotomies between 1939 and 1967.[49] However, later research found that following this irreversible operation only one-third of patients showed stable improvement, while another one-third became worse off. The development of new antipsychotic and antidepressant drugs in the 1950s made the widespread use of lobotomies unnecessary.[49]

> **Electroconvulsive therapy (ECT)** method of treatment for mental disorders involving the administration of electric current to the scalp to induce convulsions and unconsciousness
>
> **Lobotomy** surgical severance of nerve fibers of the brain by incision
>
> **National Institute of Mental Health (NIMH)** the nation's leading mental health research agency, housed in the National Institutes of Health

Mental Health Care After World War II

In the postwar 1940s, a number of factors brought about greater federal involvement in mental health care. New feelings of optimism in the country, together with testimony before the U.S. Congress by both military and civilian experts, soon resulted in the passage of the National Mental Health Act of 1946, which established the **National Institute of Mental Health (NIMH)**. Modeled after the National Cancer Institute, NIMH came under the umbrella of the National Institutes of Health. The purposes of NIMH were (1) to foster and aid research related to the cause, diagnosis, and treatment of neuropsychiatric disorders; (2) to provide training and award fellowships and grants for work in mental health; and (3) to aid the states in the prevention, diagnosis, and treatment of neuropsychiatric disorders.[47]

The Effects of War

In the wake of both World Wars I and II, mounting evidence became unavoidable that soldiers were arriving home in a very different mental state than when they deployed.[50] Initially called "shell shock,"[51] the

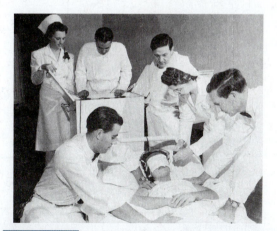

FIGURE 11.5 A team of doctors and nurses prepares to demonstrate the procedures involved in electroconvulsive therapy (shock treatment), 1942.

© AP/Shutterstock

Deinstitutionalization
the process of discharging, on a large scale, patients from state mental hospitals to less-restrictive community settings

constant exposure to violent death, alongside bearing witness to the death of other men in their unit, caused soldiers to show signs of what we now call Post-Traumatic Stress Disorder (PTSD).[9] In 1941, Abram Kardiner published his first clinical study on the effects of combat titled, *The Traumatic Neuroses of War*, which was revised in 1947 to include discussions of factors that would protect soldiers from psychological breakdown and how to speed up their recovery.[52] Large-scale, systematic study of PTSD would not begin until after the Vietnam War.[50]

Deinstitutionalization

During the early 1950s, public distress about the conditions in state mental hospitals continued to grow until the necessity of finding a new approach to caring for those with mental illness was clear and inescapable.[45] The term **deinstitutionalization** has been used to describe the discharging of tens of thousands of patients from state-owned mental hospitals and the resettling and maintaining of these discharged persons in less-restrictive community settings. To show the magnitude of deinstitutionalization, in 1955, 322 state psychiatric hospitals served 558,922 resident patients. By 1990, the number of patients had dropped to less than 120,000 (**Figure 11.6**), and by 2004 to under 30,000.[53,54]

Deinstitutionalization was not a preplanned policy. Rather, it was propelled by four forces that had been building up for more than half a century: (1) economics, (2) idealism, (3) legal considerations, and (4) the development and marketing of antipsychotic drugs.[45] Economically, the states needed to reduce expenditures for mental hospitals so more money was available for other major state budgetary items, such as education, health care, and criminal justice. Meanwhile, Medicare and Medicaid legislation provided federal funds to reimburse the costs of outpatient and inpatient services for eligible people with mental illness who were not residing in a state institution. (For more information about Medicare and Medicaid, see Chapter 14.)

By the early 1960s, questions arose about the legality of institutionalizing people against their will who had not been convicted of any crime, but simply because they had mental illness. The American Bar Association pointed out that people with mental disorders, even when institutionalized, had certain rights, including the right to treatment.[53] Over the ensuing decade, courts began to show more concern for the rights of individuals with mental illness—who were viewed as needing the courts' protection from inappropriate involuntary commitment—and less concern for society's right to be protected from these individuals.[45] Eventually, the test for

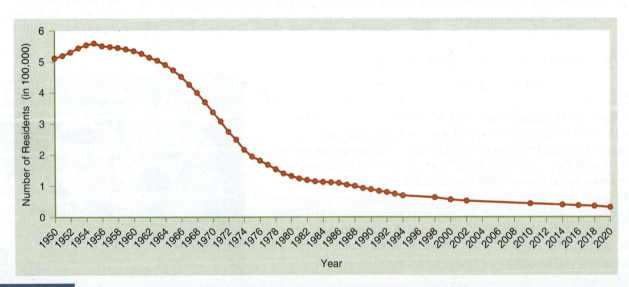

FIGURE 11.6   Number of resident patients in state and county mental hospitals, 1950–2020.

Data from Frank, R. G., & Glied, S. A. (2006). Better but not well. Johns Hopkins University Press; 55; National Association of State Mental Health Program Directors. (2022). Trends in Psychiatric Inpatient Capacity, United States and Each State, 1970 to 2018. Available at https://www.nasmhpd.org/sites/default/files/2023-01/Trends-in-Psychiatric-Inpatient-Capacity_United-States%20_1970-2018_NASMHPD-2.pdf

involuntary civil commitment became one of whether these individuals could be considered dangerous to themselves or others.

Although economics, idealism, and legal considerations all helped to launch deinstitutionalization, new medications expedited it. One of the first was **chlorpromazine (Thorazine)**, introduced in 1954 and characterized as a **neuroleptic drug** because it appeared to reduce nervous activity. Used first in hospitals, chlorpromazine and the other phenothiazines introduced later produced a remarkably calming effect in psychotic patients, and in many cases, became the only form of treatment provided. In these situations, a **chemical straitjacket** was said to have been substituted for a physical one, and unfortunately, some of the drugs' acute and chronic side effects were overlooked. Acute side effects (such as blurred vision, weight gain, and constipation) can cause compliance failures, resulting in relapses or in attempts to self-medicate with other drugs, including drugs of abuse. Long-term use of chlorpromazine can impair the central nervous system and produce **tardive dyskinesia**, the irreversible, involuntary, and abnormal movements of the tongue, mouth, arms, and legs.[55] Despite these deleterious effects, phenothiazines are still used extensively to treat patients with severe disorders.

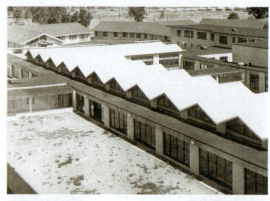

FIGURE 11.7   Between 1966 and 1989, 750 community mental health centers were established.

© Denver Post/Getty images

Community Mental Health Centers

In 1963, mental illness and its treatment gained national attention when President John F. Kennedy addressed Congress on the subject of mental health care.[43] The resulting **Community Mental Health Act** promised funding to establish one fully staffed, full-time **community mental health center (CMHC)** in each of 1,499 designated catchment areas covering the entire United States (**Figure 11.7**). These centers were to provide five core services: (1) inpatient care, (2) outpatient services, (3) 24-hour emergency care, (4) day treatment or other partial hospitalization services, and (5) consultation and education. Hundreds of CMHCs were established in the 1960s and 70s, but for a number of years after that they fell short of the lofty expectations outlined in Kennedy's speech. One problem was that many older patients with chronic mental illness never returned to the community and instead simply underwent **transinstitutionalization** to nursing homes. CMHCs also struggled to serve deinstitutionalized persons living in the community, because no effective services had been developed to supplement the use of medications with this population.[56]

The federal government responded to the problems of deinstitutionalization and transinstitutionalization in 1977 by creating the Community Support Program, which was the first recognition that the problems of people with chronic mental illness are, first and foremost, social welfare problems. This program offered grants to communities to help people with chronic mental illness find the resources necessary for successful independent living, namely, income, housing, food, medical care, transportation, vocational training, and opportunities for recreation.[57] Despite the many problems resulting from deinstitutionalization, surveys indicate that most people with chronic mental illness prefer life in the community over life in an institution. Most communities now have appropriate services in place, and inpatient care is more effective and requires less time because community support is available following discharge.

Mental Health Care Concerns in the United States Today

For the most part, the experience of people with serious mental illness has improved in the 60 years since passage of the Community Mental Health Act. Today, nearly all of them live in the community, receive at least some treatment, have disability income, and enjoy civil liberties; some of them also lead productive lives.[54] However, specific challenges remain, including: (1) how to help people who are homeless with serious mental illness and/or co-occurring substance use disorders, (2) what to do about the perception that mental illness is linked to extreme

Chlorpromazine (Thorazine) the first and most famous antipsychotic drug, introduced in 1954

Neuroleptic drug a drug that reduces nervous activity; another term for antipsychotic drugs

Chemical straitjacket a drug that subdues a psychiatric patient's behavior

Tardive dyskinesia irreversible condition of involuntary and abnormal movements of the tongue, mouth, arms, and legs, which can result from long-term use of certain antipsychotic drugs

The Community Mental Health Act a law that made the federal government responsible for assisting in the funding of mental health facilities and services

Community mental health center (CMHC) a fully staffed center originally funded by the federal government that provides comprehensive mental health services to local populations

Transinstitutionalization transferring patients from one type of public institution to another, usually as a result of policy change rather than improved treatment effectiveness

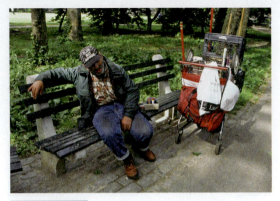

FIGURE 11.8 As many as two-thirds of all people with serious mental illness have experienced homelessness or been at risk for homelessness at some point in their lives.

© Photos.com.

violence, (3) resolving the problem of people with mental illness becoming involved with the criminal justice system and too often ending up in jail or prison, (4) domestic and intimate partner violence, (5) suicide, and (6) the mental health effects of the COVID-19 pandemic.

Serious Mental Illness in People Who Are Homeless

On any given night, approximately 582,500 people experience homelessness in the United States,[58] 25% of whom experience mental illness.[59] (see **Figure 11.8**). People who are homeless are exposed to more environmental stressors and threats than people with homes, and about one-half of all adults who are homeless have substance use disorders, major depression, and other co-occurring mental illness.[60] These individuals tend to remain homeless and (except for emergency rooms and the police) disengaged from services, and their rates of criminal behavior and victimization are higher than among housed adults with severe mental illness.[61]

Veterans are an often-ignored subset of the homeless population in the United States. Homeless veterans make up approximately 7% (33,129) of adults experiencing homelessness on any given night.[62] The majority of homeless veterans are men. Many of these veterans are living with the effects of Post-Traumatic Stress Disorder (PTSD), substance use disorders, and other diagnosable mental illnesses.[63]

Although the problems of people who are homeless with mental illness are complex, their most pressing needs are for safe, affordable housing that they choose and actually want to live in, and services they need.[64] If available at all, services to people who are homeless are often fragmented, although integration of medical, mental health, substance use, and housing services is possible.[65]

Mental Illness and Violence

Recent mass shootings at schools, theaters, places of worship, and other everyday settings by young men alleged to have mental illness have drawn extensive media coverage and reinforced an already widely held connection in the minds of Americans between serious mental illness and violence.[66] It is misleading, however, to draw conclusions from individual cases in isolation. Mass shootings are a small percentage of all gun violence; the majority of people with serious mental illnesses are never violent,[67] and histories of prior violence, substance use, and early trauma are more likely to contribute to subsequent violence than mental illness per se.[68]

Furthermore, the actions that should be taken to prevent violence by people with mental illness are not clear, in light of the individual rights granted to all Americans by the U.S. Constitution and the nature of serious mental illness. Legally, authorities can act to prevent potential violence only when someone voluntarily seeks assistance or has made frank threats. Relaxing these criteria so that more people believed to have a propensity for violence are detained could discourage individuals with mental illness from seeking help or being candid with their families and the authorities. Detaining larger numbers of people is also unlikely to prevent violence, because mental health experts do little better than chance in predicting who will be violent.

In addition, people with the most severe mental illnesses, especially if they are angry and alienated, do not often seek treatment voluntarily, and those who do may not be fully engaged or cooperative. Many of those who perpetrated mass shootings had received psychotherapy and other forms of treatment beforehand, but a lack of motivation to change and the fact that some psychiatric disorders are not particularly responsive to therapy make successful treatment difficult and expensive.

People with serious mental illness are frequently marginalized individuals who, for the most part, are unemployed, economically impoverished, live in disadvantaged neighborhoods, misuse alcohol and illicit drugs, and are regularly victimized and traumatized. Most violent behavior is due to factors stemming from marginalization rather than mental illness, although psychiatric disorders, such as depression are strongly implicated in suicide, which accounts for over half of firearm-related fatalities in the United States.[69]

Some public health authorities advocate restricting advertising and sales and increasing taxation on guns and ammunition, as well as mandatory licensing, locking devices, and safety inspections, citing the reduction of health problems related to poisoning, motor vehicle crashes, and tobacco use following the adoption of similar measures.[70] The difficulty facing society is that, like mental illness itself, gun violence results from many causes, invokes deeply held values (public safety versus civil liberties), and, in today's sociocultural context, leaves policymakers with no easy options.

The New Asylums: Mental Health Care in Jails and Prisons

Cognitive and emotional deficits imposed by mental illness, coupled with intense stressors like homelessness and victimization, increase the risk that people with serious mental illness will commit criminal acts.[71] Before 1820 in the United States, it was common to find people with mental illness in jails or prisons. Efforts by Dorothea Dix and others eventually convinced most state legislatures that people with mental illness belonged in hospitals rather than prisons, and by 1880, only 0.7% of U.S. prisoners had serious mental illness. Since that time, and largely out of public view, we have reversed this policy completely and in effect have recriminalized mental illness. Today, a person with mental illness is 10 times more likely to be in jail than in a psychiatric hospital, and the three largest psychiatric inpatient facilities in the United States are its three largest jails, the Los Angeles County Jail, Chicago's Cook County Jail, and Rikers Island in New York City[72] (**Figure 11.9**). The fact that people with mental disorders are jailed more often than hospitalized reveals more about how our society operates than about any criminal tendencies intrinsic to mental illness. In contrast to other health-related emergencies, law enforcement personnel are usually the first responders in a mental health crisis, and the decision about whether a person in custody belongs in jail or in the hospital is made by the gatekeepers of the legal system: police officers, prosecutors, and judges.[56,73]

Up to 20% of police calls nationally involve individuals with mental illness or substance use issues,[74] and police officers write one-third of emergency mental health referrals.[75] Control and arrest techniques that are used routinely in other types of calls may inadvertently escalate a mental health crisis, leading to injuries to officers and subjects and the unnecessary arrest of persons whose only clear "crime," in some cases, is displaying symptoms of mental illness. Officers can learn alternative methods of policing, but managing serious mental illness in the community is beyond the scope of a police intervention alone and must become a community issue. Mental health services need to be better integrated with law enforcement to increase the availability of services and reduce the burden on the police of being the primary, and often sole, responders. One option, known as the **Crisis Intervention Team**, involves special training for police and direct collaboration with mental health authorities to remove barriers that interfere with immediate access to mental health services (for example, lack of beds and insurance processing delays).[76]

Once incarcerated, inmates with mental illness must be closely monitored and may require medical treatment, yet the fundamental purpose of correctional facilities is to confine and punish, not treat. Harsh and socially isolating conditions in jail or prison can exacerbate mental illness, and courts have interpreted the U.S. Constitution as ensuring a right to treatment to protect prisoners who have

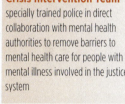

Crisis Intervention Team specially trained police in direct collaboration with mental health authorities to remove barriers to mental health care for people with mental illness involved in the justice system

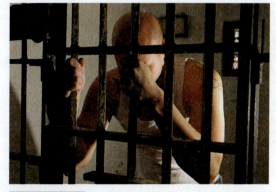

FIGURE 11.9 Many prison inmates with mental illness remain in prison years beyond their original sentence because they are unable to conform to good conduct requirements of the prison system.

© Tim Harman/Shutterstock

Legal leverage when service providers control disability income or other benefits received by a person with mental illness to enforce participation in treatment in return for suspending a criminal sentence imposed by a court of law

Mental health courts where judges have special training and use nonadversarial procedures that mandate treatment and rehabilitation rather than incarceration if a person with mental illness is found guilty of a crime

medical and psychiatric needs against cruel and unusual punishment. However, U.S. prisons are seriously overcrowded, and effective treatment requires adequate space, a sufficient number of qualified treatment personnel, and timely access to services.[77] Some of the worst conditions are in juvenile justice centers, where adolescents from diverse cultural backgrounds and with a variety of disorders, criminal convictions, and family problems receive little or no treatment, and sometimes only multiple forms of medication.[78] Furthermore, even when treatment is available, severe mental illness (paranoid schizophrenia, bipolar disorder, or other serious mental disorders)[79] may hinder inmates' cooperation with their prescribed medication schedules, and without medication, these inmates may be incapable of "good behavior," a prerequisite for parole or release.

Individuals with criminal involvement and serious mental illness who do not receive treatment are more likely to commit another offense than are justice-involved people without mental disorders. Although they constitute a small proportion of the people with mental illness, these individuals often resist participating in treatment and may pose a danger to themselves or the public, resulting in frequent psychiatric hospitalizations. In response, many communities have resorted to the use of mandatory commitment to outpatient treatment, "legal leverage" to compel cooperation, and special mental health courts.

Using **legal leverage** to force a patient to accept treatment may involve service providers taking control of the patient's disability income and/or suspending the patient's eligibility for subsidized housing.[78] While controversial, legal leverage attempts to balance the values of civil rights and normalization with those of patient welfare and public safety.

Mental health courts use judges who have special training and nonadversarial procedures that mandate treatment and rehabilitation rather than incarceration for defendants found guilty when mental illness was a significant contributing factor in their arrest. In such cases, the court will suspend the guilty person's sentence and work with local mental health professionals to develop treatment plans that the patient agrees to follow. If participants do not adhere to the agreement, the court can revoke the suspended sentence or charge the patient with violating the terms of probation. Hundreds of these courts now operate across the country, and evidence indicates that their use can help to lower recidivism, improve mental health outcomes,[79] and reduce the risk of violence by justice-involved persons with mental disorders.[80]

We should note that legal leverage and mental health courts do not just commit patients to participate in treatment; they also involuntarily commit the community mental health system to provide it. Both policies are more successful when paired with effective services, including case management and supports for work and housing, and when mental health and criminal justice staff work together on what they recognize is a shared community problem. Such comprehensive programs are expensive, taking resources from other mental health priorities. They are also coercive, straining the patient's relationships with providers and family members.[56] These efforts are easiest to justify when the goals include not just fewer arrests or days in jail but meaningful steps toward genuine recovery from mental illness or addiction.

Issues at home: Domestic Violence (DV) and Intimate Partner Violence (IPV)

Both domestic violence (DV) and intimate partner violence (IPV) are significant issues affecting individuals across the United States daily. While the terms are often used interchangeably, DV includes physical or psychological harm, sexual assault, stalking, or the threat of harm between two parties in a household.[81] In contrast, IPV is the intentional intimidation through physical, sexual, verbal, financial, or mental abuse as part of a systemic power differential perpetrated by one intimate partner over another. IPV can result in mental and physical trauma and in some cases, death.[82] Approximately 47% of women and 44% of men indicate they've been the victim of physical or sexual violence or stalking by an intimate partner in their lifetime.[83] Of those individuals, one in three women and one in seven men had symptoms of PTSD. Other common mental health effects for victims of intimate partner violence are increased depression, anxiety, risk of self-harming behaviors (including substance use), and suicide.[84] Contrary to popular belief, the most dangerous time for victims of intimate partner violence is when the victim makes the final decision to leave.[85]

The Suicide Epidemic

According to the Centers for Disease Control and Prevention (CDC), suicide is one of the leading causes of death in the United States. In 2021, 48,183 people died by suicide in the United States and men were almost four times as likely to die by suicide as women.[86] A variety of factors contribute to suicide risk, including: a history of depression or other mental illness, previous suicide attempts, job loss or financial problems, substance use or abuse, current or prior history of interpersonal victimization or adverse childhood experiences (ACEs). There are additional community issues that are also risk factors for suicide, such as exposure to violence in the community, lack of access to health care, historical trauma, and discrimination.[87]

On the other hand, there are protective factors that can reduce the likelihood that an individual will die by suicide. Protective factors include: being a caretaker (of a family member or pet); having effective coping and problem-solving skills; feeling connected to institutions in the community (for example, school); support and a feeling of connection to peers, family, or friends; and having a value system that objects to suicide.[87] Within the community, there are many strategies for suicide prevention that would benefit society as a whole. For example, increasing access to quality mental health care through insurance and increased providers in underserved areas, providing immediate access to help via telehealth. Additionally, starting in elementary school by teaching social-emotional learning and problem-solving skills.

Mental Health and the COVID-19 Pandemic

The onset of the COVID-19 pandemic in March of 2020 brought with it not only insurmountable physical health concerns, but mental health concerns as well. There are two lenses through which to view the mental health effects of the pandemic for the purposes of this text: (1) the effects on the general population, and (2) the effects on healthcare professionals. Initially, fear and the uncertainty of the pandemic itself, supply shortages, and "stay-at-home" orders lasting for an indeterminate amount of time wreaked havoc on people around the world. While it became increasingly important for healthcare professionals to monitor the mental health of their patients, the professionals themselves suffered greatly. Many doctors and nurses lacked testing materials and shortages of personal protective equipment (PPE), and they were subjected to increasingly unrealistic workloads.[88] The World Health Organization (WHO) estimates that in the first year of the COVID-19 pandemic, anxiety and depression increased by 25% worldwide.[89]

Meeting the Needs of People with Mental Illness

The legal and moral obligation to provide cost-effective prevention, treatment, and rehabilitation services to people with mental illness is an important challenge facing every community today.[36]

Prevention

The concepts of primary, secondary, and tertiary prevention (see Chapter 4) are also applicable to mental disorders. Primary prevention in community mental health is important due to its heavy socioeconomic burden, low number of effective treatments, and potential for intergenerational transmission. The COVID-19 pandemic led to an increase in reported mental illnesses, which incentivized public health officials to explore primary prevention of this class of diseases. Although the issue of mental illness and its impact was already increasing in the

Psychopharmacology
treatment for mental illness that
involves medications

United States before the pandemic, the COVID-19 pandemic is expected to accelerate the social and economic cost, which will require innovative approaches by public health officials and policy makers to alter the projected trajectory of mental illness in the coming decade.[90] Secondary prevention, although not reducing the incidence of mental illness, can reduce its prevalence by shortening the duration of episodes through prompt intervention. Examples of secondary prevention include employee assistance programs, juvenile delinquency diversion programs, and crisis intervention. These programs can be provided by licensed professionals in private clinics, clinical mental health counseling centers, hospital emergency rooms, and other social-service agencies. Tertiary prevention, treatment, and rehabilitation ameliorate the symptoms of illness and prevent further problems for the individual and the community. Intensive community treatment programs, discussed later in connection with psychiatric rehabilitation, are examples of tertiary prevention.[91] Healthcare professionals should be aware that the (primary, secondary, tertiary) framework does not inherently address health inequities (e.g., unjust health disparities based on race inequities, socioeconomic status, or geographic location), which not only can occur with treatment but also access to primary and secondary prevention.[92]

Treatment Approaches

Treatment goals for mental disorders are to (1) reduce symptoms, (2) improve personal and social functioning, (3) develop and strengthen coping skills, and (4) promote behaviors that make a person's life better. The basic approaches to treating mental disorders include psychopharmacology, psychotherapy, peer support, technology, self-help groups, and psychiatric rehabilitation.

Psychopharmacology

Psychopharmacology involves treatment with medications. This approach regards mental disorders as medical illnesses just like hypothyroidism or diabetes, and as such, are treatable with drugs. The development of the currently licensed psychotropic drugs began in the 1950s and has seen huge advances in the last 70 years. In the late 19th century and into the early 20th century, drugs, such as paraldehyde, chloral hydrate, and bromides were being used as treatments for anxiety disorders. The discovery of barbiturates in the early 20th century is often considered the start of psychopharmacology. The origins of all major classes of drugs used to treat psychiatric disorders stem from clinical observations made when investigating treatments for other unrelated illnesses or conditions. In 1937, Dr. Charles Bradley discovered the beneficial effects of benzedrine (racemic amphetamine) in what is now known as attention deficit hyperactivity disorder (ADHD). Dr. Bradley had been administering the drug to children who suffered from severe headaches and during his observations of the children, noted that the drug improved their behavior and school performance. This eventually led to the use of stimulant drugs to treat ADHD.[93] Common psychological disorders that include psychotropic drugs in their treatment plans include, but are not limited to: depressive disorders, anxiety disorders, psychotic and related disorders, bipolar-related disorders, neurodevelopmental disorders, substance use disorders, and neurocognitive disorders. However, it is important to keep in mind that not everyone who has these disorders responds to medication.[94] At this time, there are no drugs licensed for the treatment of personality disorders, but it still remains a common practice.[95] This reflects both the shortcomings of the diagnostic process and our limited understanding of the biological basis of mental disorders. Furthermore, because some of these drugs have serious side effects, and because of the nature of mental illness itself, almost half of patients may not cooperate fully in taking their medications.

Another form of biomedical therapy is ECT, which was discussed earlier in this chapter. In ECT, alternating electric current passes through the brain while the patient is under general anesthesia to produce a convulsive seizure. ECT is used for severe depression, selected cases of schizophrenia, or overwhelming suicide ideation, especially when the need for treatment is seen as urgent. Contemporary ECT methods use low doses of electric shock to the brain and general anesthetics to reduce the unpleasant side effects.[48]

Psychotherapy

Psychotherapy is a collaborative treatment approach based on the relationship between an individual and a therapist (i.e., a trained mental health professional, such as a psychologist, social worker, or counselor). It provides a supportive environment where an individual can speak openly with someone who is objective, neutral, and nonjudgmental[96] (see **Figure 11.10**). There are numerous approaches to psychotherapy, including interpersonal, couple, group, and family formats. Psychodynamic psychotherapy examines current problems as they relate to earlier experiences, even from childhood, while cognitive psychotherapy focuses on current thinking patterns that are faulty or distorted. **Cognitive-behavioral therapy** focuses on how maladaptive feelings and behaviors are the result of distorted thinking, and uses exercises, role playing, and other structured procedures to promote new thought patterns and regular homework between sessions to practice more effective coping responses. In general, psychotherapy is most likely to be successful in less-severe cases of emotional distress or when used in conjunction with other approaches (such as psychopharmacology).[97]

Support Groups & Peer Support

Most U.S. communities face a severe shortage of mental health providers.[98] Group therapy can provide a solution to this problem by allowing for the treatment of multiple people at the same time. Using this method can help healthcare providers to reduce wait times and increase accessibility. Group therapy is often necessary to meet the needs of rural and low-income areas where clinics are understaffed and have a high volume of patients. There are various types of support groups: psychoeducational groups, which are led by a trained mental health professional and provide participants with education about their diagnosis and work on instilling positive behavior change; interpersonal process groups (therapy groups), which are led by a therapist and focused on helping participants process their presenting issues and work toward change;[99] support groups, which are led by a trained professional and are often less directive—they always have a clearly stated purpose but meet clients where they are; peer support groups, which are led by a trained individual who shares a lived experience with the group members;[100] and self-help groups, which are informal groups of people who come together to address their common problems and are sometimes connected to an organization like Alcoholics Anonymous (AA).[101] Whether delivered online or in person, "natural" support from other people who themselves are coping with mental illness has become a valuable resource in community-based care. Such support reduces people's social isolation and loneliness, can effectively engage people who are struggling and convince them to enroll in services, and provides genuine empathy regarding the challenges of serious mental illness and useful advice for coping with these challenges.[89]

Telemental Health

Telemental health (also referred to as telehealth or online psychotherapy) is the use of telecommunications or videoconferencing technology to provide mental health services.[102] Even though the technology for telehealth has been available since the 1990s, the mental healthcare industry did not embrace it until the COVID-19 pandemic.[103] The pandemic forced most mental health providers to see clients remotely. In 2021, the COVID-19 Advisory Committee of the American Psychoanalytic Association conducted a survey to understand the differences in their members' practices before and after the pandemic. Before the pandemic, 35% of mental health practitioners had no use for technology in their practice, and another

Psychotherapy a treatment that involves verbal communication between the patient and a trained clinician

Cognitive-behavioral therapy treatment based on learning new thought patterns and adaptive skills, with regular practice between therapy sessions

Peer support support from other people who themselves are coping with mental illness; it reduces people's social isolation, improves their access to services, and provides useful advice for managing the disorder

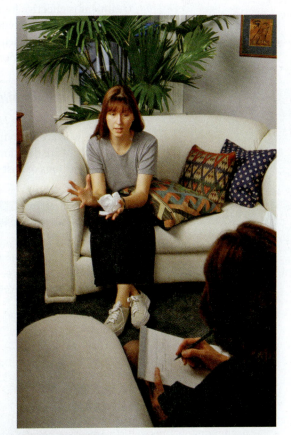

FIGURE 11.10 Psychotherapy is usually only one of the services needed by persons who are suffering from mental illness.

© David Buffington/Photodisc/Getty Images

55% used technology for less than 20% of their sessions. Only 10% were using technology regularly in their professional practice. After the pandemic, 55% of the mental health professionals surveyed reported only doing online therapy, and another 25% reported doing between 60% and 99% of their practice online. All respondents reported doing some form of online therapy and slightly under 40% were doing some form of hybrid practice.[104] This transition to offering more mental health services online has many benefits (e.g., less travel required, a broader reach, more flexibility in scheduling). However, telehealth also has drawbacks that must be considered. Most mental health professionals practice with a state license and the state licensing boards have often made practicing across state lines very difficult.[104] During the pandemic, some of these restrictions were lifted to accommodate the overwhelming need for mental health services, but after the pandemic, most of those exceptions were retracted, leaving many practitioners who were new to telehealth unsure of best practices. More research is needed on the topic of telemental health, which could help create consistent standards of practice similar to the ones that have been created for in-person therapy.[104] In terms of effectiveness, teletherapy was researched even before the pandemic and compared with in-person therapy and both were found to be equally effective.[105] Technology has been uniquely helpful under conditions of enforced social separation and isolation, such as during disasters or infectious disease pandemics like COVID-19.

Finally, for certain individuals, who may have severe cognitive or language impairments or social anxiety, communicating with a therapist using a visual display of words on a screen can be more effective than face-to-face conversation.[106] Computer therapy and in-person therapy are about the same in overall effectiveness and, with greater convenience and more flexible use of client and therapist time, drop-out from computer treatments may occur less often than in face-to-face therapy.[107] The many advantages of digital methods notwithstanding, no form of treatment is effective for everyone, and the same will likely be true of these new options, even as they continue to proliferate rapidly.

Examples of self-help groups are the **National Alliance on Mental Illness (NAMI)**, Recovery, Inc., and Alcoholics Anonymous (AA). For more information on NAMI, see **Box 11.2**.

Psychiatric Rehabilitation

One of the objectives of *Healthy People 2030* is to increase the proportion of adults with mental disorders who are receiving treatment (see **Box 11.3**). With financial considerations influencing most health care decisions today, the treatment of mental disorders is driven more and more by considerations of cost-effectiveness.

BOX 11.2   National Alliance on Mental Illness

Serious mental illness has devastating effects not just on individuals who experience it but also their family members.[108] NAMI is an important resource for reducing the loneliness, isolation, and stigma felt by caregivers and family members of people with mental disorders.[56] NAMI is "the nation's largest grassroots mental health organization dedicated to improving the lives of persons living with serious mental illness and their families. Founded in 1979, NAMI has become the nation's voice on mental illness, a national organization, including NAMI organizations in every state and in over 1,100 local communities across the country who join together to meet the NAMI mission through advocacy, research, support, and education."

According to its mission statement, "NAMI is dedicated to the eradication of mental illnesses and to the improvement of the quality of life of all whose lives are affected by these diseases." NAMI members, leaders, and friends share the agency's mission of "support, education, advocacy, and research for people living with mental illness through various activities" that include maintaining a website and a toll-free help line, sponsoring a Mental Illness Awareness Week, and maintaining a public education speakers bureau.

NAMI also provides a cadre of educational programs and a network of support groups. NAMI "advocates on the federal level to ensure nondiscriminatory and equitable federal and private-sector policies are in place as well as a commitment to research for the treatment and cures for mental illness."[109] As with other voluntary health organizations, NAMI is involved in fundraising, and does so with events, such as NAMI Walks and an annual black-tie event, the Unmasking Mental Illness Science and Research Gala, held in Washington, D.C.

More information about NAMI is available on their website: www.NAMI.org.

BOX 11.3   *Healthy People 2030:* Mental Health and Mental Disorder Objectives

Health Care: Increase the proportion of adults with mental disorders who receive treatment.

Targets and Baselines:

Objective	Demographic	2018 Baseline	2030 Target
MHMD-04	Adults aged 18 years and older with serious mental illness	64.1%	68.8%
MHMD-05	Adults aged 18 years and older with major depressive episode	64.8%	69.5%

Target-setting method: Percentage point improvement.

Data source: National Survey on Drug Use and Health (NSDUH), Substance Abuse and Mental Health Services Administration (SAMHSA).

For Further Thought

Just over 60% of adults with serious mental illness received treatment in 2018. What factors do you think contributed to this statistic? One-third of adults with major depressive episodes do not receive treatment. How would reaching the *Healthy People 2030* target (a small increase in the proportion of adults with major depression who receive treatment) affect the overall adult suicide rate?

Data from U.S. Department of Health and Human Services, Office of Disease Prevention and Health Promotion. (2020). *Healthy People 2030*. Available at https://health.gov/healthypeople/objectives-and-data/browse-objectives/mental-health-and-mental-disorders

Mental disorders are widely prevalent and can begin in adolescence, or even earlier. They entail not only neurobiologic lesions that produce distortions in thinking and feeling but also deficits in coping skills that damage relationships, and stigma that interferes with social acceptance. Mental disorders can last a lifetime, and most who have them simply live with their symptoms (e.g., people with schizophrenia learn to tolerate voices in their head) just as people with chronic arthritis or diabetes live with their disabilities. Thus, today the primary objective is most often **recovery** rather than cure. Recovery relies on self-directed coping using cognitive and behavioral strategies to prevent symptoms from occurring or to lessen their impact, as well as reduced dependence on the formal mental health system.[110] When formal medical intervention is needed for psychiatric rehabilitation and recovery there are a few different treatment options available to individuals who may be struggling with issues like substance use, suicidal ideation, mental health disorders, or any combination of the three.

Assisted outpatient treatment (AOT) refers to court-ordered treatment for individuals who do not have pending criminal charges but have resisted engaging in treatment despite past histories of hospitalization and often arrest. The justification for involuntary treatment is that these individuals do not understand their illness and need protection from imminent harm through suicide or self-neglect, while the public needs protection from acts of violence these individuals might perpetrate. Use of AOT has been associated with reductions in rehospitalization, criminal recidivism, violence, and victimization, and with increases in quality of life.[111]

Intensive Outpatient Programs (IOP) are direct services for individuals with substance use issues or co-occurring mental and substance use disorders who do not require medical detoxification or 24-hour surveillance. They are used as alternatives to inpatient and residential treatment and are designed to establish psychosocial support as well as provide coping strategies to avoid relapse.[112]

Partial Hospitalization Program (PHP) is an outpatient program specifically designed for the diagnosis or active treatment of a serious mental disorder when there is reasonable expectation for improvement or it is necessary to maintain a patient's functional level and prevent relapse or full hospitalization (definition approved by Congress).[113] Partial hospitalization can help some individuals avoid full hospitalization or can be a transition from inpatient to outpatient care.

Because people who lack satisfying friendships and activities, good health, and hope for the future have little incentive to manage their illnesses, recovery from mental illness needs to be social and economic as well as psychiatric. It means progress toward financial and residential

Recovery outcome sought by most people with mental illness; includes increased independence, effective coping, supportive relationships, community participation, and sometimes gainful employment

Assisted outpatient treatment (AOT) laws mandating involuntary psychiatric treatment for individuals who do not understand their illness, to protect the individual from harm and safeguard the public

Neurodiversity the idea that unique differences in brain function and behavior are not necessarily pathological and can represent strengths, and are perceived negatively primarily because of social factors like ignorance or stigma

Psychiatric rehabilitation intensive, individualized services encompassing treatment, rehabilitation, and support delivered by a team of providers over an indefinite period to individuals with severe mental disorders to help them maintain stable lives in the community

Evidence-based way of delivering services to people using scientific evidence that shows that the services actually work

Assertive community treatment (ACT) service that uses active outreach by a team of providers over an indefinite period of time to deliver intensive, individualized services

Individual placement and support (IPS) an evidence-based model of employment services emphasizing real work opportunities, integrated mental health services, and individualized job supports

independence, satisfaction with life, and basic "personhood"—that is, mental and physical well-being, supportive relationships, opportunities to spend time productively (e.g., pursuing education, employment, volunteer work, or hobbies), and self-determination in exercising the adult rights and privileges that come with community life.[114]

People in recovery thus know how to live satisfying and fulfilling lives regardless of their symptoms or diagnoses. Broader still is the idea of **neurodiversity**, the view that extensive individual variability in brain functioning, and in personality differences like sociability or attention, reflects natural human heterogeneity more than pathology or defect. Because everyone's brain is unique, being different from others in any number of ways is normal. Anomalies or peculiar sensitivities can even be assets, and any disabling aspects of these differences are mostly attributable to societal factors, such as stigma, poverty, or lack of understanding.

Recovery from mental illness requires change, such as community participation in the form of work, volunteer activities, the forming of new relationships, and sometimes parenthood. Change is difficult and brings added stress, making daily pursuit of recovery a challenge to persons with mental illness and the providers who work with them. The current recovery-oriented services are collectively known as **psychiatric rehabilitation**.[115] Psychiatric rehabilitation is modeled on rehabilitation practices for people with physical and developmental disabilities (e.g., independent living, gainful employment) and its services often carry the modifier "supported" (as in supported employment, supported housing, supported education) in keeping with patient self-determination. Services include medication, therapy, and adaptive skills (e.g., helping a patient learn to use an online dating service) as needed, but also changing the environment through accommodations at work or school (e.g., extended time to complete tests and other assignments, use of aids, such as audio recorders, and frequent breaks). In addition, practices are **evidence-based**, which means there is consistent evidence showing that they improve patient outcomes. The providers of psychiatric rehabilitation services typically represent diverse professional backgrounds (psychiatry, nursing, addictions, social work, and vocational services) and work collaboratively as an integrated team. Sometimes these team members are themselves recovering from mental illness, which brings a different perspective to the team's efforts.[116]

One of the best-known psychiatric rehabilitation services is **assertive community treatment (ACT)**, which uses active outreach by a team of providers over an indefinite period of time to deliver intensive, individualized services (e.g., help finding a place to live, learning self-care skills needed for independence, using public transportation).[57] While ACT has been shown to reduce hospital use, it is expensive and not always available.[117] Critics have also questioned its reliance on "legal leverage" and other coercive techniques that undermine privacy and autonomy of people in recovery.[118]

Another challenge of community life for people with serious mental illness is lack of employment, and over one-third have annual incomes below $10,000.[119] Supported employment services help those wanting to work secure paid employment, and with it, a higher quality of life and greater community integration. For example, **individual placement and support (IPS)** is an evidence-based model that emphasizes real work opportunities matched to the individual's interests and values, integrated mental health and employment services, and individualized job supports. Even with such helpful resources, however, gainful employment for people with serious mental illness is usually part time and makes only a small difference in how much they earn and in their overall quality of life.[120] These modest recovery outcomes for adults with chronic histories of mental disorder have intensified the search for interventions to help younger people grappling with the earliest stages of mental illness. Besides medications and traditional treatment, these newer efforts offer help with jobs and school, as well as family counseling.[121]

Regardless of the effectiveness of formal services, recovery remains the overarching goal so that families and treatment providers do not underestimate what a person with mental illness can achieve in the world. Interestingly, recovery from disorders like schizophrenia tends to be better (with longer remissions and fewer relapses) in the developing world, including Africa, India, and Indonesia, than in developed countries, such as the United States.[122] Rather than being socially isolated, homeless, or in jail, for example, people in India who have schizophrenia are usually married and living with their families.[123] Nonwestern cultures use less-stigmatizing explanations for mental illness and prescribe a recovery process that includes collaborative roles for everyone—patient, family, and community. In Tanzania, for example, supernatural spirits are believed to cause mental illness, which is seen as a stern test by God that a faithful person should accept with patience and grace. A person with mental illness is not a source of embarrassment needing coercion but a family member or neighbor whose odd behavior is dealt with gently and, if possible, without confrontation.[124] The lesson in recovery provided by these "less-developed" parts of the world is that mental disorders like schizophrenia are not just "broken brains," but also culturally determined social and moral phenomena that involve all of us.

Mental health care in the United States faces a number of serious challenges. Multiple services are needed by people with severe or comorbid disorders, and lack of some services (such as for addictions) limits the effectiveness of others (e.g., ACT). Staff turnover is relatively high in behavioral health care,[125] and successful psychosocial rehabilitation requires sustained commitment by staff to the principles of evidence-based practice and patient recovery.[126] People with serious mental illness still face high rates of poverty, social disadvantage, and stigma, and substantial recovery (e.g., stable, gainful employment) is achieved by relatively few of them.[54] Related to all these problems are the immediate and longer-term needs of family members of people with mental illness for information, financial help, coping with stigma, and sometimes therapeutic support for themselves.[127]

The mental health care system is decentralized and fragmented, with many different kinds of providers.[54] General medical practitioners treat the largest number of people with mental disorders, with specialty mental health providers, human services, self-help groups, and various combinations serving the rest.[128] In 2006, there were about 350,000 licensed providers of mental health services (including psychiatrists, psychologists, social workers, psychiatric nurses, licensed counselors, and marital/family therapists) in the United States, but relatively few of them served rural and low-income counties[98] (**Figure 11.11**). Patient sex, ethnicity, geography,

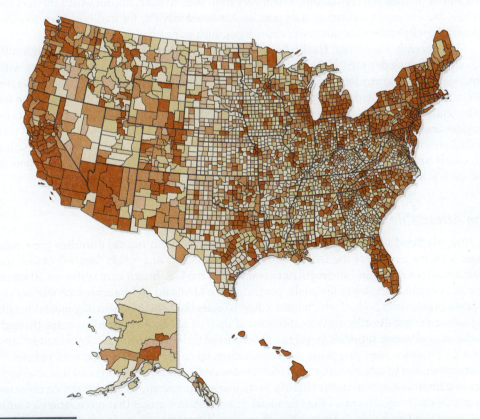

FIGURE 11.11   Number of mental health professionals, by county, for counties with mental health professionals (the darker the shading, the higher the number of mental health professionals per 10,000 population).

Data from Ellis, A., Konrad, T., Thomas, K., & Morrissey, J. (2009). County-level estimates of mental health professional supply in the United States. Psychiatric Services, 60, 1315–1322. Reprinted with permission from *Psychiatric Services* (Copyright 2009). American Psychiatric Association.

immigration status, sexual orientation, and income are all related to the likelihood of receiving help. For example, racial-ethnic minorities are less engaged in therapy than Whites with respect to whether formal treatment is sought, the number of visits, retention in treatment, follow-up with aftercare, and adherence to medication.[129] The problem may not be overt discrimination but rather a lack of cultural competence on the part of providers regarding their multicultural patients' attitudes toward medications and medication side effects (such as weight gain), and patients' misguided expectations of treatment in the context of particular religious, and spiritual or folk beliefs.

Finally, in addition to their often pronounced deficits in thinking and coping, people with serious mental disorders tend to be among the poorest members of society and typically live in neighborhoods where crime, illicit drugs, victimization, homelessness, unemployment, and social disorganization are rampant.[130] It may be too much to expect that medications, psychotherapy, psychosocial rehabilitation, self-help, and other circumscribed supports and services are enough to overcome these systemic problems. From this vantage point, it is not the people with mental disorders who fail, but rather the communities and social systems in which they live that have failed.

Government Policies and Mental Health Care

Until deinstitutionalization began in the 1950s, the state hospital system served as the de facto social insurance program for mental illness in the United States.[54] Following deinstitutionalization, the federal government's role in mental health funding and policy became substantial. For example, the federal Medicaid program now pays more than half of publicly funded mental health care, and its policies and regulations, which vary from state to state, impact which services are covered. Depending on individual state policies, Medicaid may pay for traditional services like inpatient hospitalization but not newer approaches, such as psychiatric rehabilitation.

More recently, the Mental Health Parity and Addiction Act of 2008 requires that if health care coverage includes mental health or substance use disorders there must be parity with physical disorders in any limitations or restrictions (i.e., any limits on the number of visits per year, annual or lifetime dollars spent, and deductibles or copayments must be the same for both mental and physical disorders). In combination with aggressive management of costs by provider organizations, **parity** has succeeded in removing previous insurance limitations that applied only to behavioral health care without unintended consequences, such as eliminating behavioral health coverage.[131] In so doing, it has reduced consumers' out-of-pocket expenses and made it less likely they will be bankrupted by psychiatric treatment costs.[58,56]

The Affordable Care Act

In 2010, Medicaid's important role in covering individuals with mental disorders grew even larger with the passage of the federal **Patient Protection and Affordable Care Act (ACA)**, the most ambitious expansion and regulatory overhaul of the U.S. health care system in 50 years. The ACA expands eligibility for public programs like Medicaid and increases the availability of private insurance, both of which must cover 10 essential benefits, including mental health and substance use disorder services. Millions of individuals have obtained coverage through Medicaid expansions, subsidies for private plans offered through state insurance exchanges, and the ACA provision requiring plans to cover children up to age 26 on their parents' policies.[132] Outcome studies to date have reported increased access to health care, reduced financial burden, and improvements in mental health, particularly depression.[133] More insurance coverage for people under age 26 years offers financial protection to a group that often struggles with low income and high debt. It also enables them to seek treatment in early adulthood, a critical point in the onset of mental illness.[56]

For adults with serious mental illness, comorbidity between mental and medical disorders and premature mortality are the rule rather than the exception, yet historically, healing of

Parity the concept of equality in health care coverage for people with mental illness and those with other medical illnesses or injuries

Patient Protection and Affordable Care Act (ACA) federal legislation that expands eligibility for Medicaid and increases access to private insurance for low-income Americans not covered by employer-provided health insurance

mind and body was divided, with separate treatment and reimbursement systems leading to both high costs and excess mortality. Parity and the ACA forged an opportunity to integrate mental health and general medical care by making it advantageous to deliver primary care and behavioral health services in the same conveniently located community settings. In this way, recovery from mental illness becomes an integral part of physical well-being and overall wellness.

Integrative care is care a patient receives from a team of primary care and behavioral health clinicians, working together with patients and families, using shared, cost-effective care plans that incorporate patient goals.[134] Integrative care reduces racial-ethnic disparities in mental health services[135] and also increases opportunities for prevention through primary care practices, such as screening for depression, substance use, and domestic violence.[136]

Because individuals with mental disorders tend to have low incomes and are unlikely to be insured, they stand to be heavy consumers of care under the ACA, which could exacerbate the shortcomings of mental health services and the scarcity of professionals. In addition, the U.S. The Supreme Court has allowed states to opt out of expanding Medicaid, giving state Medicaid policy makers considerable discretion in what coverages to provide and putting in doubt the status of costly services, such as ACT and supported employment. Continuing evidence of unmet need, especially for people caught up in the criminal justice system, made it clear that although health insurance coverage is necessary it is not sufficient for stable recovery from mental illness.[137]

As a result, in 2016, the **21st Century Cures Act** launched new funding for a number of priorities covered in this chapter, from suicide screening and intervention to expanded support for Crisis Intervention Teams, assisted outpatient treatment, and mental health courts to divert people with mental illness from the criminal justice system. The 21st Century Cures Act also prioritizes assertive community treatment; promotes strategies to improve the recruitment, training, and retention of professional care providers; and funds new models of integrated care for primary care and behavioral healthcare services.

All of these recent changes make it difficult to determine how the nation, states, and local communities will respond to the needs of those with mental illness in the future. The response will depend on economics, the degree to which taxpayers have been personally touched by mental illness, and the degree to which they are willing to tolerate the spectacle of people who are homeless with mental illness in their communities and in their jails and prisons. A key task facing communities is to find ways to unite formal services and informal supports to promote social inclusion and recovery by people who are coping with mental disorders.

> **Integrative care** care a patient receives from a team of primary health care and behavioral health clinicians, working together with patients and families, using shared, cost-effective care plans that incorporate patient goals
>
> **21st Century Cures Act** legislation that funds comprehensive programs for addressing challenges to recovery, including the criminalization of mental illness, gaps in community-based services, and inadequate numbers of service providers

Chapter Summary

- Mental illness constitutes a major community health concern because of its prevalence and chronicity, its effects on individual and community well-being, and the social, cultural, and economic attention and resources it demands from all of us.

- Americans are afflicted with a variety of mental disorders, caused by genetic factors, environmental factors, or a combination. These disorders, which can range from mild to severe, are often chronic and may limit the ability of some of those afflicted to live independently. The *Diagnostic and Statistical Manual of Mental Disorders, Fifth Edition Text Revision (DSM-5-TR)*, the most significant revision of the diagnostic system in over 20 years, was published in 2022.

- Stress, resulting from social and environmental forces, can have a detrimental influence on both physical and mental health. Combat-zone military veterans and survivors of and responders to natural and human-made disasters and pandemics are at especially high risk for developing mental disorders.

- Over the years, society's response to the needs of those with mental illness has been characterized by long periods of apathy interrupted by enthusiastic movements for new and enlightened approaches to care.

- Deinstitutionalization, in which hundreds of thousands of psychiatric patients housed in state and county hospitals were discharged and returned to their communities, was the most prominent movement of the twentieth century. The origins of many of the current problems in community mental health care, such as a large number of people who are homeless with mental illness, can be traced to this movement.

- Mass shootings have sometimes been linked to mental illness in media accounts and public perceptions, although most people with mental disorders are never violent and other factors (such as substance use and early trauma) also affect the likelihood of violence.

- Having serious mental illness can increase the risk that a person will become involved with the criminal justice system, raising a number of concerns about the use of incarceration and other traditional law enforcement practices in such cases.

- The COVID-19 pandemic, which began in 2020, has had serious and long-term ramifications for the mental health of people across the globe. Specifically, increases in both depression and anxiety, and feelings of isolation and loneliness.

- The basic concepts of prevention in community health (primary, secondary, and tertiary prevention) can be applied to reducing the incidence and prevalence of mental disorders.

- Among the most common approaches to treating mental disorders are psychopharmacology, which is based on the use of medications; and psychotherapy, including cognitive-behavioral therapy. Peer support and the use of technology assume an increasingly significant role in today's mental health services, and self-help groups provide additional help to people at risk for relapse.

- People with severe mental illness generally pursue recovery rather than cure. Recovery entails adaptive change, including increased independence, effective coping, supportive relationships, community participation, and sometimes gainful employment.

- Psychiatric rehabilitation programs for those with serious mental illness, such as assertive community treatment and supported employment, represent the current "best practices" in support of recovery and community integration.

- The federal government now dominates overall mental health policy in the United States, with its distribution of Medicaid funds and the enactment of the Affordable Care Act and the 21st Century Cures Act.

- Important issues face those concerned about people with mental disorders. The most daunting challenge is finding ways to provide a variety of easily accessible prevention and treatment services to people from culturally diverse backgrounds, who have multiple problems and few resources, in a climate where both the effectiveness of services and the cost of care are paramount concerns.

Scenario: Analysis and Response

1. Let us assume that Shari Sanders is not alone in her concerns about Alejandra, her new neighbor. Another neighbor, Paul, has called for a meeting of the residents to discuss this "new" resident. You are also a resident, and he is expecting you to attend. What is your response?

2. What worries might residents express regarding their new neighbor?

3. Would it make any difference to you whether Alejandra found a job and was away at work during a good part of the day?

4. Do you suppose the landlord knew about Alejandra's medical, and military history when they rented the unit to her? Can landlords refuse to rent to someone like Alejandra?

5. Are you aware of any federal laws, such as the Fair Housing Act or the Americans with Disabilities Act (ADA), which could bear on this matter?

6. If you were Shari, what would be your response? What would you do?

7. Do you feel the preconceived notions held about veterans helps or harms community perceptions of Alejandra's situation?

Review Questions

1. How prevalent is the problem of mental disorders in the United States?

2. How are mental disorders related to chronological age, and to other chronic illnesses and overall life expectancy?

3. What is meant by the term *mental health*?

4. What are the characteristics of a mentally healthy person?

5. What is a mental disorder?

6. What is the *Diagnostic and Statistical Manual of Mental Disorders, Fifth Edition, Text Revision* (*DSM-5-TR*)? How do issues of comorbidity and cultural competence affect the use of the *DSM-5-TR*?

7. Give examples of the many different causes of mental disorders.

8. What is stress? Give some examples of stressors.

9. What is the relationship between stress and mental health? For example, how is mental health affected by acute stresses like traumatic events? How is it affected by chronic stresses, such as being an immigrant or a member of a racial minority group?

10. How were people with mental illness cared for in Colonial America?

11. What was included in Tuke's therapy known as "moral treatment"?

12. What role did Dorothea Dix play in the care of indigent people with mental illness?

13. How would you characterize the treatment of those with mental illness in state hospitals prior to World War II?

14. What piece of legislation resulted in the establishment of the National Institute of Mental Health, and what were the purposes of the Institute?

15. Define the word *deinstitutionalization*. When did it start in the United States? What caused it?

16. Why was there a movement to establish community mental health centers in the 1960s?

17. What services were originally provided by community mental health centers?

18. Why was the community support program considered a novel approach to helping people with mental disorders?

19. Approximately what percentage of people who are homeless are living with mental illness?

20. What legal and practical concerns limit society's options for dealing with the potential for serious violence among people who have mental illness?

21. Why are people with serious mental illness more likely to be in jail or prison today than in a psychiatric hospital?

22. How are assisted outpatient treatment, legal leverage, and mental health courts used to manage the risks that a person's mental illness will lead to self-harm and/or an adverse relationship with the criminal justice system?

23. Describe primary, secondary, and tertiary prevention of mental illness, and give an example of a service for each level of prevention.

24. What is involved in psychotherapy for mental illness? In cognitive-behavioral therapy? In psychopharmacological therapy?

25. How is technology being used to improve the accessibility and flexibility of treatment services?

26. What are support groups? How do they supplement people's individual efforts to cope with long-term disorders?

27. What is meant by "recovery" from serious mental illness? How do psychiatric rehabilitation services like assertive community treatment and supported employment promote recovery?

28. What kinds of clinical, multicultural, practical, and political challenges do mental health care efforts face early in the twenty-first century?

29. What role does federal government policy play in supporting care for people with mental illness in the United States?

Activities

1. Make a list of all of the stressors you have experienced in the last 2 weeks. Select two of the items on the list and answer the following questions about them:
   - Did you realize the stressor was a stressor when you first confronted it? Explain.
   - What physiologic responses did you notice in yourself when confronted with the stressor?
   - Have you confronted the stressor before? Explain your answer.
   - What stress mediators (coping responses) do you have to deal with each of the stressors?

2. Using the Internet, identify the organizations in the community that you believe would provide mental health services. Then create a list of the agencies/organizations. Divide the list into three sections based on the type of service (primary, secondary, tertiary prevention) offered. If you are not sure what type of services are offered, call the agency/organization to find out. After you have completed your list, write a paragraph or two about what you feel to be the status of mental health care in your community.

3. Make an appointment with someone in the counseling and psychological service center on your campus for an

orientation to the services offered by the center. Most mental health services range from stress management to test anxiety to individual counseling. Find out what your school has to offer and write a one-page summary of available services.

4. Call agencies or service groups in your community to find out what services are needed for people who are homeless. Also find out how serious the homeless situation is in the community and what plans there are to deal with the problem. Summarize your findings in a two-page paper. Agencies or services to call include the American Red Cross, the local police department, the Salvation Army, the local soup kitchen, a community mental health center, local hospitals, local homeless shelters, and other shelters.

5. Look online or call the community information/crisis center to locate a mental health or substance use self-help group. Call the group's number and find out what kinds of open meetings or public education activities they have.

References

1. World Health Organization. (2022). *Mental Disorders.* Retrieved from https://www.who.int/news-room/fact-sheets/detail/mental-disorders

2. Chesney, E., Goodwin, E., & Fazel, S. (2014). Risks of all-cause and suicide mortality in mental disorders: A meta-review. *World Psychiatry, 13*(2), 153–160.

3. Prince, M., Patel, V., Saxena, S., Maj, M., Maselko, J., & Phillips, M. (2007). Global mental health 1: No health without mental health. *Lancet, 370*(9590), 859–877.

4. Substance Abuse and Mental Health Services Administration. (2023). *National report on drug use and health.* Retrieved from https://www.samhsa.gov/data/release/2022-national-survey-drug-use-and-health-nsduh-releases

5. Meyer, H. C., & Lee, F. S. (2019). Translating developmental neuroscience to understand risk for psychiatric disorders. *American Journal of Psychiatry, 176*(3), 179–185.

6. American College Health Association. (2023). *Undergraduate student reference group executive summary.* Retrieved from https://www.acha.org/documents/ncha/NCHA-III_SPRING_2023_UNDERGRAD_REFERENCE_GROUP_EXECUTIVE_SUMMARY.pdf

7. Lipson, S. K., Lattie, E. G., & Eisenberg, D. (2019). Increased rates of mental health service utilization by U.S. college students: 10-year population-level trends (2007–2017). *Psychiatric Services, 70*(1), 60–63.

8. U.S. Department of Health and Human Services. (1999). *Mental health: A report of the surgeon general.* Substance Abuse and Mental Health Services Administration.

9. American Psychiatric Association. (2022). *Diagnostic and statistical manual of mental disorders* (5th ed., text revision.). American Psychiatric Association.

10. Harrington, A. (2019). *Mind fixers: Psychiatry's troubled search for the biology of mental illness.* W. W. Norton.

11. Smid, G. E., Groen, S., de la Rie, S. M., Kooper, S., & Boelen, P. A. (2018). Toward cultural assessment of grief and grief-related psychopathology. *Psychiatric Services, 69*(10), 1050–1052.

12. Gara, M., Vega, W., Arndt, S., Escamilla, M., Fleck, D., Lawson, W. B., Lesser, I., Neighbors, H. W., Wilson, D. R., Arnold, L. M., & Strakowski, S. M. (2012). Influence of patient race and ethnicity on clinical assessment in patients with affective disorders. *Archives of General Psychiatry, 69*(6), 593–600.

13. Coleman, K. J., Stewart, C., Waitzfelder, B. E., Zeber, J. E., Morales, L. S., Ahmed, A. T., . . . Simon, G. E. (2016). Racial-ethnic differences in psychiatric diagnoses and treatment across 11 health care systems in the mental health research network. *Psychiatric Services, 67*(7), 749–757.

14. Skammeritz, S., Sari, N., Jiménez-Solomon, O., & Carlsson, J. (2019). Interpreters in transcultural psychiatry. *Psychiatric Services, 70*(3), 250–253.

15. Seedat, S., Scott, K., Angermeyer, M., Berglund, P., Bromet, E. J., Brugha, T. S., , . . . Kessler, R. C. (2009). Cross-national associations between gender and mental disorders in the World Health Organization world mental health surveys. *Archives of General Psychiatry, 66*(7), 785–795.

16. Corrigan, P. W. (2015). Challenging the stigma of mental illness: Different agendas, different goals. *Psychiatric Services, 66,* 1347–1349.

17. Geschwind, D. H., & Flint J. (2015). Genetics and genomics of psychiatric disease. *Science, 349*(6255), 1489–1494.

18. Estes, M. L., & McAllister, A. K. (2016). Maternal immune activation: Implications for neuropsychiatric disorders. *Science, 353,* 772–777.

19. Nosarti, C., Reichenberg, A., Murray, R., Cnattingius, S., Lambe, M. P., Yin, L., MacCabe, J., Rifkin, L., & Hultman, C. M. (2012). Preterm birth and psychiatric disorders in young adult life. *Archives of General Psychiatry, 69*(6), 610–617.

20. Hamer, M., Stamatakis, E., & Batty, G. (2010). Objectively assessed secondhand smoke exposure and mental health in adults. *Archives of General Psychiatry, 67*(8), 850–855.

21. Orlovska, S., Pedersen, M., Benros, M., Mortensen, P., Agerbo, E., & Nordentoft, M. (2014). Head injury as risk factor for psychiatric disorders: A nationwide register-based follow-up study of 113,906 persons with head injury. *American Journal of Psychiatry, 171,* 463–469.

22. Centers for Disease Control and Prevention. (2013). Mental health surveillance among children — United States, 2005–2011. *Morbidity and Mortality Weekly Report, 62*(Suppl 2), 1–35.

23. Costello, E. J., He, J.-P., Sampson, N. A., Kessler, R. C., & Merikangas, K. R. (2014). Services for adolescents with psychiatric disorders: 12-month data from the National Comorbidity Survey–Adolescent. *Psychiatric Services, 65,* 359–366.

24. Lee, F. S., Heimer, H., Giedd, J. N., Lein, E. S., Sestan N., Weinberger, D. R., & Casey, B. J. (2014). Adolescent mental health—opportunity and obligation. *Science, 346*(6209), 547–549.

25. Brent, D., & Silverstein, M. (2013). Shedding light on the long shadow of childhood adversity. *Journal of the American Medical Association, 309*(17), 1777–1778.

26. Gilbert, R., Widom, C., Browne, K., Fergusson, D., Webb, E., & Janson, S. (2009). Burden and consequences of child maltreatment in high-income countries. *Lancet, 373*(9657), 68–81.

27. Copeland, W., Wolke, D., Angold, A., & Costello, E. (2013). Adult psychiatric outcomes of bullying and being bullied by peers in childhood and adolescence. *JAMA Psychiatry, 70*(4), 419–426.

28. Haidt, J. (2020). Digital technology under scrutiny. *Nature, 578,* 226–227.

29. Shim, R. S., & Compton, M. T. (2018). Addressing the social determinants of mental health: If not now, when? If not us, who? *Psychiatric Services, 69*(8), 844–846.

30. Charles, S. T., Piazza, J. R., Mogle, J., Sliwinski, M. J., & Almeida, D. M. (2013). The wear and tear of daily stressors on mental health. *Psychological Science, 24*(5), 733–741.

31. Harvard Health Publishing. (2024). Understand the stress response. Harvard Health Publishing. Retrieved from https://www.health .harvard.edu/staying-healthy/understanding-the-stress-response

32. Sederer, L. I. (2016). The social determinants of mental health. *Psychiatric Services, 67*, 234–235.

33. House, J. S., Landis, K. R., & Umberson, D. (1988). Social relationships and health. *Science, 241*, 540–545.

34. Payne, W. A., Hahn, D. B., & Lucas, E. B. (2006). *Understanding your health* (9th ed.). McGraw-Hill Higher Education.

35. Galea, S., Ahern, J., Resnick, H., Kilpatrick, D., Bucuvalas, M., Gold, J., & Vlahov, D. (2002). Psychological sequelae of the September 11 terrorist attacks in New York City. *New England Journal of Medicine, 346*(13), 982–1087.

36. Reardon, S. (2015). Hurricane Katrina's psychological scars revealed. *Nature, 524*, 395–396.

37. Kessler, R. C., Heeringa, S. G., Stein, M. B., Volpe, L. J., Fullerton, C. S., Hwang, I., . . . Army STARRS Collaborators. (2014). Thirty-day prevalence of *DSM-IV* mental disorders among nondeployed soldiers in the US Army. *JAMA Psychiatry, 71*(5), 504–513.

38. Czeisler, M. E., Lane, R. I, Petrosky, E., . . . Rajaratnam, S. M. (2020). Mental health, substance use, and suicidal ideation during the COVID-19 pandemic—United States, June 24–30, 2020. *Morbidity and Mortality Weekly Report, 69*, 1049–1057.

39. Derr, A. S. (2016). Mental health service use among immigrants in the United States: A systematic review. *Psychiatric Services, 67*(3), 265–274.

40. Case, A., & Deaton, A. (2015). Rising morbidity and mortality in midlife among white non-Hispanic Americans in the 21st century. *Proceedings of the National Academy of Sciences, 112*(49), 15078–15083.

41. Olfson, M., Carlos Blanco, C., Wall, M., Liu, S. M., Saha, T. D., Pickering, R. P., & Grant, B. F. (2017). National trends in suicide attempts among adults in the United States. *JAMA Psychiatry, 74*(11), 1095–1103.

42. Grob, G. N. (1994). *The mad among us: A history of the care of America's mentally ill.* The Free Press.

43. Johnson, A. B. (1990). *Out of Bedlam: The truth about deinstitutionalization* (pp. 306). Basic Books.

44. Gerhart, U. C. (1990). *Caring for the chronic mentally ill.* F. E. Peacock; 5.

45. Mosher, L. R., & Burti, L. (1989). *Community mental health.* W. W. Norton.

46. Foley, H. A., & Sharfstein, S. S. (1983). *Madness and government.* American Psychiatric Press.

47. Kellner, C. H., Greenberg, R. M., Murrough, J. W., Bryson, E. O., Briggs, M. C., & Pasculli, R. M. (2012). ECT in treatment-resistant depression. *American Journal of Psychiatry, 169*(12), 1238–1244.

48. El Hai, J. (2005). The lobotomist. Wiley.

49. Herman, J. (2015). *Trauma and recovery: The aftermath of violence – From domestic abuse to political terror.* Basic Books.

50. Myers, C. S. (1940). *Shell shock in France.* Cambridge University Press.

51. Kardiner, A., & Spiegel, H. (1947). *The traumatic neuroses of war.* Hoeber.

52. Grob, G. N. (1991). *From asylum to community.* Princeton University Press.

53. Frank, R. G., & Glied, S. A. (2006). *Better but not well.* Johns Hopkins University Press.

54. Marder, S. R., & Cannon, T. D. (2019). Schizophrenia. *New England Journal of Medicine, 381*(18), 1753–1761.

55. Rosenberg, K. P. (2019). *Bedlam: An intimate journey into America's mental health crisis.* Avery.

56. Levine, M., Toro, P. A., & Perkins, D. V. (1993). Social and community interventions. *Annual Review of Psychology, 44*, 525–558.

57. Green Doors. (n.d.). *General homelessness facts.* Retrieved from https://greendoors .org/facts/general-data.php

58. Schanzer, B., Boanerges, D., Shrout, P. E., & Caton, L. M. (2007). Homelessness, health status, and health care use. *American Journal of Public Health, 97*(3), 464–469.

59. Roy, L., Crocker, A. G., Nicholls, T. L., Latimer, E. A., & Ayllon, A. R. (2014). Criminal behavior and victimization among homeless individuals with severe mental illness: A systematic review. *Psychiatric Services, 65*, 739–750.

60. The U.S. Department of Housing and Urban Development. (2022). *The 2022 annual homelessness assessment report (AHAR) to Congress.*

61. Tsai, J., & Rosenheck, R. A. (2015). Risk factors for homelessness among US Veterans. *Epidemiologic Reviews, 37*, 177– 195.

62. Gulcer, L., Tsemberis, S., Stefancic, A., & Greenwood, R. M. (2007). Community integration of adults with psychiatric disabilities and histories of homelessness. *Community Mental Health Journal, 43*(3), 211–228.

63. Gilmer, T., Stefancic, A., Ettner, S., Manning, W., & Tsemberis, S. (2010). Effect of full-service partnerships on homelessness, use and costs of mental health services, and quality of life among adults with serious mental illness. *Archives of General Psychiatry, 67*(6), 645–652.

64. McGinty, E., Webster, D., & Barry, C. (2013). Effects of news media messages about mass shootings on attitudes toward persons with serious mental illness and public support for gun control policies. *American Journal of Psychiatry, 170*, 494–501.

65. Metzl, J. M., & MacLeish, K. T. (2015). Mental illness, mass shootings, and the politics of American firearms. *American Journal of Public Health, 105*, 240–249.

66. Steadman, H. J., Monahan, J., Pinals, D. A., Vesselinov, R., & Robbins, P. C. (2015). Gun violence and victimization of strangers by persons with a mental illness: Data from the MacArthur Violence Risk Assessment Study. *Psychiatric Services, 66*, 1238–1241.

67. Swanson, J. W. (2018). Redirecting the mental health and gun violence conversation from mass shootings to suicide. *Psychiatric Services, 69*(12), 1198–1199.

68. Mozaffarian, D., Hemenway, D., & Ludwig, D. (2013). Curbing gun violence: Lessons from public health successes. *Journal of the American Medical Association, 309*(6), 551–552.

69. Edalati, H., Nicholls, T. L., Crocker, A. G., Roy, L., Somers, J. M., & Patterson, M. L. (2017). Adverse childhood experiences and the risk of criminal justice involvement and victimization among homeless adults with mental illness. *Psychiatric Services, 68*(12), 1288–1295.

70. Torrey, E. F., Zdanowicz, M. T., Kennard, A. D., Lamb, H. R., Eslinger, D. F., Biasotti, M. C., & Fuller, D. A. (2014). *The treatment of persons with mental illness in prisons and jails: A state survey.* National Institute of Corrections. Retrieved from https:// nicic.gov/resources/nic-library/all-library-items/treatment -persons-mental-illness-prisons-and-jails-state

71. Montross, C. (2016). Hard time or hospital treatment? Mental illness and the criminal justice system. *New England Journal of Medicine, 375*(15), 1407–1409.

72. Westervelt, E. (Host). (2020). Mental health and police violence: How crisis intervention teams are failing. In *All Things Considered.* National Public Radio. Retrieved from https://www.npr .org/2020/09/18/913229469/mental-health-and-police-violence-how -crisis-intervention-teams-are-failing

73. Compton, M. T., Bakeman, R., Broussard, B., Hankerson-Dyson, D., Husbands, L., Krishan, S., . . . Watson, A. C. (2014). The police-based crisis intervention team (CIT) model: I. Effects on officers' knowledge, attitudes, and skills. *Psychiatric Services, 65*(4), 517–522.

74. Cross, A. B., Mulvey, E. P., Schubert, C. A., Griffin, P. A., Filone, S., Winckworth-Prejsnar, K., DeMatteo, D., & Heilbrun, K. (2014). An agenda for advancing research on crisis intervention teams for mental health emergencies. *Psychiatric Services, 65*, 530–536.

75. Metzner, J. L. (2012). Treatment for prisoners: A U.S. perspective. *Psychiatric Services, 63*, 276.

76. Moore, S. (2009). Mentally ill offenders strain juvenile system. *The New York Times*, A1.

77. Fovet, T., Geoffroy, P. A., Vaiva, G., Adins, C., Thomas, P., & Amad, A. (2015). Individuals with bipolar disorder and their relationship with the criminal justice system: A critical review. *Psychiatric Services, 66*, 348–353. *Psychiatric Services, 67*(6), 630–635.

78. Swanson, J., Van Dorn, R., Monahan, J., & Swartz, R. (2006). Violence and leveraged treatment for persons with mental disorders. *American Journal of Psychiatry, 163*, 1404–1411.

79. Hiday, V. A., Ray, B., & Wales, H. (2016). Longer-term impacts of mental health courts: Recidivism two years after exit. *Psychiatric Services, 67*(4), 378–383.

80. McNiel, D. E., Sadeh, N., Delucchi, K. L., & Binder, R. L. (2015). Prospective study of violence risk reduction by a mental health court. *Psychiatric Services, 66*, 598–603.

81. Moorer, O. (2021). Intimate partner violence vs. domestic violence. Retrieved from https://ywcaspokane.org/what-is-intimate-partner-domestic-violence/

82. National Coalition Against Domestic Violence. (n.d.). Learn more: What is domestic violence? Retrieved from https://ncadv.org/learn-more

83. Centers for Disease Control and Prevention. (2022). The national intimate partner and sexual violence survey: 2016/2017 report on intimate partner violence. Retrieved from https://www.cdc.gov/violenceprevention/pdf/nisvs/NISVSReportonIPV_2022.pdf

84. National Domestic Violence Hotline. (2020). General domestic violence statistics. Retrieved from https://www.thehotline.org/stakeholders/domestic-violence-statistics/

85. National Coalition Against Domestic Violence. (n.d.). Learn more: Why do victims stay? Retrieved from https://ncadv.org/why-do-victims-stay

86. The Centers for Disease Control and Prevention (CDC). (2023). Suicide data and statistics. Retrieved from https://www.cdc.gov/suicide/suicide-data-statistics.html

87. The Centers for Disease Control and Prevention (CDC). (2023). Risk and protective factors. https://www.cdc.gov/suicide/factors/index.html

88. Pfefferbaum, B. & North, C. S. (2020). Mental health and the COVID-19 pandemic. *New England Journal of Medicine, 383*(6), 510– 512.

89. World Health Organization. (2022). COVID-19 pandemic triggers 25% increase in prevalence of anxiety and depression worldwide. Retrieved from https://www.who.int/news/item/02-03-2022-covid-19-pandemic-triggers-25-increase-in-prevalence-of-anxiety-and-depression-worldwide

90. Waechter, R., Gallant, C., De Wilde, K., Arens, G., Brady, T., Custodio, J., . . . & Bhagat, A. (2023). Prevention of mental illness within public health: An analysis of progress via systematic literature review and a pathway forward. *Preventive Medicine Reports, 34*, 1–11. Retrieved from https://doi.org/10.1016/j.pmedr.2023.

91. Levine, M., Perkins, D. D., & Perkins, D. V. (2004). *Principles of community psychology: Perspectives and applications* (3rd ed.). Oxford University Press.

92. Compton, M. T., & Shim, R. S. (2020). Mental illness prevention and mental health promotion: When, who, and how. *Psychiatric Services, 71*, 981– 983.

93. Robinson, E. (2018). Psychopharmacology: From serendipitous discoveries to rationale design, but what next? *Brain and Neuroscience Advances, 2*. Retrieved from https://doi.org/10.1177/2398212818812629

94. Gaynes, B., Warden, D., Trivedi, M., Wisniewski, S. R., Fava, M., & Rush, J. (2009). What did STAR*D teach us? Results from a large-scale, practical, clinical trial for patients with depression. *Psychiatric Services, 60*, 1439–1445.

95. American Psychological Association. (2008). Clinical psycho-pharmacology. Retrieved from https://www.apa.org/ed/graduate/specialize/clinical-psychopharmacology

96. American Psychological Association. (2023). Understanding psychotherapy and how it works. Retrieved from https://www.apa.org/topics/psychotherapy/understanding

97. Dunlop, B. W., LoParo, D., Kinkead, B., Mletzko-Crowe, T., Cole, S. P., Nemeroff, C. B., Mayberg, H. S., & Craighead, W. E. (2019). Benefits of sequentially adding cognitive-behavioral therapy or antidepressant medication for adults with nonremitting depression. *American Journal of Psychiatry, 176*(4), 275–286.

98. Thomas, K., Ellis, A., Konrad, T., Holzer, C. E., & Morrissey, J. P. (2009). County-level estimate of mental health professional shortage in the United States. *Psychiatric Services, 60*, 1323–1328.

99. Substance Abuse and Mental Health Services Administration. (2015). Substance abuse treatment: Group therapy. U.S. Department of Health and Human Services. Retrieved from https://www.ncbi.nlm.nih.gov/books/NBK64220/pdf/Bookshelf_NBK64220.pdf

100. Shalaby, R. A., & Agyapong, V. I. (2020). Peer support in mental health: Literature review. *JMIR Mental Health, 7*(6), e15572. Retrieved from https://doi.org/10.2196/15572

101. Khasnabis, C., Heinicke Motsch K., Achu K., et al., eds. (2010). Community-Based Rehabilitation: CBR Guidelines. World Health Organization. Retrieved from https://www.ncbi.nlm.nih.gov/books/NBK310972/

102. National Institutes of Mental Health. (2021). What is telemental health? Retrieved from https://infocenter.nimh.nih.gov/sites/default/files/2022-01/what-is-telemental-health.pdf

103. Calkins, H. (2021). Online therapy is here to stay. *Monitor on Psychology, 52*(1). Retrieved from https://www.apa.org/monitor/2021/01/trends-online-therapy

104. Scharff, D. (2021). The data are in: Telehealth is here to stay. *Psychology Today,* Retrieved from https://www.psychologytoday.com/us/blog/psychoanalytic-exploration/202111/the-data-are-in-telehealth-is-here-stay#:~:text=Now%2C%2055%25%20are%20practicing%20only,differentiate%20between%20online%20or%20phone

105. Giordano, C., Ambrosiano, I., Graffeo, M. T., Di Caro, A., & Gullo, S. (2022). The transition to online psychotherapy during the pandemic: A qualitative study on patients' perspectives. *Research in psychotherapy (Milano), 25*(3), 638. Retrieved from https://doi.org/10.4081/ripppo.2022.638

106. Rotondi, A. J., Anderson, C. M., Haas, G. L., Eack, S. M., Spring, M. B., Ganguli, R., Newhill, C., & Rosenstock, J. (2010). Web-based psychoeducational intervention for persons with schizophrenia and their supporters: One-year outcomes. *Psychiatric Services, 61*, 1099–1105.

107. Thase, M. E., Wright, J. H., Eells, T. D., Barrett, M. S., Wisniewski, S. R., Balasubramani, G., McCrone, P., & Brown, G. K. (2018). Improving the efficiency of psychotherapy for depression: Computer- assisted versus standard CBT. *American Journal of Psychiatry, 175*(3), 242–250.

108. Lerner, D., Chang, H., Rogers, W. H., Benson, C., Lyson, M. C., & Dixon, L. B. (2018). Psychological distress among caregivers of individuals with a diagnosis of schizophrenia or schizoaffective disorder. *Psychiatric Services, 69*(2), 169–178.

109. National Alliance on Mental Illness (NAMI). n.d. What does NAMI do? Retrieved from http://namiccmd.org/about-us/

110. Cohen, A. N., Hamilton, A. B., Saks, E. R., Glover, D. L., & Glynn, S. M. (2017). How occupationally high-achieving individuals with a diagnosis of schizophrenia manage their symptoms. *Psychiatric Services, 68*(4), 324–329.

111. Meldrum, M. L., Kelly, E. L., Calderon, R., Brekke, J. S., & Braslow, J. T. (2016). Implementation status of assisted outpatient treatment programs: A national survey. *Psychiatric Services, 67*(6), 630–635.

112. McCarty, D., Braude, L., Lyman, D. R., Dougherty, R. H., Daniels, A. S., Ghose, S. S., & Delphin-Rittmon, M. E. (2014). Substance abuse intensive outpatient programs: Assessing the evidence. *Psychiatric*

services, 65(6), 718–726. Retrieved from https://doi.org/10.1176/appi.ps.201300249

113. Definition of partial hospitalization. The National Association of Private Psychiatric Hospitals and the American Association for Partial Hospitalization. (1990). The *Psychiatric Hospital, 21*(2), 89–90.

114. Ware, N., Hopper, K., Tugenberg, T., Dickey, B., & Fisher, D. (2007). Connectedness and citizenship: Redefining social integration. *Psychiatric Services, 58*, 469–474.

115. Corrigan, P., Mueser, K., Bond, G., Drake, R., & Solomon, P. (2008). *Principles and practice of psychiatric rehabilitation: An empirical approach*. Guilford.

116. Austin, E., Ramakrishnan, A., & Hopper, K. (2014). Embodying recovery: A qualitative study of peer work in a consumer-run service setting. *Community Mental Health Journal, 50*, 879–885.

117. Spivak, S., Cullen, B. A., Green, C., Firth, T., Sater, H., & Mojtabai, R. (2019). Availability of assertive community treatment in the United States: 2010 to 2016. *Psychiatric Services, 70*(10), 948–951.

118. Manuel, J. I., Appelbaum, P. S., Le Melle, S. M., Mancini, A. D., Huz, S., Stellato, C. B., & Finnerty, M. T. (2013). Use of intervention strategies by assertive community treatment teams to promote patients' engagement. *Psychiatric Services, 64*, 579–585.

119. Luciano, A., & Meara, E. (2014). Employment status of people with mental illness: National survey data from 2009 and 2010. *Psychiatric Services, 65*, 1201–1209.

120. Drake, R. E., Frey, W., Bond, G. R., Goldman, H. H., Salkever, D., Miller, A., Moore, T. A., Riley, J., Karakus, M., & Milfort, R. (2013). Assisting social security disability insurance beneficiaries with schizophrenia, bipolar disorder, or major depression in returning to work. *American Journal of Psychiatry, 170*, 1433–1441.

121. Kane, J. M., Robinson, D. G., Schooler, N. R., Mueser, K. T., Penn, D. L., Rosenheck, R. A., . . . Heinssen, R. K. (2016). Comprehensive versus usual community care for first-episode psychosis: 2-year outcomes from the NIMH RAISE early treatment program. *American Journal of Psychiatry, 173*(4), 362–372.

122. Hopper, K. (2004). Interrogating the meaning of 'culture' in the WHO international studies of schizophrenia. In J. Jenkins & R. Barrett (Eds.), *Schizophrenia, culture, and subjectivity: The edge of experience* (pp. 62–86). Cambridge University Press.

123. Miller, G. (2006). A spoonful of medicine—and a steady diet of normality. *Science, 311*, 464–465.

124. McGruder, J. (2004). Madness in Zanzibar: An exploration of lived experience. In J. Jenkins & R. Barrett (Eds.), *Schizophrenia, culture, and subjectivity: The edge of experience* (pp. 255–281). Cambridge University Press.

125. Woltmann, E. M., Whitley, R., McHugo, G. J., Brunette, M., Torrey, W. C., Coots, L., Lynde, D., & Drake, R. E. (2008). The role of staff turnover in the implementation of evidence-based practices in mental health care. *Psychiatric Services, 59*, 732–737.

126. Marshall, T., Rapp, C. A., Becker, D. R., & Bond, G. R. (2008). Key factors for implementing supported employment. *Psychiatric Services, 59*, 886–892.

127. Drapalski, A. L., Marshall, T., Seybolt, D., Medoff, D., Peer, J., Leith, J., & Dixon, L. B. (2008). Unmet needs of families of adults with mental illness and preferences regarding family services. *Psychiatric Services, 59*, 655–662.

128. Wang, P., Demler, O., Olfson, M., Pincus, H. A., Wells, K. B., & Kessler, R. C. (2006). Changing profiles of service sectors used for mental health care in the United States. *American Journal of Psychiatry, 163*, 1187–1198.

129. Interian, A., Lewis-Fernández, R., & Dixon, L. B. (2013). Improving treatment engagement of underserved U.S. racial-ethnic groups: A review of recent interventions. *Psychiatric Services, 64*, 212–222.

130. Byrne, T., Bettger, J. P., Brusilovskiy, E., Wong, Y.-L. I., Metraux, S., & Salzer, M. S. (2013). Comparing neighborhoods of adults with serious mental illness and of the general population: RESEARCH implications. *Psychiatric Services, 64*, 782–788.

131. Hodgkin, D., Horgan, C. M., Stewart, M. T., Quinn, A. E., Creedon, T. B., Reif, S., & Garnick, D. W. (2018). Federal parity and access to behavioral health care in private health plans. *Psychiatric Services, 69*(4), 396–402.

132. Mark, T. L. (2019). The effect of the affordable care act on uninsured rates among individuals with mental and substance use disorders. *Psychiatric Services, 70*, 343.

133. Fry, C. E., & Sommers, B. D. (2018). Effect of Medicaid expansion on health insurance coverage and access to care among adults with depression. *Psychiatric Services, 69*(11), 1146–1152.

134. Raney, L. E. (2015). Integrating primary care and behavioral health: The role of the psychiatrist in the collaborative care model. *American Journal of Psychiatry, 172*(80), 721–728.

135. Lee-Tauler, S. Y., Eun, J., Corbett, D., & Collins, P. Y. (2018). A systematic review of interventions to improve initiation of mental health care among racial-ethnic minority groups. *Psychiatric Services, 69*(6), 628–647.

136. Shim, R. S., Koplan, C., Langheim, F. J., Manseau, M., Oleskey, C., Powers, R. A., & Compton, M. T. (2012). Health care reform and integrated care: A golden opportunity for preventive psychiatry. *Psychiatric Services, 63*, 1231–1233.

137. Howell, B. A., Wang, E. A., & Winkelman, T. N. (2019). Mental health treatment among individuals involved in the criminal justice system after implementation of the Affordable Care Act. *Psychiatric Services, 70*(9), 765–771.

CHAPTER 12

Alcohol, Tobacco, and Other Drugs: A Community Concern

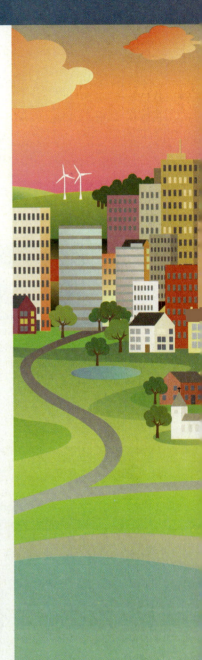

Chapter Objectives

After studying this chapter, you will be able to:

1. Identify personal and community consequences of alcohol and other drug abuse.
2. Describe the trends of alcohol and other drug use by high school students.
3. Define drug use, misuse, and abuse.
4. Define drug dependence.
5. List and discuss the risk factors for the abuse of alcohol and other drugs.
6. Explain why alcohol is considered the number one drug use problem in the United States.
7. Describe the health risks of cigarette smoking.
8. Define the terms *over-the-counter* and *prescription* drugs, and explain the purposes of these drugs and how they are regulated.
9. Define the terms *controlled substances* and *illicit (illegal) drugs*, and provide examples.
10. Characterize recent trends in the prevalence of drug use among American high school seniors.
11. List and explain four elements of drug abuse prevention and control.
12. Give an example of primary, secondary, and tertiary prevention activities in drug abuse prevention and control programs.

Chapter Objectives

13. Summarize the federal government's drug abuse control efforts.

14. List and describe an effective community and an effective school drug use prevention program.

15. List the five facets of a typical workplace substance use prevention program.

16. Name some voluntary health agencies and self-help support groups involved in the prevention, control, and treatment of alcohol, tobacco, and other drug use.

Scenario

Andy is 36 years old. He lives in the suburbs with his wife, Sara, and their twin boys. Andy and Sara have been married for 10 years. Andy works full time as a sales consultant for a midsize company, where he has been employed since he graduated with his MBA 8 years ago. He also leads the local chamber of commerce. Andy plays soccer in a local adult coed league, and he coaches his boys' soccer team on the weekends. He and Sara are very social and spend a lot of time out in the community with friends.

Last year, Andy hurt his knee playing soccer. He had reconstructive knee surgery to repair a torn ligament. His doctor prescribed an opioid pain reliever to help with pain management following surgery. Andy was given a 2-week supply. The medication helped, and Andy looked forward to starting physical therapy the week after surgery. The first physical therapy appointment went well, but Andy was in a lot of pain. The pain was so bad that he thought of little else, had trouble sleeping, and was very discouraged. The physical therapist recommended an over-the-counter pain reliever, rest, elevation, and ice. Andy followed this regimen and continued to take the opioid pain reliever as prescribed. After 2 weeks, he ran out of his medication, just 2 days before his postoperative checkup with his surgeon. During those 2 days, Andy took over-the-counter pain relievers, but he felt he could not get a handle on his pain. He also felt depressed and repeatedly thought, "If only I had the opioid medication, I would be fine."

At Andy's checkup with his surgeon, he talked about his high level of pain, how well the opioid pain reliever was working, and how much progress he was able to make in physical therapy when he was taking it. He also told the surgeon that he tried over-the-counter pain relievers but they did not help. He asked for a refill of the opioid pain reliever, and the surgeon agreed to prescribe another 2-week supply. They would re-evaluate things in 2 weeks at the next appointment. At first, Andy took the opioid pain reliever as prescribed. As he continued with physical therapy, though, he realized that he needed to take more of the medication to get the same effect. This led to him taking the medication more times per day than prescribed. After a week, Andy ran out of the medication. He quickly noticed a change in how he was feeling—when he was on the medication, he felt great about himself and had little pain, but when he was off the medication, he felt awful. He knew he could not tell his doctor that he ran out, and so he turned to over-the-counter medications, taking and misusing a combination of ibuprofen, acetaminophen, and naproxen as soon as he felt any twinge of pain. However, he could not recapture the sense of well-being he felt when he was taking the opioid pain reliever.

At his next checkup, Andy asked the surgeon for another refill. At first, the surgeon said no and recommended over-the-counter pain relievers from that point on. After Andy stated his case, however, the surgeon relented, giving him another 2-week supply. The surgeon made it clear that this would be the last opioid pain reliever prescription he would receive.

Andy finished the prescription in less than a week and was consumed with dread for how he would feel without it. Andy had a friend at work who recently had back surgery and who had been prescribed the same opioid pain reliever. The friend did not respond well to the medication and never finished the prescription. Andy asked him if he could have his extra pills, and the friend gave them to him.

Over the next 6 months, Andy became addicted to opioid pain relievers, needing more and more to achieve the same sense of well-being. Andy desperately sought more pills through legal and illegal channels. He intermittently took money out of the joint savings account that he and Sara shared, hoping that Sara would not notice, to pay for his expensive addiction. She knew something was wrong but when she asked him about it, he yelled at her, lied that everything was fine, and started pushing her away. Andy stopped showing up to his boys' soccer games and started dropping out of social obligations. His work was affected too as he became unreliable, especially if he ran out of pills and experienced withdrawal. He met someone who told him that heroin had the same effect as opioid pain relievers but was a much cheaper option. Andy agreed to try it one time. He overdosed but did not die. The paramedics who found him administered naloxone, which saved his life. He is now in a drug rehabilitation program and on long-term disability from his job.

Introduction

The use, misuse, and abuse of mind-altering substances undoubtedly predate our recorded history. Early civilizations may have used drugs as a vehicle to communicate with spirits. Even today, drugs are used for this purpose in some cultures.

For many Americans, drug-taking is experimental or social, a temporary departure from a natural, nondrugged physical and mental state. For many others, it is a misguided attempt to self-medicate or to cope with personal problems, such as depression, loneliness, guilt, or low self-esteem. For a small but significant segment of the population, drug-taking ceases to be a matter of conscious choice; these people have become chronic drug users, or drug dependent. In most cultures, chronic alcohol or other drug use or dependence is regarded as destructive behavior, both to oneself and to the surrounding community. Community members whose lives center around drug acquisition and use usually provide little benefit to their communities and often detract from their communities.

Scope of the Current Drug Problem in the United States

More deaths, illnesses, and disabilities can be attributed to the use/misuse of alcohol, tobacco, and other drugs than to any other preventable health condition.[1] About one-fourth of the approximately 3.5 million deaths each year are due to alcohol, tobacco, or illicit drug use (see **Table 12.1**). In 2011, 2.4 million emergency department visits were due to drug use and misuse.[2] In 2022, drug-related emergency department visits rose exponentially to 7.7 million.[3] The top five drugs involved in drug-related ED visits in 2021 were alcohol (39.33% of all drug-related ED visits), opioids (14.07%), methamphetamine (11.02%), marijuana (10.78%), and cocaine (4.71%).[4] The economic cost of substance use/misuse in the United States [5-7] include direct costs (such as healthcare expenditures, premature death, and impaired productivity) and indirect costs, which include the costs of crime and law enforcement, courts, jails, and social work. The cost of alcohol abuse and alcoholism is estimated at $249 billion, drug use/misuse at $193 billion, smoking at $300 billion, with prescription opioid increasing to an alarming $1 trillion (see Table 12.1).[5-7] Clearly, the use/misuse of alcohol and other drugs is one of the United States' most expensive community and public health problems.

The global COVID-19 pandemic in 2020 had a profound impact on societies, healthcare systems, public health, and individual health. The pandemic had the potential to create even worse health outcomes for people with substance use disorders, as they are more susceptible to the virus and the stress associated with COVID-19.[8] Studies indicate that the use of alcohol and other substances increased during the early stages of the pandemic, especially among those with clinical anxiety, depression, and COVID-related stress.[8] During the COVID-19 pandemic, drug overdoses

TABLE 12.1 Annual Cost in Lives and Dollars Attributable to Alcohol, Tobacco, and Illicit Drug Abuse in the United States

Type of Drug	Estimated Number of Deaths Each Year	Economic Cost to Society
Alcohol	140,000	$249 billion
Tobacco	480,000	$600 billion
Illicit drugs (not including opioids)	106,699	$115 billion
Opioids	80,411	$1.02 trillion

Data from Centers for Disease Control and Prevention. (2024). Alcohol and Public Health: Alcohol-Related Disease Impact. Annual average for United States 2015–2019 alcohol-attributable deaths due to excessive alcohol use, all ages; U.S. Department of Health and Human Services. The Health Consequences of Smoking—50 Years of Progress: A Report of the Surgeon General. Atlanta: U.S. Department of Health and Human Services, Centers for Disease Control and Prevention, National Center for Chronic Disease Prevention and Health Promotion, Office on Smoking and Health, 2014; U.S. Department of Health and Human Services. (2024). Addiction and Substance Misuse Reports and Publication; National Institute on Drug Abuse. (2021). *Trends and statistics*. Available at https://www.drugabuse.gov/related-topics/trends-statistics/overdose-death-rates; Centers for Disease Control and Prevention. (2024). *Injury Prevention & Control*. The Economic of Injury and Violence Prevention. Available at https://www.cdc.gov/injury/features/health-econ-cost-of-injury/

Physical dependence
a physiologic state in which discontinued drug use results in clinical illness

increased, leading to more than 110,000 deaths from drug overdose in 2022—the highest number recorded to date. Other factors related to the pandemic, such as social isolation, stress, decreased access to treatment, and emergency services may have contributed to the upward trend. However, there was also a concurrent rise of potent fentanyl in the drug supply during the pandemic, so the exact causes are difficult to determine.[9] However, there were some positive outcomes during and after the pandemic. Drug and alcohol use among adolescents and young adults had the largest decrease since the 1970s.[10] In addition, the need for remote options in health care, support systems, and treatment led to increased opportunities for services to reach more people.[10]

Those abusing alcohol and other drugs represent serious health threats to themselves, their families, and their communities. They are a threat to themselves and their families because they put themselves and their families at risk for physical, mental, and financial ruin. The drug user may develop a psychological and/or **physical dependence** on the drug and thus experience great difficulty in discontinuing use, even in the face of deteriorating physical and mental health and erosion of financial resources. If the drug is an illegal one, its use constitutes criminal activity and may carry with it the added risks of arrest and incarceration.

People with alcohol and other drug addictions have greater health care needs, suffer more injuries, and are less productive than those who do not. Community consequences range from loss of economic opportunity and productivity to social and economic destruction (see **Table 12.2**). Additionally, those who use or misuse drugs may perpetrate more violent acts that result in economic loss, injury, and death.

The Monitoring the Future surveys on drug use among high school and college students have been carried out annually since 1975.[11] Two themes have emerged from the Monitoring the Future surveys between 1975–2022. The first theme is the 1990s drug relapse due to the quick rise in drug use in the early 1990s. The second theme is the cohort effect in which groups of youth born at the same time experience similar drug trends as they age.[12] Several factors can influence cohort-specific pattern of drug use, whether increasing or decreasing: perceived risk,

TABLE 12.2 Personal and Community Consequences of Drug Abuse	
Personal Consequences	**Community Consequences**
Absenteeism from school or work	Loss of productivity and revenue
Underachievement at school or work	Lower than average SAT scores
Scholastic failure/interruption of education	Loss of economic opportunity
Loss of employment	Increase in public welfare load
Marital instability/family problems	Increase in number of broken homes
Risk of infectious diseases	Epidemics of sexually transmitted diseases
Risk of chronic or degenerative diseases	Unnecessary use of healthcare system resources
Increased risk of accidents	Unnecessary deaths and economic losses
Financial problems	Defaults on mortgages/loans; bankruptcies
Criminal activity	Increased cost of insurance and security
Arrest and incarceration	Increased cost for police/courts/prisons
Risk of adulterated drugs	Increased use of medical care system resources
Adverse drug reactions or "bad trips"	Greater need for emergency medical services
Drug-induced psychoses	Unnecessary drain on mental health services
Drug overdose	Unnecessary demand for medical services
Injury to fetus or newborn baby	Unnecessary use of expensive neonatal care
Loss of self-esteem	Increase in mental illness, underachievement
Suicide and death	Damaged and destroyed families

TABLE 12.3   Percentage of High School Seniors Who Have Used Drugs

Drug	Class of 2012, %			Class of 2022, %		
	Ever Used	Past 30 Days	Daily Use	Ever Used	Past 30 Days	Daily Use
Alcohol	69.4	41.5	2.5	61.6	28.4	1.5
Cigarettes	39.5	17.1	9.3	16.8	4.0	1.6
Marijuana	45.2	22.9	6.5	38.3	20.2	6.3
Amphetamines	12.0	3.3	0.3	5.3	1.3	0.2
Methamphetamine	1.7	0.5	Less than 0.05	1.1	0.4	0.0
Inhalants	7.9	0.9	0.1	5.8	0.7	0.1
Cocaine	4.9	1.1	0.1	2.4	0.8	0.2
Tranquilizers	6.0	1.0	—	6.1	2.0	0.0
	8.5	2.1	0.1	3.3	0.7	
LSD	3.8	0.8	0.1	4.4	0.2	0.1
MDMA	7.2	0.9	0.1	3.0	0.9	0.1
Crack	2.1	0.6	0.1	1.3	0.6	0.2
PCP	1.6	0.5	0.1	—	—	—
Heroin	1.1	0.3	0.1	—	0.3	0.1
Vaping Nicotine	—	—	—	38.8	20.7	6.2
Vaping Marijuana	—	—	—	27.5	14.8	2.1

Data from Johnston, L. D., Miech, R. A., O'Malley, P. M., Bachman, J. G., Schulenberg, J. E., & Patrick, M. E. (2022). *Monitoring the Future national survey results on drug use, 1975–2022: Overview, key findings on adolescent drug use.* Institute for Social Research, The University of Michigan. Available at. https://monitoring thefuture.org/wp-content/uploads/2023/01/mtfoverview2022.pdf

peer norms concerning acceptability, change in legal status of the drug, and level of addictiveness. Trends at the lower grade levels can be a predictor of future levels. One notable trend is the perceived risk of marijuana use, which was 79% in 1991 and 28% in 2022.[12] Decreases in perceptions of risk of harm from regular use have been associated with increases in usage.[12]

Use levels for specific drugs have fluctuated since 1992. For most drugs, use levels peaked in the mid to late 1990s and early 2000s. Some drugs are currently at their lowest reported levels. Over a 10-year period from 2012 to 2022, decreases in 30-day prevalence of use have been seen in alcohol consumption and more significantly in cigarette use among high school seniors (see **Table 12.3**).[11] Marijuana and illicit drug use have decreased slightly or remained the same.[11] However, there is a major upward trend in vaping marijuana and vaping nicotine.[11]

When the words *drug abuse* are mentioned, most people think of illicit drugs, such as heroin, LSD, cocaine, and other illegal substances. Although the use of illicit drugs is certainly a major problem in the United States, use of alcohol and tobacco products are also serious challenges to American's health. Although the rate of cigarette smoking and alcohol consumption has declined among those in grades 8, 10, and 12 since 1992, use levels remain high (see **Figure 12.1**). In 2022, 16.8% of high school seniors reported having been drunk during the past 30 days, while 28.3% of high school seniors reported any alcohol use during the past 30 days.[11] For grades 8, 10, and 12 combined, the 30-day prevalence for any alcohol use in 2022 was 15.6%.[11] In that same year, the 30-day prevalence for cigarette use among those in grades 8, 10, and 12 was about 2.1%, while 4.0% of high school seniors reported cigarette use during the past 30 days.[11] Data on vaping was

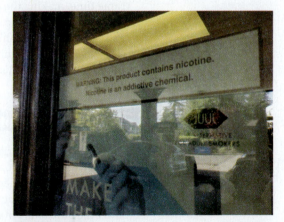

FIGURE 12.1   The prevalence of alcohol use among American high school seniors remains high and vaping has risen dramatically since 2015.

© Tomsmith585/iStock/Getty Images

first collected in 2015 by Monitoring the Future surveys. The 30-day prevalence for vaping any product nearly doubled from 12.8% in 2015 to 22.5% in 2019, but went down to 17.0% for the combined grades of 8, 10, and 12.[11] Vaping was highest among high school seniors, rising from 16.3% in 2015 to 30.9% in 2019 but decreased to 25.6% in 2022.[11] Although cigarette use among those in grades 8, 10, and 12 is declining, vaping is increasing at an alarming rate.

The United States has been trying to solve the problem of drug addiction for decades. Most adults who use drugs eventually "mature out" of the behavior, but there is a constant supply of potential drug users among U.S. children. This "generational forgetting" means that drug prevention education is never finished. Instead, drug prevention efforts must become a permanent part of our culture. That is, we must teach our children about the dangers of experimental drug use in the same way we teach them to look both ways before they cross the street.

Definitions

We begin a discussion of alcohol, tobacco, and other drugs as a community health problem by defining some terms. A **drug** is a substance, other than food or vitamins, that, upon entering the body in small amounts, alters one's physical, mental, or emotional state. **Psychoactive drugs** are substances that alter sensory perceptions, mood, thought processes, or behavior.

In this chapter, the term **drug use** is a nonevaluative term referring to drug-taking behavior in general, regardless of whether the behavior is appropriate. **Drug misuse** refers primarily to the inappropriate use of legally purchased prescription or nonprescription drugs. For example, drug misuse occurs when one discontinues the use of a prescribed antibiotic before the entire prescribed dose is completed or when one takes four aspirin rather than two as specified on the label. **Drug abuse** can be defined in several ways, depending on the drug and the situation. Drug abuse occurs when one takes a prescription or nonprescription drug for a purpose other than that for which it is medically approved. For example, drug abuse occurs when one takes a prescription diet pill for its mood-altering effects (stimulation). The abuse of legal drugs, such as nicotine or alcohol is said to occur when one is aware that continued use is detrimental to one's health. Because illicit drugs have no approved medical uses, any illicit drug use is considered drug abuse. Likewise, the use of alcohol and nicotine by those under the legal age is considered drug abuse.

Drug (chemical) dependence occurs when a user feels that a particular drug is necessary for normal functioning. It may be **psychological dependence**, in which case the user experiences a strong emotional or psychological desire to continue use of the drug even though clinical signs of physical illness may not appear, or it can be physical, in which discontinuation of drug use results in clinical illness. Usually, both psychological and physical dependence are present at the same time, making the discontinuation of drug use very difficult. Such is frequently the case with cigarette smoking. **Substance use disorder (SUD)** is the disorder defined by the American Psychiatric Association's *Diagnostic and Statistical Manual of Mental Disorders, fifth edition (DSM-5-TR; 2022)*, combines substance abuse and substance dependence into a single condition called substance use disorder.

Factors That Contribute to Alcohol, Tobacco, and Other Drug Abuse

The factors that contribute to the abuse of alcohol, tobacco, and other drugs are many, and the decision to use drugs lies ultimately with the individual; it is a matter of choice. However, studies have determined that individuals are differentially at risk for engaging in drug-taking behavior.[13] Factors that increase the probability of drug use are called *risk factors*; those that lower the probability of drug use are called *protective factors*. People with a high number of risk factors are said to be vulnerable to drug abuse or dependence, while those who have few risk factors and more protective factors are said to be resistant to drug abuse.

Risk and protective factors can be either genetic (inherited) or environmental. Numerous studies have concluded that inherited traits can increase one's risk of developing dependence on alcohol, and it is logical to assume that susceptibility to other drugs might also be inherited. Environmental risk factors, such as one's home and family life, school and peer groups, and society and culture, have also been identified.

Inherited Risk Factors

The vast majority of the data supporting the notion that the risk of drug dependence can be inherited comes from studies on alcoholism. Evidence for the heritability of risk for alcoholism is provided by numerous studies,[14-17] which have been reviewed by Tabakoff and Hoffman[18] and in the *Tenth Special Report to the U.S. Congress on Alcohol and Health*, from the Secretary of Health and Human Services.[19] Studies of alcoholics' families have found that there are at least two types of inherited alcoholism,[15] referred to as Type I (or milieu-limited) and Type II (or male-limited) alcoholism.[19] These observational studies of alcoholics' families are supported by research using genetic and biological markers in animal models. Some of these markers predispose an individual biochemically to increased susceptibility to developing alcohol-related problems, while others may actually be protective in nature. For example, genes that code for enzymes that inhibit the normal metabolism of alcohol could cause one to respond positively to the effects of alcohol and thus to drink more, or respond negatively to alcohol and thus drink less or not at all.[18] Studies provided evidence in support of the idea that genes also influence cigarette smoking.[20-22] The heritability of susceptibility to other drugs is still under investigation. The combination of genetics, environmental influence, and social factors can affect risks for alcohol dependence.[23]

Environmental Risk Factors

There are a great many environmental factors, both psychological and social, that influence the use and misuse of alcohol and other drugs. Included are personal factors, such as the influences of home and family life, school and peer groups, and other components of the social and cultural environment. A study conducted by the National Institute on Alcohol Abuse and Alcoholism (NIAAA), part of the National Institutes of Health (NIH), researchers identified subtypes of alcoholism based on family history, age of onset, patterns of dependence and abuse, and other substance abuse and mental disorders. The subtypes are: (1) adult alcoholic (31.5%), (2) young antisocial alcoholic (21%), (3) functional alcoholic (19.5%), (4) intermediate familial alcoholic (19%), and (5) chronic severe alcoholic (9%).[24]

Personal Factors

Personal factors include personality traits, such as impulsiveness, depressive mood, susceptibility to stress, or possibly personality disturbances. Some of these factors have been reviewed by Needle and colleagues.[25] Although models that involve personal factors provide frameworks for research and theorizing about the etiology of alcohol and drug use/misuse, they have their limitations. It is difficult to determine the degree to which these factors are inherited or are simply the product of the family environment. For example, one's choice to use alcohol or drugs in response to a stressful situation (and the outcome of that decision) could be the result of either inherited characteristics or learned behavior, or a combination of these factors.

Home and Family Life

The importance of home and family life on alcohol and drug use/misuse has been the subject of numerous studies, some of which have been reviewed by Meller[26] and by Needle and colleagues.[25] Research demonstrates that not all family-associated risk is genetic in origin. Family structure, family dynamics, quality of parenting, and family problems can all contribute to drug experimentation by children and adolescents (see **Figure 12.2**). Family turmoil (deaths and divorces) have been associated with the initiation of alcohol and other drug use.[25,27] In this sense, alcohol and drug use is a symptom of personal and/or family problems, not a cause.[28]

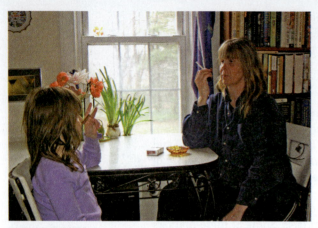

FIGURE 12.2   Influences of home and family life can affect one's decisions about alcohol, tobacco, and other drugs.

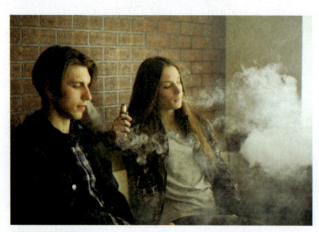

FIGURE 12.3   Peers can influence one's expectations of the effects of a drug.

© Aleksandr Yu/Shutterstock

The development of interpersonal skills, such as communication skills, independent living skills, and learning to get along with others, is nurtured in the home. The failure of parents to provide an environment conducive to the development of these skills can result in the loss of self-esteem and increase in delinquency, nonconformity, and sociopathic behavior, all personal risk factors for alcohol and drug use/misuse.[29]

Finally, family attitudes toward alcohol and drug use influence adolescents' beliefs and expectations about the effects of drugs. These expectations have been shown to be important factors in adolescents' choices to initiate and continue alcohol use.[29] The age of first use of alcohol, tobacco, and illicit drugs is correlated to later development of alcohol and drug problems, especially if use begins before age 15.[30]

School and Peer Groups

Perceived and actual drug use by peers influences attitudes and choices by adolescents (see **Figure 12.3**). Some studies have shown that perceived support of drinking by peers is the single most important factor in an adolescent's choice to drink.[29] Peers can also influence expectations for a drug. Alcohol may be perceived as "a 'magic elixir' that can enhance social and physical pleasure, sexual performance and responsiveness, power and aggression and social competence."[29] It is interesting to note that these are precisely the mythical qualities about alcohol portrayed in advertisements for beer and other alcoholic beverages.

Sociocultural Environment

The notion of environmental risk includes the effects of sociocultural and physical settings on drug-taking behavior. The study of the effects of the physical and social environment upon the individual is termed *social ecology*.[31] Environmental risk for drug-taking can stem from one's immediate neighborhood or from society at large. For example, living in an inner city—in which citizens are exposed to crime, the city's physical decay, and threats to personal safety—could set into motion a variety of changes in values and behaviors, including some related to alcohol or drug use.

Opportunities for community interventions exist, however. For example, federal, state, and local drug-prevention education programs, law enforcement successes, and treatment availability can improve the social environment and reduce the prevalence of drug use/misuse. Also, increasing taxes on tobacco products and alcoholic beverages and developing zoning ordinances that limit the number of bars and liquor stores in certain neighborhoods can be effective in reducing the alcohol, tobacco, and other drug problems in a community.

Types of Drugs Abused and Resulting Problems

Almost any psychoactive drug available is subject to abuse by at least some segment of the population. Classification systems of drugs of abuse are many, and none of them is perfect. Problems of classification arise because all drugs have multiple effects and because the legal status of a drug can depend on its formulation and strength and, in some cases, on the age of the user. In this chapter, our classification system includes legal drugs and illegal drugs. Legal (licit) drugs include alcohol, nicotine, and nonprescription and prescription drugs. Illegal (illicit) drugs can be classified further on the basis of physiologic effects as stimulants, depressants, narcotics, hallucinogens, marijuana, and other drugs.

Legal Drugs

Legal drugs are drugs that can be legally bought and sold in the marketplace, including those that are closely regulated, like morphine; those that are lightly regulated, like alcohol and tobacco; and still others that are not regulated at all, like caffeine.

Alcohol

Alcohol is a major drug issue in the United States by almost any standard of measurement—the number of those who abuse it, the number of injuries and injury deaths it causes, the amount of money spent on it, and its social and economic costs to society through broken homes and lost wages. Alcohol is consumed in a variety of forms, including beer, wine, fortified wines and brandies, and liquor. Although many people view liquor as the most dangerous form of alcohol, it is now recognized that the form of alcohol involved in most heavy-episodic drinking is beer. High school and college students are at risk for **binge drinking** (consuming five or more drinks on a single occasion for males and four or more drinks for females).

A major community health concern is underage drinking, that is, drinking by those younger than 21 years. Underage drinkers, many of them children and teenagers, can destroy their own lives and the lives of others through reckless driving, risky sexual behavior that can lead to disease transmission and unintentional pregnancies, and the commission of other violent and injurious acts. Of all of the alcoholic beverages sold in the United States, underage youth consumed 11.73% in 2011 and 8.6% in 2016. Underage consumption was responsible for 10% of the total sales revenue for alcohol in 2011 and 7.4% in 2016.[32] The alcohol industry would take a huge hit if underage drinking were to stop. The industry relies on underage drinkers for two reasons: the amount of alcohol they consume and the fact that many pathological underage drinkers will become pathological adult drinkers, a group that accounts for $25.8 billion, or 20.1%, of the consumer expenditures for alcohol.[33,34] According to the CDC, more than 3,900 deaths and 225,000 years of potential life are lost to excessive drinking by underage people.[35]

Drinking by high school and college students continues to be widespread, despite the fact that it is illegal for virtually all high school students and for most college students to purchase these beverages. In 2022, 61.% of high school seniors reported having drunk alcohol (more than a few sips) at least once in their lifetime, with 51.9% in the past year, and 28.4% in the past 30 days.[11] In that same year, 16.8% of high school seniors reported having been drunk during the past 30 days.[11] Another analysis showed that nearly 26% of all underage drinkers meet clinical criteria for alcohol abuse or dependence, compared with 9.6% of adult drinkers.[34,36,37] College students reported an even higher prevalence of drinking. Among college students in 2022, 49.6% consumed any alcohol during the past 30 days; 24.1% reported binge drinking in the past 2 weeks.[38] The rate of binge drinking among all college students has fluctuated over the recent years, from 31.4% (2011), to 30.3% (2013), to 33.7% (2014), to 30.4% (2015), to 32.9% (2016), to 29.7%, (2017), and to 29.8% (2018).[39-47]

Most of those who experiment with alcohol begin their use in a social context and become light or moderate drinkers. Alcohol use is reinforcing in two ways: It lowers anxieties and produces a mild euphoria. For many people, alcohol use does not become a significant problem, but about 6.7% will develop **Alcohol Use Disorder (AUD)**.[48] Alcohol use disorder (AUD) is a medical condition in which an individual has an impaired ability to discontinue or control the use of alcohol, even when adverse social, occupational, or health consequences occur.[49] AUD includes conditions referred to as alcohol abuse, alcohol dependence, alcohol addiction, and alcoholism. Some people become **problem drinkers**; that is, they begin to experience personal, interpersonal, legal, or financial problems because of their alcohol consumption. Still others lose control of their drinking and develop a dependence on alcohol. Physical dependence on alcohol and the loss of control over one's drinking are two important characteristics of **alcoholism**. According

Binge drinking consuming five or more alcoholic drinks in a row for males and four or more for females in a 2-hour period

Alcohol use disorder (AUD) a medical condition characterized by an impaired ability to stop or control alcohol use despite adverse social, occupational, or health consequences

Problem drinkers people for whom alcohol consumption results in a medical, social, or other type of problem

Alcoholism a disease characterized by impaired control over drinking, preoccupation with drinking, and continued use of alcohol despite adverse consequences

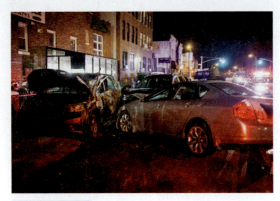

FIGURE 12.4   The risk of a motor vehicle crash increases progressively with alcohol consumption.

© Photo Spirit/Shutterstock

Blood alcohol concentration (BAC) the percentage concentration of alcohol in the blood

to the National Council on Alcoholism and Drug Dependence and the American Society of Addiction Medicine:

> Alcoholism is a primary, chronic disease with genetic, psychosocial, and environmental factors influencing its development and manifestations. The disease is often progressive and fatal. It is characterized by impaired control over drinking, preoccupation with the drug alcohol, use of alcohol despite adverse consequences, and distortions in thinking, most notably denial. Each of these symptoms may be continuous or periodic.[50]

The cost of alcohol abuse and alcoholism in the United States is estimated to be $249 billion.[6] That is $774.69 for every U.S. citizen.[40] Binge drinking accounts for three-quarters of that total.[6] More than 72% of the cost is due to lost productivity, 11% is due to healthcare costs, and 9.4% is from criminal justice costs.[51] Healthcare costs for alcoholics are about twice those for nonalcoholics.[1]

Alcohol and other drugs are contributing factors to a variety of unintentional injuries and injury deaths. The risk of a motor vehicle crash increases progressively with alcohol consumption and **blood alcohol concentration (BAC)** (see **Figure 12.4**).

Risk of a fatal crash is much higher among drivers 16–20 years old compared with drivers 21 and older. The likelihood of a fatal crash for drivers with a BAC of 0.08% compared with those with a zero BAC are: 10 times higher for 16–20 year olds, seven times higher for 21–34 year olds, and six times higher for 35 and older. For male and female drivers, the fatal crash risk is the same in any given age group.[52]

Young drivers are particularly at risk because they are inexperienced drivers and inexperienced drinkers. This combination can be deadly. One study found that that in 2016, 24% of young drivers (15 to 20 years old) who were killed in crashes had blood alcohol concentrations (BACs) of 0.01 g/dL or higher.[53]

Despite these grim statistics, some progress has been made in reducing the overall rate of alcohol-related vehicle deaths. In 1994, 38% of all persons killed in traffic fatalities had a BAC of 0.01 or greater. That figure decreased to 36% in 2014 and to 31% in 2021.[54] The *Healthy People 2030* objective is to reduce the proportion of motor vehicle crash deaths involving an alcohol-impaired driver with a BAC of 0.08 grams/deciliter (g/dL) or higher (see **Box 12.1**).[55] Past success and the promise of future achievement of the target came through public policy changes—raising the minimum legal drinking age, strengthening and enforcing state license revocation laws, and lowering the BAC tolerance levels from 0.10 to 0.08 in some states—stricter law enforcement, and better education for those cited for driving while intoxicated.[54] In October of 2000, President Clinton signed a bill that made 0.08 BAC the national standard. States that refused to impose the standard by October of 2004 would lose millions of dollars of federal highway construction money.[56] By the end of 2004, all 50 states, Puerto Rico, and the District of Columbia had adopted the 0.08 standard. In May of 2013, the National Transportation Safety Board (NHTSA) released new recommendations to states to reduce the legal BAC limit from 0.08 to 0.05.[57]

Alcohol has also been found to increase one's risk for other types of unintentional injuries, such as drowning, falls, fires, and burns. Associations between unintentional injuries and the abuse of other drugs are less well documented, but given knowledge of the effects of such drugs, one can assume that they increase neither the alertness nor the coordination of users.

Alcohol also contributes to intentional violence in the community. For example, alcohol consumption is associated with child abuse, rape and other sexual assault, homicide, assault, suicide, and spouse and partner abuse. Among college students aged 18 to 24, alcohol has been associated with sexual assault, assault, suicide, vandalism, and property damage.[58-60] Studies published between 2002 and 2009 indicated that alcohol is a factor in 50% to 70% of sexual

---

BOX 12.1   *Healthy People 2030*: Objectives

Objective SU-11: Reduce the proportion of motor vehicle crash deaths that involve a drunk driver.
Target-setting method: Minimal statistical significance.
Data source: Fatality Analysis Reporting System (FARS), Department of Transportation (DOT)/NHTSA.
Baseline: 29.3% of motor vehicle crash deaths involved a driver with a BAC of 0.08 g/dL or higher in 2017.
Target: 28.3%.

For Further Thought

The reduction of alcohol-related vehicle deaths is one of the greatest success stories of public health during the twentieth century. What are some factors that have contributed to decreasing alcohol-related vehicle deaths? Similar success has not been achieved for substance abuse–related deaths or drug abuse–related emergency department visits overall. What explanation can you offer for this difference?

Data from U.S. Department of Health and Human Services, Office of Disease Prevention and Health Promotion. (2020). Healthy People 2030. Available at https://health.gov/healthypeople/objectives-and-data

---

assaults on college campuses.[60-62] In 2006, Wisconsin became the 50th state to enact a law designed to protect women at risk of sexual assault by acquaintances at social gatherings where alcohol is served. A person convicted under the law can be fined up to $100,000 and sentenced up to 25 years in prison.[60]

Another community health problem resulting from drinking is **fetal alcohol spectrum disorder (FASD)**. FASDs can result in a range of intellectual and behavioral problems, appearing at any time during childhood and last a lifetime.[63] FASDs are caused by drinking during pregnancy and include diagnoses, such as fetal alcohol syndrome (FAS), alcohol-related birth defects (ARBD), and alcohol-related neurodevelopmental disorders (ARND). Prevalence of FASD in the United States is difficult to determine because there is no universal method for tracking individual cases. Estimates vary greatly, from 0.3 cases of FASD per 1,000 live births to 9.0 cases per 1,000 live births.[64,65] FASD costs society thousands of dollars over a diagnosed person's lifetime. Costs can be attributable to medical treatment for pre- and postnatal growth defects requiring surgery; services for developmentally disabled children; home health care, special education, social services, training and supervision, and institutional care for affected individuals; and lost productivity. It is estimated that the lifetime cost for one individual with FASD is $2 million.[66] For FAS cases alone, the annual cost to the United States is estimated at over $4 billion.[66]

> **Fetal alcohol spectrum disorder (FASD)** a range of disorders caused by prenatal exposure to alcohol. FASD refers to conditions, such as fetal alcohol syndrome (FAS), fetal alcohol effects (FAE), alcohol-related neurodevelopmental disorder (ARND), and alcohol-related birth defects (ARBD)

Nicotine

Nicotine is the psychoactive and addictive drug present in tobacco products, such as cigarettes, e-cigarettes, cigars, smokeless or "spit" tobacco (chewing tobacco and snuff), and pipe tobacco. An estimated 41 million Americans aged 12 or older, or 14.6% of persons in that age group, used a tobacco product in the past 30 days.[67] Among young adults aged 19–30, cigarette smoking has been declining steadily since 2004 and reached new historic lows in 2022. Significant decreases were seen in cigarette usage rates in the past 12 month use, past 30 day use, daily use, and smoking a half pack or more per day over the past 5 years and 10 years[67]

The use of electronic cigarettes, or e-cigarettes, is emerging as a concern. An estimated 23.5 million (8.3%) Americans aged 12 or older vaped nicotine in the last 30 days.[67] E-cigarettes are categorized as electronic nicotine delivery systems (ENDS). Through the use of ENDS, a liquid that contains nicotine and other ingredients is heated into an aerosol that is then inhaled by the user.[68] The rate of vaping nicotine in the past 30 days was 17.2% for young adults in 2022 with the highest rates at ages 21–24 (22.1–22.8%); however, e-cigarettes have the highest use of all tobacco products among high school students.[11] In recent years, nicotine vaping has become the more common way for teens to use nicotine,[10] The most popular e-cigarette among teenagers is JUUL, which is shaped like a USB drive and does not produce visible emissions; this makes it more discreet and desirable to teenagers.[69] Some JUUL "pods" have about the same amount of nicotine as an entire pack of cigarettes, making the product highly dangerous and highly addictive.[69] Rates of vaping in high school students have nearly doubled between 2015 and 2019, an alarmingly sharp rise in a short period of time.[11] However, the percentage of

12th grade students who vaped nicotine within the last 12 months in 2022 was 27%, as it was in 2021.[10] In both of these years, the survey took place after the onset of the pandemic. These levels are significantly lower than they were during the pre-pandemic years of 2020 and 2019, when the prevalence level was 35% in both years.[10] The decline from 35% in 2020 to 27% in 2021 is the largest 1-year decline recorded for 12th grade students since the survey began tracking nicotine vaping in 2017.[10] Because the health effects of e-cigarette use is still evolving, usage is a major health concern.

The consequences of tobacco use on individuals and communities are devastating. Tobacco use is the single most preventable cause of disease, disability, and death in the United States. The health consequences of tobacco use are familiar to all (see **Box 12.2**). They include increased risks for heart disease, lung cancer, chronic obstructive lung disease, stroke, emphysema, and other conditions. Each year in the United States, smoking results in approximately 480,000 premature deaths and 5.1 million years of potential life lost.[70-72] Worldwide, tobacco use results in approximately 6 million premature deaths each year; by 2030, this number is expected to rise to 8 million per year.[73] After a multistate outbreak of severe lung illnesses in 2019, the CDC created a new term—e-cigarette or vaping product use-associated lung injury (EVALI).[74] In 2020, there were over 2,800 EVALI hospitalizations and 68 deaths in the United States.[74] Preliminary laboratory data indicated that tetrahydrocannabinol (THC) and vitamin E acetate are strongly linked to the EVALI outbreak.[74] As a result, the CDC and U.S. Food and Drug Administration (FDA) recommended that e-cigarettes or vaping products containing THC not be used by anyone, especially youth, young adults, and pregnant women and that vitamin E acetate not be added to e-cigarettes.[65,74]

The economic cost of tobacco smoking in the United States is estimated at more than $300 billion per year.[5] More than half of this total, $156 billion, is due to lost productivity; the remainder is due to healthcare costs.[5] A significant portion of the healthcare costs attributed to smoking (43%) are paid with government funds, including Medicaid and Medicare.[1] Inasmuch as tobacco use and nicotine addiction increase the cost of these programs, they clearly add to the economic burden on society.

BOX 12.2   Eleven Great Public Health Achievements, 2000–2020: Tobacco Control

Less Smoke, More Prevention

During the last century, smoking went from being an accepted norm to being recognized as the number one preventable cause of death and disability in the United States. The first decade of the twenty-first century saw an increase in the adoption of policies at the federal, state, and local levels designed to prevent and reduce tobacco use. Major achievements include the following:

- Adoption of the Family Smoking Prevention and Tobacco Control Act (Tobacco Control Act) in 2009, which gives the U.S. Food and Drug Administration (FDA) the authority to regulate tobacco
- Adoption of comprehensive smoke-free laws by 25 states and the District of Columbia by 2010 and 30 states by 2012
- The largest federal cigarette tax increase in history

- Increased restrictions on advertising and marketing of tobacco products to youth
- The T21 tobacco legislation, which raised the federal minimum age for the sale of tobacco products from 18 to 21 years

Although substantial progress has been made, and millions of lives have been saved, increased prevention efforts are needed to reduce the impact of tobacco use on public health. Each year, smoking still kills more people than all of the following health hazards combined:

- HIV
- Alcohol abuse
- Drug use/misuse
- Motor vehicle crash injuries
- Murders
- Suicides

Data from U.S. Food and Drug Administration. (2013). *Overview of the Family Smoking Prevention and Tobacco Control Act: Consumer fact sheet.* Available at https://www.fda.gov/tobacco-products/rules-regulations-and-guidance/family-smoking-prevention-and-tobacco-control-act-overview; Centers for Disease Control and Prevention. (2011). Ten great public health achievements—United States, 2001-2010. *Morbidity and Mortality Weekly Report, 60*(19), 619–623. Available at https://www.cdc.gov/mmwr/preview/mmwrhtml/mm6019a5.htm; Murphy S. L., Xu, J. Q., & Kochanek, K. D. (2013). Deaths: Final data for 2010. *National Vital Statistics Reports, 61*(4). National Center for Health Statistics. Available at http://www.cdc.gov/nchs/data/nvsr/nvsr61/nvsr61_04.pdf; U.S. Food and Drug Administration. (2020, January 15). *Newly signed legislation raises federal minimum age of sale of tobacco products to 21.* Available at https://www.fda.gov/tobacco-products/retail-sales-tobacco-products/tobacco-21#:~:text=On%20Dec.,from%2018%20to%2021%20years

Well-established research findings have demonstrated that one does not have to use tobacco products to be adversely affected. The 1986 U.S. Surgeon General's report on the effects of **environmental tobacco smoke (ETS; secondhand smoke)** indicated that adults and children who inhale the tobacco smoke of others (passive smoking) are also at increased risk for cardiac and respiratory illnesses.[75] These findings resulted in new smoking regulations in many public indoor environments. Then, in December 1992, the U.S. Environmental Protection Agency (EPA) released the report titled, *Respiratory Health Effects of Passive Smoking: Lung Cancer and Other Disorders.*[76] This report stated that ETS is a human class A carcinogen (the same class that contains asbestos) and that it is responsible for 42,000 deaths annually among nonsmoking Americans.[76] Furthermore, it stated that ETS exposure is causally associated with as many as 150,000 to 300,000 cases of lower respiratory infections (such as bronchitis and pneumonia) in infants and young children up to 18 months of age. The EPA study also found that ETS aggravates asthma in children and is a risk factor for new cases of childhood asthma.[76,78] From 2013 to 2014, approximately 58 million Americans were exposed to secondhand smoke and 37.9% were between the ages of 3 and 11 years old.[78] There has been a decrease in the last 60 years in the percentage of nonsmokers exposed to secondhand smoke.[79] Potential reasons for the decline in secondhand smoke exposure include: laws that prohibit smoking in the workplace, restaurants, and bars; decreased prevalence of smoking; increased public awareness of the health risks of secondhand smoke, and people voluntarily not smoking in homes.[79]

For many years, the enforcement of state laws prohibiting the sale of cigarettes and other tobacco products to minors was varied and inconsistent. In other cases, cigarettes could easily be purchased by youth from vending machines. The problem of uneven state tobacco laws regarding sales to minors and the lack of enforcement of these laws was remedied in 1992 by the **Synar Amendment**, a federal law that requires all states to adopt legislation that prohibits the sale and distribution of tobacco products to people under age 18. States that do not comply with this regulation lose federal dollars for alcohol, tobacco, and other drug prevention and treatment programs.[80] States may choose to adopt stricter regulations regarding the sale of tobacco products to minors. For example, in late 2013, New York state passed a law that raised the legal age to purchase tobacco products from 18 to 21. In 2016, California became the second state to enact such legislation. In December of 2019, legislation was signed to raise the federal minimum age of sale of tobacco products from 18 to 21 years with a movement called Tobacco 21 or T21. It is illegal for any retailer to sell any tobacco product, including cigarettes, cigars, and e-cigarettes to any person under the age of 21.[81] Raising the age limit of the sale of tobacco is designed to make tobacco products less accessible and less attractive to youth. Every day, nearly 2,500 children smoke their first cigarette, with more than 400 becoming daily cigarette smokers.[82] In addition, about one in five people over the age of 12 who vaped were underage.[67] Children can become addicted before they are old enough to understand the risks.

On June 22, 2009, President Obama signed the Family Smoking Prevention and Tobacco Control Act into law, giving the FDA oversight over tobacco products.[83] The law also banned deceptive marketing practices by the tobacco industry, specifically the use of the words "light," "low," or "mild" on cigarette packaging. The sale of candy-, fruit-, and liquor-flavored cigarettes was banned in 2006. It remains to be seen how effective this new law will be in lowering smoking rates among young Americans. The tobacco industry spends billions of dollars each year on advertising and promotions to sell its products. Another proven way to reduce smoking rates is to increase taxes on cigarettes, thereby increasing the financial cost of smoking. Nationally, every 10% increase in cigarette prices reduces youth smoking by about 7% and total cigarette consumption by about 4%.[84] Cigarettes are taxed at the federal level, state level, and, in some jurisdictions, at the county or city level. In 2009, the federal tax increased to $1.01 per pack. In 2023, the average state tax was $1.93, up from the 2016 rate of $1.61 per pack.[84] Perhaps raising the cost of cigarettes in this manner will reduce smoking rates among young people.

In May of 2016, the FDA extended its authority to regulate tobacco products to ENDS, including e-cigarettes, in response to the significant rise in e-cigarette use.[72] Prior to this date, retailers could sell e-cigarettes to people under the age of 18.[72]

Environmental tobacco smoke (ETS; secondhand smoke) tobacco smoke in the environment that is a mixture of mainstream and sidestream smoke, and that can be inhaled by nearby or transient nonsmokers

Synar Amendment federal law that requires states to set the minimum legal age for purchasing tobacco products at 18 years and requires states to enforce this law

Over-the-counter (OTC) drugs (nonprescription drugs) drugs (except tobacco and alcohol) that can be legally purchased without a physician's prescription

U.S. Food and Drug Administration (FDA) a federal agency within the U.S. Department of Health and Human Services charged with ensuring the safety and efficacy of all prescription and nonprescription drugs

Over-the-Counter Drugs

Over-the-counter (OTC) drugs are those legal drugs, with the exception of tobacco and alcohol, which can be purchased without a physician's prescription. Included in this category are internal analgesics, such as aspirin, acetaminophen (Tylenol), and ibuprofen (Advil); cough and cold remedies (Robitussin); emetics; laxatives; mouthwashes; vitamins; and many others. Thousands of different OTC products are sold by pharmacies, supermarkets, convenience stores, and in vending machines. These products are manufactured and sold to those who self-diagnose and self-medicate their own illnesses.

Over-the-counter drugs are carefully regulated by the **U.S. Food and Drug Administration (FDA)**, an agency of the U.S. Department of Health and Human Services (HHS). The FDA ensures the safety and effectiveness of these products when they are used according to their label directions. There is no person or agency that supervises the actual sale or use of these substances.

Naturally, some of these substances are misused and abused. Examples of misuse are not following the dosage directions or using the drugs after their expiration date. A specific example of OTC drug misuse is the taking of laxatives or emetics to lose weight or to avoid gaining weight. Other OTC drugs that are often misused are sedative antihistamines, laxatives, and decongestants. Examples include dextromethorphan (DXM), a cough suppressant and loperamide, an anti-diarrheal. Common cold OTC products that contain pseudoephedrine were the target of people whose intent was to manufacture methamphetamine, which led to tighter regulation by the FDA. In 2006, the Combat Methamphetamine Epidemic Act of 2005 was signed into law. The law requires, among other things, that retailers limit the sale of pseudoephedrine products and place pseudoephedrine products where customers do not have direct access to such products before a sale is made, such as behind the pharmacy counter.[85]

Most OTC drugs provide only symptomatic relief and do not provide a cure. For example, cough and cold remedies relieve the discomfort that accompanies a cold but do not in any way rid a person of the cold virus that is causing these symptoms. Therefore, a real danger of OTC drug misuse is that symptoms that should be brought to the attention of a physician remain unreported. Another danger is that those who misuse these drugs may become dependent, thus unable to live normally without them. Finally, misuse of OTC drugs may establish a pattern of dependency that predisposes the user to developing dependent relationships with prescription drugs or illicit drugs.

Prescription Drugs

Because all prescription drugs have serious side effects for some people, they can be purchased only with a physician's (or dentist's) written instructions (prescription). Like OTC drugs, prescription drugs are carefully regulated by the FDA. The written prescription connotes that the prescribed drugs are being taken by the patient under the prescribing physician's supervision. Each prescription includes the patient's name, the amount to be dispensed, and the dosage. The percentage of people in the United States using at least one prescription drug during the past month is estimated at 48.6.[86] Nonetheless, prescription drugs are also subject to misuse. Types of misuse include those previously cited for the OTC drugs and also the giving of one person's prescription drug to another. Furthermore, certain prescription drugs, such as stimulants (amphetamines), depressants (Valium), and prescription opioid pain relievers (fentanyl, morphine, codeine) have a higher potential for misuse than others. Because prescription drugs are usually stronger or more concentrated than OTC drugs, there is a greater risk of developing dependence or taking an overdose from these drugs. Those who develop dependence may try to obtain duplicate prescriptions from other physicians or steal the drugs from hospital dispensaries or pharmacies.

In recent years, the number of deaths from unintentional drug overdoses has risen to unprecedented levels. The misuse of opioid pain relievers, in particular, has risen to epidemic proportions. Between 2000 and 2014, the rate of overdose deaths in the United States involving opioids, including heroin and prescription opioid pain relievers, increased by 200%.[85] During that time period, more than 165,000 overdose deaths involving prescription opioids occurred, and overdose deaths involving prescription opioids quadrupled.[86-89] Drug overdose deaths for just the year 2017 totaled 70,237, about half of the amount of the 14-year time period of 2000–2014.[90] In 2021, opioids were involved in 75.4% of all drug overdose deaths, an increase from 67.8% in 2017.[91] A drug that can reverse the effects of opioid overdose called Naloxone (brand name Narcan or Evzio) is being used increasingly throughout communities and can be life-saving if administered in time.[88]

The increase in overdoses involving prescription opioids is influenced by several factors. First, prescription opioids are potent pain relievers, with similar effects to heroin.[92] Their potency makes them highly addictive. Second, when mixed with illicit drugs, such as cocaine and heroin, they can be lethal. Third, they have been increasingly available. The primary factor contributing to overdoses is an increase in prescriptions for opioid pain relievers.[93] Prescription opioid misuse can lead to dependency. Use of prescription opioids is a risk factor for heroin use; some prescription opioid users may progress to heroin.[92] There were six times as many people dying from drug overdose in 2021 compared with 1999.[94] Opioid overdose deaths numbered nearly 645,000 between 1999-2021.[94] In 2021, over 75% of all drug overdose deaths involved opioids.[94]

Since the 1990s, there have been three waves of overdose deaths involving opioids (**Figure 12.5**). The categories depicted in Figure 12.5 are: Any Opioid, Other Synthetic Opioids (tramadol, fentanyl, prescribed or illicitly manufactured), and Commonly Prescribed Opioids (natural and semi-synthetic opioids and methadone).

Wave 1: 1990s: prescriptions of opioids increased as well as deaths involving prescription opioids.

Wave 2: 2010: rapid increase of overdose deaths involving heroin

Wave 3: 2013: rise in overdose deaths involving synthetic opioids, particularly those manufactured with fentanyl.

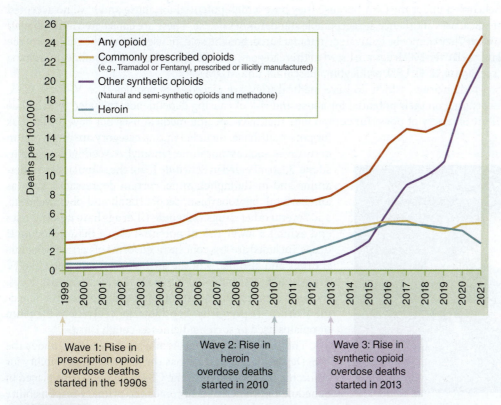

FIGURE 12.5   Three waves of opioid overdose deaths.

Reproduced from CDC. (2024, February 10). Three waves of opioid overdose deaths. Available at https://www.cdc.gov/overdose-prevention /media/images/sharable-graphics/OverdosePrevention-3-waves-opioid-overdose-deaths-1999-2021.png

The CDC's efforts to combat the opioid epidemic includes monitoring trends; advancing research; building state, local, and tribal capacity; supporting providers and healthcare systems; partnering with public safety officials and community organizations; and increasing public awareness.[94] Collaboration and coordinated efforts are essential to prevent opioid misuse and overdose deaths. Prescription drug misuse leads to other serious consequences. Prescription drug misuse puts an additional strain on our already overburdened emergency departments. There were an estimated total of 7,714,521 drug-related ED visits in the United States in 2022. In that year, 21.2% of all drug-related ED visits were polysubstance, meaning involving more than one substance.[95] Table 6 presents each substance's frequency of polysubstance drug-related ED visits. Prescription drug misuse can also lead to the development of drug-resistant strains of pathogens. When patients fail to complete the entire antibiotic treatment (e.g., 3 days of a 10-day prescription), some of the bacteria survive and multiply, reinfecting the body with drug-resistant organisms. Thus, succeeding treatments are less effective. When this strain of the disease is transmitted to another, the antibiotic treatment fails. New drugs are then needed to treat these patients. As drug misuse continues to occur, bacteria become resistant to multiple drugs. Multidrug-resistant tuberculosis (MDR-TB) is an example. Another example is the growing number of reports of community-associated methicillin-resistant *Staphylococcus aureus* (CA-MRSA) infections. These are bacterial infections of the skin or other organs that are resistant to some antibiotics. The prevalence of MDR-TB and the increase in the incidence of CA-MRSA point both to the dangers of drug misuse and the need to continue to develop new antibiotics for the treatment of bacterial infections.

Controlled Substances and Illicit (Illegal) Drugs

Controlled substances are those regulated by the **Controlled Substances Act of 1970 (CSA; Comprehensive Drug Abuse Control Act of 1970)**. Many of the drugs discussed next belong to Schedule I under the CSA because they have a high potential for abuse and have no accepted medical uses and, hence, no acceptable standards of safe use. These are considered **illicit (illegal) drugs**. They cannot be cultivated, manufactured, bought, sold, or used within the confines of the law. Well over 150 drugs are listed in this category, including heroin, methaqualone, marijuana (see **Figure 12.6**), LSD, psilocybin, mescaline, and MDMA.[93]

Other drugs, which do have medical uses, are placed in Schedules II to V of the CSA, depending on their potential for abuse and risk of causing dependence. Included in Schedule II are a variety of powerful compounds that have specific medical uses but have a high risk for potential abuse. Included in this category are many opium derivatives, such as morphine, fentanyl, oxycodone, and methadone. Also included in Schedule II are the stimulants amphetamine and methamphetamine, certain depressants, such as amobarbital, pentobarbital, secobarbital, and phencyclidine, and several other drugs. Schedule III drugs have medical uses and exhibit a lower risk of potential abuse than Schedule II drugs. Included are less concentrated forms of certain Schedule II drugs and also many of the anabolic steroids. Schedule IV drugs exhibit less potential for abuse than Schedule III drugs. Included are many milder stimulants and depressants. Schedule V drugs are primarily very dilute concentrations of opium or opiates used in such medicines as cough syrups.[96]

The **Drug Enforcement Administration (DEA)**, under the U.S. Department of Justice, has the primary responsibility for enforcing the provisions of the CSA. Once a drug is placed in Schedule I of the CSA, it becomes the primary responsibility of the DEA to interdict the trafficking (manufacturing, distribution, and sales) of the substance. The only sources of these drugs are illegal growers and manufacturers. Schedule II to V

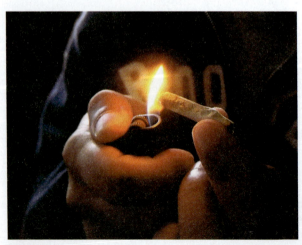

FIGURE 12.6   Marijuana is the nation's most popular drug.

© Tiburon Studios/Shutterstock

substances often reach the street illegally, either by illegal production (in clandestine labs) or by diversion of legally manufactured prescription drugs.

Marijuana

After alcohol, **marijuana** is the most commonly used psychotropic drug used in the United States.[82] Twenty-three states, two territories, and the District of Columbia have legalized small amounts of cannabis (marijuana) for adult recreational use.[97] The legal status of marijuana at the state level, as well as how it is talked about in the literature and society at large, is changing. The term "marijuana" is increasingly being replaced with the term "cannabis."[38] Laws are continually changing and it is important to understand the health effects and impact of marijuana use. "Pot" and the related products, hashish and hash oil, are derived from the hemp plant, *Cannabis sativa* or *Cannabis indica*. These plants contain THC, a mind-altering chemical, along with other compounds.[82] The products are most commonly used by smoking but can also be ingested. Although marijuana abuse has declined, it remains a concern for several reasons. The act of smoking is detrimental to one's health, and marijuana smoking often occurs in conjunction with the drinking of alcohol or the use of other drugs. The effects of **polydrug use** (the use of more than one drug at a time) may be more serious than those of single-drug use. Finally, as is true of all drugs, the adolescent who uses marijuana is delaying the accomplishment of developmental tasks, such as attaining an adult self-identity, achieving independence, and developing the interpersonal skills necessary for successful independent living.

In a 2022 survey, the percentage of high school seniors who reported having smoked marijuana at least once in their lives was 38.3%, down from 43.7% in 2019.[10] Also, 20.2% reported having smoked marijuana in the past 30 days, a slight decrease from 22.3% in 2019.[10] As with many of the other drugs, the prevalence of marijuana use has waxed and waned over the past 30 years. The perceived risk of use is one of the factors that seems to contribute to the level of use. In 1992, when 76.5% of high school seniors felt there was great risk associated with regular marijuana use, the 30-day use prevalence was 11.9%. In 2022, when 27.6% of seniors felt there was great risk associated with regular marijuana use, the 30-day use prevalence was 20.2%.[10] One of the objectives of *Healthy People 2030* is to increase the proportion of adolescents who think substance abuse is risky. Another measurement of students' attitudes is disapproval rates. From 2009 to 2019, disapproval rates among high school seniors for trying marijuana once or twice, smoking marijuana occasionally, or regularly using marijuana have steadily declined. Another objective of *Healthy People 2030* is to reduce the proportion of adolescents reporting use of marijuana during the past 30 days (see **Box 12.3**).

The acute health effects of marijuana use include reduced concentration, slowed reaction time, impaired short-term memory, and impaired judgment. Naturally, these effects can have serious consequences for someone operating a motor vehicle or other machinery or can even result in a medical emergency. Marijuana use in combination with other drugs can be especially

Marijuana dried plant parts of the hemp plant, *Cannabis sativa* or *Cannabis indica*

Polydrug use concurrent use of multiple drugs

BOX 12.3   *Healthy People 2030:* Objectives

Objective SU-06: Reduce the proportion of adolescents reporting use of marijuana during the past 30 days.
Baseline: 6.7% of adolescents aged 12 to 17 years reported use of marijuana in the past 30 days in 2018.
Target: 5.8%
Target-setting method: Projection
Data source: National Survey on Drug Use and Health (NSDUH), Substance Abuse and Mental Health Services Administration (SAMHSA)

For Further Thought

Attitudes and beliefs are often key factors influencing drug-taking behavior among adolescents. Studies have shown that when there is a high level of disapproval of marijuana use by adolescents, the prevalence of marijuana use declines. Conversely, an increase in marijuana use occurs when there is an apparent decline in those expressing strong disapproval of use. How strong are prevailing feelings of disapproval of marijuana use in your community? Do adolescents in your community feel that it is "OK" to try marijuana once or twice?

Data from U.S. Department of Health and Human Services, Office of Disease Prevention and Health Promotion. (2020). *Healthy People 2030.* Available at https://health.gov/healthypeople/objectives-and-data

Amotivational syndrome a pattern of behavior characterized by apathy, loss of effectiveness, and a more passive, introverted personality

dangerous because drugs in combination may affect the brain differently. Marijuana, used alone or with one or more other drugs, was involved in an estimated 455,668 emergency department visits in 2011 and slightly declined to 407,995 in 2022.[98]

The chronic effects of smoking marijuana include damage to the respiratory system by the smoke itself and, for some, the development of a controversial condition known as **amotivational syndrome**. Amotivational syndrome has been described as a chronic apathy toward maturation and the achievement of the developmental tasks listed previously (e.g., developing skills for independent living, setting and achieving goals, and developing an adult self-identity). In addition, there is now evidence that long-term marijuana users experience physiologic and psychological withdrawal symptoms. Although these "unpleasant behavioral symptoms are less obvious than those for heroin or alcohol, they are significant and do perhaps contribute to continued drug use."[99] Further evidence of the dependence-producing nature of marijuana is the number of persons seeking admission to treatment programs. Admissions to treatment programs for marijuana use peaked in 2009 with 405,400 admissions, to an all-time low of 129,343 in 2021, down from 250,786 in 2017.[98] Admissions due to marijuana were surpassed by admissions due to opiates, alcohol, and stimulants. In 2021, marijuana was reported as the primary drug of abuse for approximately 8.7% of those aged 12 and older who entered drug treatment programs in the United States, a decrease from 13% in 2017.[67,100] Finally, one of the chief concerns with marijuana is that those who use marijuana are more likely to use other licit and illicit drug and develop addictions to other substances.[101]

Synthetic Marijuana

Another cause for concern is the manufacture, distribution, and use of synthetic marijuana or synthetic cannabinoids. Synthetic marijuana is a category of drugs that are chemically produced and have properties similar to THC, the psychoactive ingredient found in marijuana.[102] These drugs are typically sold in the form of small packets of plant material that are laced with synthetic THC-like compounds.[102] They may be labeled as incense or potpourri and have been sold at convenience stores, gas stations, and online. Street names include K2 or "Spice." Synthetic marijuana has been deceptively marketed as a "safe," legal alternative to marijuana.[102] Among 8th, 10th, and 12th grade students, use of synthetic marijuana steadily declined from 8% in 2012 to 2.3% in 2022.[10] However, attitudes about the perceived harmfulness of synthetic marijuana pose a risk, with 29.0% of 10th graders seeing perceived occasional use as harmful.[10]

Despite safety claims by sellers, synthetic marijuana poses a serious threat to public health. It has the potential for abuse and other adverse health effects, and its long-term effects are still unknown. Some users have reported immediate effects similar to those of marijuana, while others have reported symptoms, such as rapid heart rate, increased blood pressure, hallucinations, agitation, and vomiting.[102]

To protect the public against these harms, in March of 2011, five chemicals used to produce synthetic marijuana were temporarily placed into Schedule I of the Controlled Substances Act, in accordance with the CSA's emergency scheduling provision.[103] In July of 2012, President Obama signed the Synthetic Drug Abuse Prevention Act of 2012 (SDAPA). The SDAPA permanently places specific known classes of cannabimimetic agents, the chemicals used to produce synthetic marijuana, into Schedule I of the CSA.[104] It also expands the list of temporarily scheduled chemicals. States also have taken steps to ban synthetic drugs. Since 2011, all 50 states have banned synthetic marijuana.[105] In 2012, the DEA initiated Project Synergy, a collaborative international effort to target and take down synthetic drug traffickers. In June of 2013, it was announced that the effort resulted in more than 227 arrests and the seizure of 1,252 kilograms of synthetic marijuana.[106]

Despite these efforts, synthetic marijuana laws are difficult to enforce. One challenge lies in identifying synthetic marijuana. Products are labeled as incense or potpourri, or as legal, not as synthetic, marijuana. They must be tested in a lab to determine whether they contain any banned cannabimimetic agents. Another challenge is that manufacturers are discovering and utilizing new classes of cannabimimetic agents that are not already banned by federal or state laws, thus finding ways to get around the law to produce synthetic marijuana.

Narcotics: Opium, Morphine, Heroin, and Others

Opium and its derivatives, morphine and heroin, come from the oriental poppy plant, *Papaver somniferum*. These **narcotics** numb the senses and reduce pain. As such, they have a high potential for abuse. The sharp increase in narcotic use has been fueled, in part, by the prescription opioid epidemic. Heroin is a less-expensive alternative to prescription opioids, while users experience a similar effect. Users who become dependent on prescription opioids may seek out heroin because it is a less expensive option. In 2022, 0.3%, of 12th grade students reported using heroin in the past year, up from 0.1% in 2021.[107]

Opium poppies do not grow in the continental United States. Heroin arrives in the United States from four geographic areas: Southwest Asia, Southeast Asia, Mexico, and South America. Most of the heroin available in the United States now enters across the southwestern border. Although significant amounts of heroin reaching the United States originate in South America, the proportion of heroin seizures in which the heroin originated in Mexico has grown. Mexican heroin production has increased in recent years, and the influence of Mexican drug trafficking organizations is expanding.[108] Deaths involving heroin overdose rose from 1,960 in 1999 to 15,482 in 2017, then decreased to 13,165 deaths in 2020 and 9,173 deaths in 2021.[108]

Narcotics produce euphoria, analgesia, and drowsiness. They reduce anxiety and pain without affecting motor activity the way alcohol and barbiturates do. If use continues, the body makes physiologic adjustments to the presence of the drug. This **tolerance** means that larger and larger doses are required to achieve the same euphoria and numbing as the initial dose. Whereas tolerance develops rapidly to the euphoric effects, the depressing effects on respiration may continue to increase with dose level, increasing the risk of a fatal overdose. As the cost of the drug addiction becomes higher, the user may attempt to quit. Because the body has become physically dependent on the drug, this results in withdrawal symptoms. People addicted to heroin have a difficult time changing their lifestyle for several reasons. First, there is the addiction itself, both physical and psychological. Often, there are underlying psychosocial problems as well, such as poor self-image, lack of job skills, and absence of supporting family and friends. People with substance use disorder usually mistrust official programs set up to help them. They are usually in poor health mentally and physically. Because the duration of action of heroin is only 4 to 5 hours, the user is usually too concerned with finding the next dose or recovering from the previous one to be productive in the community.

The community is affected by more than just the loss of productivity. The user must obtain money to purchase heroin, and the price of the addiction can be high—as much as $200 per day. The money is usually obtained illegally through burglaries, thefts, robberies, muggings, prostitution (male and female), and selling drugs. The result is not only a deteriorating community but also epidemics of sexually transmitted diseases, such as gonorrhea, syphilis, chlamydia, herpes, and HIV. Because most people addicted to heroin inject the drug, there are also epidemics of bloodborne diseases, such as those caused by HIV and hepatitis viruses. In 2015, a rural county in Indiana experienced an outbreak of HIV that was associated with the use of heroin that was taken intravenously.[109]

In this way, drug abuse requires many community and public health resources. People who turn to dealing drugs to support their addiction increase the availability of the drug and may introduce it to first-time users. When a person's drug use leads to criminal activity, it requires the resources of the criminal justice system when they are arrested, prosecuted, incarcerated, and rehabilitated.

Cocaine and Crack Cocaine

Cocaine is the psychoactive ingredient in the leaves of the coca plant, *Erythroxylon coca*, which grows in the Andes mountains of South America. Cocaine is a **stimulant**; that is, it increases the activity of the central nervous system. For centuries, natives of the Andes mountains have chewed the leaves to improve stamina during work and long treks. In its more purified forms, as a salt (white powder) or dried paste (crack), cocaine is a powerful euphoriant/stimulant and highly addictive. The effects of cocaine occur almost immediately and can last from several

---

Narcotics drugs derived from or chemically related to opium that reduce pain and induce stupor, such as morphine

Tolerance physiological and enzymatic adjustments that occur in response to the chronic presence of drugs, which are reflected in the need for ever-increasing doses

Cocaine the psychoactive ingredient in the leaves of the coca plant, *Erythroxylon coca*, which, when refined, is a powerful stimulant/euphoriant

Stimulant a drug that increases the activity of the central nervous system

minutes to an hour.[110] When cocaine is taken in combination with other substances like alcohol, heroin, and marijuana, the risk of harm greatly increases.[110]

Cocaine use among high school seniors peaked in 1985, when 13.1% reported use within the past year. By 1992, the annual prevalence dropped to only 3.1%, but by 1999, the figure had doubled to 6.2%.[11] In 2022, the annual prevalence was 1.5%, with 5.3 million Americans aged 12 and older using cocaine.[67] Cocaine remains a serious drug problem in the United States.

Hallucinogens

Hallucinogens are drugs that produce illusions, hallucinations, and other changes in one's perceptions of the environment. These effects are due to the phenomenon known as **synesthesia**, a mixing of the senses. Hallucinogens include both naturally derived drugs, such as mescaline, from the peyote cactus; and psilocybin and psilocin, from the psilocybin mushroom; and synthetic drugs, such as lysergic acid diethylamide (LSD). In some cases, hallucinogens can be addictive and tolerance does occur. Although overdose deaths are rare, "bad trips" (unpleasant experiences) do occur, and a few people have experienced permanent visual disturbances. Because there are no legal sources for these drugs, users are always at risk for taking fake, impure, or adulterated drugs.

Stimulants

As previously mentioned, stimulants are drugs that increase the activity level of the central nervous system. Examples include the amphetamines, such as amphetamine itself (bennies), dextroamphetamine (dexies), methamphetamine (meth), dextromethamphetamine (ice); methylphenidate (Ritalin); and methcathinone (cat). These drugs cause the release of high levels of the neurotransmitter dopamine, which stimulates brain cells. Tolerance builds quickly, so users must escalate their doses rapidly. Chronic users can develop tremors and confusion, aggressiveness, and paranoia. The long-term effects include memory loss and permanent brain damage.[102]

Amphetamines are Schedule II prescription drugs that have been widely misused for many years. Increased regulatory efforts in the 1970s probably contributed to the rise in the cocaine trade in the 1980s. When cocaine use declined in the late 1980s, there was a resurgence of amphetamine use, primarily **methamphetamine**, also known as "crystal," "crank," "speed," "go fast," or just "meth." At first, the clandestine labs that produced methamphetamine, and those abusing the substance, were concentrated primarily in the southwestern states. However, by 1995, production and use had spread to the Midwest, and by 1999 methamphetamine use had become the fastest growing drug threat in the United States. Methamphetamine is a highly addictive substance in which the effects come and go quickly, often causing a "binge and crash" cycle.[111] The popularity of amphetamines has been in decline. In 2019, 4.6% of those in grades 8, 10, and 12 reported any amphetamine use in the past year, trending down in 2022 to 3.0%.[10] Annual prevalence of methamphetamine use among those in grades 8, 10, and 12 declined from 4.1% in 1999 to 0.5% in 2022, the lowest reported level.[10] For young adults, the methamphetamine use has stayed between 0.5 and 1.0% since 2008, with a rate of 0.8% in 2022.[10]

Methylphenidate (Ritalin) is a Schedule II drug used to treat attention-deficit/hyperactive disorder. Although not produced in clandestine labs, the drug is often diverted from its intended use and abused by those for whom it was not prescribed.

Depressants

Barbiturates, **benzodiazepines**, **methaqualone**, and other **depressants** slow down the central nervous system. They are attractive to some people because, like alcohol, among the first effects of taking these drugs are the lowering of anxiety and the loss of inhibitions. These effects produce the feeling of a "high," even though these drugs depress the central nervous system. As one continues to use these drugs, like Xanax, tolerance develops, and the user experiences the need for greater and greater doses to feel the same effects that the previous dose provided. Strong physical dependence develops so that abstinence results in severe clinical illness; thus, users of these substances must often rely on medical assistance during detoxification and recovery.

Club Drugs and Designer Drugs

Club drugs is a term for a number of illicit drugs, primarily synthetic, that are most commonly encountered at nightclubs, bars, and parties. These drugs include MDMA, ketamine, GHB, GBL, Rohypnol, LSD, PCP, methamphetamine, and others. They are often taken in combination with alcohol or other drugs. Because these drugs are illegal, there is no guarantee of their safety or even their identity. Long-term effects of club drugs are still under evaluation, but there is evidence that these drugs may cause brain damage.[111,112] MDMA, also known as "Ecstasy" or "Molly," is the most popular of the club drugs. MDMA was initially popular among teens and young adults at raves (all-night dance parties). In recent years, use has spread to a broader audience beyond the nightclub scene.[112] Annual use of MDMA among those in grades 8, 10, and 12 peaked at 6% in 2001, declined to 1.6% in 2019 and to 0.9% in 2022.[10] The prevalence among young adults for MDMA was 3.2% in 2022 with no significant changes from the 5 years prior.[10]

Rohypnol (flunitrazepam) is a powerful depressant in the benzodiazepine group that has achieved notoriety as a date-rape drug because its amnesic and sedative effects, when combined with alcohol, can last up to 8 hours. This drug is a legal prescription drug in more than 50 countries. In the United States, the drug is regarded as more dangerous and less medically useful than other sedatives and is classified Schedule IV substance.

Designer drugs is a term coined in the 1980s to describe drugs synthesized by amateur chemists in secret laboratories. By constantly changing the design of their drugs, these chemists hoped to stay one step ahead of law enforcement. Examples of designer drugs included MDMA (3,4-methylenedioxy-methamphetamine), synthetic narcotics, and dissociative anesthetics, such as PCP (angel dust) and ketamine. Under the Controlled Substance Act of 1970, only those drugs that were listed as illegal were illegal, whereas similar, but slightly altered, drugs were not. The Controlled Substances Analogue Act of 1986 was enacted to reduce the flow of designer drugs into the market and make it easier to prosecute those involved in manufacturing and distributing these drugs. Designer and club drugs are still a problem.

Anabolic Drugs

Anabolic drugs are protein-building drugs. Included are the anabolic/androgenic steroids (AS), testosterone, and human growth hormone (HGH). These drugs have legitimate medical uses, such as the rebuilding of muscles after starvation or disease and the treatment of dwarfism. However, they are sometimes misused by athletes and bodybuilders as a shortcut to increasing muscle mass, strength, and endurance. Misuse of steroids is accompanied by numerous acute and chronic side effects for men, including acne, gynecomastia (the development of breasts), baldness, reduced fertility, and reduction in testicular size. Side effects for women are masculinizing: development of a male physique, increased body hair, failure to ovulate (menstrual irregularities), and a deepening of the voice. Long-term misuse of anabolic steroids can result in psychological dependence, making the discontinuation of use very difficult.[113]

In the late 1980s, it became apparent that increasing numbers of boys and young men of high school and college age were taking anabolic steroids as a shortcut to muscle building or to maturity (see **Figure 12.7**). Because of these trends in the misuse of anabolic steroids, in 1990 the drugs were placed in Schedule III of the Controlled Substance Act. Misuse of steroids increased during the 1990s but has leveled off recently. As with other drugs discussed earlier, "steroids" sold on the Internet may not be authentic. Purchasing such substances online is certainly an example of the phrase "Buyer, beware."

Club drugs a general term for those illicit drugs, primarily synthetic, that are most commonly encountered at night clubs and "raves" (examples include MDMA, GHB, GBL, LSD, PCP, ketamine, Rohypnol, and methamphetamine)

Rohypnol (flunitrazepam) a powerful depressant in the benzodiazepine group that has achieved notoriety as a date-rape drug because it has amnestic and sedative effects, when combined with alcohol, can last up to 8 hours

Designer drugs drugs synthesized illegally that are similar to, but structurally different from, known controlled substances

Anabolic drug compounds, structurally similar to the male hormone testosterone, that increase protein synthesis and thus muscle building

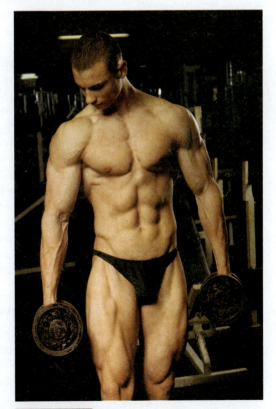

FIGURE 12.7   Misuse of anabolic drugs carries the risk of serious acute and chronic health problems.

© Skydive Erick/Shutterstock

Inhalants

Inhalants are a collection of psychoactive, breathable chemicals. They include paint solvents, motor fuels, cleaners, glues, aerosol sprays, cosmetics, and other types of vapor. Because of their easy availability and low cost, they are often the drug of choice for the young. The primary effect of most of the inhalants is depression. As with alcohol, the user may at first experience a reduction of anxieties and inhibitions, making the user feel high. Continued use may result in hallucinations and loss of consciousness. Many of these chemicals are extremely toxic to the kidneys, liver, and nervous system. Annual use of inhalants among those in grades 8, 10, and 12 peaked at 10.2% in 1995 and was at a low of 2.6% in 2022.[10]

Prevention and Control of Drug Abuse

The prevention and control of alcohol and other drug abuse require a knowledge of the causes of drug-taking behavior, sources of illicit drugs, drug laws, and treatment programs. Also required are community organizing skills, persistence, and cooperation among a vast array of concerned individuals and official and unofficial agencies.

From a community health standpoint, drug abuse tends to be a chronic condition. Thus, the activities of drug abuse and prevention agencies and organizations can be viewed as chronic disease prevention activities. This approach, involving three different levels of prevention, is discussed next in relation to drug abuse prevention and control.

Levels of Prevention

Drug abuse prevention activities can be viewed as primary, secondary, or tertiary, depending on the point of intervention. *Primary prevention* programs are aimed at those who have never used drugs, and their goal is to prevent or forestall the initiation of drug use. Drug education programs that stress primary prevention of drug and alcohol use are most appropriate and successful for children at the elementary school age. In a broader sense, almost any activity that would reduce the likelihood of primary drug use could be considered primary prevention. For example, raising the price of alcohol, increasing cigarette taxes, arresting a neighborhood drug pusher, or destroying a cocaine crop in Bolivia could be considered primary prevention if it forestalled primary drug use in at least some individuals.

Secondary prevention programs are aimed at those who have begun alcohol or other drug use but who have not become chronic users and have not suffered significant physical or mental impairment from their drug or alcohol abuse. Alcohol and other drug abuse education programs that stress secondary prevention are often appropriate for people of high school or college age. They can be presented in educational, workplace, or community settings.

Tertiary prevention programs are designed to provide drug abuse treatment and aftercare, including relapse prevention programs. As such, they are usually designed for adults. More tertiary programs for teenagers are needed. Tertiary prevention programs may receive clients who "turn themselves in" for treatment voluntarily, but more often than not, clients are referred by the courts.

Elements of Prevention

Four basic elements play a role in drug abuse prevention and control. These are (1) education, (2) treatment, (3) public policy, and (4) enforcement. The goals of education and treatment are the same: to reduce the demand for drugs. Likewise, setting effective public policy and law enforcement share the same goal: to reduce the supply and availability of drugs in the community.

Education

The purpose of **drug abuse education** is to limit the demand for drugs by providing information about drugs and the dangers of drug abuse, changing attitudes and beliefs about drugs, providing the skills necessary to abstain from drugs, and ultimately changing drug abuse behavior. Education, principally a primary prevention activity, can be school-based or community-based. Examples of school-based drug abuse prevention programs are Project ALERT, LifeSkills Training (LST), and Class Action.[114] For these programs and other school-based programs to be successful, community members, such as parents, teachers, local business people, and others must visibly support the program. Examples of community-based programs are the American Cancer Society's Great American Smokeout; Race Against Drugs (RAD), a nationwide program that links drug abuse prevention with motor sports; and the Reality Check Campaign, a program to boost awareness of the harmful effects of marijuana smoking among youth.

Treatment

The goal of **treatment** is to remove the physical, emotional, and environmental conditions that have contributed to drug dependency. Like education, treatment aims to reduce demand for drugs. It also aims to save money. Consider the money saved on law enforcement, medical costs, and lost productivity when treatment is successful. Treatment for drug abuse occurs in a variety of settings and involves a variety of approaches. Treatment may be residential (inpatient) or nonresidential (outpatient). Under managed care, "behavioral health care" guidelines usually limit inpatient care to 28 days, after which the care may continue on an outpatient basis. In drug abuse treatment, what happens after the initial treatment phase is critical. **Aftercare**, the continuing care provided to the recovering former drug user, often involves peer group or self-help support group meetings, such as those provided by Alcoholics Anonymous (AA) or Narcotics Anonymous (NA). Despite frequent relapses, treatment for drug dependence is viewed as an important component of a community's comprehensive drug abuse prevention and control strategy.

Beginning January 1, 2010, the Paul Wellstone and Pete Domenici Mental Health Parity and Addiction Equity Act of 2008 (MHPAEA) took effect. This law "requires health insurers and group health plans to provide the same level of benefits for mental and/or substance use treatment and services that they do for medical/surgical care."[115] In 2010, the Patient Protection and Affordable Care Act (Affordable Care Act) was signed into law. The Affordable Care Act bars insurance companies from establishing eligibility rules based on pre-existing conditions, including history of addiction and substance use treatment. It also defines essential health benefits that must be covered, which include services and treatment for substance use disorders. Implementation of the provisions of these laws should improve substance use treatment options for many people.

Public Policy

Public policy embodies the guiding principles and courses of action pursued by governments to solve practical problems affecting society. Examples include passing drunk-driving laws or zoning ordinances that limit the number of bars in a neighborhood and enacting laws that regulate the type and amount of advertising for such legal drugs as alcohol and tobacco. Public policy should guide the budget discussions that ultimately determine how much a community spends for education, treatment, and law enforcement. Further examples of public policy decisions are restrictions of smoking in public buildings, setting a BAC of 0.08 as the point at which driving becomes illegal, and zero tolerance laws for BACs for minors. Setting the level of state excise taxes on alcohol and tobacco is also a public policy decision.

Law Enforcement

Law enforcement in drug abuse prevention and control is the application of federal, state, and local laws to arrest, jail, bring to trial, and sentence those who break drug laws or break laws because of drug use. The primary roles of law enforcement in a drug abuse prevention and control program are to (1) control drug use; (2) control crime, especially crime related to drug use and drug trafficking—the buying, selling, manufacturing, or transporting of illegal drugs; (3) prevent the establishment of crime organizations; and (4) protect neighborhoods. Law enforcement is concerned with limiting the supply of drugs in the community by interrupting

Treatment with respect to drug abuse and dependence, care that removes the physical, emotional, and environmental conditions that contributed to drug abuse and/or dependence

Aftercare the continuing care provided to the recovering former drug user

Public policy the guiding principles and courses of action pursued by governments to solve practical problems affecting society

Law enforcement the application of federal, state, and local laws to arrest, jail, bring to trial, and sentence those who break drug laws or break laws because of drug use

the source, transit, and distribution of drugs. There are law enforcement agencies at all levels of government. The principal agencies are discussed next.

Governmental Drug Prevention and Control Agencies and Programs

Government agencies involved in drug-abuse prevention, control, and treatment include a multitude of federal, state, and local agencies. At each of these levels of government, numerous offices and programs aim to reduce either the supply of or the demand for drugs.

Federal Agencies and Programs

The nation's antidrug efforts are headed up by the White House **Office of National Drug Control Policy (ONDCP)**, which annually publishes a report detailing the nation's drug control strategy and budget. The 2022 National Drug Control Strategy focuses on seven priority areas[116]:

1. Expanding access to evidence-based treatment, particularly medication for opioid use disorder
2. Advancing racial equity in our approach to drug policy
3. Enhancing evidence-based harm reduction efforts
4. Supporting evidence-based prevention efforts to reduce youth substance use
5. Reducing the supply of illicit substances
6. Advancing recovery-ready workplaces and expanding the addiction workforce
7. Expanding access to recovery support services

The ONDCP developed a National Drug Control Strategy with a focus on reducing overdose deaths by enhancing the substance use treatment infrastructure and increasing law enforcement efforts to reduce the supply of illicit drugs.[116] The strategic goals and objectives are to reduce illicit substance use and increase efforts of prevention, harm reduction, treatment, and recovery.[116]

The National Drug Control Strategy budget request for the fiscal year (FY) 2023 was about $42.5 billion, the largest amount ever requested and reflects an increase from $34.6 billion in FY 2020.[116] The budget funds the national drug control functions of prevention, treatment, interdiction, international operations, and law enforcement.[116]

U.S. Department of Health and Human Services

HHS receives the largest portion of the federal drug budget, more than $21 billion in FY 2022.[116] This money is spent on drug prevention education, treatment programs, and research into the causes and physiology of drug abuse. The preponderance of these funds is spent to reduce the demand for drugs. The approach of HHS to the drug problem is broad and includes research, treatment, and educational activities.

The misuse of tobacco, alcohol, and other drugs are addressed primarily as lifestyle problems, that is, as health promotion issues—like physical fitness and nutrition. As such, HHS recognizes that the problems of drug misuse and abuse are complex—involving inherited, environmental, social, and economic causes. Therefore, the solutions are also viewed as being complex. The typical approach involves the application of the three levels of prevention—primary, secondary, and tertiary. It also recognizes the importance of incorporating the three primary prevention strategies of education, regulation, and automatic protection.

HHS has published health status, risk reduction, and service and protection objectives on the use of tobacco, alcohol, and other drugs in *Healthy People 2030* (refer to Box 12.1 and Box 12.3). These are but two examples of objectives that set the direction and standards for success of all of national drug control efforts.

The lead agency within HHS is the **Substance Abuse and Mental Health Services Administration (SAMHSA)**. Within SAMHSA, there are four centers: the Center for Substance Abuse Prevention (CSAP), the Center for Substance Abuse Treatment (CSAT), the Center for Mental Health Services (CMHS), and the Center for Behavioral Health Statistics and Quality

(CBHSQ). In addition to SAMHSA, two other important agencies deal with the problems of alcohol and other drugs: the National Institute on Drug Abuse and the FDA.

The **National Institute on Drug Abuse (NIDA)** is the largest institution in the world devoted to drug abuse research. At NIDA, research efforts are aimed at understanding the causes and consequences of drug abuse and evaluating prevention and treatment programs. Within NIDA are several important divisions and centers, such as the Division of Clinical Neuroscience and Behavioral Research; Division of Neuroscience and Behavior; Division of Epidemiology, Services, and Prevention Research; and Division of Therapeutics and Medical Consequences. These agencies conduct research and publish articles on the causes, prevention, and treatment of tobacco, alcohol, and other drug abuse.

Another important agency within HHS is the Food and Drug Administration (FDA). As stated earlier, the FDA is charged with ensuring the safety and efficacy of all prescription and nonprescription drugs. The FDA dictates which drugs reach the market and how they must be labeled, packaged, and sold. The FDA is more concerned with drug misuse than abuse.

U.S. Department of Justice

The second-largest portion of federal spending for drug control, $8.5 billion in FY 2020, goes to the U.S. Department of Justice (DOJ).[117] The DOJ addresses the supply side of the drug trade most directly by identifying, arresting, and prosecuting those who break drug laws. It tries to protect the welfare of society by incarcerating the most serious offenders, deterring others from becoming involved in drug trade, and providing a clear picture to all of the cost of drug trade and abuse. Regarding the latter, the DOJ indirectly contributes to reducing the demand for drugs.

The DOJ's budget is large because, in addition to its enforcement responsibilities, the department maintains prisons and prisoners. The DOJ not only employs those who manage the penal system but also many marshals, attorneys, and judges. The single largest portion of the DOJ's budget goes to the Bureau of Prisons. The DOJ also operates treatment, education, and rehabilitation programs in these prisons.

Within the DOJ are several important drug-fighting agencies. The lead agency in this respect is the Drug Enforcement Agency (DEA), which investigates and assists in the prosecution of drug traffickers and their accomplices in the United States and abroad and seizes the drugs as well as the assets on which they depend. The DEA employs more than 5,000 special agents and support personnel.

Three other important agencies in the DOJ that are involved in the prevention and control of drug abuse are the Federal Bureau of Investigation (FBI), the Office of Justice Programs (OJP), and the **Bureau of Alcohol, Tobacco, Firearms, and Explosives (ATF)**. The FBI investigates multinational organized crime networks that control the illegal drug market. The OJP provides leadership to federal, state, local, and tribal justice systems by disseminating knowledge and practices and providing grants for the implementation of these crime-fighting strategies. The OJP does not directly carry out law enforcement and justice activities, but it works with the justice community to identify crime-related challenges and to provide information, training, coordination, and innovative strategies and approaches for addressing these challenges.[111] The ATF has a wide range of responsibilities. One of its responsibilities is to protect communities from the illegal diversion of alcohol and tobacco products. ATF partners with communities, industries, law enforcement, and public safety agencies to safeguard the public through information sharing, training, research, and use of technology.[118]

U.S. Department of Homeland Security

Shortly after the terrorist attacks on the World Trade Center and the Pentagon on September 11, 2001, President George W. Bush authorized the establishment of the DHS. Subsequently, a number of federal agencies involved in drug control activities were transferred into this new department, which received the third-largest portion of funding from the National Drug Control Budget ($6.1 billion).[117] Those agencies receiving funds are Immigration and Customs Enforcement (ICE), Customs and Border Protection (CBP), Counternarcotics Enforcement, and the U.S. Coast Guard. In the current environment, in which protection from terrorist acts

National Institute on Drug Abuse (NIDA) the federal government's lead agency for drug abuse research; part of the National Institutes of Health

Bureau of Alcohol, Tobacco, Firearms, and Explosives (ATF) the federal agency in the U.S. Department of Justice that regulates alcohol and tobacco

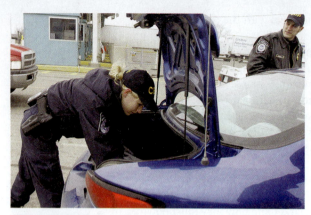

FIGURE 12.8   Customs agents assist in the arrest and prosecution of those involved in drug trafficking.

Courtesy of Gerald L. Nino/U.S. Customs and Border Protection.

is DHS's primary concern, the prevention and control of drug trafficking seem somewhat less urgent by comparison. Nonetheless, it is part of the mission of these agencies. For example, ICE works to prevent the immigration to this country of criminals, including those involved in drug trafficking. CBP works with ICE to protect our borders from external threats, including illegal drugs (see **Figure 12.8**). The Coast Guard helps to interdict illegal drug trafficking in our coastal waters.

Other Federal Agencies

Other federal agencies involved in drug abuse prevention and control are the U.S. Departments of State, Defense, Veterans Affairs, and Education. The U.S. State Department, through various diplomatic efforts, including "drug summits," attempts to achieve a reduction in the production and shipment of illicit drugs into this country. The U.S. Defense Department assists foreign allies to control the cultivation of illegal drug crops and the production of illegal drugs. Funding slated for the U.S. Department of Veteran Affairs is aimed primarily at the treatment of drug-related health problems of veterans.

The U.S. Department of Education (DOE) launched a program to support drug-free schools and communities in the late 1980s. The effort was aimed at encouraging schools to adopt clear "no drug use" policies and to provide a message that both communities and schools do not condone or approve of alcohol or drug use by minors. A handbook titled, *What Works: Schools Without Drugs*, was prepared and distributed to schools and communities.[119] The DOE continues to participate in the federal drug prevention effort. The national drug control budget for the DOE for FY 2022 is $59 million.[116]

State and Local Agencies and Programs

Whereas considerable economic resources can be brought to bear on the drug problem at the federal level, it is becoming increasingly clear that to achieve success, the drug war in the United States must be fought at the local level—in homes, neighborhoods, and schools. State support usually comes in the form of law enforcement expertise in education and mental health, the coordination of local and regional programs, and sometimes funding initiatives. It is usually up to local citizens to put these state initiatives into action or to begin initiatives of their own.

State Agencies

State agencies that address drug-abuse prevention and control issues include the offices of the governor, as well as state departments of health, education, mental health, justice, and law enforcement. Sometimes an umbrella agency coordinates the activities of the various offices and departments. To review agencies involved in the prevention and control of drug abuse and drug dependence problems in your state, visit your state government's homepage and search using the terms "drug abuse prevention agencies" or "drug abuse prevention programs." (You can usually find your state government's homepage by typing "www.nameofyourstate.gov." For example, www.texas.gov will take you to the Texas government's homepage; www.in.gov will take you to the homepage of the Indiana state government.) Searching these sites in this way will reveal the agencies involved in drug abuse prevention at the state level.

The role of these state-level agencies is evident from their titles. Some state agencies provide actual services; others provide statistics or other information. Still others provide expertise or serve as a conduit for federal funding aimed at local (city or county) governments.

The role of state government is to promote, protect, and maintain the health and welfare of its citizens. Thus, each state has its own laws regulating the sale of tobacco, alcohol, and prescription drugs. States issue licenses to doctors, dentists, pharmacists, liquor stores, and taverns.

Each state also passes laws and sets the penalties for the manufacture, sale, and possession of illicit drugs, such as marijuana. For example, in California, possession of 28.5 grams (1 ounce) of marijuana or fewer is legal, whereas possession of more than 28.5 grams is a misdemeanor, punishable by 6 months in jail and a $500 fine.[120]

In some cases, states have passed laws that conflict with federal laws. For example, some states have decriminalized marijuana cultivation and possession for medical or recreational use. In 2023, 38 states have legalized marijuana for medical purposes.[97] As of 2023, the possession and recreational use of small amounts of marijuana for recreational purposes is legal in 24 states.[97] States that have legalized marijuana, either for recreational or medical purposes, maintain laws that regulate its use.[121] Even so, these people could still be arrested by the DEA and prosecuted under federal law. Although marijuana use still violates federal law, the U.S. Department of Justice announced that it would rely heavily on states to enforce their own marijuana laws.[122]

Local Agencies

Agencies of local governments that are involved in drug-abuse prevention and control include mayors' offices, police and sheriffs' departments, school corporations, health departments, family services offices, mental health services, prosecutors' offices, the juvenile justice system, judges and courts, drug task forces, and so on. In some communities, there is a community drug task force or coordinating council that includes both government officials and representatives of nongovernmental agencies. Such task forces or councils might include local religious leaders, representatives from local industry (both labor and management), healthcare providers, and members from local voluntary agencies. The task of these organizations is usually to prioritize problems faced by the community and decide on approaches to solving them. The goal is to develop a coordinated and effective effort to resolve the issue. Sometimes, a solution might involve selecting an approach that has been used with success in another community or school system.

Nongovernmental Drug Prevention and Control Agencies and Programs

Many nongovernmental programs and agencies make valuable contributions to the prevention and control of drug abuse in the United States. Among these are community- and school-based programs, workplace programs, and voluntary agencies.

Community-Based Drug Education Programs

Community-based drug education can occur in a variety of settings, such as child care facilities, public housing, religious institutions, businesses, and healthcare facilities. Information about the abuse of alcohol, tobacco, and other drugs can be disseminated through television and radio programs, movies, newspapers, and magazines.

Community-based drug education programs are most likely to be successful when they include six key features[123]:

1. A comprehensive strategy
2. An indirect approach to drug abuse prevention
3. The goal of empowering youth
4. A participatory approach
5. A culturally sensitive orientation
6. Highly structured activities

Community-based drug education programs that address broader issues (e.g., coping and learning skills) are most effective, as are those embedded in other existing community activities (see **Figure 12.9**). Participation can be increased by planning drug education programs around sporting or cultural events.

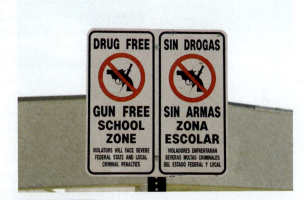

FIGURE 12.9 Use of appropriate language can be the difference between success and failure of a community drug-prevention program.

© Lisa C. McDonald/Shutterstock

Culturally sensitive programs are crucial for reaching minorities in the community. Use of the appropriate language, reading level, and spokespersons can mean the difference between success or failure of a program.

In the past 30 years, a great many drug abuse prevention education programs have been conceived and tested. Some of these have been scientifically proven to be effective. SAMHSA has a searchable database of successful programs linked to its website.[114]

An example of a community-based program is the Drug-Free Communities (DFC) support program. The DFC program is aimed at the community level, focusing on mobilizing local leaders to address issues unique to their area. The two goals of the DFC program are: to establish and strengthen collaboration among local, state, and federal agencies, as well as public and non-profit sectors and to prevent and reduce substance use among youth.[124]

School-Based Drug Education Programs

Most health educators believe that a strong, comprehensive school health education program—one that occupies a permanent and prominent place in the school curriculum—is the best defense against all health problems, including drug abuse. However, many schools lack these strong programs and, in their absence, substitute drug education programs developed specifically for school use.

One such program is the Botvin LifeSkills Training program, which has shown to reduce drug use by up to 70%, alcohol use by up to 60%, and tobacco use by up to 87%.[125] The program is designed to accommodate flexible schedules with a recommendation of multiyear programming with a curriculum designed specifically for elementary school, middle school, and high school students. There is also a program for students moving on to the workforce or higher education and a program for parents.

Another evidence-based school program shown to be effective is Project ALERT. Project ALERT reduced students' current marijuana use by 60%, reduced the likelihood of alcohol use by 24%, and substantially reduced students' pro-drug-use attitudes and beliefs.[126]

Student assistance programs (SAPs) are school-based programs modeled after employee assistance programs in the workplace. They are aimed at identifying and intervening in cases of drug problems. **Peer counseling programs** are also present in some schools. In these programs, students talk about mutual problems and receive support and perhaps learn coping skills from peers who have been trained in this intervention activity and do not use drugs.

Workplace-Based Drug Education Programs

In September of 1986, concern about widespread drug use in the workplace led then-President Ronald Reagan to sign Executive Order 12564, proclaiming a Drug-Free Federal Workplace.[127] The rationale for the order signed in September of 1986 was cited in the document itself: the desire and need for the well-being of employees, the loss of productivity caused by drug use, the illegal profits of organized crime, the illegality of the behavior itself, the undermining of public confidence, and the role of the federal government as the largest employer in the nation to set a standard for other employers to follow in these matters. It had also become apparent to all that drug abuse is not only a personal health problem and a law enforcement problem but that it is also a behavior that affects the safety and productivity of others, especially at work. Studies have shown that substance users (1) are less productive, (2) miss more workdays, (3) are more likely to injure themselves, and (4) file more workers' compensation claims than their non-substance-abusing counterparts.

The Drug-Free Federal Workplace order required federal employees to refrain from using illegal drugs, and it required agency heads to develop plans for achieving drug-free workplaces for employees in their agencies. The order further required the setting up of drug-testing programs and procedures and employee assistance programs that would include provisions for rehabilitation.[127] Similar workplace substance-abuse programs, which include drug testing, soon spread to the private sector so that by the mid-1990s, such programs were in place in more than 80% of American companies.[128]

CHAPTER 13

Healthcare Delivery in the United States

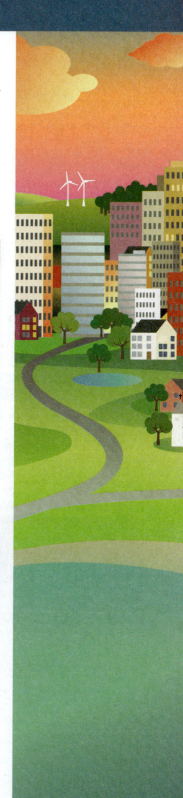

Chapter Outline

Chapter Objectives

After studying this chapter, you will be able to:

1. Define the term *healthcare system*.
2. Trace the history of healthcare delivery in the United States from colonial times to the present.
3. Discuss and explain the concept of the spectrum of healthcare delivery.
4. Distinguish between the different kinds of health care, including population-based public health practice, medical practice, long-term practice, and end-of-life practice.
5. List and describe the different levels of medical practice.
6. Name and characterize the various groups of healthcare providers.
7. Explain the differences among allopathic, osteopathic, and nonallopathic providers.
8. Define complementary and alternative medicine.
9. Explain why there is a need for healthcare providers.
10. Prepare a list of the different types of facilities in which health care is delivered.
11. Explain the differences among private, public, and voluntary hospitals.
12. Explain the difference between inpatient and outpatient care facilities.
13. Briefly discuss the options for long-term care.
14. Explain what The Joint Commission does.
15. Identify the major concerns with the healthcare system in the United States.
16. Discuss the various means of reimbursing healthcare providers.
17. Briefly describe the purpose and concept of insurance.
18. Define the term *insurance policy*.

Chapter Objectives *(continued)*

19. Explain the insurance policy terms *deductible, coinsurance, copayment, fixed indemnity, exclusion,* and *pre-existing condition.*
20. Explain what is meant when a company or business is said to be self-insured.
21. List the different types of medical care usually covered in a health insurance policy.
22. Briefly describe Medicare, Medicaid, and Medigap insurance.
23. Briefly summarize the Children's Health Insurance Program (CHIP).
24. Briefly explain long-term care health insurance.
25. Define managed care.
26. Define the terms *health maintenance organization* (HMO), *preferred provider organization* (PPO), and *point-of-service option.*
27. Identify the advantages and disadvantages of managed care.
28. Define consumer-directed health plans and give several examples.
29. Provide a brief overview of the Affordable Care Act passed in 2010.
30. Summarize the four cases that have been heard by the U.S. Supreme Court that have had an impact on the Affordable Care Act.

Scenario

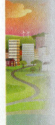

Technology has changed the way we utilize health care. The COVID-19 pandemic has certainly increased its use even more. Mirra is currently in college and has been feeling unwell for the past few days. She knows from the COVID-19 pandemic that she should stay in the dorm and not get others sick. She is in desperate need of some symptom relief because nothing over-the-counter has worked for her. Since she is in the student dorms and living on campus, she currently does not have transportation to get to the local clinic. Currently, there is a Student Health Center on campus, but she doesn't know if she would be covered to see a provider there. She's not sure if it would be the right place to go since she currently has a fever and is worried about out-of-pocket costs. She logs on to her computer and tries to determine which is the best option for her. She could find transportation and go to a local urgent care center but is not quite sure of the medical costs. She also knows that she could wait in the ER to get seen but it might take a while. Another option would include a video appointment with her parents' insurance coverage back home and she could speak to her family physician and only pay her co-payment. While looking at her options she noticed there was also a telephone appointment with her campus Student Health Center. With all of these options to choose from, Mirra decides that a video appointment would be best.

Introduction

The process by which health care is delivered in the United States is unlike the processes used in other countries of the world. Other developed countries have national health insurance run or organized by the government and paid for, in large part, by general taxes. Also, in these countries, almost all citizens are entitled to receive healthcare services, including routine and basic health care.[1] Even with the changes that were made to the U.S. healthcare system in 2010 through the Patient Protection and Affordable Care Act, the healthcare delivery system is still uniquely American.[2] Health care is still delivered by an array of **providers**, in a variety of settings, under the watchful eye of regulators, and paid for in a variety of ways. Because of this process, the United States healthcare delivery system is very complex. (see **Figure 13.1**). "these various individuals and organizations are generally referred to collectively as "the healthcare delivery system," the phrase suggests order, integration, and accountability which is something the United States healthcare delivery system strives for. Communication, collaboration, or systems

Providers healthcare facilities or health professionals that offer healthcare services

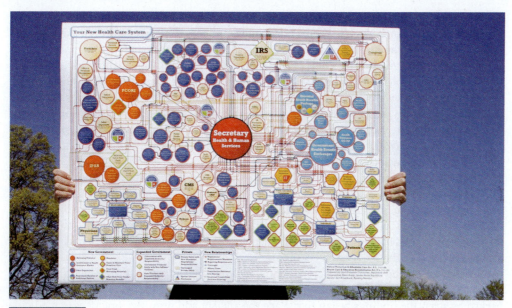

FIGURE 13.1   The United States' complex healthcare delivery system.

© J. Scott Applewhite/AP Photo

planning among these various entities is limited and is almost incidental to their operations."[3] Whether or not healthcare delivery in the United States should be called a "system," there is a process in place in which healthcare professionals, located in a variety of facilities, provide services to deal with disease and injury for the purpose of promoting, maintaining, and restoring health to the citizens. In this chapter, we provide a brief history of healthcare delivery in the United States, examine the structure of health care, and describe how our unique system functions. Finally, we discuss healthcare reform in the United States.

A Brief History of Healthcare Delivery in the United States

For as long as humankind has been concerned with disease, injury, and health, there has always been a category of health care in which people have tried to help or treat themselves. This category of care is referred to as *self-care* or *self-treatment*. For example, in most American homes, there are usually provisions to deal with minor emergencies, nursing care, and the relief of minor pains or ailments. This type of care continues today. The following discussion of the history of healthcare delivery in the United States does not include self-care because it is assumed that most people would engage in some type of self-care prior to seeking professional help. Instead, we review the development of professional care provided by those trained to do so.

As might be assumed with the birth of a new country, from colonial times through the latter portion of the nineteenth century, health care and medical education in the United States lagged far behind their counterparts in Great Britain and Europe. During this period of time, anyone, trained or untrained, could practice medicine. Much of the early health care was provided by family members and neighbors and consisted of home and folk remedies that had been handed down from one generation to another. When a person did receive training as a physician, it was nothing like the rigorous training that a physician goes through today. The early medical education in the colonies was not grounded in science. Prior to 1870, medical education was provided primarily through an apprenticeship with a practicing physician who may have been trained in the same way.[4] Consequently, medical care was primitive and was considered to be more a trade than a profession.[1] In addition, most of the health care was provided in the patient's home and not in an office or clinic.

There were some hospitals during these early years, but they were located primarily in large cities and seaports, such as New York, Philadelphia, and New Orleans. However, the hospitals were very different from the hospitals of today and served more in a social welfare function than as places to receive health care. They were not very clean, and unhygienic practices prevailed. The forerunner of today's hospitals and nursing homes was the *almshouse* (also called a *poorhouse*).[1] Almshouses were run by the local government primarily to provide food, shelter, and basic nursing care for indigent people (i.e., people who are homeless, ill, orphaned, or disabled) who could not be cared for by their own families.[1] In addition to almshouses, local government also operated *pesthouses*, which served as a place to isolate people who had contracted an infectious disease, such as cholera, smallpox, or typhoid.[1]

In the late nineteenth century, formal health care gradually moved from the patient's home to the physician's office and into the hospital. The primary reason for this change was the building and staffing of many new hospitals. It was felt that patients could receive better care in a setting designed for patient care, staffed with trained people, and equipped with the latest medical supplies and instruments. In addition, physicians could treat more patients in a central location because of the reduced travel time.

It was also during the latter portion of the nineteenth century that the scientific method began to play a more important role in medical education and health care. Medical procedures backed by scientific findings began to replace the ancient and primitive practices of medicine as the standards for medical care. With the acceptance of the germ theory of disease and the identification of infectious disease agents, there was real hope for the control of communicable diseases, which were the leading health problems of that period.

At the beginning of the twentieth century, communicable diseases were still the leading causes of death; however, mortality rates were beginning to decline. Most of the decline can be attributed to improved public health measures. Yet, at the end of World War I, mortality rates not only spiked in the United States but also worldwide because of the 1918–1919 influenza pandemic. This deadliest pandemic in history killed as many as 100 million people. Shortly after the pandemic, in the early 1920s, a major shift took place in the United States as chronic diseases moved past communicable diseases as the leading causes of death.

At the same time that chronic diseases were pushing to the top of the list of causes of death, much change was taking place in health care. New medical procedures, such as X-ray therapy, specialized surgical procedures, and chemotherapy were developed, group medical practices were started, and new medical equipment and instruments (such as the electrocardiograph to measure heart function) were invented. The training of doctors and nurses also improved and became more specialized.

By 1929, the United States was spending approximately 3.9% of its gross domestic product (GDP) on health care, which means that 3.9% of all goods and services produced by the nation that year were associated with health care. During this time, the development of the modern health insurance system began with what was considered the first employer-sponsored plan that started with a group of teachers at Baylor University, known as the **Baylor Plan**.[5]

Even with some of these "new" advances in the practice of medicine, U.S. medicine was still limited pretty much to two parties—patients and physicians. "Diagnosis, treatment, and fees for services were considered confidential between patients and physicians. Medical practice was relatively simple and usually involved long-standing relationships with patients and, often, several generations of families. Physicians set and often adjusted their charges to their estimates of patients' ability to pay and collected the payments. This was the intimate physician–patient relationship the profession held sacred."[6]

By the early 1940s, the United States was again at war. World War II affected health care in the United States in a variety of ways. One consequence of the war that would have a lasting impact on health care was employers' use of health insurance to lure workers to their companies. Because of the large number of men and women in the armed services, there was a shortage of workers to fill the jobs back home. Also, because of the need for resources for the war effort, the U.S. government put restrictions on the wages that companies could pay their employees. However, there were no restrictions on the healthcare insurance that employers could provide

Baylor Plan Established in 1929 by Baylor administrators during the Great Depression to help area citizens afford hospital care. It is the first prepaid hospital insurance plan in the United States and the predecessor of Blue Cross.

for their employees. Thus, companies began using health insurance to recruit and retain workers, and as a result, employer-provided health insurance took a foothold at this time.

Also, as a result of World War II, huge technical strides were made in the late 1940s and 1950s as medical procedures and processes developed during the war found applications in civilian medicine. However, adequate health facilities to treat long-term diseases were lacking in many areas of the country. The **Hospital Survey and Construction Act of 1946 (Hill-Burton Act)**, which was named after the authors of the legislation, provided substantial funds for hospital construction. The infusion of federal funds helped to remedy the serious hospital shortage caused by the lack of construction during the Depression and World War II. The Hill-Burton Act was primarily a federal–state partnership. State agencies were given grants to determine the need for hospitals and then were provided with seed money to begin construction of the facilities.[7] However, the major portion of construction dollars came from state and local sources.[8] Through the years, the Hill-Burton Act has been amended several times to help meet healthcare needs in the United States. Funds have been made available for additional construction, modernization, and replacement of other healthcare facilities, and for comprehensive health planning.

With improved procedures, equipment, and facilities, and the increase in noncommunicable diseases, the cost of health care began to rise. As the cost of health care rose, it became too expensive for some people. Concerns were expressed about who should receive health care and who should pay for it. The debate over whether health care is a basic right or a privilege in the United States began in earnest. By the end of the 1950s, there remained an overall shortage of quality health care in the United States. There was also a maldistribution of healthcare services—metropolitan areas were being better served than the less-developed rural areas.

In the 1960s, there was an increased interest in health insurance, and it became common practice for workers and their bargaining agents to negotiate for better health benefits (see **Figure 13.2**). Undoubtedly, some employers preferred to increase benefits rather than to raise wages. Few then could foresee the escalation in healthcare costs for Americans. Thus, the **third-party payment system** for health care became solidified as the standard method of payment for healthcare costs in the United States. The third-party payment system gets its name from the fact that the insurer—government, private insurance company, or a self-insured organization (third party)—reimburses (pays the bills) to the provider (second party) for the health care given to the patient (first party).[9] (A detailed explanation of the third-party payment system is presented later in this chapter.) More recently, when some speak of the third-party payment system, they add a fourth party— the purchaser of the insurance, often an employer. It should be noted that the government and private insurers pay the medical bills with tax dollars and collected premiums, respectively—not with their own funds.

With the growth of the third-party system of paying for health care, the cost of health care rose even more rapidly than before, because patients enjoyed increased access to care without or with little out-of-pocket expenses. However, those without insurance found it increasingly more difficult to afford care. When the Democrats regained the White House in the 1960s, they introduced a series of legislation to increase citizen access to health care, which culminated in 1965 with the authorization of Medicare and Medicaid by Titles XVIII and XIX, respectively, of the Social Security Act. (These programs, which were enacted to help provide care for people who are elderly, disabled, and living in poverty, are also discussed later in this chapter.) Also in

Hospital Survey and Construction Act of 1946 (Hill-Burton Act) federal legislation that provided substantial funds for hospital construction

Third-party payment system a health insurance term indicating that bills from a healthcare provider for services rendered to a patient are paid by the insurer

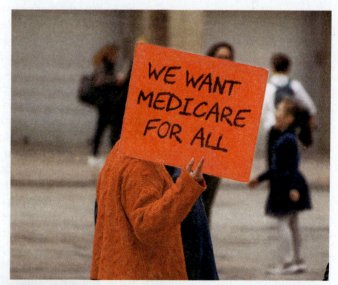

FIGURE 13.2   Health benefits have become an important part of the total compensation package for workers.
© No-Mad/Shutterstock

the 1960s, the federal government increased funding for medical research and technology to support transplants and life extension.

By the late 1960s and early 1970s, it had become apparent that the Hill-Burton Act had not only stimulated the growth of healthcare facilities but also the demand for healthcare services. With this growth came a continuing rise in healthcare costs and a need for better planning in healthcare delivery.

Among the early attempts at planning were the 1964 amendments to the Hill-Burton Act. The amendments called for comprehensive planning on a regional level. Their purpose was to make more efficient use of federal funds by preventing the duplication of facilities. However, they depended on good faith efforts and could not be enforced. It soon became evident that more legislation was needed to control costs and to coordinate and control rapid growth in healthcare facilities.

Another attempt was made to encourage better planning 2 years later. The Comprehensive Health Planning and Public Service Amendments of 1966 authorized funds for state- and area-wide comprehensive health planning agencies. The assumption was at the time that this would facilitate a more consumer-oriented medical care industry and would greatly benefit from planning technology.[10] However, it failed because it did not deliver what was widely anticipated.[10] In 1974, Public Law 93-641 was passed. This law, known as the National Health Planning and Resources Development Act of 1974, combined several pieces of previous legislation to provide robust comprehensive planning efforts. There were high hopes and expectations that these pieces of legislation would provide reason and order to the development and modification of healthcare services.[11] This legislation led to the formation of health system agencies throughout the entire country. Their purpose was to cut costs by preventing the building of "unnecessary" facilities or the purchase of unnecessary equipment. Although some money may have been saved, the health system agencies were viewed by some as yet another unnecessary government bureaucracy, and when the late President Reagan took office in 1980, he, along with Congress, eliminated this program.

Before leaving our healthcare discussion of the 1970s, it should be noted that another piece of legislation was passed that did not seem all that important at the time but that would have a profound impact on the way health care was delivered later. This legislation was the Health Maintenance Organization (HMO) Act of 1973. This act "provided both loans and grants for the planning, development, and implementation of combined insurance and healthcare delivery organizations and required that a minimum prescribed array of services be included in the HMO arrangement."[6]

The 1980s brought many changes to the healthcare industry, the most notable of which was probably the deregulation of healthcare delivery. In 1981, with Ronald Reagan in the White House, it was announced that the administration would let the competitive market, not governmental regulation, shape healthcare delivery.[12] Open competition is a philosophy of allowing consumers to regulate delivery by making choices about where and from whom they receive their care. In theory, those who provide good care would get more patients, and in turn be able to offer the care at a lower price. In other words, the resulting competition would help squeeze out costly waste and ineffective care.[13]

Some economists, however, do not believe that the healthcare system behaves like a normal market. For example, it is not likely that an ill patient seeking medical care will shop for a less expensive physician. Physicians do not advertise the cost of their services. Also, it is the physician who tells the patient which hospital to go to and when to check in and out, due to the admitting privileges that physicians have. In addition, providers tend to offer more and more services to entice the market to "shop with us," the effect of which is to drive up healthcare spending. For these reasons, the competitive market approach is of questionable value in lowering healthcare costs.

The 1980s also saw a proliferation of new medical technology (e.g., magnetic resonance images [MRIs] and ultrasound). Along with this new technology have come new healthcare issues, such as medical ethics (e.g., prolonging life, ending life, and gene therapy) and more elaborate health insurance programs (e.g., policies that cover specific diseases, such as cancer and AIDS, home care, and rehabilitation).

Many of the concerns of the 1980s continued into the 1990s. The 1992 presidential campaign again brought attention to the United States' problems with healthcare delivery. Bill Clinton, then governor of Arkansas, based his election campaign strategy on being a new kind of Democrat—one who could take on the nation's domestic ills. He saw health care as one of those ills because the present system failed to cover everyone, and its spiraling costs threatened to bankrupt the government and damage American industry.

Shortly after being elected president, Mr. Clinton appointed the first lady, Hillary Rodham Clinton, to head a committee to develop a plan to overcome the shortcomings of the healthcare system. By the fall of 1993, the committee had completed a plan that the president then presented to a joint session of the U.S. Congress in front of a national television audience. This detailed plan, referred to informally as the president's Health Security Plan and formally as the **American Health Security Act of 1993**, was over 1,500 pages in length. The focal point of the plan was to provide universal coverage. President Clinton's healthcare plan was much discussed in Congress in 1994; however, opposition kept it from ever reaching the floor for a vote before Congress adjourned. This was the sixth time in U.S. history that the concept of universal coverage was defeated. (The other attempts at universal coverage are discussed later in this chapter.) Although the plan was never approved, the pressures generated by the plan transformed the private healthcare system in the United States.

In the mid- to late 1990s, rapid changes occurred in the organization and financing of health care. These changes can be summed up in two words—managed care. **Managed care** "is a system of health care delivery that (1) seeks to achieve efficiency by integrating the four functions of healthcare delivery, (2) employs mechanisms to control (manage) utilization of medical services, and (3) determines the price at which the services are purchased, and consequently, how much the providers get paid."[14]

In the mid-1990s, with the advent of managed care, the increase of healthcare costs slowed; in fact, the actual growth for several years was almost flat. Even so, both the percentage of the GDP and the dollars spent on health care continued to inch up. Health care is the one segment of the U.S. economy that continues to grow consistently faster than the cost of inflation (see **Table 13.1**). Ever-newer technology, ever-increasing demands for the best care, growing medical liability, new diagnostic procedures, the lengthening of life spans, the development of new drugs, and newly identified diseases put great demands on the system.

By the mid- to late 1990s, managed care had become the dominant form of healthcare financing and delivery, but it became apparent that support for it, with some exceptions, was not deep.[15] In addition, it was obvious that the slowdown in healthcare costs, which was attributed to managed care, would be a one-time savings if other measures were not taken. President Clinton saw this as an opportunity to again seek healthcare reform. This time, President Clinton treaded carefully, offering small but politically popular programs. The most notable of these was the State Children's Health Insurance Program (SCHIP), healthcare

American Health Security Act of 1993 the comprehensive healthcare reform introduced by then President Clinton, but never enacted

Managed care a system that integrates the functions of financing, insurance, delivery, and payment and uses mechanisms to control costs and utilization of services

TABLE 13.1 Consumer Price Index and Average Annual Percentage of Change for All Items and Selected Items: United States, Selected Years 1960–2020

Year	All Items	Medical Care	Food	Apparel	Housing	Energy
1960	29.6	22.3	30.0	45.7	—	22.4
1980	82.4	74.9	86.8	90.0	81.1	86.0
2000	172.2	260.8	167.8	129.6	169.6	124.6
2010	218.0	388.4	219.6	119.5	216.3	192.9
2015	236.5	451.1	247.5	122.8	239.5	186.4
2020	258.6	555.56	261.8	124.4	324.3	208.3

Notes: Data are based on reporting by samples of providers and other retail outlets; —, data not available; 1982–1984 = 100.

Data from U.S. Department of Labor, Bureau of Labor Statistics. (2020). Consumer price index. Available at http://www.bls.gov/cpi/

coverage for uninsured children (SCHIP is now known as CHIP; see the discussion of CHIP later in this chapter).

The most notable change to U.S. health care during the presidency of George W. Bush was the passage of the Medicare Prescription Drug, Improvement, and Modernization Act of 2003 (MMA). The most visible components of the MMA have been the voluntary outpatient prescription drug benefit for people on Medicare, known as Part D (see the discussion of Medicare Part D later in the chapter), and health savings accounts (HSAs). HSAs are tax-free savings accounts that can be used to pay for near-term medical expenses incurred by individuals, spouses, and dependents and would save for future long-term costs. (HSAs are also discussed in greater detail later in the chapter.)

Throughout the early part of the twenty-first century, both consumers and healthcare providers agreed that healthcare delivery in the United States needed to be changed. The Institute on Medicine (IOM) claimed "health care today harms too frequently and routinely fails to deliver its potential benefits."[16] Furthermore, the healthcare system suffered from lack of coordinated, comprehensive services, resulting in both the wasteful duplication of efforts and unaccountable gaps in care.[16] In its reports, the IOM outlined a number of recommendations for changing healthcare delivery in the United States. These recommendations, combined with the release of the World Health Organization's report, *The World Health Report 2000—Health Systems: Improving Performance*, in which the U.S. health system was ranked thirty-seventh out of 191 countries,[17] provided some direction for changing the way health care was delivered.

Because of the great concern for healthcare reform, much attention was given to the topic during the presidential debates in 2008. In fact, all major candidates outlined plans for change if elected. When President Obama took office in 2009, one of the top issues on his agenda for change was healthcare reform. The first piece of legislation signed into law by President Obama was the Children's Health Insurance Program (CHIP) Reauthorization Act of 2009 (CHIP was formerly known as SCHIP). This law expanded CHIP to approximately 4.1 million uninsured children and was funded by a $0.62 increase in the federal tax on cigarettes.

It took another year before a more comprehensive healthcare reform was passed. In 2010, President Obama signed into law two bills—the Patient Protection and Affordable Care Act (Public Law 111-148) and the Health Care and Education Reconciliation Act of 2010 (Public Law 111-152). These two acts were consolidated with other approved legislation and are now referred to as the Affordable Care Act (ACA). Portions of this act went into effect in 2010, and the last portion is scheduled to go into effect in 2025. The road for ACA implementation has not been smooth. As of the writing of this text, the start dates for some portions of the ACA have been pushed back, a number of technical difficulties were encountered with the health insurance exchange website, the U.S. Congress has voted to repeal the ACA 62 times,[18] and on four occasions, parts of the ACA have been litigated in the U.S. Supreme Court. A more complete presentation of the act comes in the last part of this chapter.

Healthcare System: Structure

The structure of the healthcare system of the United States is unique in the world. In the sections that follow, we examine the *spectrum of healthcare delivery* and describe the various types of healthcare providers and the facilities in which health care is delivered.

The Spectrum of Healthcare Delivery

Because health care in the United States is delivered by an array of providers in a variety of settings, reference is sometimes made to the spectrum of healthcare delivery (see **Table 13.2**). The spectrum of healthcare delivery refers to the various types of care. Within this spectrum, four levels of practice have emerged: population-based public health practice, medical practice, long-term practice, and end-of-life practice.

TABLE 13.2 The Spectrum of Healthcare Delivery

Level of Practice	Description	Examples of Delivery Settings
Public health practice	Practice aimed at the development and application of preventive interventions to promote and protect the health of populations	Community and school health programs; public health clinics
Medical practice		
Primary care	Clinical preventive services, first-contact treatment services, and ongoing care for commonly encountered medical conditions; emphasizes prevention, early detection, and routine care	Primary care provider offices; public clinics; managed care organizations; community mental health centers
Secondary care	Specialized attention and ongoing management for common and less frequently encountered medical conditions, including support services for people with special challenges due to chronic or long-term conditions	
Acute care	Short-term, intense medical care that may require hospitalization	Emergency rooms; urgent/emergency care centers; outpatient/inpatient surgical centers; hospitals
Subacute care	Convalescence after acute care, need for more nursing intervention	Special subacute units in hospitals (e.g., transitional care units); skilled nursing facilities; home health care
Tertiary care	Subspecialty referral care requiring highly specialized personnel and facilities	Specialty hospitals (e.g., psychiatric, chronic disease); general hospitals with highly specialized facilities
Long-term practice		
Restorative care	Intermediate follow-up care, such as surgical postoperative care	Home health; progressive and extended care facilities; rehabilitation facilities that specialize in therapeutic services; halfway houses
Long-term care or chronic care	Care for chronic conditions; personal care	Nursing homes; facilities for people with intellectual disabilities or are emotionally disturbed; geriatric day care centers
End-of-life practice	Care provided to those who have less than 6 months to live	Hospice services provided in a variety of settings

Data from Cambridge Research Institute. (1976). *Trends affecting the U.S. health care system*. U.S. Government Printing Office; U.S. Public Health Service. (1994). *For a healthy nation: Return on investments in public health*. USPHS; Pratt, J. R. (2016). *Long-term care: Managing across the continuum* (4th ed.). Jones & Bartlett Learning; Turnock, B. J. (2016). *Public health: What it is and how it works* (6th ed.). Jones & Bartlett Learning; Shi, L., & Singh, D. A. (2017). *Essentials of the U.S. health care system* (4th ed.). Jones & Bartlett Learning.

Public Health Practice

Public health practice incorporates "the development and application of preventive strategies and interventions to promote and protect the health of populations."[19] A primary component of public health practice is education. If people are going to behave in a way that will promote their health and the health of their community, they first must know how to do so. Health education not only provides such information but also attempts to empower and motivate people to put this information to use by discontinuing unhealthy behaviors and adopting healthy ones. Although much of public health practice takes place in governmental health agencies, it also takes place in a variety of other settings (such as voluntary health agencies, social service agencies, schools, businesses and industry, and even in some traditional medical care settings).[19]

Pulic Health empowers communities to take action toward their own health outcomes.

Public health practice incorporates the development and application of preventive strategies and interventions to promote and protect the health of populations

Primary care clinical preventive services, first-contact treatment services, and ongoing care for commonly encountered medical conditions

Secondary medical care specialized attention and ongoing management for common and less frequently encountered medical conditions, including support services for people with special challenges due to chronic or long-term conditions

Tertiary medical care specialized and technologically sophisticated medical and surgical care for those with unusual or complex conditions

Restorative care that is provided after successful treatment or when the progress of an incurable disease has been arrested

Medical Practice

Medical practice means "those services usually provided by or under the supervision of a physician or other traditional health care provider."[19] Such services are offered at several different levels. You may recall that we use the terms *primary, secondary,* and *tertiary* as they related to levels of prevention. These terms have a similar meaning here, but they are now applied to healthcare delivery rather than prevention.

Primary Medical Care

Primary care is "front-line" or "first-contact" care. "The unique characteristic of primary care is the role it plays as a regular or usual source of care for patients and their families."[3] Formally, **primary care** has been defined as "clinical preventive services, first-contact treatment services, and ongoing care for commonly encountered medical conditions."[19] Eighty percent of necessary medical care is provided by primary care.[19] Primary care includes routine medical care to treat common illnesses or to detect health problems in their early stages, and thus, includes such things as semiannual dental checkups; annual physical exams; health screenings for hypertension, high blood cholesterol, and breast or testicular cancer; and sore throat cultures. Physicians, nurse practitioners, physician assistants, and an array of other individuals on the primary care team usually provide primary care in practitioners' offices, clinics, and other outpatient facilities. Primary care is the most difficult to obtain for people who live below the federal poverty line and are uninsured (see **Box 13.1**).

Secondary Medical Care

Secondary medical care is "specialized attention and ongoing management for common and less-frequently encountered medical conditions, including support services for people with special challenges due to chronic or long-term conditions."[19] This type of care is usually provided by physicians, ideally upon referral from a primary care provider.[19]

Tertiary Medical Care

Tertiary medical care "is even more highly specialized and technologically sophisticated medical and surgical care for those with unusual or complex conditions (generally no more than a few percent of the need in any service category)."[19] This care is not usually performed in smaller hospitals; however, it is provided in specialty hospitals, academic health centers, or on specialized floors of general hospitals. Such facilities are equipped and staffed to provide advanced care for people with illnesses, such as cancer and heart disease, as well as procedures like heart bypass surgery.

Long-Term Practice

Long-term practice can be divided into two subcategories—restorative care and long-term care.

Restorative Care

Restorative care is the health care provided to patients after surgery or other successful treatment, during remission in cases of an oncogenic (cancerous) disease, or when the progression of an incurable disease has been arrested. This level of care includes follow-up to secondary

---

BOX 13.1 *Healthy People 2030:* Objectives

Access to Health Services

Goal: Improve access to comprehensive, quality healthcare services

Objective: AHS-07, Increase the proportion of persons with a usual primary care provider

Target: 84%

Baseline: 76% of persons had a usual primary care provider in 2017

Target-setting method: Percentage point improvement

Data source: Medical Expenditure Panel Survey (MEPS), Agency for Healthcare Research and Quality (AHRQ)

For Further Thought

Why is it so important for the United States to reach the objectives stated here? What impact would reaching these objectives have on the cost of health care in the United States? Provide a rationale for your response.

Data from U.S. Department of Health and Human Services, Office of Disease Prevention and Health Promotion. (2020). *Healthy People 2030.* Available at https://health.gov/healthypeople/objectives-and-data/browse-objectives/health-care-access-and-quality

and tertiary care, rehabilitative care, therapy, and home care (see **Figure 13.3**). Typical settings for this type of care include inpatient and outpatient rehabilitation units, nursing homes, assisted-living facilities, halfway houses, and private homes.

Long-Term Care

Long-term care includes the different kinds of help that people with chronic illnesses, disabilities, or other conditions that limit them physically or mentally need. In some situations, time-intensive skilled nursing care is needed, whereas some people just need help with basic daily tasks like bathing, dressing, and preparing meals. Long-term services and supports (LTSS) assist people in maintaining or improving an optimal level of functioning and quality of life and can include help from other people, special equipment, and assistive devices.[20] LTSS "should (1) fit the needs of different individuals, (2) address their changing needs over time, and (3) suit their personal preferences."[14] This type of care is provided in various settings, such as nursing homes, facilities for individuals with mental and emotional disorders, assisted-living facilities, and adult and senior daycare centers. However, long-term care is used to help people live at home rather than in institutions.

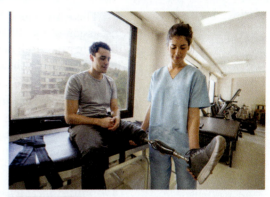

FIGURE 13.3   Restorative care can follow either secondary or tertiary care.

© Andresr/Getty Images

End-of-Life Practice

The final level of practice in healthcare delivery is end-of-life practice. **End-of-life practice** is usually thought of as those healthcare services provided to individuals shortly before death. The primary form of end-of-life practice is hospice care. **Hospice care** is "a cluster of special services for the dying, which blends medical, spiritual, legal, financial, and family support services. The venue can vary from a specialized facility, to a nursing home, to the patient's own home."[14] The most common criterion for admission to hospice care is being terminally ill with a life expectancy of less than 6 months. The first hospice program in the United States was established in 1974[21]; in 2023, there were 6,000 Medicare-certified providers and suppliers of hospice services in the United States.[20]

Types of Healthcare Providers

To offer comprehensive health care that includes services at each of the levels just mentioned, a great number of healthcare workers are needed. In 2022, the number of civilians employed in the health service industry was 14.7 million. These 14.7 million represented approximately one of every 12 employed civilians in the United States.[22]

Despite the large number of healthcare workers, the demand for more is expected to continue to grow. During the peak years of COVID-19 in 2019 and 2020, the American Hospital Association indicated that the need for nursing personnel increased by 30%. Healthcare workers are projected to be the fastest growing occupational group during the 2018 to 2028 projections decade. This group is expected to contribute 1.8 million new jobs, representing about one in four of all new jobs during that 10-year period.[22] Due to the continuing geographic maldistribution of healthcare workers, the need will be greater in some settings than in others. The settings of greatest need will continue to be the rural and inner-city areas.

About two-fifths (39%) of all healthcare employees work in hospitals, more than one-fourth (26%) work in offices of health practitioners (i.e., offices and clinics), one-fifth (20%) work in nursing and residential care facilities, and 8% each work in home health services and outpatient, laboratory, and other ambulatory care services.[23] As changes have come to the way health care is offered, the proportions of healthcare workers by setting have also changed, with fewer persons working in hospitals (in 1970, 63% worked in hospitals) and more employed in nursing homes and ambulatory care settings (such as surgical and emergency centers). This trend is expected to continue in the future, with special needs in the area of long-term care workers to meet the needs of the aging baby boom generation.

Long-term care different kinds of help that people with chronic illnesses, disabilities, or other conditions that limit them physically or mentally need

End-of-life practice healthcare services provided to individuals shortly before death

Hospice care a cluster of special services for the dying which blends medical, spiritual, legal, financial, and family support services. The venue can vary from a specialized facility, to a nursing home, to the patient's own home.

There are about 250 different careers in the healthcare industry. To help simplify the discussion of the different types of healthcare workers, they have been categorized into six different groups—independent providers, limited-care providers, nurses, nonphysician practitioners, allied healthcare professionals, and public health professionals.

Independent Providers

An **independent provider** is a healthcare workers who has the specialized education and legal authority to treat any health problem or disease that an individual has. This group of workers can be further divided into allopathic, osteopathic, and nonallopathic providers.

Allopathic and Osteopathic Providers

An **allopathic provider** is a provider who uses a system of medical practice in which specific remedies for illnesses, often in the form of drugs or medication, are used to produce effects different from those of diseases. The practitioners who fall into this category are those who are referred to as doctors of medicine (MDs). The usual method of practice for MDs includes the taking of a health history, a physical examination—perhaps with special attention to one area of the complaint—and the provision of specific treatment, such as antibiotics for a bacterial infection or a tetanus injection and sutures for a laceration.

Another type of physician who provides services similar to those of MDs is the **osteopathic provider**, or doctor of osteopathic medicine (DO). At one time, MDs and DOs would not have been grouped together because of differences in their formal education, methods, and philosophy of care. While the educational requirements and methods of treatment used by MDs have remained essentially consistent over the years, those of DOs have not. The practice of osteopathy was started in 1874 by Andrew Taylor Still, MD, DO, who was dissatisfied with the effectiveness of nineteenth-century medicine.[24] The distinctive feature of osteopathic medicine is the recognition of the reciprocal interrelationship between the structure and function of the body. The actual work of DOs and MDs is very similar today. Both types of physicians use all available scientific modalities, including drugs and surgery, in providing care to their patients. Both can also serve as primary-care physicians (approximately 30% of MDs[25] and 56% of DOs are primary care physicians)[26] or as board-certified specialists. Their differences are most notably the greater tendency of DOs to use manipulation in treating health problems and the DOs' perception of themselves as being more holistically oriented than MDs. DOs constitute 7% of all physicians today.[27] Few patients today would be able to tell the difference between the care given by a DO and an MD.

The educational requirements for MD and DO degrees are very similar. Both complete a bachelor's degree, 4 years of medical education, and 3 years (such as in family medicine) to 7 years (such as neurosurgery) of medical specialty training known as a *residency*. The first year of a residency is referred to as the *internship year*, and the physician is referred to as an **intern** or first-year **resident**. During this year, the interns can only practice medicine under the guidance of a licensed physician. Upon successful completion of the internship year, the interns are then eligible to sit for the third part of the licensing examination (the first two parts are taken during medical school). If they pass the exam, they are then entitled to practice medicine without the supervision of another licensed physician. At this point, almost all interns will complete the remaining years of residency (and are referred to generically as residents) to be eligible to sit for the board specialty examinations. Passing this examination will make them "board certified" in their specialty.

The American Medical Association (AMA) Physician Masterfile lists more than 200 specialty categories.[28] With so many specialties and subspecialties, even though primary care specialties (which include family medicine/general practice, internal medicine, internal medicine/pediatrics, and pediatrics) make up the largest percentage of physicians, healthcare experts are worried that not enough primary care physicians will be trained. This became an even bigger concern in 2010 with the passage of the ACA because of the emphasis the ACA placed on prevention and primary care.

Nonallopathic Providers

Nonallopathic providers are identified by their nontraditional means of providing health care. Some have referred to much of the care provided by these providers as complementary/alternative medicine (CAM) or complementary/integrative medicine. Included in this group of providers are chiropractors, acupuncturists (see **Figure 13.4**), naturopaths (those who use natural therapies), herbalists (those who use herbal brews for treating illness), and homeopaths (those who use small doses of herbs, minerals, and even poisons for therapy).

The best-known and most often used type of nonallopathic provider in the United States is the **chiropractor**. The underlying premise of the care provided by chiropractors is that all health problems are caused by misalignments of the vertebrae in the spinal column. The chiropractic (done by hand) approach to the treatment is (1) the identification of the misalignment through X-rays and (2) the realignment of the bones through a series of treatments called "adjustments."

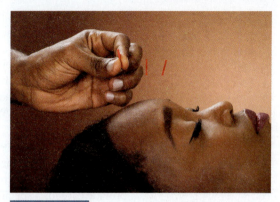

FIGURE 13.4 Many people seek out nontraditional means of health care, such as acupuncture.

© Andrey_Popov/Shutterstock

Chiropractors are educated in 4-year chiropractic colleges. The Council on Chiropractic Education accredits colleges of chiropractic medicine in the United States. As with allopathic and osteopathic programs, students usually enter chiropractic programs after earning a bachelor's degree. Those who graduate from chiropractic colleges earn a doctor of chiropractic (DC) degree. Chiropractors are licensed in all 50 states and must pass either a state licensing examination or an examination given by the National Board of Chiropractic Examiners. There are approximately 37,740 chiropractors in the United States today.[29]

As noted earlier, much of the care provided by nonallopathic providers is referred to as **complementary/alternative medicine (CAM)**, or *complementary/integrative medicine.* CAM has been defined as "a group of diverse medical and health care systems, practices, and products that are not presently considered to be a part of conventional medicine."[30] When using a nonmainstream approach together with conventional medicine, it is identified as *complementary.*[30] An example of a complementary medicine is using acupuncture in addition to conventional medicine to help lessen pain. When using a nonmainstream approach in place of conventional medicine, it is labeled as *alternative.*[30] An example of alternative is using a special diet to treat cancer instead of undergoing surgery, radiation, or chemotherapy that has been recommended by a conventional doctor. When mainstream medical therapies are combined with CAM therapies for which there is some high-quality scientific evidence of safety and effectiveness, it is referred to as *integrative medicine.*[31] CAM is one of the fastest growing areas of health care today. Data indicate that approximately 38% of adults and 12% of children in the United States reported using CAM in 2017,[30] although the percentage changes, depending on what is considered CAM. Whereas natural products (i.e., dietary supplements other than vitamins and minerals) were the most commonly used complementary approach, pain was the condition for which most people used a complementary approach.[32] The percentage of use is highest when the definition of CAM includes prayer specifically for health reasons. Americans paid for most CAM out of pocket. A nationwide government survey showed that U.S. adults spent $33.9 billion out of pocket in 1 year on CAM.[33] Nearly two-thirds of that total was spent on self-care purchases of CAM products, classes, and materials, whereas the remaining portion was spent on practitioner visits. Despite this emphasis on self-care therapies, adults made more than 354 million visits to CAM practioners.[33] "Insurance coverage for complementary health approaches is often complex and varies widely based on factors, such as state laws, regulations, and differences among specific plans. Many individuals' decisions to use these practices are influenced by the type of health insurance they have. To determine whether a particular approach is covered, it is essential to review the specifics of the insurance plan. Contacting the insurance provider is a practical first step in obtaining accurate and detailed information."[34]

Nonallopathic providers independent providers who provide nontraditional forms of health care

Chiropractor a nonallopathic, independent healthcare provider who treats health problems by adjusting the spinal column

Complementary/alternative medicine (CAM) a group of diverse medical and healthcare systems, practices, and products that are not presently considered to be a part of conventional medicine

Limited (restricted) care providers healthcare providers who provide care for a specific part of the body

Licensed practical nurse (LPN) one who is prepared in 1- to 2-year programs to provide nontechnical bedside nursing care under the supervision of physicians or registered nurses

Registered nurse (RN) one who has successfully completed an accredited academic program and a state licensing examination

There are literally hundreds of systems, approaches, and techniques that fall within the CAM rubric. CAM practices are often grouped into broad categories, such as natural products (e.g., herbal medicines also known as botanicals); mind-body medicine (e.g., meditation, yoga, acupuncture, hypnotherapy, tai chi); manipulative and body-based practices (e.g., spinal manipulation and massage therapy); and other CAM practices (movement therapies [e.g., Pilates, Rolfing], traditional healers, manipulation of energy fields [i.e., magnet therapy], and whole medical systems [e.g., Ayurvedic medicine, homeopathy, naturopathy]).[30]

Limited (or Restricted) Care Providers

Much health care is provided by **limited (or restricted) care providers** who have advanced training, usually a doctoral degree, in a healthcare specialty. Their specialty enables them to provide care for a specific part of the body. This group of providers includes but is not limited to dentists (teeth and oral cavity), optometrists (eyes, specifically refractory errors), podiatrists (feet and ankles), audiologists (hearing), and psychologists (mental health).

Nurses

We have categorized nurses into a group of their own because of their unique degree programs, the long-standing tradition of nursing as a profession, and their overall importance in the healthcare industry. It has been estimated that there are between 4 and 5 million individuals who work in the nursing profession. These include registered nurses, licensed practical nurses, and ancillary nursing personnel, such as nurse's aides.[35–37] Nurses outnumber physicians, dentists, and every other single group of healthcare workers in the United States. Even with such numbers, the need for nurses will continue[35–37] (see **Figure 13.5**).

Future of Nursing

During the COVID-19 pandemic, nurses faced exhausting hours and excessive workloads, causing significant mental and physical stress. In order to meet the demands of the healthcare system in the United States, nurses need to address the ongoing pandemic, patient demographics, and their needs. Each year, there are about 193,100 nursing job opportunities within the United States. An increase in nursing jobs will be needed in areas of home health, long-term care, telehealth, and outpatient services.[37]

Training and Education of Nurses

Nurses can be divided into subcategories based on their level of education and type of preparation. The first are those who are prepared as licensed practical nurses. Once they complete their 1 to 2 years of education in a vocational, hospital, or associate-degree program and pass a licensure examination, this type of nurse is referred to as a **licensed practical nurse (LPN)**, or licensed vocational nurse (LVN) in some states. LPNs care for people who are sick, injured, convalescent, or disabled under the supervision of physicians or registered nurses.[38] "The nature of the direction and supervision required varies by state and job setting."[38] Not too many years ago, it was thought that LPNs would be phased out and replaced with more qualified nurses. In 2018, there were 728,900 LPNs or LVNs working in the United States, and that number was projected to grow by 11% to 807,100 by 2028.[35]

A second group of nurses is *registered nurses*. A **registered nurse (RN)** is one who has successfully completed an accredited academic program and a state licensing (registration) examination. The three typical educational paths to registered nursing are a bachelor's degree (BSN), an associate degree (ADN), and a diploma from an approved nursing program.[36] ADN programs take approximately 2 to 3 years to complete and are typically offered by community or junior colleges. Diploma programs are offered by hospitals and last about 3 years. RNs holding BSN

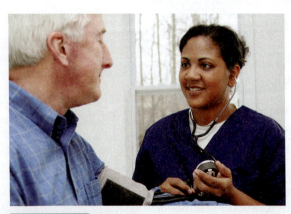

FIGURE 13.5 There is still a need for more nurses.

© Rob Marmion/Shutterstock

degrees are considered to have been more thoroughly prepared for additional activities involving independent judgment. Of the employed registered nurses, 60% worked in hospitals, about 18% in ambulatory healthcare services, 7% in nursing and residential care facilities, 5% in government, and 3% in educational services.[36] In 2018, there were 3.1 million RNs working in the United States, and that number was projected to grow by 12% to 3.4 million by 2028.[36]

Advanced Practice Registered Nurses

With advances in technology and the development of new areas of medical specialization, there is a growing need for specialty-prepared advanced practice registered nurses (APRNs). Many professional nurses continue their education and earn master's and doctoral degrees in nursing. The master's degree programs are aimed primarily at specialties, such as nurse practitioners (NPs; e.g., pediatric nurse practitioners and school nurse practitioners), clinical nurse specialists (CNSs), certified registered nurse anesthetists (CRNAs), and certified nurse midwives (CNMs). The largest portion of APRNs is nurse practitioners (NPs). NPs "assess patients, order and interpret diagnostic tests, make diagnoses, and initiate and manage treatment plans—including prescribing medications."[39] Not only do they provide high-quality care in a cost-effective manner, but they are also considered primary care providers in chronically medically underserved inner-city and rural areas. Close to 90% of all NPs are prepared in primary care.[39] The authors of the ACA saw the value of NPs to the U.S. healthcare system and as such included funding to increase both the number of those trained as NPs and the number of clinics in which NPs practice.

Even though there is evidence to show the value of NPs, regulatory barriers prevent many NPs from practicing to their full potential. Currently, NPs in 28 states and the District of Columbia have full practice authority. "Most states with full practice authority for NPs allow them to practice without formal oversight immediately upon licensure. These states are Alaska, Arizona, Hawaii, Idaho, Iowa, Montana, New Hampshire, New Mexico, North Dakota, Oregon, Rhode Island, Utah, Washington, and Wyoming, plus the District of Columbia." Fourteen states with full practice authority require that NPs practice in collaboration with physicians or experienced NPs for a transitional period before they are allowed to practice and prescribe without formal oversight.[40]

Like other nurses, the demand for NPs is also expected to increase, especially as a greater portion of the population gains access to health care and more of the population becomes enrolled in managed care. In 2023, there were 385,000 NPs licensed in the United States, and that number was projected to grow to 242,400 employed NPs by 2028.[39]

The relatively few nurses who hold doctorate degrees in nursing are highly sought after as university faculty. Nurses with doctorates teach, conduct research, and otherwise prepare other nurses or hold administrative (leadership) positions in healthcare institutions.

Physician Assistants

The **physician assistant (PA)** is a healthcare professional who practices medicine with physician supervision.[41] They are considered midlevel providers with training and skills beyond those of RNs and less than those of physicians.[38] Physician assistant programs began in response to the shortage of primary care physicians. Most PAs have a bachelor's degree and then complete a 2-year accredited educational program for PAs that typically leads to a master's degree.[35] After completion of the program or degree, PAs must pass a national certifying examination. PAs always work under the direct supervision of a licensed physician (thus the name *physician extenders*). They carry out many of the same duties that are thought of as the responsibilities of physicians, such as taking medical histories, examining patients, ordering and interpreting laboratory tests and X-rays, counseling patients, making preliminary diagnoses, treating minor injuries, and, in most states, prescribing medications.[38] The specific duties of a PAs would depend on (1) the setting in which they work, (2) their level of experience, (3) their specialty, and (4) the laws in the state where they practice.[42] In 2022, there were 140,910 PAs working in the United States, and that number was projected to grow by 27% to 187,300 between 2018 and 2028.[43]

Physician assistant (PA)
healthcare professional who practices medicine with physician supervision

Allied healthcare professionals healthcare workers who provide services that assist, facilitate, and complement the work of physicians and other healthcare specialists

Public health professionals healthcare workers who work in a public health organization

Allied Healthcare Professionals

Allied health describes a large group of health-related professions that fulfill necessary roles in the healthcare delivery system. These **allied healthcare professionals**, who constitute approximately 60% of the healthcare workforce, assist, facilitate, and complement the work of physicians, dentists, and other healthcare specialists. These healthcare workers provide a variety of services that are essential to patient care. Often they are responsible for highly technical services and procedures. Allied healthcare professionals can be categorized into several groups. They include (1) laboratory technologists and technicians (e.g., medical technologists, emergency medical technicians, nuclear medicine technicians, operating room technicians, dental technicians and hygienists, and radiographers [X-ray technicians]); (2) therapeutic science practitioners (e.g., occupational, physical, radiation, and respiratory therapists and speech pathologists); (3) behavioral scientists (e.g., health education specialists, social workers, and rehabilitation counselors); and (4) support services (e.g., medical record keepers and medical secretaries). The educational backgrounds of allied health workers range from vocational training to clinical doctoral degrees. Many of these professionals must pass a state or national licensing examination before they can practice.

The demand for allied healthcare workers in all of the areas previously noted is expected to continue. The primary reasons for this are the growth of the entire healthcare industry and the continuing arrival of the baby boomers as senior citizens.

Public Health Professionals

A discussion about healthcare providers would be incomplete without the mention of a group of health workers who provide unique healthcare services to the community—**public health professionals**. They support the delivery of health care by such hands-on providers as public health physicians, dentists, nurses, and dietitians who work in public health clinics sponsored by federal, state, local, and voluntary health agencies (see **Figure 13.6**). Examples of other public health professionals are environmental health workers, public health administrators, epidemiologists, health education specialists, public health nurses and physicians, biostatisticians, the U.S. Surgeon General, and the research scientists at the Centers for Disease Control and Prevention. Public health professionals often make possible the care that is practiced in immunization clinics, nutritional programs for women, infants, and children (WIC), dental health clinics, and sexually transmitted infection clinics. School nurses are also considered public health professionals. Public health services are usually financed by tax dollars and, although available to most taxpayers, primarily serve the economically disadvantaged. During public health emergencies like COVID-19, public health had to rely heavily on its workforce to respond rapidly to continuous threats and, at the same time, continue with the fundamentals of public health services. The United States public health infrastructure consists of 2,800 local health departments, 51 health departments in each state, including the district of Columbia, and eight territorial or freely associated state public health agencies, and 300 regional and district offices.[20]

Healthcare Facilities and Their Accreditation

Health care is provided in a variety of settings in the United States. The major settings and the accreditation of these facilities are discussed in the sections that follow.

Healthcare Facilities

Healthcare facilities are the physical settings in which health care is actually provided. They include a wide variety of settings but can be divided into two large categories: inpatient care and outpatient care. *Inpatient care facilities* include any in which a

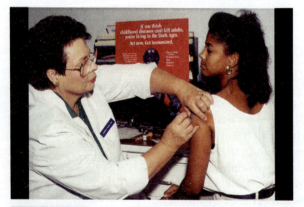

FIGURE 13.6   Public health professionals, such as this public health nurse, make up a key component of the healthcare system.

Courtsey of Barbara Rice/CDC.

patient stays overnight, such as a hospital. *Outpatient care facilities* refer to any facility in which the patient receives care and does not stay overnight.

Inpatient Care Facilities

The primary inpatient care facilities are hospitals, nursing homes, and assisted-living facilities. Because nursing homes and assisted-living facilities are discussed elsewhere, we discuss only hospitals here. In 2015, there were 564 hospitals in the United States,[25] and they varied in size, mission, and organizational structure. The major purpose of hospitals is to provide a place for secondary and tertiary care.

Hospitals can be categorized in several different ways; one way is by hospital ownership (see **Figure 13.7** and **Table 13.3**). A **private (proprietary or investor-owned) hospital** is one that is owned as a business for the purpose of making a profit. "Most for-profit hospitals belong to one of the large hospital management companies that dominate the for-profit hospital network."[6] One type of private hospital is the **specialty hospital**. These hospitals are stand-alone, single-specialty (e.g., women's health, surgery, cardiac, or orthopedic) facilities not within the walls of a full-service hospital.[44] Most are owned, at least in part, by the physicians who practice in them.[6] When this is the case, such hospitals have been referred to as physician-owned hospitals (POHs). A lot of controversy surrounds these hospitals. Larger general hospitals, which are losing patients and revenue to the specialty hospitals, say that these specialty hospitals are just a "grab for money" by the physicians who own them. Physicians say specialty hospitals allow them to practice medicine the way that it should be practiced, without answering to a hospital administrator who is trying to cut corners to make a profit. Because of the controversy surrounding POHs, a section of the ACA placed a ban on building new or expanding POHs. However, a recent study concluded that "[a]lthough POHs may treat slightly healthier patients, they do not seem to systematically select more profitable or less disadvantaged patients, or to provide lower value care."[45] In addition, ratings of POHs by the Centers for Medicare and Medicaid Services (CMS) and the U.S. Department of Health and Human Services (HHS) have shown that POHs have fared well compared with general hospitals in quality, costs, and consumer satisfaction.[46] Because of these data, several attempts have been made to amend the ACA to lift the ban, but to no avail, in part because of the controversy in the U.S. Congress on the best way to offer health care.

A second type is a **public hospital**. These hospitals are supported and managed by governmental jurisdictions and are usually found in larger cities. Public hospitals can be operated by agencies at all levels of government. Hospitals operated by the federal government include military hospitals (e.g., Walter Reed National Medical Center in Bethesda, Maryland) and the

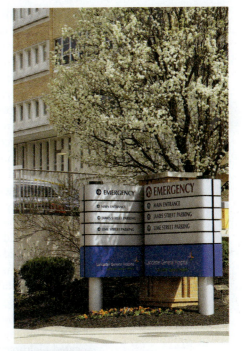

FIGURE 13.7   Hospitals are often categorized by ownership.

© James F. McKenzie

Private (proprietary or investor-owned) hospital a for-profit hospital

Specialty hospital a stand-alone, single-specialty (e.g., women's health, surgery, cardiac, or orthopedic) facility not within the walls of a full-service hospital

Public hospital a hospital that is supported and managed by governmental jurisdictions

TABLE 13.3   Number of Beds and Hospitals According to Ownership— United States, 2019

Type	Number	Beds
All hospitals	6120	916,752
Federal	207	38,768
Nonfederal community hospitals	5,129	784,112
Private or proprietary or investor-owned (for-profit)	1,219	136,365
Public (state or local)	923	115,300
Voluntary (not-for-profit)	2,987	531,907

Data from National Center for Health Statistics. (2019). *Health, United States, 2019: With special feature on Mortality.* Hyattsville, MD: Author.

Voluntary hospital
a nonprofit hospital administered by a not-for-profit corporation or charitable community organization

Full-service hospital
a hospital that offers services in all or most of the levels of care defined by the spectrum of healthcare delivery

Limited-service hospital
a hospital that offers only the specific services needed by the population served

many hospitals run by the Veterans Administration and Indian Health Service. There are also hospitals that are owned or partially financed by state and local governments. Examples include university hospitals, state mental hospitals, and local city and county hospitals.

The **voluntary hospital** makes up the third category of hospitals. These are nonprofit hospitals administered by not-for-profit corporations or religious, fraternal, and other charitable community organizations. These hospitals make up about one-half of all hospitals in the United States. Examples of this latter group are the Southern Baptist hospitals, the Shriners' hospitals, and many community hospitals. In recent years, voluntary hospitals have been expanding their scope of services and many now include wellness centers, stress management centers, chemical dependency programs, and a variety of satellite centers.

A second way of classifying hospitals is by dividing them into *teaching* and *nonteaching* hospitals. Teaching hospitals have, as a part of their mission, the responsibility to prepare new healthcare providers. These hospitals are typically aligned with medical schools, universities, and medical residency programs. However, a number of hospitals not affiliated with medical schools provide medical residency programs and clinical education for nurses, allied health personnel, and a wide variety of technical specialties.

A third means of categorizing hospitals is by the services offered. A **full-service hospital**, or general hospital, is one that offers care at all or most of the levels of care discussed earlier in the chapter. These are the most expensive hospitals to run and are usually found in metropolitan areas. A **limited-service hospital** offers the specific services needed by the population served, such as emergency, maternity, general surgery, and so on, but they lack much of the sophisticated technology available at full-service hospitals. This type of hospital is more common in rural areas. Many limited-service hospitals were once full-service hospitals but have become limited-service hospitals because of the low volume of patients, a shortage of healthcare personnel, and financial distress.

Outpatient Care Facilities

An *outpatient care facility* is one where a patient receives ambulatory care (i.e., patients voluntarily leave their home to seek care) without being admitted as an inpatient.[1,47] Because of the variety of outpatient care services offered throughout the United States and the variety of arrangements for ownership of the services (e.g., hospitals, hospital systems, physician groups, and for-profit or not-for-profit chains), it is difficult to identify all possible outpatient care facilities. "For example, agencies providing home health services can be freestanding, hospital based, or nursing home based. In many instances, physician group practices are merging with hospitals, and hospitals and freestanding surgical centers often compete against each other for various types of surgical procedures."[1]

What is known is that today, care and procedures that once were performed only on an inpatient basis are increasingly being performed in a variety of outpatient settings.[21] In fact, today, the majority of all surgical procedures are performed on an outpatient basis.[6] The growth and movement of services to outpatient care facilities have resulted from a combination of new medical and diagnostic procedures, technological advances, consumer demand for user-friendly environments, the reimbursement process, and financial mandates from insurance companies and the government.[6] The types of outpatient care facilities found in communities are healthcare practitioners' offices, clinics, primary-care centers, retail clinics, urgent/emergent care centers, ambulatory surgery centers, and freestanding service facilities.

Probably, the outpatient care facilities with which people have the most familiarity are healthcare practitioners' offices that house private practices. In 2012, there were more than 883.7 million patient visits to physician offices in the United States,[48] with the average person having a little under three visits per year.[48]

Because it is expensive to set up a private practice, it is increasingly common to see more than one practitioner sharing both an office and staff. These practices are often referred to as *group practices*, to distinguish them from *solo* (single practitioner) *practices*. Also, when two or more physicians practice as a group, the facility in which they provide medical services is called a *clinic*. Some clinics are small, with just a few providers, while others are large, with many providers, such as the Mayo Clinic in Rochester, Minnesota, or the Cleveland Clinic in Cleveland, Ohio. Some clinics provide care only for individuals with special health needs, such as treatment of cancer or diabetes or assistance in family planning; others accept patients with a wide range of problems. A misconception held by many is that clinics are not very different from hospitals. One big difference is that clinics do not have inpatient beds, and hospitals do. Some clinics do have an administrative relationship with inpatient facilities so that if a person needs to be admitted to a hospital, it is a relatively simple process; other clinics may be freestanding, or independent of all other facilities.

Although many clinics are run as either for-profit or not-for-profit facilities, some are funded by tax dollars. These clinics have been created primarily to meet the needs of the **medically indigent**—people who lack the financial ability to pay for their own medical care. Most of these clinics are located in large urban areas or rural areas that are underserved by the private sector. Two examples of this type of clinic are *public health clinics* and *community health centers* (CHCs). The former are usually a part of a local health department (LHD). The scope of healthcare services offered by LHDs varies greatly. These services can range from prevention-oriented programs, such as immunizations and well-baby care, to complete personal health services, such as those offered at private-sector clinics. CHCs have been around since the late 1960s and were known initially as *neighborhood health centers*. A CHC that receives funding under Section 330 of the Public Health Service Act is known as a **Federally Qualified Health Center (FQHC)**. FQHCs operate under the auspices of the Bureau of Primary Health Care, which is part of HHS.[49] Today, there are over 1,200 FQHCs, which are located in every state and territory.[49] The importance of FQHCs to the primary healthcare needs of the underserved populations in the United States is huge.[6]

In 2018, FQHCs served almost 27 million patients nationally, many from racial and ethnic minority groups. Of those patients, 92% had family incomes at or below the poverty level, 23% were uninsured, and another 49% depended on Medicaid.[49] The importance of FQHCs was reinforced when additional funding for them was included in the ACA.[50]

Some of the most recent additions to outpatient care facilities are retail clinics found in pharmacies (e.g., CVS, Walgreens), supermarkets (e.g., Kroger), and retail stores (e.g., Walmart, Target). The concept was born in 2000 when the first retail clinic opened in a grocery store in Minnesota.[51] In 2014, the number was approximately 1,800.[52] The services offered are limited, but they "represent an entrepreneurial response to consumer demand for fast, affordable treatment of easy-to-diagnose, acute conditions."[6] The facilities are often operated by an outside company, maybe even a hospital, and are generally staffed by nurses, nurse practitioners, and physician assistants. Initially, payment at these clinics was out of pocket for the consumer, but the concept has caught the eye of insurers as a less-expensive way of providing acute care, and thus many insurers now have contracts with the clinics, allowing patients to pay only copays.[6] Employers also like the idea and waive the copay when employees use them.[6] Some employers have even set up similar "quick clinics" within their own facilities. Response to these clinics has been good from both insurers and consumers, but some in the medical community question the quality of care received.

Urgent/emergent care centers have been around in the United States since the early 1970s. They "fill gaps in the delivery system created by the rigidity of private physician appointments and unavailability during nonbusiness hours. The centers also provide a much more convenient and user-friendly alternative to a hospital emergency department during hours when private physicians are not available."[6] Urgent/emergent care centers often provide quicker service with less paperwork, particularly for those with cash or credit cards. These facilities (often not much larger than a fast-food restaurant) have sometimes been referred to as "doc-in-a-box"! These facilities are not appropriate for all emergency cases. A majority of patients with life-threatening conditions are still taken to hospital emergency rooms, which have top-of-the-line advanced life support equipment and emergency physicians are on staff. Although emergency rooms are expensive for hospitals to maintain, they obviously perform a needed service (see **Figure 13.8**).

Medically indigent people who lack the financial ability to pay for their own medical care

Federally Qualified Health Center (FQHC) community health center that receives funding under Section 330 of the Public Health Service Act

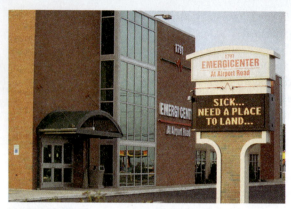

FIGURE 13.8   Many outpatient care facilities provide medical services safely and efficiently without the overhead of a hospital.

© James F. McKenzie

Ambulatory surgery centers do not perform major surgery, such as heart transplants. They do, however, perform same-day surgeries where a hospital stay following the surgery is not needed. As noted earlier, today, the majority of all surgical procedures are performed in these types of facilities.[5] Factors that have promoted the increase in ambulatory surgical procedures as alternatives to inpatient surgery include the development of new, safe, and faster-acting general anesthetics; advances in surgical equipment and materials; development of noninvasive or minimally invasive surgical and nonsurgical procedures; and reduced coverage by insurance companies for hospital stays.

One area of tremendous growth in outpatient care facilities in recent years has been in the development of freestanding, nonhospital-based specialty facilities. These facilities frequently offer a single service, such as dialysis for individuals with kidney failure, or similar services, such as those available in a diagnostic imaging center. In the latter example, the services often included are simple radiograph technology (X-rays), computed tomography (CT), and magnetic resonance imaging (MRI), which are used for viewing the body's anatomical structures in several planes. These technologies are ideal for outpatient facilities because of their noninvasive nature and profitability.

Even though convenience and cost are often the reasons for the development of new outpatient care facilities, the establishment of a new outpatient care facility in a community is not always received with enthusiasm. In previously underserved communities, fast-growing communities, or communities with many temporary residents such as resort communities, they have been well received. However, in stable or shrinking communities where an adequate number of health providers exists, the arrival of a new freestanding ambulatory care facility is sometimes viewed as unfriendly competition. In some of these cases, the "unfriendly competition" has come from outside for-profit healthcare companies; however, a more recent trend has been physicians breaking away from voluntary (independent or not-for-profit) hospitals, where they once performed the procedures in the hospital's outpatient facility, to create their own facilities in which to perform the procedures. The primary reasons for this trend are physicians wishing to have control over how the facility is run (e.g., the times and days procedures are scheduled, who is hired to work in the facilities) and to receive a greater share of the profits.

Rehabilitation Centers

A **rehabilitation center** is a healthcare facility in which patients work with healthcare providers to restore functions lost because of injury, disease, or surgery. These centers are sometimes part of a clinic or hospital but may also be freestanding facilities. Rehabilitation centers may operate on both an outpatient and an inpatient basis. Providers who commonly work in a rehabilitation center include physical, occupational, and respiratory therapists as well as exercise physiologists.

Long-Term Care Options

Not too many years ago, when the topic of long-term care was mentioned, most people thought of nursing homes and state hospitals for people with mental illness and emotional disabilities. Today, however, the term *long-term care* not only includes the traditional institutional residential care but also special units within these residential facilities (such as for Alzheimer's disease patients), halfway houses, group homes, assisted-living facilities, transitional (step-down) care in a hospital, daycare facilities for patients of all ages with health problems who require special care, and personal home health care. Older adults are the biggest users of long-term care, but other users include those with disabilities or chronic conditions, and those with acute and subacute conditions who are unable to care for themselves.

Rehabilitation center a facility in which restorative care is provided following injury, disease, or surgery

One area of long-term care that has received special attention in recent years is home health care. The demand for home health care has been driven by the restructuring of the healthcare delivery system, technological advances that enable people to be treated outside of a hospital and to recover more quickly, and the cost containment pressures that have shortened hospital stays. **Home health care** involves providing health care via health personnel and medical equipment to individuals and families in their places of residence, for the purpose of promoting, maintaining, or restoring health or maximizing the level of independence while minimizing the effects of disability and illness, including terminal disease. Home health care can be either long-term, to help a chronically ill patient avoid institutionalization, or it can be short term to assist a patient following an acute illness and hospitalization until the patient is able to return to independent functioning. Home health care can be provided either through a formal system of paid professional health caregivers (e.g., home healthcare agency) or through an informal system where the care is provided by family, friends, and neighbors.[6] Medicare is the largest single payer for home health care, accounting for about one-third of the total annual expenditures.[6]

The need for professional health caregivers will continue into the future because of the "increase in the number of older persons and their expressed desire to remain in their homes for care whenever possible."[6] As of 2021, there were 11,474 Medicare-certified home health agencies in the United States. That number is almost four times as many as existed in 1980.[18] There are approximately 3 million Medicare fee-for-service beneficiaries using home healthcare service. In 2020, 8.3% of all fee-for-service utilized home healthcare.[53] Even though Medicare and Medicaid are the largest payers for home healthcare services, the amounts spent are relatively small compared with the total dollars spent on the Medicare and Medicaid programs.[25]

Accreditation of Healthcare Facilities

One way of determining the quality of a healthcare facility is to find out if it is accredited by a reputable organization. **Accreditation** is the process by which an agency or organization evaluates and recognizes an institution as meeting certain predetermined standards. The predominant organization responsible for accrediting healthcare facilities is **The Joint Commission**, formerly known as the Joint Commission on Accreditation of Healthcare Organizations (JCAHO). The Joint Commission is an independent, not-for-profit organization that accredits and certifies more than 21,000 healthcare organizations and programs in the United States. The healthcare facilities/organizations that can be accredited by The Joint Commission include ambulatory healthcare centers, behavioral healthcare organizations, independent or freestanding laboratories, homecare agencies/organizations, hospitals (e.g., general, children's, psychiatric, rehabilitation, and critical access), and long-term care facilities (e.g., nursing homes and rehabilitation centers). To earn and maintain The Joint Commission accreditation, a facility or organization must complete an application and undergo an on-site survey (visit) by a Joint Commission survey team. The Joint Commission surveyors conduct an unannounced visit to accredited healthcare organizations a minimum of once every 39 months (2 years for laboratories) to evaluate standards compliance.[54] Only those organizations that are in compliance with all standards at the time of the on-site survey are accredited. The Joint Commission feels that compliance with its standards is not an every 3-year process but rather an ongoing process.

Joint Commission accreditation does not begin and end with the on-site survey. It is a continuous process. Every time a nurse double-checks a patient's identification before administering a medication, every time a surgical team calls a "time out" to verify they agree they are about to perform the correct procedure, at the correct site, on the correct patient, they live and breathe the accreditation process. Every quarter, hospitals submit performance data to The Joint Commission on conditions, such as cardiac care and stroke The Joint Commission accreditation is woven into the fabric of a healthcare organization's operations.[54]

(© The Joint Commission, 2023. Reprinted with permission.)

Home health care care that is provided in the patient's residence for the purpose of promoting, maintaining, or restoring health

Accreditation the process by which an agency or organization evaluates and recognizes an institution as meeting certain predetermined standards

The Joint Commission the predominant organization responsible for accrediting healthcare facilities

Healthcare System: Function

Like the structure of the healthcare system, the function of the U.S. healthcare system is also unique, compared with the healthcare systems of other developed countries. The ACA is most notable for the transformations it made "to health insurance—both access to it and its contents—rather than for structural reforms made to the delivery system."[2] The purpose of the ACA was to (1) expand health insurance coverage, (2) hold insurance companies accountable, (3) lower healthcare costs, (3) guarantee more choice, and (5) enhance the quality of care for all Americans.[55] Some parts of the ACA went into effect shortly after the legislation was signed (e.g., Patient Bill of Rights), some of its biggest parts (e.g., individual mandate for health insurance) were rolled out in 2014, implementation of other parts has been postponed or delayed (e.g., employer responsibility provision). Some parts have been repealed (e.g., the unsustainable Community Living Assistance Services and Supports [CLASS] program of government-subsidized long-term care insurance),[56] and the final portions were implemented in 2020. The remainder of the chapter includes some of the structure from the past that led to the new law, and what can be expected in terms of the change in structure as the laws are always being introduced.

Understanding the Structure of the Healthcare System

To begin, it must be understood that the healthcare system of the United States is enormous and complicated. It is enormous from the standpoint of cost—it is extremely expensive (see **Figure 13.9**)—and because of the many stakeholders that include, but are not limited to, healthcare consumers, healthcare providers, healthcare administrators, politicians, policymakers, government regulators, insurance companies, and professional and trade associations. It is complicated because healthcare policy is intertwined with other policies (e.g., the U.S. tax code, where credits for employers who provide health insurance for employees and healthcare consumers who get deductions on their income taxes if their healthcare spending reaches certain levels in a year), and because of the politics and ideologic viewpoints of the decision makers.

The major issues of the healthcare system in the United States can be represented by the cost containment, access, and quality triangle noted by Kissick[57] (see **Figure 13.10**). In Kissick's equilateral triangle, the equal 60-degree angles represent equal priorities. That is, access is just as important as quality and cost containment, and vice versa. However, an expansion of any one of the angles compromises one or both of the other two. For example, if we were interested in increasing the quality of our already good services, it would also increase the costs and decrease access. Or, some feel, if we increase access, costs will go up, and the quality will decrease. Or, if we concentrate on containing costs, both quality of care and access will decrease. With such dilemmas, the United States continues to struggle to find the right combination of policy and accountability to deal with these shortcomings. Concerns associated with each of the three sides of the cost containment, access, and quality triangle are discussed later in this chapter.

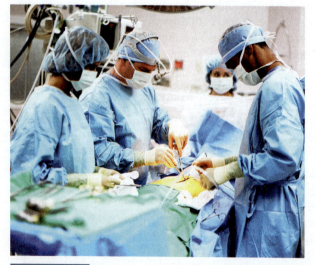

FIGURE 13.9   Healthcare services offered by U.S. providers are perhaps the best in the world, but at what cost?
© Photos.com

Access to Health Care

Even with several different means of gaining access to healthcare services, access has been and continues to be a major health policy issue in the United States. Health insurance coverage and the generosity of coverage are major determinants of access to health care.[58] Decreasing the number of uninsured Americans was a key goal of the ACA. Since the major coverage provisions of the ACA went into effect in January of 2014, the number of uninsured has declined.[59] In 2015, 28.8 million persons of all ages (9.1%) were uninsured—16.0 million fewer persons than in 2013 and 17.5 million fewer than in 2011.[60] Stated another way, almost 91% of Americans now have health insurance. This number represents a historic increase in the number of insured Americans. However, 28.8 million uninsured is still too many. Most uninsured people are adults in low-income working families, with minorities being at higher risk of being uninsured than non-Hispanic White populations[59] (see **Box 13.2**). The uninsured numbers are greatest in states that did not expand Medicaid eligibility under the ACA.[59] In 2018, The U.S. Census reported that the number of Americans without health insurance rose in a decade by 2 million people.[61]

Matching a record low, the U.S. Census found that 7.9% of the U.S. population went without medical insurance for all of 2022, down from 8.3% in 2021.[62] Interestingly enough, the uninsured do not lack emergency or urgent care because no one needing such care and willing to go to a hospital emergency room may be turned away. However, studies repeatedly demonstrate that the uninsured are less likely than those with insurance to receive preventive care (i.e., checkups, screenings, and prenatal care) and services for major health conditions and chronic diseases[59] (see Box 13.1). Without adequate primary care, many patients eventually find themselves in need of more costly and often less-effective medical treatment.

A brief summary of the most notable steps of ACA to increase the number of Americans with health insurance is presented in **Box 13.3**. Among these steps, the one that has had the biggest impact on allowing the uninsured to gain access to insurance, and in turn, access to care, is the *Health Insurance Marketplace*. The **Health Insurance Marketplace** (or exchange) is an organization that was set up to create more organized and competitive markets for buying health insurance.[63] A marketplace simplifies the search for health coverage by gathering the available options for consumers in one place. The marketplaces, which can be run by a state or the federal government, were created primarily for two groups: individuals buying insurance on their own and small businesses with up to 50 employees (some states may use different employee maximums to define small businesses). The marketplace for small businesses is called the Small Business Health Options Program (SHOP) Marketplace.[64]

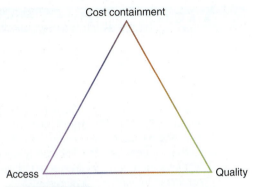

FIGURE 13.10   The cost containment, access, and quality triangle of health care.

Reproduced from Kissick, W. L. (1994). *Medicine's dilemmas: Infinite needs versus finite resources.* Yale University Press. © 1994. Reprinted by permission of Yale University Press.

Health Insurance Marketplace organization established to create more organized and competitive markets for purchasing health insurance

---

BOX 13.2   *Healthy People 2030:* Objectives

Access to Health Services

Goal: Improve access to comprehensive, quality healthcare services.

Objective: AHS-01, Increase the proportion of persons with health insurance.
Target: 92.1%
Baseline: 89% of persons under 65 years had medical insurance in 2018.
Target-setting method: Projection
Data source: National Health Interview Survey (NHIS), CDC/National Center for Health Statistics (NCHS)
Objective: AHS-02 Increase the proportion of persons with dental insurance.
Target: 59.8%
Baseline: 54.4%

Target-setting method: Projection
Potential data source: NHIS, CDC/NCHS
Objective: AHS-03 Increase the proportion of persons with prescription drug insurance.
Target: 70.6%
Baseline: 61.1%
Target-setting method: Percentage point improvement
Potential data source: NHIS, CDC/NCHS

For Further Thought

Do you think the ACA was the best way to go about reaching these objectives? Defend your response. Do you think the United States should adopt a national health insurance plan like the other developed countries of the world to make sure all persons have health insurance? Why or why not?

Data from U.S. Department of Health and Human Services, Office of Disease Prevention and Health Promotion. (2020). *Healthy People 2030.* Available at https://health.gov/healthypeople/objectives-and-data/browse-objectives/health-insurance

BOX 13.3   Components of the Affordable Care Act to Increase Access to Care

1. *Individual mandate.* In 2014, all individuals were required to have health insurance or pay a fee. The fee was phased in from 2014 to 2016. The fee for 2016 was the higher of 2.5% of household income or $695 per adult ($347.50 per child), up to a maximum of $2,085. The fee is paid through the federal income tax return. There are some exceptions to this requirement that include financial hardship, religious objections, incarcerated individuals, and for American Indians.*

2. *Expansion of public programs.* Medicaid expanded to cover non–Medicaid-eligible individuals under the age of 65 up to 133% (because of the way it is calculated, it turns out to be 138%) of the federal poverty level based on modified adjusted gross income (under current law, undocumented immigrants are not eligible for Medicaid except for the state of California, which became the first state in the nation to offer health insurance to undocumented immigrants in 2024). In 2023, the federal poverty level for a family of four was $27,750, making the 133% level $41,496. This expansion created a national uniform eligibility standard across states if states accepted the expansion.* The federal government pays for most of the expansion.

3. *Health Insurance Marketplace* (i.e., exchange). For people who do not receive employer-sponsored insurance and who make more than 133% of the federal poverty level, health insurance is available through new exchanges created by states.** (*Note*: States that did not create exchanges could have either partnered with the federal government to operate an exchange, or used a federally facilitated exchange.) Plans in the exchanges must provide benefits that meet a minimum set of standards. Insurers offer four levels of coverage (bronze, silver, gold, and platinum) that vary based on premiums, out-of-pocket costs, and benefits beyond the minimum required plus a catastrophic coverage plan (*Note*: A catastrophic plan is available to those up to age 30 and people of any age with a hardship exemption from mandate to purchase coverage). The silver plan has become the most popular. Various premium credits and cost-sharing subsidies are available to those with incomes between 100 and 400% of the federal poverty level.

4. *Changes to private insurance.* New health insurance regulations changed the way insurers must operate. Insurers: (1) cannot deny coverage to people because of health status (i.e., preexisting condition); (2) cannot charge people more because of health status or gender; (3) with all new health plans, have to provide comprehensive coverage that includes a minimum set of services, caps out-of-pocket spending, does not impose cost-sharing for preventive services, and does not impose annual or lifetime limits on coverage; (4) have to allow young adults to remain on their parents' health insurance up until age 26; and (5) have to limit waiting periods to no longer than 90 days on employer-sponsored plans.

5. *Employer responsibility provision.* Employers with 50 or more full-time employees, or full-time equivalents, must offer health insurance that is affordable (i.e., ≤9.66% of an employee's W-2 wages in 2016) and provides minimum value (i.e., 60%+ of the costs of covered services) to their full-time employees and their children up to age 26 or be subject to a penalty. Employers who failed to offer health insurance were assessed a fee of $2,160 per full-time employee (in excess of 30 employees) in 2016 if they had at least one full-time employee who received a premium tax credit (i.e., subsidy) through a marketplace. Employers who did provide insurance but did not offer health insurance that was affordable and provided a minimum value and had at least one employee who received a premium tax credit from marketplace coverage were required to pay the lesser of $3,240 per employee in 2016 who received a premium tax credit or $2,160 per employee (in excess of 30 employees). If employees offer coverage and have workers who do not sign up for the plan or do not opt out of a plan, the employer must automatically enroll employees in the lowest cost premium plan. The employer provision penalty for employers with 100 or more employees went into effect in January of 2015; for employers with 50 to 99 employees, it went into effect in January of 2016.

*As of February of 2024, 41 states (including the District of Columbia) had expanded Medicaid and the remaining 10 had not adopted expansion.

**As of January of 2016, 13 states had state-based marketplaces, six states had federally supported marketplaces, seven had a state-partnership marketplace, and 32 used federally facilitated marketplaces.

Data from Families USA. (2016). *Federal poverty guidelines*. Available at http://familiesusa.org/product/federal-poverty-guidelines; The Henry J. Kaiser Family Foundation. (2013). *Summary of the Affordable Care Act*. Available at http://kff.org/health-reform/fact-sheet/summary-of-new-health-reform-law/; The Henry J. Kaiser Family Foundation. (2020). *State health facts*. Available at http://kff.org/statedata/; Kaiser Family Foundation. (2020). Health insurance exchange. Available at https://www.kff.org/health-reform/state-indicator/state-health-insurance-marketplace-types/?currentTimeframe=0&sortModel=%7B%22colId%22:%22 Location%22,%22sort%22:%22asc%22%7D

BOX 13.4   Essential Health Benefits Included in Health Insurance Available Through the Marketplaces

The essential health benefits that all private health insurance plans must offer include the following:

- Ambulatory patient services (outpatient care you get without being admitted to a hospital)
- Emergency services
- Hospitalization
- Maternity and newborn care (care before and after your baby is born)
- Mental health and substance use disorder services, including behavioral health treatment, counseling, and psychotherapy

- Prescription drugs
- Rehabilitative and habilitative services and devices (services and devices to help people with injuries, disabilities, or chronic conditions gain or recover mental and physical skills)
- Laboratory services (i.e., laboratory tests)
- Preventive and wellness services, including counseling, screenings, and vaccinations, and chronic disease management
- Pediatric services

Note: Plans may offer more than the benefits listed here. Specific healthcare benefits may vary by state. Even within the same state, there can be small differences among health insurance plans.

Data from Centers for Medicare and Medicaid Services. (2013). *10 health care benefits covered in the health insurance marketplace.* Available at https://www.healthcare.gov/blog/10-health-care-benefits-covered-in-the-health-insurance-marketplace/

By using the marketplaces, consumers can compare plans based on price, benefits, quality, and other features important to them before making a choice. Consumers can also get help online, by phone, by chat, or in person.[64] The insurance plans in marketplaces are offered by private companies and must meet the set of benefits called the essential health benefits[64] (see **Box 13.4**). Marketplaces became available to consumers via the federal website (Healthcare.gov) or a state website, if a state had its own state-based marketplace on October 1, 2013, with health insurance policies purchased before December 15, 2013, going into effect on January 1, 2014. The initial rollout of the Healthcare.gov website was not without problems. Most, but not all, of the problems dealt with technical glitches. Now that the website has been up and running for several years, online enrollment has run much more smoothly.

Quality of Health Care

All people are entitled to and should receive quality health care. Yet several different reports, including one that compared U.S. health care with that of Australia, Canada, France, Germany, the Netherlands, New Zealand, Norway, Sweden, Switzerland, and the United Kingdom,[65] indicate that the U.S. healthcare system underperforms relative to other countries on most dimensions of performance, and people in the United States could be receiving better care. *Quality health care* has been defined as, "the degree to which health services for individuals and populations increase the likelihood of desired health outcomes and are consistent with current professional knowledge."[66] The Institute of Medicine has further delineated that quality health care should be as follows[67]:

- *Effective.* Delivering health care based on scientific evidence to all who could benefit based on need
- *Safe.* Delivering health care to patients that avoids injuries to patients from the care that is intended to help them
- *Timely.* Delivering health care in a way that reduces waits and sometimes harmful delays
- *Patient-centered.* Providing health care that is respectful of and responsive to individual patient preferences, needs, and values
- *Equitable.* Delivering health care that does not vary in quality because of personal characteristics of patients
- *Efficient.* Delivering health care that maximizes resources and avoids waste

Although the definitions of quality health care are easily understood, operationalizing quality health care is not as easy, yet a number of groups have created measures for healthcare quality. Since 2003, the Agency for Healthcare Research and Quality (AHRQ), together with

HHS and some private sector partners, has annually reported on progress and opportunities for improving healthcare quality as mandated by the U.S. Congress by publishing the National Healthcare Quality Report (NHQR) and the National Healthcare Disparities Report (NHDR). Beginning in 2014, the findings on healthcare quality and healthcare disparities was integrated into a single document—*National Healthcare Quality and Disparities Report* (QDR).[68] Both the NHQR and the NHDR are built on, for the most part, the same dimensions. The QDR "is based on 250 measures of quality and disparities covering a broad array of healthcare services and settings."[68]

Another group that measures healthcare quality is the National Committee for Quality Assurance (NCQA).[69] The NCQA is a private, not-for-profit organization that has been assessing and accrediting healthcare plans since 1990. It assesses how well a health plan manages and delivers health care in four different ways: (1) through accreditation (a rigorous on-site review of key clinical and administrative processes); (2) through certification (a rigorous review of certain functions—for example, credentialing or utilization management—that health plans or employers have delegated to another organization); (3) through the Healthcare Effectiveness Data and Information Set (HEDIS—a tool that consists of 90 measures across six domains that is used to measure performance in key areas, such as immunization and mammography screening rates) and members' satisfaction with their care in areas, such as claims processing, customer service, and getting needed care quickly[70]; and (4) through physician recognition programs that identify physicians who provide quality care in areas, such as diabetes, back pain, and heart/stroke care. Although participation with NCQA is voluntary, NCQA-accredited health plans cover 173 million people enrolled in health plans.[69] The data from NCQA's assessments are available on its website. Employers, consultants, and consumers use HEDIS data, along with the accreditation, certification, and recognition information to help them select the best-managed care programs for their needs.[70]

Regardless of what method is used to measure the quality of health care delivered in the United States, the results have been similar. The general consensus is that the quality of health care has been getting better at a modest pace, but that it is not as good as it could or should be.

Dealing with the problem of "less than desirable quality in health care" is not easy, because it runs through every aspect of care. That is why there are not just a few items in the ACA that deal with quality—there are many. Examples include (1) requiring healthcare plans to offer preventive services (e.g., screenings and vaccinations) without charging a copay, coinsurance, or deductible; (2) providing information about the quality of nursing homes and making it easier to file complaints about the quality of care in nursing homes; (3) linking payments to physicians and hospitals based on the quality of care provided; and (4) incentivizing healthcare providers to use electronic medical records. Other activities aimed at improving quality of health that have gained much attention are the National Quality Strategy, accountable care organizations (ACOs), and the patient-centered medical home program. These programs are discussed in the following sections.

National Quality Strategy

The National Quality Strategy (NQS)[71] was mandated by the ACA to serve as a catalyst and compass for a nationwide focus on quality improvement efforts and measuring quality. The NQS was developed by a broad-based group of more than 300 organizations and individuals representing all sectors of the healthcare industry. In addition, the general public was given an opportunity to provide comments on it. The NQS is guided by a set of three overarching aims: to provide better care, to make care more affordable, and to promote healthy people and communities. These aims are also used to assess the efforts to improve the quality of care. To achieve the three aims, the NQS applies six priorities that address the most common health concerns that affect most Americans. "Achievement of the National Quality Strategy can only occur if individuals, family members, payers, providers, employers, and communities work together."[72] To assist these stakeholders with their work for improving quality, the NQS includes nine levers that can be used by the stakeholders to align their work to the NQS (see **Box 13.5**). The NQS also provides the basis for the annual report to Congress on quality improvement in health care.[73]

BOX 13.5   National Quality Strategy: Aims, Priorities, and Levers

Aims

The NQS pursues three broad aims. These aims will be used to guide and assess local, state, and national efforts to improve health and the quality of health care.

- *Better care.* Improve the overall quality by making health care more patient-centered, reliable, accessible, and safe.
- *Healthy people/healthy communities.* Improve the health of the U.S. population by supporting proven interventions to address behavioral, social, and environmental determinants of health, in addition to delivering higher quality care.
- *Affordable care.* Reduce the cost of quality health care for individuals, families, employers, and government.

Priorities

- Make care safer by reducing harm caused in the delivery of care.
- Ensure that each person and family is engaged as a partner in their care.
- Promote effective communication and coordination of care.
- Promote the most effective prevention and treatment practices for the leading causes of mortality, starting with cardiovascular disease.
- Work with communities to promote wide use of best practices to enable healthy living.

- Make quality care more affordable for individuals, families, employers, and governments by developing and spreading new healthcare delivery models.

Levers

- *Measurement and feedback.* Provide performance feedback to plans and providers to improve care.
- *Public reporting.* Compare treatment results, costs, and patient experience of consumers.
- *Learning and technical assistance.* Foster learning environments that offer training, resources, tools, and guidance to help organizations achieve quality improvement goals.
- *Certification, accreditation, and regulation.* Adopt or adhere to approaches to meet safety and quality standards.
- *Consumer incentives and benefit designs.* Help consumers adopt healthy behaviors and make informed decisions.
- *Payment.* Reward and incentivize providers to deliver high quality, patient-centered care.
- *Health information technology.* Improve communication, transparency, and efficiency for better coordinated health and health care.
- *Innovation and diffusion.* Foster innovation in healthcare quality improvement and facilitate rapid adoption within and across organizations and communities.
- *Workforce development.* Invest in people to prepare the next generation of healthcare professionals and support lifelong learning for providers.

Reproduced from U.S. Department of Health and Human Services, Agency for Healthcare Research and Quality. (2015). *About the National Quality Strategy (NQS)*. Available at http://www.ahrq.gov/workingforquality/about.htm

Accountable Care Organizations

An **accountable care organization (ACO)** is a group of doctors, hospitals, and other healthcare providers, which comes together voluntarily as a legal entity to give coordinated high-quality care to Medicare patients. "The goal of coordinated care is to ensure that patients, especially the chronically ill, get the right care at the right time, while avoiding unnecessary duplication of services and preventing medical errors"[74] and, therefore, reduce costs for care. ACOs were not created by the ACA, they have been around since 2006,[75] but provisions for ACOs were included in the ACA. The ACA authorized Medicare to contract with ACOs in a Medicare Shared Savings Program.[76] The incentive for providers to form an ACO is financial. "The ACA enables ACOs to share in savings to the federal government based on ACO performance in improving quality and reducing health care costs."[6]

Patient-Centered Medical Home

Like ACOs, the concept of the *patient-centered medical home* (PCMH) is not new; early forms of it can be traced back to the 1960s as a response to try to improve the way care was offered. Like ACOs, the PCMH is a model of care that reorganizes the way care is offered. The **patient-centered medical home**, which applies to patients of all ages, has been defined as "a care delivery model whereby patient treatment is coordinated through their primary care physician to ensure they receive the necessary care when and where they need it, in a manner they can understand."[77] The PCMH is responsible for providing all of the patient's healthcare needs (i.e., preventive services, treatment of acute care and chronic illnesses, and assistance with end-of-life issues) or appropriately arranging a patient's care with other qualified providers.[5] AHRQ has identified five functions and attributes of a medical home: (1) comprehensive care,

Accountable care organization (ACO) a group of doctors, hospitals, and other healthcare providers, which comes together voluntarily as a legal entity to give coordinated high-quality care to Medicare patients

Patient-centered medical home a care delivery model whereby patients' treatment is coordinated through their primary care physician to ensure they receive the necessary care when and where they need it, in a manner they can understand

(2) patient-centered care, (3) coordinated care, (4) accessible services, and (5) quality and safety.[78] The PCMH has gained momentum in the medical community in recent years, and in 2006 the Patient-Centered Primary Care Collaborative (PCPCC), a not-for-profit organization, was created. The PCPCC "is dedicated to advancing an effective and efficient health system built on a strong foundation of primary care and the patient-centered medical home."[79] The ACA supports provisions for the continuing development of the PCMH model as it relates to Medicaid expansion, payment rates for primary care, primary care provider shortages, and the Center for Medicare and Medicaid Innovation to test various service delivery and payment models. For the PCMH to be fully accepted, some changes will be needed in the way physicians are reimbursed in order to compensate them for the time spent organizing patients' care.

The Cost of and Paying for Health Care

The cost of health care and paying for health care continue to be burdens on both individuals and the U.S. population as a whole. In 2022, health expenditures grew from 4.1% to $4.5 trillion and consumed 17.3% of the gross domestic product (GDP). That amounted to $13,493 per person. It is estimated that healthcare spending will continue to grow at 5.5% per year through the next decade. With such growth, spending is expected to reach $6.0 trillion and 19.4% of the GDP by 2028.[80] These figures confirm the U.S. healthcare system as the most costly in the world.[65] In fact, the United States spends "more on health care than the next 10 biggest spenders combined: Japan, Germany, France, China, United Kingdom, Italy, Canada, Brazil, Spain, and Australia."[81] Under the U.S. system, the actual cost of the service, for the most part, is usually not known until after the service has been provided, unless the consumer is bold enough to inquire ahead of time. However, starting in 2013, and continuing each year since, in an effort to make the U.S. healthcare system more affordable and accountable, the Centers for Medicare and Medicaid Services has released data and information comparing the charges for the 100 most common inpatient services, 30 common outpatient services, all physician and other supplier procedures and services, and all Part D prescriptions for Medicare patients. These data showed that there were significant variations across the country and within communities in what providers charged for common services.[82] Many journalists picked up on this information and confronted providers, making providers respond to why their charges may be different from other parts of the country. Such transparency is needed if health care is to become a true market system.

Even with more transparency, the cost of health care continues to go up and is growing at an unsustainable rate.[81] In 2020, the COVID-19 pandemic had an impact on national health spending. The pandemic showed growth of 9.7% in national healthcare spending, bringing spending in the United States to $4.1 trillion.[80] There are several other reasons[83–86] for this growth. They include, but are not limited to (1) major coverage expansions of Medicaid and private health insurance under the ACA; (2) paying providers and hospitals in ways that reward doing more, rather than being efficient; (3) an aging U.S. population with many chronic health conditions; (4) the demand for medical advances in the form of new drugs, technologies, services, and procedures; (5) relatively price-insensitive patients who have limited out-of-pocket costs; (6) the lack of evidence to make decisions on which medical care is best; (7) hospital and providers that are increasingly gaining market share and are better able to demand higher prices; (8) supply and demand issues (e.g., restricting the practices of nurse practitioners and physician assistants when there is a need for more primary care); and (9) legal issues (e.g., malpractice premiums) that complicate efforts to slow spending

So who pays the healthcare bill? Payments for the U.S. healthcare bill come from four sources. The first is consumers themselves. In 2018, these direct or out-of-pocket payments represented approximately one-tenth (10%) of all payments. The remaining portion of healthcare payments, nine-tenths (90%), comes almost entirely from indirect, or third-party, payments. Of the third-party payments, the first source is private insurance companies. Private insurance companies paid about one-third (34%) of the healthcare bill in 2014. These payments were made from premiums paid to the insurance company by employees and/or their employers. The second source of third-party payments is governmental insurance programs (e.g., Medicare, Medicaid, Veterans Administration, CHIP, or military). These government programs are funded

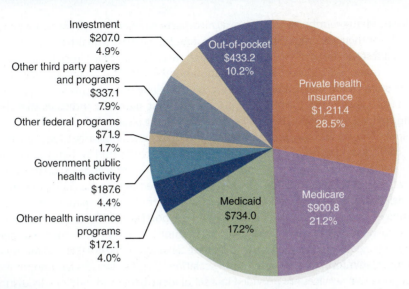

FIGURE 13.11   Health expenditures by source of funds—United States, 2021.

Modified from *Centers for Medicare and Medicaid Services. National Health Expenditure Accounts: Methodology Paper, 2020 Definitions, Sources, and Methods (PDF). Centers for Medicare & Medicaid Services. December 2021.

**Health Resources and Services Administration. About the Provider Relief Fund and Other Programs. Health Resources and Services Administration, November 2021.

***U.S. Small Business Administration. Paycheck Protection Program: An SBA-backed loan that helps businesses keep their workforce employed during the COVID-19 crisis. U.S. Small Business Administration, 2022.

by a combination of federal and state taxes and premiums (as in the case of Part B Medicare coverage). In 2014, about two-fifths (41%) of the healthcare bill was paid for by governmental insurance programs. The third source, for the remainder (13%) of the healthcare bill was paid by other third-party payers[87] (see **Figure 13.11**).

It is clear that the cost of health care is going to continue to rise. One of the major selling points of the ACA was to try to slow down the rise in the cost of health care, thus the title "Affordable Care." The Congressional Budget Office (CBO) and the Joint Committee on Taxation (JCT) estimated that the ACA's coverage provisions will result in a net cost to the federal government of $41 billion in 2014 and $1,487 billion over the period from 2015 to 2024."[86] In 2017, the Trump administration repealed the individual mandate through the Tax Cuts and Jobs Act, and the CBO and JCT have updated their estimates based on the effects of repealing the mandate. Repealing the mandate would eliminate the penalty of people who have no health insurance; those who are not exempt from the mandate must pay under current law. According to CBO and JCT estimates, repealing the mandate, which started in 2019, would reduce federal budget deficits by about $338 billion between 2018 and 2027. The number of people with health insurance would decrease by 4 million in 2019 and by 13 million in 2027. When Biden became President in 2021, the tax mandate was put back into place. As a disclaimer, the CBO and JCT's baseline projections are also uncertain, and revisions to them would alter interactions and change the estimates, such as the effects of eliminating the mandate and/or placing the mandate back in place.[88] These costs are financed through a combination of savings from Medicare and Medicaid and new taxes and fees. The savings from Medicare and Medicaid come mostly from how the government pays providers. Examples of new taxes include taxes on high-cost health insurance and tanning bed use, whereas examples of new fees include those that have to be paid by those individuals who chose not to purchase health insurance. Many believe that in addition to the cost savings from Medicare and Medicaid, healthcare costs have the potential to be lower because millions of people who were uninsured before the law will now be paying premiums, and many of them are young and healthy and will not use a lot of health care.

The monetary value that healthcare providers and facilities receive for providing services to patients is referred to as **reimbursement**.[87] As noted earlier, third-party payers (i.e., insurance companies, government entities) provide most of the reimbursement for health services. The

Reimbursement the monetary value that healthcare providers and facilities receive for providing services to patients

Fee-for-service a method of paying for health care in which after the service is rendered, a fee is paid

Packaged pricing several related health services are included in one price

Resource-based relative value scale (RBRVS) reimbursement to physicians according to the relative value of the service provided

process for receiving reimbursement from a third-party payment usually begins when a health-care provider or their staff requests information about the patient's health insurance plan. They normally request the name of the insuring company (e.g., Aetna, Blue Cross/Blue Shield, Cigna), the policy number, and a personal identification number (PIN). The insurer usually provides this information to the insured on a wallet-sized card. The provider may then ask the patient to sign an insurance claim form in two places. The first signature indicates that the service has been provided and authorizes the provider to submit patient information with the claim for payment. The second signature instructs the insurance company to make the payment directly to the provider. Upon receiving and reviewing the completed and signed form, the insurance company then issues payments to the provider for services based on the provisions of the insurance policy. Depending on the level of reimbursement for the claim, the provider will either consider the bill paid in full or will request payment from the patient for the amount of the difference between the provider's full fee and the portion paid by the insurance company.

In recent years, the methods by which the amount of the reimbursement has been determined have changed. Traditionally, providers have favored the **fee-for-service** method, but it is not used much anymore because of the cost escalation.[1] The fee-for-service amount is based on the assumption that services are provided in a set of identifiable and individually distinct units, such as a doctor's office visit or a specific medical procedure.[1] Under the fee-for-service format, consumers select a provider, receive care (service) from the provider, and incur expenses (a fee) for the care. The provider is then reimbursed for covered services in part by the insurer and in part by the consumer, who is responsible for the balance unpaid by the insurer. Initially, the providers set the fees and insurers would pay the claim. But because of increased costs, insurers started to limit the amount they would pay for "usual, customary, and reasonable charges." The biggest drawback of the fee-for-service format is that providers have a greater incentive to provide more services, some of which may not be essential.

Under the fee-for-service format, consumers are obligated to pay their fee at the time the service is rendered. In the past, before health insurance was common, some physicians provided care when needed and worried about payment later. Others often accepted "in kind" payment, such as farm produce or other products or services, as payment in full for a medical service rendered. Today, for patients to receive care via fee-for-service, they are often required to demonstrate the ability to pay (to assume financial responsibility for the fee) before the service is rendered. A provider's receptionist may ask, "How do you plan to settle your bill?" In other cases, providers have signs placed around the waiting room that state, "Payment is expected when service is rendered, unless other arrangements have been made prior to the appointment."

The more recent methods of reimbursement for health services have included *packaged pricing, resource-based relative value scale, capitation, prospective reimbursement,* and *pay-for-performance.* In **packaged pricing**, also referred to as *bundled charges,* several related services are included in one price. For example, optometrists will bundle the cost for an eye exam, frames, and lenses into a single charge.[1]

Resource-based relative value scale (RBRVS) was created for Medicare as part of the Omnibus Budget Reconciliation Act of 1989 to reimburse physicians according to the *relative value* of the service provided. The relative value units (RVUs) are derived through a complex formula based on time, skill, and intensity to provide the service. Also included in the RVU is an overhead charge to run a practice.[14] Each year, Medicare publishes the Medicare Physician Fee Schedule, adjusted for geographic parts of the country, which provides the reimbursement amount for services and procedures under the Current Procedural Terminology (CPT) code.[1]

Managed care organizations (MCOs; see information about managed care later in this chapter) use several different approaches for reimbursement. Preferred provider organizations (PPOs) use a variation of the fee-for-service method. The variation is that the PPOs "establish fee schedules based on discounts negotiated with providers participating in its network."[1] Health maintenance organizations (HMOs), depending on their structure, have either paid providers a salary if they are employed by the HMO or have reimbursed them using a mechanism called *capitation.*

Under **capitation**, insurers make arrangements with healthcare providers to provide agreed-upon covered healthcare services to a given population of consumers for a (usually discounted) set price—the per-person premium fee—over a particular time period. Often, the arrangements are set up on a per-member, per-month (PMPM) rate called a *capitated fee*. The provider receives the capitated fee per enrollee regardless of whether the enrollee uses healthcare services and regardless of the quality of services provided. The provider is responsible for providing all needed services determined to be medically necessary and covered under the plan. In addition to the capitated fee, consumers may pay additional fees (copayments) for office visits and other services used. The insurer organizes the delivery of care by building an infrastructure of providers and implementing the systems to monitor and influence the cost and quality of care.

Prospective reimbursement has been around since 1983 when it was first used in the form of diagnosis-related groups (DRGs) for hospital stays under Medicare Part A (see discussion of Medicare and DRGs later in the chapter). It replaced *retrospective reimbursement*, which was based on the length of stay and services provided. Under retrospective reimbursement, providers were rewarded for longer stays and more services, which increased costs. **Prospective reimbursement**, referred to as the prospective pricing system (PPS), "uses certain pre-established criteria to determine in advance, the amount of reimbursement."[1] Because of the success of DRGs, the Balanced Budget Act of 1997 mandated implementation of a Medicare PPS for hospital outpatient services and postacute providers, such as skilled nursing facilities, home health agencies, and inpatient rehabilitation facilities.[14] Thus, the four primary prospective reimbursement methods used today are (1) DRGs (used for Medicare Part A), (2) ambulatory payment classifications (APCs; used for payment to hospital outpatient departments), (3) resource utilization groups (RUGs; used for payment to skilled nursing facilities), and (4) home health resource groups (HHRGs; used for payment of home health care).[1]

Pay-for-performance (P4P) or "value-based purchasing" is a payment system that offers financial rewards to providers and facilities for meeting, improving, or exceeding quality measures (i.e., process, outcome, patience experience, and structure) or other performance goals.[89,90] Thus, its purpose is to improve the quality, efficiency, and overall value of health care.[91] For example, providers can receive incentives for achieving a quality measure goal, such as the reduction in hemoglobin A1c in patients with diabetes.[89] In addition to incentives, P4P payment systems can also include disincentives or penalties for not providing quality care. An example of a penalty incorporated within the ACA is the Medicare Hospital Readmissions Reduction Program, which took effect in 2012. With this program, Medicare "can reduce payments by 1% to hospitals that have excessively high rates of avoidable readmissions for patients experiencing heart attacks, heart failure, or pneumonia."[90] For FY 2023, CMS calculates the payment adjustment factor and component results for each hospital, based on their performance during the 3-year performance period of July 1, 2018, through June 30, 2021.

In addition, ACOs, which we noted earlier, are mandated in the ACA; they are the best-known P4P programs. To date, P4P programs have received mixed reviews regarding their effectiveness.[91] Time will tell if this type of payment system can be improved and, in turn, improve the quality of care.

Health Insurance

Health insurance, like all other types of insurance, is a risk- and cost-spreading process. That is, the cost of one person's injury or illness is shared by everyone in the group. Each person in the group has a different chance (or risk) of having a problem and thus needing health care. Some members of the group, for example, those who experience chronic and/or congenital health problems, will probably need more care, whereas others in the group will need less. The concept of insurance requires everyone in the group, regardless of their individual risk, to help pay for the collective risk of the group. The risk of costly ill health is spread in a reasonably equitable fashion among all persons purchasing insurance, and everyone is protected from having to pay an insurmountable bill for a catastrophic injury or illness.

Capitation a method of paying for covered healthcare services on a per-person premium basis for a specific time period prior to the service being rendered

Prospective reimbursement a system that uses pre-established criteria to determine the amount of reimbursement in advance

Pay-for-performance (P4P) a payment system that offers financial rewards to providers and facilities for meeting, improving, or exceeding quality measures or other performance goals

There are some exceptions to the "equitable fashion." If someone in the group knowingly engages in a behavior that increases their risk, such as smoking cigarettes or driving in a reckless manner, that person may have to pay more to cover the increased risk. In short, the greater the risk (or probability of using the insurance), the more the individual or group must pay for insurance.

The concept of health insurance is not a new one in this country. Group health and life insurance are considered American inventions of the early twentieth century. In 1911, Montgomery Ward and Company sold health insurance policies based on the principles still used today in the business. Currently, hundreds of companies in the United States sell health and life insurance policies.

The Health Insurance Policy

A **health insurance policy** is a contract between an insurer (i.e., private insurance company or the government) and an individual (known as the insured or policyholder) that outlines in exact terms what healthcare services are covered, how the insured will be compensated, the cost of the policy to the insured (i.e., **premium**), and any associated information, for example, the mode of premium payment or deductibles. The insurance company benefits in that it anticipates collecting more money in premiums than it must pay out for services; hence, it anticipates a profit. The insured benefits by not being faced with medical bills they cannot pay, because the insurance company is obligated to pay them according to the terms of the contract. The added benefit for those insured as a group is that group premiums are less expensive than premiums for individuals.

The expectations of both insurers and insured are not always met. An insurer occasionally has to pay out more than it collects in premiums. Alternatively, the insured often purchases insurance that is never used.

Although the language of health insurance policies can be confusing, everyone needs to understand several key terms. One of the most important is **deductible**. The deductible is the amount of money that the beneficiary (insured) must incur (pay out of pocket), generally up to an annual limit before the insurance company begins to pay for covered services. A common yearly deductible level is $500 per individual policyholder, or a maximum of $1,000 per family. This means that the insured must pay the first $500/$1,000 of medical costs before the insurance company begins paying. The higher the deductible of a policy, the lower the premiums will be.

Usually, but not always, after the deductible has been met, insurance companies will pay a percentage of what they consider the "usual, customary, and reasonable" charge for covered services. The insurer generally pays 80% of the usual, customary, and reasonable costs, and the insured is responsible for paying the remaining 20%. This 20% is referred to as **coinsurance**. If the healthcare provider charges more than the usual, customary, and reasonable rates, the insured will have to pay both the coinsurance and the difference. One form of coinsurance, often associated with managed care programs, is **copayment** (or *copay* for short). A copayment is a negotiated, set amount a patient pays for certain services—for example, $20 for an office visit and $15 for a prescription. Some insurance policies may require both coinsurance and copayments. The greater the proportion of coinsurance paid by the insured, the lower the premiums.

A fourth key term, **fixed indemnity**, refers to the maximum amount an insurer will pay for a certain service. For example, a policy may state that the maximum amount of money paid for orthodontia is $2,000. Depending on the language of a policy, the fixed indemnity benefit may or may not be subject to the provisions of the deductible or coinsurance clause. Costs above the fixed indemnity amount are the responsibility of the insured.

Another key term related to health insurance is **exclusion**. When an exclusion is written into a policy, it means that a specified health condition is excluded from coverage. That is, the policy does not pay for service to treat the condition. Common exclusions include a pregnancy that began before the health insurance policy went into effect or a chronic disease or condition, such as diabetes or hypertension that has been classified as a pre-existing condition.

Health insurance policy a contract between an insurer and the insured that outlines what health services are covered and what will be compensated

Premium a regular periodic payment for an insurance policy

Deductible the amount of expenses that the beneficiary must incur before the insurance company begins to pay for covered services

Coinsurance the portion of the insurance company's approved amounts for covered services that a beneficiary is responsible for paying

Copayment a negotiated, set amount that a patient pays for certain services

Fixed indemnity the maximum amount an insurer will pay for a certain service

Exclusion a health condition written into the health insurance policy indicating what is not covered by the policy

A **pre-existing condition** is a medical condition that had been diagnosed or treated, usually within the 6 months before the date the health insurance policy went into effect. Prior to the mid-1990s, because of such exclusions, people who had a serious condition or disease were often unable to obtain health insurance coverage for the condition/disease or in general. Some health insurance policies also excluded a condition/disease for a specified period of time, such as 9 months for pregnancy or 1 year for all other exclusions.

The rule that a pre-existing condition could be an exclusion "trapped" many people in jobs, because the employees were afraid of losing their health insurance for the condition if they changed employers. To deal with this issue, Congress passed the Health Insurance Portability and Accountability Act of 1996 (Public Law 104-102, known as HIPAA). This law was created, in part, to ensure that people would not have to wait for health insurance to go into effect when changing jobs. More specifically, a pre-existing condition had to be covered without a waiting period when a person joined a new plan if the person had been insured for the previous 12 months. If a person had a pre-existing condition and it had not been covered during the previous 12 months before joining a new plan, the longest that person had to wait before being covered for that condition is 12 months.

Even with HIPAA, many people, mostly older Americans, were unable to get health insurance because of pre-existing conditions. Thus, pre-existing conditions were addressed in the ACA. Beginning in 2014, insurance companies were required to cover all individuals regardless of health status and charge the same premium regardless of pre-existing conditions.[92]

Types of Health Insurance Coverage

As has been noted in the previous discussions, there are a number of different types of services that health insurance policies cover. The more common types of coverage are hospitalization, surgical, regular medical, major medical, dental, and disability. **Table 13.4** presents a short overview of each of these coverage types.

Although the types of health insurance coverage remain constant, several trends associated with health insurance plans and the products they offer are emerging. The trends that characterize health insurance plans today are (1) the plans are becoming more complex and are concentrated among fewer companies; (2) there is an increase in the diversity of products,

TABLE 13.4   Types of Health Insurance Coverage

Insurance	Coverage
Dental	Dental procedures
Disability (income protection)	Income when insured is unable to work because of a health problem
Hospitalization	Inpatient hospital expenses, including room, patient care, supplies, and medications
Long-term care	Umbrella term for an array of supportive services to help people function in their daily lives, including but not limited to: nursing care, home health care, personal care, rehabilitation, adult daycare, case management, social services, assistive technology, and assisted-living services; services may be provided at home or in another place of residence like a nursing home
Major medical	Large medical expenses usually not covered by regular medical or dental coverage
Optical (vision)	Nonsurgical procedures to improve vision
Regular medical	Nonsurgical service provided by healthcare providers. Often uses set amounts (fixed indemnity for certain procedures)
Surgical	Surgeons' fees (for inpatient or outpatient surgery)

© James F. McKenzie

so consumers have many more options in the type of plan they select, especially with the passage of the ACA; (3) there is an increased focus on delivering care through a network of providers rather than independent providers; (4) there is a movement toward shifting to financial structures and incentives among purchasers, health plans, and providers; and (5) more health insurance plans are developing clinical infrastructures to manage utilization and to improve the quality of care. Such trends will make understanding health insurance plans more challenging for consumers. These trends will require a greater investment in education and information to help consumers understand how insurance products differ, how best to navigate managed care systems, and what differences exist in structure or performance across the plans.

The Cost of Health Insurance

Over the years, the cost of health insurance has pretty much mirrored the cost of health care. From the early 1970s through the early 1990s, healthcare costs and the costs of health insurance grew in the neighborhood of 10% to 12% per year.[80] Since that time, there have been some years when the cost of premiums slowed. One example was when there was a shift in the health insurance marketplace away from traditional fee-for-service indemnity insurance to managed care in the mid- to late-1990s. The rate of growth of premiums slowed again in the early years after the passage of the ACA. Even with the slower growth, the cost of health insurance continues to outpace the cost of inflation and growth in salaries. In the period between 2002 and 2012, premiums increased by 97%.[93] The burden of the cost of health insurance for those who are working falls primarily on the employer and, to a lesser but a growing extent, on the employee. In 2014, 56% of Americans younger than age 65 years received their health insurance through their employer or the employer of their parent or spouse/partner.[94] In 2020, 57.1% received health insurance through their employer.[95] In 2023, the cost of the average yearly health insurance premium for an individual was $8,435; employers contributed $7,034 of that amount and the employee contributed $1,401.[96] The average yearly health insurance premium for a family in that same year was $23,698; employers contributed $17,123 of that amount and the employee contributed $6,575.[96] Because of the increasing costs of health insurance and its impact on the "bottom line" of companies, employers are shifting more of the cost onto their employees by (1) increasing the workers' share of the premium, (2) raising the deductibles that workers must pay, (3) increasing the copayments for prescription drugs, and (4) increasing the number of items on the exclusion list. A vivid example of the cost of health insurance comes from coffee store giant Starbucks. This company spends more money on health insurance than it does on coffee beans.[97]

The cost of health insurance for those who purchase it through a marketplace created by the ACA varies greatly, depending on a number of factors, including (1) the state in which you live, (2) your location within the state, (3) your age, (4) the yearly family income, (5) whether you smoke or not, (6) whether health insurance coverage is available via your employer or a spouse's employer, (7) the number of people in your family, (8) the breakdown of the number of adults and children, and (9) the type of plan (i.e., bronze, silver, gold, or platinum) purchased. Based on this information, it will be determined if the person applying would qualify for either a *premium tax credit* or a *cost-sharing subsidy*. Premium tax credits for people who buy coverage through the marketplace are available to those with family incomes between 100% (in 2016 for a family of four it was $24,300) and 400% (in 2016 for a family of four it was $97,200) of the poverty level.[98] "These individuals and families will have to pay no more than 2.03% to 9.66% of their incomes for a mid-level plan ("silver") premium. Anything above that is paid by the government."[98] Cost-sharing subsidies help people with their costs when they use health services, such as when seeing a physician or for a hospital stay.[98] Cost-sharing subsidies are only available to people purchasing their own insurance and who make between 100% and 250% of the poverty level. These subsidies are also available to some Native Americans.[98]

In the end, the actual cost of a policy is determined by two major factors—the risk of those in the group and the amount of coverage provided. An increase in either risk or coverage will result in an increase in the cost of the policy.

Self-Funded Insurance Programs

Because of the high cost of health care, since the 1970s, some employers (or other group, such as a union or trade association)[6] that provide health insurance for their employees have decided to cut their costs by becoming self-insured. In such an arrangement, a **self-funded insurance program** pays the healthcare costs of its employees with the premiums collected from the employees and the contributions made by the employer instead of using a commercial carrier.[6] Self-funded insurance programs "often use the services of an actuarial firm to set premium rates and a third-party administrator to administer benefits, pay claims, and collect data on utilization. Many third-party administrators also provide case management services for potentially extraordinarily expensive cases to help coordinate care and control employee risk of catastrophic expenses."[6]

There are several benefits to being self-funded. First, the organization gets to set most of the parameters of the policy—deductibles, coinsurance, fixed indemnities, and exclusions. If the organization wants to exclude some services and include others, it can. For example, if the organization has an older workforce, it may wish to delete obstetrics from the policy but include a number of preventive health services. Second, the organization holds onto the cash reserves in the benefits account instead of sending them to a commercial carrier, and thus gets to accrue interest on them. Third, the self-funded organizations have been exempt from the Employee Retirement and Income Security Act of 1974 (ERISA), which mandates minimum benefits under state law.[6] However, self-insured employer plans do need to meet the 10 essential health benefits required in the ACA.[99] And fourth, generally the administrative costs of self-funded organizations have been less than those of traditional commercial carriers and, in general, health insurance costs to these groups have risen at a slower rate.[6] Other than the need to meet the ACA 10 essential benefits requirement, these four points have not been affected by the ACA; however, the law did include language that indicates that the Secretary of the U.S. Department of Labor is required to provide an annual report about self-funded insurance programs to the appropriate committees of Congress so that they can study their workings. In addition, the law requires the Secretary of HHS to conduct a study of self-funded insurance programs to determine if there are any adverse effects on the components of healthcare reform.[100]

For self-funded insurance to work, there must be a sizable group of employees over which to spread the risk. Larger organizations usually find it more useful than smaller ones. However, if a small workforce is composed primarily of low-health-risk employees, say, for example, younger employees, self-funded programs make sense.

> **Self-funded insurance program** type of insurance that pays the healthcare costs of its employees with the premiums collected from the employees and the contributions made by the employer
>
> **Medicare** a national health insurance program for people 65 years of age and older, certain younger people who are disabled, and people with permanent kidney failure

Health Insurance Provided by the Government

Although there are some in the United States who would like to see all health insurance provided by the government—a national health insurance plan—at the present time, government health insurance plans are only available to select groups in the United States. The only government health insurance plans—those funded by governments at federal, state, and local levels—that exist today are Medicare, Medicaid, CHIP, Veterans Administration (VA) benefits (see **Figure 13.12**), Indian Health Service, and healthcare benefits for the uniformed services (military and U.S. Public Health Service or TRICARE), federal employees (Federal Employees Health Benefits Program), and people who are incarcerated. Our discussion here is limited to Medicare, Medicaid, and CHIP. Medicare and Medicaid were created in 1965 by amendments to the Social Security Act and were implemented for the first time in 1966. CHIP was created in 1997 and codified as Title XXI of the Social Security Act.

Medicare

Medicare, is a federal health insurance program for people 65 years of age or older, people of any age with permanent kidney failure, and certain people under 65 who are disabled. It is administered

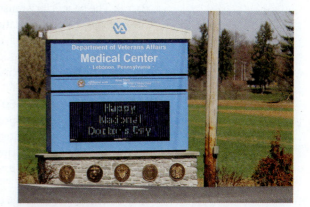

FIGURE 13.12   Insurance provided for veterans is one of several insurance plans paid for by the U.S. government.

© James F. McKenzie

by the Centers for Medicare and Medicaid Services (CMS) within HHS. The Social Security Administration provides information about the program and handles enrollment. Medicare is considered a contributory program, in that employers and employees are required to contribute a percentage of each employee's wages/salaries through Social Security (FICA) tax to the Medicare fund. Medicare has four parts: hospital insurance (Part A), medical insurance (Part B), Medicare Advantage plans (Part C), and prescription drug plans (Part D).

The Medicare hospital insurance (Part A) portion is mandatory and is provided for eligible persons with no further cost. Some are not eligible for premium-free Part A because they or their spouses did not pay into Social Security at all or paid only a limited amount, may be able to purchase Part A coverage. In 2024, for those premiums, a person will pay either $278 or $505 each month for Part A. In addition, you'll also have to sign up for Part B to buy Part A.[101] Although Medicare Part A has a deductible of $1,632 in 2024 and coinsurance provisions, it helps pay for inpatient care in a hospital and in a skilled nursing facility after a hospital stay, hospice care, and some home health care.[102]

In 2024, the premium for Part B is $174.70 per month.[101] Most Part A enrollees are also enrolled in Part B and have their premium deducted directly from their Social Security check. Part B of Medicare helps cover physicians' and other healthcare providers' services, outpatient care, durable medical equipment, home health care, and some preventive services. Part B also has a deductible of $204 per year in 2024 and coinsurance (80/20 coverage). Whereas most Medicare beneficiaries pay the standard premium rate, a small percentage pay a higher rate based on their income. In 2024, the higher rates ranged from $244.60 to $599.00 per month, depending on the extent to which an individual beneficiary's income exceeded $103,000 (or $206,000 for those filing a joint tax return), with the highest rates paid by those whose incomes were more than $500,000 (or $750,000 for those filing a joint tax return).[101]

Part C of Medicare is formally called Medicare Advantage and was added to Medicare as part of the Balanced Budget Act (BBA) of 1997. It was introduced primarily as a means to try to reduce costs compared with the original fee-for-service Medicare plan. Medicare Advantage plans provide all of the coverage provided in Parts A and B and must cover medically necessary services except for hospice care. They generally offer extra benefits; thus, there is no need to purchase a separate supplemental Medigap policy (see the discussion on Medigap later in this chapter), and many include Part D prescription drug coverage. Part C plans are offered by private insurance companies and are not available in all parts of the country. Because private companies offer them, the specifics of the plans are not consistent from plan to plan. Some are set up on a fee-for-service arrangement, whereas others are offered as managed care plans (i.e., PPOs, HMOs, and medical savings accounts). Most have an annual deductible and require a monthly premium in addition to premiums paid for Part B.[102] In 2023, 31.6 million people were enrolled in Part C plans.[103] To participate in Part C, a beneficiary must first be enrolled in both Part A and Part B. The beneficiary must pay Part B premiums to Medicare and an additional premium to the managed care organization, although some plans with high deductibles have no premium.[1]

Medicare Part D, which currently covers more than 50.5 million people,[103] is the prescription drug program. Part D is optional and run by insurance companies and other private companies approved by Medicare. To use it, eligible people must sign up for it and pay a monthly premium (most range from $20 to $60 per month). The premium varies based on the plan selected (most states offer approximately 50 different plans). Like Part B, there is an additional fee for those with higher incomes. A special provision in Part D—"extra help"—offers drug coverage at low cost for qualified people with limited incomes and resources. Although Part D has provided welcome help with the cost of prescription drugs to those who are eligible, the process of using Part D has been difficult for many to understand. It is complicated for several reasons. The first is the large number of plans available. The plans vary in drugs covered and costs. For example, one drug may be on the list of drugs covered (called the formulary) by one plan but not another. Many plans cover only generic drugs, whereas others cover both generic and brand-name drugs. Most plans have copayments or coinsurance. In addition, there is the coverage gap, or what has become known as the donut hole. The Biden administration passed a new drug law on January 1, 2023, that will help save money with people on Medicare. The new drug law lowers costs of insulin and more vaccines are covered. It will also cap out the out-of-pocket cost to $2,000 starting in 2025. The consumer also has the option to pay out-of-pocket costs monthly instead of when it occurs. In addition, Medicare will negotiate directly with manufacturers for high brand names. If manufacturers do not follow the negotiations, they will have to pay a tax and penalties.[103]

In 2023, Medicare Part D patients paid $505 deductible. Once this deductible was met, the plans covered the costs of drugs up to $4,660. However, some plans lower this limit to $2,000 or even $1,850 (lower limits are used to lower monthly premiums for people with minimal medication needs). Then at $4,660, the enrollees had to pay out of pocket 25% for both brand-name and generic drugs until they had spent $7,400.[101] This does not include the plan's premium. Once enrollees reached the plan's out-of-pocket limit, the donut hole closed and the enrollees had catastrophic coverage. This means that those covered paid a small coinsurance amount or a copayment for the rest of the calendar year.[101] Some of the complexity of Part D will be resolved by the ACA. As part of that legislation, the confusing donut hole (i.e., coverage gap) will be gradually reduced, and by 2025, it will be eliminated.[100]

It should be noted that when healthcare providers take assignment (are willing to accept Medicare patients) on a Medicare claim, they agree to accept the Medicare-approved amount as payment in full. These providers are paid directly by the Medicare carrier, except for the deductible and coinsurance amounts, which are the patient's responsibility.

Finally, Medicare, like private health insurance programs, is affected by the high costs of health care and, therefore, the government is always looking for ways of cutting costs for these programs. As noted earlier, Medicare has used several types of prospective reimbursement to help cut costs. The oldest of these, diagnosis-related groups (DRGs), has been around since 1983. When patients with Medicare coverage are admitted to a hospital, they are assigned a DRG and the hospital is reimbursed the predetermined amount of money for the DRG as opposed to the actual cost to render care. "The correct DRG for each patient is decided by considering the patient's major or principal diagnosis, any complications or other problems that might arise, any surgery performed during the hospital stay, and other factors."[104] The amount of money assigned to each DRG is not the same for each hospital. The figure is based on a formula that takes into account the type of service, the type of hospital, the location of the hospital, and the sex and age of the patient. Using this prospective pricing system, hospitals are encouraged to provide services at or below the DRG rate. If the hospital delivers the service below the DRG rate, the hospital can retain the difference. If it is delivered above the DRG rate, the hospital incurs the extra expenses. "However, when a Medicare patient's condition requires an unusually long hospital stay or exceptionally costly care, Medicare makes additional payment to the hospital."[104] Because of DRGs, some believe that hospitals are quicker to discharge Medicare patients to keep their expenses down. This phenomenon has resulted in an increase in the need for skilled nursing care in homes, in adult daycare facilities, and in nursing homes.

In recent years, much discussion has centered around whether there are sufficient funds in Medicare (i.e., Trust Fund solvency) to pay for the healthcare costs of the 76 million baby boomers when they started to become eligible in 2011. Most projections indicate that there is enough money to begin to cover the baby boomers, but as they age, Medicare will run out of money unless changes are made. Specifically, steps need to be taken to slow the rate of spending and increase the revenue needed to fund Medicare. To deal in part with this problem, the ACA included a number of provisions that will help extend the life of Medicare by slowing the amount of "reimbursement for Medicare Advantage, hospital costs, home health services, hospices, and skilled nursing services."[105] In addition, steps have been taken to increase revenue.

Beginning in 2013, the dedicated payroll tax paid by employees and their employers that goes into the Hospital Insurance trust fund covers 88% of the cost of Part A of Medicare.[106] As of 2020, this raised the tax from 1.45% to 2.35% for people with an annual earned income of more than $200,000 ($250,000 for married couples filing jointly). Also in 2013, premiums, which fund the majority of costs for both Parts B and D of Medicare, were increased for higher income beneficiaries.[107] Based on these changes, the Medicare trustees projected that the Part A trust fund, which is the common way of measuring Medicare's financial status, will be depleted in 2031. Running deficits in 2025 and depleted by 2031.[108]

Medicaid

A second type of government health insurance is **Medicaid**, a health insurance program for low-income Americans. The option to combine the Medicaid program with CHIP (see discussion that follows) is available to states, and several have chosen to do so to provide better health care for low-income Americans. Currently, approximately 87.3 million people are covered by Medicaid and CHIP.[103] Prior to the passage of the ACA, eligibility for enrollment in Medicaid was determined by each state in consultation with the federal government. Under health reform, eligibility is based solely on income and is extended to more low-income people, including both parents and adults without dependent children. As a result of these changes, nearly everyone under the age of 65 years with income below 133% of the poverty level (in 2023 for a family of four it was $30,000) could qualify for Medicaid, significantly reducing the number of uninsured and state variations in coverage. In the previous sentence, we use the phrase "could qualify." The reason for this choice of words is the result of the 2012 Supreme Court ruling that allowed states to opt out of the Medicaid provision. As a part of that ruling, the court limited, but did not invalidate, the provision. Prior to the ruling, states had to expand Medicaid or risk losing all Medicaid funding—an option no state could afford. The Supreme Court ruled that the federal government could not force this significant change to an already-existing program on the states.[109] Thus, states could opt out of covering up to 133% of the poverty level. As noted earlier in this chapter in Box 13.3, as of December 2023, four states (including the District of Columbia) have expanded Medicaid, one state has adopted but has not implemented it, and the remaining 10 have decided not to adopt expansion. "Some health care experts said it was unthinkable that state leaders would really opt out, because the vast majority of the cost is covered by the federal government—taxes their citizens will pay, regardless of whether the state opts in or out. For the first three years, the federal government pays for 100% of the expansion. The federal government's share will gradually drop to 90% starting in 2020."[109]

Children's Health Insurance Program

The **Children's Health Insurance Program (CHIP)** was created as part of the Balanced Budget Act of 1997 and funded for 10 years. It was enacted to provide coverage to eligible low-income, uninsured children who do not qualify for Medicaid. "Uninsured children pay a heavy price: Study after study shows that they are more likely to report poor health, to see doctors less often (even when they are sick), to go without preventive care, and to turn to emergency rooms when in need of treatment. The result is needless illness, learning problems, disabilities, and sometimes even death."[110]

Like Medicaid, CHIP is a joint state–federal funded program. As of September of 2023, there were approximately 40 million children covered by CHIP.[111] In 2009, President Obama extended CHIP through 2013 by signing the 2009 Children's Health Insurance Program Reauthorization Act (CHIPRA; Public Law 111-3).[111] To help offset the cost of the reauthorization, the law included an increase in the federal excise tax on tobacco products. The ACA maintains the CHIP eligibility standards in place as of enactment through 2019 and contains provisions to increase enrollment and extend funding until 2015.[111] In 2015, President Obama signed into law H.R. 2, the Medicare Access and CHIP Reauthorization Act of 2015, which extended the funding through 2017.[112] Congress put CHIP funding on hiatus in 2017 for several months as the Trump administration authorized a public charge that led to fewer children getting health insurance (8, C.F.R § 212, 2018). The Biden administration expanded ACA coverage within the first few months of Biden taking office. The American Rescue Plan was implemented and as of September of 2022, 90 million people were enrolled in Medicare and CHIP. In February of 2020, there was an increase of 28.6%.[113]

Problems with Medicare and Medicaid

In theory, the Medicare and Medicaid programs appear to be sound programs that help provide health care to two segments of society that would otherwise find it difficult or impossible to obtain health insurance. In practice, there are two recurrent problems with these programs. One problem is that some physicians and hospitals do not accept Medicare and Medicaid patients because of the tedious and time-consuming paperwork, lengthy delays in reimbursement, and insufficient reimbursement. As a result, it is difficult, if not impossible, for some of those eligible for Medicare and Medicaid to receive health care. The second problem occurs when physicians and hospitals file Medicare and Medicaid claims for care or services not rendered or rendered incompletely. This is known as *Medicare/Medicaid fraud*.

These problems were known to Congress, so when the ACA was written, it included provisions to increase payment to physicians and hospitals and to crack down on fraud.

Medigap private health insurance that supplements Medicare benefits

Supplemental Health Insurance

Medigap

As noted earlier, Parts A and B of Medicare have deductibles and coinsurance stipulations. To help cover these out-of-pocket costs and some other services not covered by Medicare, people can purchase supplemental policies from private insurance companies. These policies have come to be known as **Medigap** (Medicare Supplement Insurance) policies because they cover the "gaps" not covered by Medicare (see **Figure 13.13**). Federal and state laws mandate national standardization of Medigap policies. Since their inception, 14 different standardized

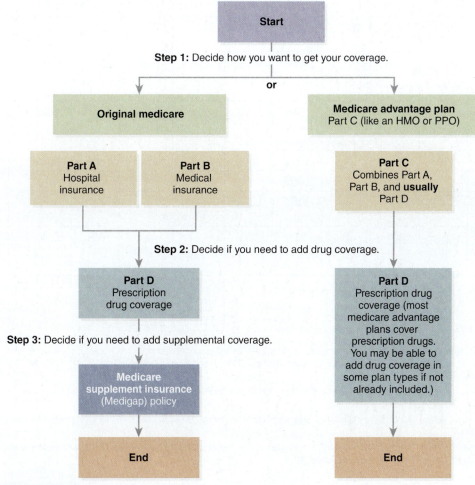

FIGURE 13.13   Your Medicare coverage choices at a glance.

CRS analysis of National Health Expenditure Account (NHEA) data obtained from the Centers for Medicare & Medicaid Services (CMS), Office of the Actuary, prepared November 2022.

Notes: Analysis includes Medicare post-acute care spending in an expanded definition of LTSS spending. Percentages may not sum to 100% due to rounding.

Data from Congressional Research Service. (2023). Who Pays for Long-Term Services and Supports? Available at https://crsreports.congress.gov/product/pdf/IF/IF10343

BOX 13.6   Medigap Plans

How to Read the Chart

This chart shows basic information about the different benefits that Medigap policies cover. If a percentage appears, the Medigap plan covers that percentage of the benefit. If a row is blank, the policy does not cover that benefit.

| Benefits | Medicare Supplement Insurance (Medigap) Plans | | | | | | | | | |
	A	B	C	D	F*	G*	K**	L**	M	N***
Medicare Part A coinsurance and hospital costs (up to an additional 365 days after Medicare benefits are used)	100%	100%	100%	100%	100%	100%	100%	100%	100%	100%
Medicare Part B coinsurance or copayment	100%	100%	100%	100%	100%	100%	50%	75%	100%	100%***
Blood (first three pints)	100%	100%	100%	100%	100%	100%	50%	75%	100%	100%
Part A hospice care coinsurance or copayment	100%	100%	100%	100%	100%	100%	50%	75%	100%	100%
Skilled nursing facility care coinsurance			100%	100%	100%	100%	50%	75%	100%	100%
Part A deductible		100%	100%	100%	100%	100%	50%	75%	50%	100%
Part B deductible			100%		100%					
Part B excess charges					100%	100%				
Foreign travel emergency (up to plan limits)			80%	80%	80%	80%			80%	80%
							Out-of-pocket limit in 2023**			
							$7,060	$3,530		

*Plans F and G also offer a high-deductible plan in some states. With this option, you must pay for Medicare-covered costs (coinsurance, copayments, and deductibles) up to the deductible amount of $2,340 in 2020 before your policy pays anything. (Plans C and F won't be available to people who are newly eligible for Medicare on or after January 1, 2023.)

**For Plans K and L, after you meet your out-of-pocket yearly limit and your yearly Part B deductible ($198 in 2020), the Medigap plan pays 100% of covered services for the rest of the calendar year.

***Plan N pays 100% of the Part B coinsurance, except for a copayment of up to $20 for some office visits and up to a $50 copayment for emergency room visits that don't result in an inpatient admission.

Reproduced from Centers for Medicare and Medicaid Services. (2023). *Choosing a Medigap policy:* A guide to health insurance for people with Medicare, 11. Available at https://www.medicare.gov/Pubs/pdf/02110-medicare-medigap-guide.pdf

Medigap plans (titled A through N) have been used. Currently, only 10 plans (A–D, F–G, K–N) are available[114] (see **Box 13.6**). All plans are required to have a core set of benefits referred to as basic benefits; however, some of the basic benefits of plans K through N are offered at a reduced level. By law, the letters and benefits of the individual plans cannot be changed by the insurance companies. However, they may add names or titles to the letter designations.

Companies are not required to offer all of the plans. "Cost is usually the only difference between Medigap policies with the same letter sold by different insurance companies."[114] "Insurance companies selling Medigap policies are required to make Plan A available. If they offer any other Medigap plan, they must also offer either Medigap Plan C or Plan F."[114] Three states—Minnesota, Massachusetts, and Wisconsin—have exceptions to the 10-plan setup because they had alternative Medigap standardization programs in effect before the federal legislation was enacted. Individuals should contact the state insurance office in these states if interested in these plans.

Two other variances to these Medigap rules should be noted. The first deals with individuals who are enrolled in the Medicare Advantage program. Because Medicare Advantage is more comprehensive in coverage than the traditional Medicare program, Medigap policies are not needed. In fact, it is illegal for insurance companies to sell a Medigap policy if they know a person is enrolled in Medicare Advantage.[114] Another variance in Medigap policy deals with Medicare SELECT. Medicare SELECT is a type of Medigap policy that is available in some states. This type of policy still provides one of the standardized Medigap plans (A–D, F–G, K–N), but requires policyholders to use specific hospitals and, in some cases, doctors (except in emergencies) to receive full Medigap benefits.[114]

Other Supplemental Insurance

Medigap is a supplemental insurance program specifically designed for those on Medicare. However, a number of supplemental insurance policies exist for people regardless of their age. Included are specific-disease insurance, hospital indemnity insurance, and long-term care insurance. Specific-disease insurance, although not available in some states, provides benefits for a single disease (such as cancer) or a group of specific diseases. Many policies are written as fixed indemnity policies. Hospital indemnity coverage is insurance that pays a fixed amount for each day a person receives inpatient hospital services, and it pays up to a designated number of days. Long-term care insurance, which pays cash amounts for each day of covered nursing home or at-home care, is of great concern to many people, and it is presented next.

Long-Term Care Insurance

With people living longer and the cost of health care on the rise, more and more individuals are considering the purchase of long-term care insurance. It has been estimated that "70 percent of people over age 65 can expect to use some form of long-term care during their lives."[115] About 35% will need care in a nursing home.[115] And, contrary to what many people believe, Medicare and private health insurance programs do not pay for the majority of long-term care services that most people need—such as help with bathing or for supervision (often called custodial care).[115] Women, who on average live 5 years longer than men, are more likely to live at home alone when they are older, and will have a need for care for longer than men (3.7 versus 2.2 years).[114] Whereas one-third of today's 65-year-olds may never need long-term care services, 20% of them will need care for more than 5 years.[115] Most—about 80%—of long-term care will be provided in the home by unpaid caregivers,[115] usually family and friends.

Planning for long-term care requires people to think about possible future healthcare needs and how they will pay for them. Obviously, the cost of long-term care varies based on the level of care, the length of time the care is provided, and where the care is provided. The most costly long-term care is nursing home care. Recent figures show that the median cost of residing in a nursing home was $260 per day (range $180 to $1,036) or $7,800 per month or $90,155 per year for a semiprivate room, $297 per day (range $195 to $$1,036) or $8,910 per month or $108,405 per year for a private room, whereas assisted-living facilities were $4,051 per month or $54,000 per year for care in a one-bedroom unit.[116] The costs vary by parts of the country, but such costs for long-term care have many people worried about their financial future. This cost is something that can quickly deplete a lifetime of savings. Medicare and other health insurance do not include most long-term care services. If people have fairly low income and savings, they may qualify for Medicaid, which is the primary payer for institutional and community-based, long-term services

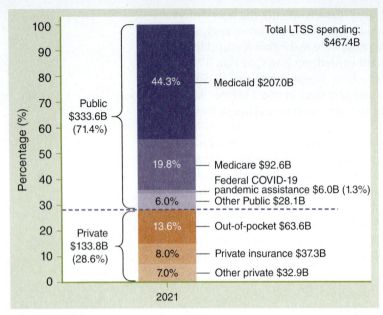

FIGURE 13.14 Long-Term Services and Supports (LTSS) Spending, by Payer, 2021 (in billions).

Reproduced from Congressional Research Service. (2023). Who Pays for Long-Term Servises and Supports? Available at https://crsreports.congress.gov/product/pdf/IF/IF10343#:~:text=Using%20 this%20definition%2C%20total%20U.S.,spent%20on%20personal%20health%20care

and supports (see **Figure 13.14**). There is a good chance that individuals will have to pay for all or some of these services out of pocket; therefore, it may be important to consider long-term care insurance.[115]

Although long-term care is expensive, not everyone needs to buy long-term care insurance. Those who do not need it are those with low incomes and few assets who could be covered by Medicaid and the very wealthy who are able to pay the cost of the care out of pocket. Those who are most likely to benefit from long-term care insurance are those in between low-income and wealthy, especially older women. However, there are several reasons why all people should consider purchasing long-term insurance. They include the following:

- To preserve financial assets
- To prevent the need for family members or friends to provide the care
- To enable people to stay independent in their homes longer
- To make it easier to get into the nursing home or assisted-living home of their choice

Managed Care

As noted earlier in this chapter, the failed attempt to adopt universal health care in the United States during the first term of President Bill Clinton led to the movement of managed care. Managed care is "a system that integrates the functions of financing, insurance, delivery, and payment and uses mechanisms to control costs and utilization of services."[14] The transition to managed care in the United States was largely driven by a desire of employers, insurance companies, and the public to control soaring healthcare costs. Although the exact number of individuals enrolled in managed care programs is constantly changing, in 2022, 80% of Americans were enrolled in some form of a managed care plan. In that same year, over 99% of employees covered by an employers' health plan was in some form of a managed care plan.[117]

Managed care plans are offered by managed care organizations (MCOs). MCOs function like insurance organizations. They offer policies, collect premiums, and bear financial risk. That is, MCOs take on the financial responsibility if the costs of the services exceed the revenue from the premiums. These organizations have agreements with certain doctors, hospitals, and other healthcare providers to give a range of services to plan members at reduced cost. MCOs have been structured in a variety of ways and are similar to the other healthcare organizations with which we are familiar (such as hospitals). Some are structured as nonprofit organizations, whereas others are for-profit and owned by a group of investors. "Regardless of their structure, their goals, however, are similar: to control costs through improved efficiency and coordination, to reduce unnecessary or inappropriate utilization, to increase access to preventive care, and to maintain or improve quality of care."[118]

The managed care plans offered by these organizations vary and are always evolving as managed care practices mature and new processes are developed to improve quality and contain costs. The plans also differ, both in cost and ease of receiving needed services. Although no plan pays for all the costs associated with medical care, some plans cover more than others. Common features in managed care arrangements include: (1) provider panels, often referred to as the network—specific physicians and other providers are selected to care for plan members; (2) limited choice—members must use the providers affiliated with the plan or pay an additional amount for providers outside the network; (3) gatekeeping—members must obtain a referral from a case manager for specialty care or inpatient services; (4) risk sharing—providers bear some of the health plan's financial risk through capitation and withholdings; and (5) **quality management and utilization review**—the plan monitors provider practice patterns and medical outcomes to identify deviations from quality and efficiency standards. The utilization review can take the form of *prospective utilization review* (as precertification), *concurrent utilization review* (i.e., during the course of healthcare utilization), or *retrospective utilization review* (completed by reviewing medical records after the care has been provided).[1] This latter type of review may involve "analysis of data to examine patterns of excessive utilization or underutilization. *Underutilization* occurs when medically necessary care is not delivered. *Overutilization* occurs when medical services that are not necessary are delivered."[1]

Types of Managed Care

As noted earlier, there are several different types of managed care arrangements. Prior to 1990, the various types of MCOs were quite distinct. Since then, the differences between traditional forms of health insurance and managed care have narrowed considerably. The following are the most commonly available arrangements.

Preferred Provider Organizations

The **preferred provider organization (PPO)** is a form of managed care closest to a fee-for-service plan. A PPO differs from the traditional fee-for-service plan in that the fee has been fixed (at a discounted rate) through a negotiation process between healthcare providers (e.g., physicians, dentists, hospitals) and the PPO, and the provider agrees to accept this discounted rate as payment in full. It works in the following manner: A PPO approaches a provider, such as a group dental practice, and contracts with the dentists to provide dental services to all those covered by the PPO's insurance plan at a fixed (discounted) rate. To the extent that the PPO succeeds in obtaining favorable prices, it can offer lower premiums, coinsurance, and copayments, and hence can attract more patients to enroll in its insurance plan. In addition to using the PPO network of providers, plan members can also use out-of-network providers. However, if they do choose to go outside the network, they will have to meet the deductible and pay higher coinsurance. In addition, they may have to pay the difference between what the provider charges and what the plan pays. "The additional out-of-pocket expenses largely act as a deterrent to going outside the network for care."[1] PPOs also control costs by requiring (1) preauthorization for hospital admissions (excluding emergencies) and expensive procedures, and (2) second opinions for major procedures, such as surgery.[6] Advantages for the providers are that they (1) do not share in any financial risk as a condition of participation,[6] (2) are reimbursed on a fee-for-service basis (but at a discounted rate) to which they are accustomed,[6] (3) are assured a certain volume of patients, and (4) are assured that the patients will pay promptly (via the PPO). Of the various types of managed care plans, PPOs enroll the largest number of Americans.[117] In 2022, this was approximately 223.1 million people.[117] Much of the increase in enrollment in PPOs was the result of people leaving HMOs (see the discussion of HMOs later) because of increased costs and the restrictions in the choice of providers.

Health Maintenance Organizations

The **health maintenance organization (HMO)** is the oldest form of managed care. Behind PPOs, HMOs enroll the second largest number of Americans.[117] Enrollment in HMOs peaked in 1999 at about 80 million and has dropped every year since then.[117] However, other types of managed care began to emerge. As HMO enrollment has been declining, PPO has been increasing. In 2022, the number of enrollees in any managed care plan was about 95 million.[117] As noted earlier, many of those leaving HMOs switched to PPOs. In an HMO, the insurance coverage and the delivery of medical care are combined into a single organization. The organization hires (through salaries or contracts) an individual doctor or group of doctors to provide care and either builds its own hospital or contracts for the services of a hospital within the community. The organization then enrolls members, usually, but not always, through the workplace.

Closed-panel HMO organization in which private physicians are contracted on an exclusive basis for services at a health maintenance organization

Open-panel HMO organization in which private practice physicians are contracted by a health maintenance organization to deliver care in their own offices

Mixed model HMO a hybrid form of health maintenance organization

Staff model HMO a health maintenance organization that hires its own staff of healthcare providers

Independent practice association (IPA) legal entity separate from the HMO that is a physician organization composed of community-based independent physicians in a solo or group practice who provide services to HMO members

Point-of-service (POS) option an option of an HMO plan that enables enrollees to be at least partially reimbursed for selecting a healthcare provider outside of the plan

Members (or their employers or the government [in the case of HMOs for Medicare and Medicaid]) make regular payments in advance on a fixed contract fee to the HMO. This contract may also include a deductible and copayment when service is provided. In return, the HMO is contractually obligated to provide the members with a comprehensive range of outpatient and inpatient services that are spelled out in the contract for a specific time period.

When members enroll in an HMO, they are given a list (network) of specific physicians/providers from which to select their primary care doctor (usually a family physician, internist, or pediatrician) and other healthcare providers. The primary care doctor (which some have referred to as the gatekeeper) serves as the member's regular doctor and coordinates the member's care, which means the member must contact their primary care doctor to be referred to a specialist. In many plans, care by a specialist is only paid for if the member is referred by the primary care doctor, thus the term *gatekeeper*. Also, if patients receive care outside the network, they must pay for all the costs, except in cases of emergency when physically not near a member of the network.

How do HMOs make a profit? An HMO's focus of care is different from that of a traditional fee-for-service provider. In an HMO, ill and injured patients become a "cost." An HMO does not make money on the ill but on keeping people healthy. The less the providers of an HMO see a patient, the lower the costs and the more profitable the organization. Therefore, most HMOs emphasize health promotion activities and primary and secondary care. "As an incentive to the enrollees to seek wellness care, HMO plans typically do not have annual deductibles, and they also have lower copayments than do other types of plans."[1]

There are two broad organizational models of HMOs—*closed-panel plans* and *open-panel plans*. A **closed-panel HMO** is one "that contracts with physicians on an exclusive basis for services and does not allow those physicians to see patients for another managed care organization."[119] Examples of closed-panel HMOs include the *staff* and *group models*. An **open-panel HMO** is one "that contracts (either directly or indirectly) with private physicians to deliver care in their own offices."[119] Examples of open-panel HMOs include *independent practice associations* (*IPAs*) and *network model HMOs*. Each of the types of HMOs noted here has spawned several hybrids. These hybrids are referred to as **mixed model HMOs**. Due to space available, we have limited our discussion to staff and IPA HMOs. Other models are defined in the glossary.

Staff Model

In a **staff model HMO** healthcare providers are employed (usually salaried) by the HMO, and they practice in common facilities paid for by the HMO. Staff model HMOs employ providers in all common specialties to provide services to their members. Special contracts are established with subspecialties for infrequently needed services. These providers are expected to follow the practice and procedures determined by the HMO. With the exception of the special contracts, the providers work only for the HMO and thus do not have their own private practices. In most instances, the HMO contracts with a hospital for inpatient services. Nationwide, the number of staff model HMOs has been declining.

Independent Practice Association Model

The **independent practice association (IPA)** is the most common type of HMO today. IPAs are legal entities separate from the HMO[119] that are physician organizations composed of community-based independent physicians in solo or group practices who provide services to HMO members.[6] Instead of establishing contracts with individual physicians or groups, the HMO contracts with the IPA for physician services. Physicians do not have contracts with the HMO, but with the IPA.[1] Thus, the IPA acts as an intermediary and is paid a capitation amount by the HMO.[1]

Other Items Related to HMOs

Point-of-Service Option

One of the major objections to HMOs is that the patients cannot freely select their provider. They are restricted to those with whom the HMO has contracted. Some HMOs have solved this problem with the **point-of-service (POS) option**, which allows for a more liberal policy of enabling patients to select providers but still retain the benefits of tight utilization management.[1] With this option, members may choose a provider from within or outside of the HMO network. Patients who obtain services outside of the network generally must pay a higher deductible and coinsurance. Initially, POSs were a good selling point for HMOs, but after reaching their peak enrollments, the numbers have gradually declined, mainly because of their high out-of-pocket expenses.[1] In 2018, the number of Americans enrolled in HMOs who had the POS option was 4.8 million.[117]

Medicare Advantage

As noted earlier, in some parts of the country, Medicare recipients may have HMO or PPO options available to them through the Medicare Advantage plan. In such plans, the Medicare recipient receives all Medicare-covered services, and often additional services not covered by Medicare, from the HMO or PPO. Some of these plans may include prescription drug coverage (Part D). If this is the case, Medigap coverage cannot be purchased. The HMO or PPO may charge the beneficiary a premium (in addition to the Medicare Part B premium) to cover coinsurance and deductibles of Medicare, but some plans that have high deductibles may have no premium.[1] In 2023, approximately 51% of the people enrolled in Medicare Advantage received their care through an HMO, 31% received their care from a PPO.[120]

Medicaid and Managed Care

As has been noted throughout this chapter, managed care plans are also available for those covered by Medicaid. The rationale for offering such plans is to improve access to care by the establishment of contracted provider networks, as well as by promoting greater accountability for quality and costs. Each state in the United States offers such a plan, and, depending on the state requirements, enrollment may or may not be voluntary. If it is mandatory, the state is required to offer a choice of managed care plans and make efforts to inform beneficiaries about their choices.[4] In 2023, more than half of the people covered by Medicaid were enrolled in managed care plans.[121]

Before leaving our discussion on managed care, we want to remind the reader that, like other aspects of the healthcare system, there have also been efforts to measure the quality of managed care. Please see the discussion of quality of health care earlier in the chapter, where we present information on the NCQA.

Other Arrangements for Delivering Health Care

Because the majority of people in the United States receive their health care through a managed care plan or a fee-for-service plan, the majority of this chapter focused on those plans. However, there are other ways of delivering health care. A few of the more highly visible arrangements are discussed next.

Healthcare Delivery in Other Countries

National health insurance, or national health care, suggests a system in which the federal government assumes the responsibility for the healthcare costs of the entire population. In such a system, the costs are primarily paid for with tax dollars. Presently, among all of the developed countries of the world, only one does not have a national healthcare plan for its citizens—the United States.

The national healthcare systems of the developed countries of the world fall into two basic models. The first is a *national health service* model with universal coverage and general tax-financed government ownership of the facilities, with doctors as public employees. Countries using this model include the United Kingdom, Spain, Italy, Greece, and Portugal. The second is a *social insurance model* that provides universal coverage under social security, financed by various means, including taxes or contributions paid by employers and employees. In Canada, contributions are made to a government entity. In France and Germany, contributions go to nonprofit funds with national negotiation on fees. Japan also has a compulsory system that relies heavily on employer-based coverage.

	AUS	CAN	FRA	GER	NETH	NZ	SWE	SWIZ	UK	US
OVERALL RANKING	1	7	5	9	2	4	6	8	3	10
Access to Care	9	7	6	3	1	5	4	8	2	10
Care Process	5	4	7	9	3	1	10	6	8	2
Administrative Efficiency	2	5	4	8	6	3	7	10	1	9
Equity	1	7	6	2	3	8	–	4	5	9
Health Outcomes	1	4	5	9	7	3	6	2	8	10

Note: SWE overall ranking calculation does not include Equity domain. See "How We Conducted This Study" for more detail.

FIGURE 13.15   Comparison of health systems: Overall ranking.

Reproduced from David Blumenthal et al., Mirror, Mirror 2024: A Portrait of the Failing U.S. Health System — Comparing Performance in 10 Nations (Commonwealth Fund, Sept. 2024). https://doi.org/10.26099/ta0g-zp66

When one considers the level of satisfaction with health care, the better access to healthcare services, the lower healthcare costs, and the superior health status indicators in these other countries, one must ask why the United States has not adopted such a program (see **Figure 13.15**). It is not because the United States has not considered such a plan—in fact, there have been seven failed attempts at addressing the issue over the past 70+ years. The first came when President Roosevelt tried to include it as part of the New Deal. President Harry Truman presented a proposal to Congress on two different occasions, only to have it defeated twice. Other unsuccessful attempts at national healthcare legislation were made during the Kennedy, Nixon, and Clinton administrations. There was also talk about a national health insurance program in the United States during the presidential campaign and debates of 2008. During that campaign, all of the front-running candidates pledged to work toward a national program, although all had different plans for getting there. As history has shown us, President Obama was unsuccessful in getting a national health insurance program; however, he was successful in getting major healthcare reform via the ACA. At the time when this edition of this book was written, the candidates vying for the Democrat nomination identified a national health insurance program as a priority, whereas most of the Republican candidates indicated they wanted to repeal the ACA and build a different healthcare delivery system.

Healthcare Reform in the United States

Prior to the passage of the ACA, the healthcare reform that has taken place in the United States in recent times has been with specific smaller, but not insignificant, portions of the healthcare system—for example, President Clinton's creation of CHIP in 1997 and the reauthorization of the program by President Obama in 2009. During President George W. Bush's term in office, reform came in the form of the Medicare Prescription Drug Improvement and Modernization Act (MMA) of 2003 (Public Law 108-173). The portion of MMA that gained the greatest publicity—that dealing with prescription drugs via Medicare Part D—was discussed earlier in the chapter. However another significant component of the MMA was health savings accounts (HSAs), sometimes referred to as the savings option. HSAs are one of several different forms of consumer-directed health plans (CDHPs). In the sections that follow, we discuss CDHPs, high deductible health plans, and the ACA.

Consumer-Directed Health Plans

A **consumer-directed health plan (CDHP)**, also called a consumer-driven health plan, consumer-directed health arrangement [CDHA], consumer choice, and self-directed health plan [SDHP])[122] is a healthcare plan that combines a high-deductible health plan (HDHP) with a pretax payment account to pay for out-of-pocket medical expenses. In theory, such plans should create more consumer responsibility for healthcare decisions. CDHPs have sought "to marshal the power of consumers making cost-conscious choices to constrain rising U.S. health care spending."[123] A critical part of CDHPs is providing those enrolled in such plans with comparative information to increase their knowledge about healthcare choices and associated costs.[6] The central idea behind CDHPs is that consumers will still have catastrophic health insurance, but because they are required to use more of their own money to pay for health care, they will be more careful about their use of services than they would be under a traditional health plan that provides greater coverage of their initial healthcare costs.[119] The options of pre-tax payment accounts available for CDHPs include health savings accounts (HSAs), health reimbursement arrangements (HRAs), and flexible spending accounts (FSAs).

The most visible option of a pretax payment account for CDHPs is the HSA. An HSA is a type of medical savings account that allows people to save money to pay for current and future medical expenses on a tax-free basis. To be eligible for an HSA, people must be covered by a high-deductible health plan (in 2023, the deductible was $1,500 for individuals and $3,000 for families),[124] not have any other health insurance (including Medicare), and not be claimed as a dependent on someone else's tax return. Those with HSAs can use this account to pay for qualified health expenses, including expenses that the plan ordinarily does not cover, such as hearing aids.[111] The law establishes a maximum amount that people with CDHPs would have to pay out of pocket for health expenses in a year. The amount is adjusted for inflation each year, but in 2023 the amount was $7,500 for individuals and $15,000 for families.[124]

During the year, those with HSAs can make voluntary contributions to the account using before-tax dollars. In 2023, the maximum amount that could be set aside was $3,850 for an individual, $7,75 for families,[124] or the amount of the deductible of the health insurance policy, whichever was lower. People aged 55 years and older can make additional "catch-up" contributions (in 2023, $1,950)[124] until they enroll in Medicare. These contributions are 100% tax deductible from gross income, thus the "pre-tax" tag. In some cases, employers may set up and help fund HSAs for their employees, but they are not required to do so. An HSA earns interest. If there is a balance in a person's HSA at the end of the year, it will roll over, allowing the person to build up a cushion against future health expenses. In addition, HSAs allow people to accumulate funds and retain them when they change plans or retire.[119] Money can be withdrawn from the account without penalty to pay for care before the deductible is met and for things not covered under the health insurance policy after the deductible is met. Money can be withdrawn and pay for anything (including nonhealth expenses) after 65 years of age, but the person must pay income tax on it. The advantages of such a plan are reduced premiums and, it is hoped, more prudent use of healthcare dollars—which should be good for both employers and employees. In addition, HSAs are portable from one employer to another. The major disadvantage for consumers is that they might have to pay more out of pocket for health care, and, therefore, might skip needed care. At the present, HSAs seem best suited for the healthy and wealthy.

As noted throughout this chapter, the ACA has made a number of changes to health care but it only made two changes to HSAs, and both went into effect in 2011. They included (1) HSAs could no longer be used tax-free for over-the-counter medications unless the medications were prescribed by a doctor; and (2) if people use their HSA funds for nonmedical expenses, they must pay a 20% penalty instead of the former 10% penalty.[125]

Although HSAs must be combined with HDHPs, HDHPs do not have to be combined with HSAs. In fact, HDHPs continue to grow in popularity because of their lower premium costs. When these plans are used, they are often accompanied by health promotion and wellness, disease management, case management, and health coaching programs to help participants

Consumer-directed health plan (CDHP) healthcare plan that combines a high-deductible health plan (HDHP) with a pretax payment account to pay for out-of-pocket medical expenses

improve and maintain health and keep medical conditions under control. One concern that has arisen with the HDHPs is that "as deductibles have grown in recent years, a surprising percentage of people with private insurance, and especially those with lower and moderate incomes, simply do not have the resources to pay their deductibles and will either have to put off care or incur medical debt."[126]

In 2019, the Trump administration expanded access to preventive care by making it easier for patients to enroll in HDHPs to get coverage for medications and drugs to treat chronic illnesses.[127]

Another type of pre-tax payment account for a CDHP is health reimbursement arrangements (HRAs). HRAs are not as flexible as HSAs. Only employers are allowed to set up HRAs for employees, and only employers can contribute to (i.e., fund) them. The employer decides how much money to put in a HRA, and the employee can withdraw funds from the account to cover allowed expenses. The ACA made some changes to the use of HRAs. In the past, HRAs were established in conjunction with a HDHP, but they could be paired with any type of health plan. Since January of 2014, HRAs can only be paired with ACA-compliant plans.[128] In addition, federal law continues to allow employers to determine whether employees can carry over all or a portion of unspent funds from year to year. Beginning in January of 2014, employers can no longer decide whether account balances will be forfeited if an employee leaves the job or changes health plans; such accounts are now forfeited upon termination of employment.[128] Also, employees must have the option to opt out of an HRA so that they can obtain health coverage via the marketplace and be eligible for premium tax credits.[128] And finally, like HSAs, as of January of 2011, HRA funds can no longer be used tax-free for over-the-counter medications unless the medications were prescribed by a doctor.[55] In 2020, the Trump administration allowed employers expanded HRA benefits by subsidizing premiums from the health insurance marketplaces.[129] Under the new rules, employers can offer an "individual coverage HRA" that gives workers and their families the ability to use tax-free employer dollars to pay for individual health coverage.

A third pre-tax payment account option for CDHPs is a flexible spending account (FSA). FSAs are set up by employers to allow employees to set aside pretax money to pay for qualified medical expenses during the year. Only employers may set up an account, and employers may or may not contribute to the account, but usually, FSAs are 100% employee funded.[130] There is a limit on the amount that employees can contribute to a flexible spending account; in 2023, that amount was $3,050. Like other CDHP options, the ACA also made changes to FSAs. First, just like HSAs and HRAs, as of January of 2011, the ACA no longer allowed FSA funds to be used tax-free for over-the-counter medications unless the medications were prescribed by a doctor.[55] Second, FSAs can now only be offered in conjunction with an employer ACA-compliant health insurance plan; they can no longer be offered on a stand-alone basis. Third, there is now a limit on the amount employers can contribute to a FSA. Employers can contribute no more than $500 or, if more, a match of up to $1 for every dollar contributed by the employee.[131] Fourth, in the past, FSAs were subject to a use-it-or-lose-it rule within the year of contributions with a 2.5-month grace period at the end of the plan year to use up funds in the account. Employers are now allowed to offer the grace period or a $500 rollover provision to the next year, but not both.[131] The tricky part of having an FSA is trying to determine how much money to place in the account in a year to avoid losing any money at year's end

Enrollment in CDHPs has been rising in recent years for three major reasons: (1) employers trying to cut healthcare costs, (2) consumers trying to reduce the cost of health insurance premiums, and (3) the tax advantages of most of the plans. Data from the 2007 National Health Interview Study (NHIS) showed that those more likely to be enrolled in a CDHP were those (1) who directly purchased private health plans, (2) had more education, and (3) had higher incomes.[132] More recent data from the 2018 NHIS show that "45.8.% of persons under age 65 with private health insurance were enrolled in an HDHP, including 20.4% who were enrolled in a CDHP [HDHP with HSA] and 25.4% who were enrolled in an HDHP without an HSA"[133] (see **Figure 13.16**). In terms of numbers, 45.8 million people were enrolled in CDHPs in 2018, up from 25.3 million in 2010.[123]

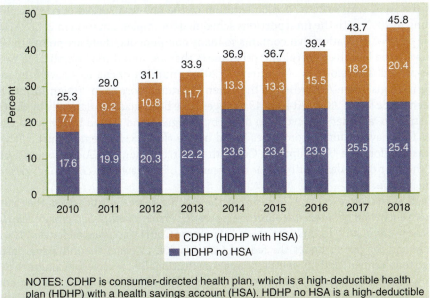

FIGURE 13.16 Percentage of persons under age 65 enrolled in HDHPs without an HSA or in a CDHP, among those with private health insurance coverage—United States, 2010 to 2018.

Reproduced from Cohen, R. A., & Martinez, M. E. (2018). *Health insurance coverage: Early release of estimates from the National Health Interview Survey.* Available at https://www.cdc.gov/nchs/data/nhis/earlyrelease/insur201905.pdf

It should be noted that CDHPs are not without critics. There are three major concerns about CDHPs. One, will consumers become educated enough to make good decisions? Since health insurance and health care are very complicated, will consumers take the time to become well educated? Two, is the healthcare field transparent enough to provide enough information to make a good decision? When was the last time that a patient received a healthcare service and knew in advance what the cost would be? Also, how do consumers know when they are receiving quality care? Who is the best physician in the community? Who is the worst? And three, because CDHPs require people to use more of their own money, will consumers seek health care in a timely manner? For example, in a traditional plan, the pneumonia vaccination is covered with a zero deductible, but with a CDHP that has a high deductible, it now costs the consumer $50 out of pocket. Will they still get the vaccine or will they save the $50 and forgo the vaccine?

Healthcare Reform in the United States

After many failed attempts to provide healthcare reform in the United States, the signing by President Obama in 2010 of the ACA was most significant in expanding access to health insurance and thus health care to many who previously did not have health insurance. As has been noted, the process to get the ACA passed was not easy. In addition to the many failed attempts, it took much discussion and much political wrangling by both Democrats and Republicans. Some called the wrangling an "ideological split." However, "[p]assage of the ACA was a historic political achievement, breaking the logjam that long stymied national progress toward equitable, quality, universal, affordable health care in the United States."[134] In the end, the Democrat members of the U.S. Senate and House of Representatives were more pleased with the results than were the Republican members. Not only was its initial passage difficult, but it has survived a number of challenges, including many votes (62 as of February of 2016)[18] in Congress to repeal or dismantle it; on four occasions, parts of the ACA have been litigated in the U.S. Supreme Court.[2]

As the ACA was written, implementation of the law was spread over multiple years beginning in 2010, with the final portions scheduled for implementation in 2025. Also, with any new piece of legislation that contains so many components, there are bound to be parts that prove to be less than useful and other parts that are found too complicated to implement as passed. Therefore, as of February of 2016, a number of changes have been made to the original legislation. According to the Galen Institute, more than 70 significant changes have been made to the ACA. At least 43 changes have been made unilaterally by the Obama administration, another 24 have been made by Congress and signed by the president, and another four have resulted from cases heard before the U.S. Supreme Court.[56] It was the three cases before the U.S. Supreme Court that worried many ACA proponents, because two of the four cases dealt with major components of the law that could have derailed its implementation.

The first challenge to the ACA heard by the U.S. Supreme Court came in the case of the *National Federation of Independent Businesses et al. versus Sebelius, Secretary of Health and Human Services, et al.*[135] In this case, the U.S. Supreme Court was asked to decide "(1) whether Congress had the power under the federal Constitution to enact the individual insurance coverage requirement, and (2) whether it was constitutionally coercive for Congress, through the ACA, to threaten to take away existing Medicaid funding from states that did not want to implement the Medicaid expansion."[2] In the former issue, the court ruled, "violating the law's mandate that Americans must purchase government-approved health insurance would not produce a 'penalty,' as stated in the legislation, but rather would result in individuals' paying a 'tax.' Paying a tax would make it, legally speaking, optional for people to comply and therefore would not violate the U.S. Constitution."[56] On the latter issue, the court ruled "that it was voluntary, rather than mandatory, for states to expand Medicaid eligibility to people with incomes up to 138% of poverty. The court rewrote the statute to say the federal government could not block funds for existing state Medicaid programs if states choose not to expand the program."[56]

The second challenge to the ACA heard by the U.S. Supreme Court came in the case of the *Burwell, Secretary of Health and Human Services, et al. versus Hobby Lobby Stores, Inc., et al.*[136] At question in this case was the portion of the ACA referred to as the contraceptive (or birth control) mandate that requires that healthcare plans must include coverage for FDA-approved contraceptive methods and counseling for all women, as prescribed by a healthcare provider.[137] The plaintiffs in the case were two private for-profit companies owned by members of a single family. The companies were the Hobby Lobby Stores, owned by a family who were Evangelical Christians, and Conestoga Wood Specialists, owned by a family who were members of the Mennonite faith. In this case, the court was asked to decide, under a federal statute called the Religious Freedom Restoration Act (RFRA) of 1993, if a closely held private for-profit corporation (i.e., one with a limited number of shareholders) had the legal right to refuse to comply with provisions of the ACA that required them to provide certain contraceptive coverage (in this case the plaintiffs objected only to the abortive Plan B drug) to which the employees would otherwise be entitled.[2] The court ruled in favor of Hobby Lobby Stores, et al., in stating that closely held private for-profit corporations cannot be forced to pay for insurance coverage for contraception for employees over their religious objections. Some think that this ruling might cause other closely held corporations to refuse all FDA-approved contraceptives for their employees,[2] whereas others believe this ruling opened the door to many more challenges from corporations over laws that they claim violate their religious liberty.[138]

The third challenge to the ACA heard by the U.S. Supreme Court came in the case of the *King et al. versus Burwell, Secretary of Health and Human Services, et al.*[139] This challenge to the ACA focused on whether or not the subsidies provided by the ACA were intended to be available to all who qualified for them and purchased their insurance through the marketplace regardless of who created the marketplace (i.e., the state or federal government). "In essence, the court case boiled down to the meaning of the four words "established by the State" or were the federal subsidies reserved only for individuals in states that established their own state-run exchange?"[2] The "court overruled the plain meaning of the ACA limiting subsidies to people living in states that created their own exchanges and instead allowed tax credits for insurance purchased through federally facilitated exchanges as well."[56]

The fourth and most recent challenge to the ACA was heard by the Supreme Court in March 2016 in the case of *Zubik et al. versus Burwell, Secretary of Health and Human Services, et al.* The challenge was brought by an order of nuns called the Little Sisters of the Poor, and consisted of seven consolidated cases brought by other nonprofit, religiously affiliated groups who lost in the lower courts. Their concern was with the ACA's requirement that group health plans provide a full range of contraceptive coverage to women at no cost because it violates a federal law meant to protect religious freedom. They were seeking an exemption to this part of the ACA that the Obama administration provided houses of worship. "In a unanimous opinion, the Supreme Court 'vacated,' meaning erased, all the lower court cases and required them to reconsider the claims brought by the Little Sisters of the Poor and others that the regulations promulgated pursuant to the ACA violate their religious exercise in light of the government's admission that it could indeed provide contraceptive coverage without the Little Sisters' collaboration.[140] This opinion included specific instructions that the government find a compromise by tweaking the contraceptive mandate so it does not include religious concerns."[140]

As noted throughout this chapter, the ACA is not a simple piece of legislation. It was almost 2,000 pages long and had many items in it that changed the way health insurance is provided in the United States. Some of the changes are obvious and easy to understand, whereas others could be skipped over by one not reading closely. Others are complicated and will take many people much time to completely understand and implement properly. In addition, the enormity of the ACA causes it to impact more than just health care. The ACA also has implications for the overall economy that may include effects on productivity and wages, the labor market, mergers in the healthcare sector (e.g., insurance companies, pharmacies, wellness companies, pharmaceutical companies),[141] commercial liability insurance,[142] and U.S. tax code, to name a few. As we move forward with the ACA, there is no indication that the rough road the ACA has experienced to date will get much smoother. As noted earlier, the law will not be fully implemented until 2025, and there are still many details that need to be worked out. In addition, there is still much hostility that many (mostly Republican) federal legislators, state governors and legislators, and citizens have for the ACA.[2] Many Americans are confused about what the law does for them.[2] Depending on the outcome of each subsequent presidential election, there may be attempts to repeal part or all of the ACA.[143] Even if the outcome of the each subsequent presidential election does not impact the ACA, there are still other lingering questions, such as: (1) Will the United States continue working toward universal health care? Will it ever reach it? (2) Will the ACA be able to control the cost of health insurance and thus the cost of health care?[2] (3) Will the 10 states that have not expanded Medicaid do so in the future? (4) Will any of the 33 states and the District of Columbia who expanded Medicaid regress to some other plan? (5) Will the functionality of the Healthcare.gov website continue to improve? (6) Will the marketplaces set up by the federal and state governments actually perform well over time?[2] (7) How many more lawsuits will there be that challenge the legality of the ACA or some of its components? (8) Will higher taxes be needed to sustain the provisions of the ACA? (9) What impact will the ACA have on medical research? All of these questions need answers, and only time will tell if and how they will be answered.

Back in 2009, prior to the passage of the ACA, President Obama stated at a joint session of Congress, "I am not the first president to take up the cause [i.e., healthcare reform], but I intend to be the last."[144] Although that was his intention, it will probably not come true. Data show that the cost of health care in the United States is too high, there are still too many Americans without health insurance, and compared with the other developed countries of the world, there is still room to improve the quality of care. The United States healthcare system will continue to require reform in the future.

Chapter Summary

- The concept of a healthcare system has been and continues to be questioned in the United States. Is it really a system or is treatment provided in an informal, cooperative manner?

- Health care in the United States has evolved from home and folk remedies, to the modest services of the independent country doctor who often visited the sick in their homes, to a highly complex, $3 trillion plus industry.

- The spectrum of health care includes four domains of practice—public health practice, medical practice, long-term care practice, and end-of-life practice.

- The following types of healthcare providers fall within the medical practice domain of health care: independent providers (allopathic, osteopathic, and nonallopathic), limited (restricted) care providers, nurses, nonphysician practitioners, allied healthcare professionals, and public health professionals.

- Complementary and alternative medicine (CAM) is "a group of diverse medical and healthcare systems, practices, and products that are not presently considered to be a part of conventional medicine."[28]

- Healthcare providers perform services in both inpatient and outpatient care facilities.

- Inpatient care facilities include hospitals, nursing homes, and assisted-living facilities.

- The types of outpatient care facilities found in communities are healthcare practitioners' offices, clinics, primary care centers, retail clinics, urgent/emergent care centers, ambulatory surgery centers, and freestanding service facilities.

- Long-term care options include traditional institutional residential care as well as special units within these residential facilities, halfway houses, group homes, assisted-living facilities, transitional (step-down) care in a hospital, daycare facilities for patients, and personal home health care.

- The predominant organization responsible for accrediting healthcare facilities is The Joint Commission.

- The major issues of concern with the healthcare system in the United States can be summed up by the cost containment, access, and quality triangle.

- Some of the barriers to access to health care in the United States have been the lack of health insurance, inadequate insurance, and poverty.

- There are a number of different methods by which the amount of reimbursement to healthcare providers is determined. They include fee-for-service, packaged pricing, resource-based relative value scale, prepaid health care, capitation, and prospective reimbursement.

- Most health care in the United States is paid for via third-party payment.

- Key health-insurance terms include *deductible, coinsurance, copayment, fixed indemnity, exclusion*, and *pre-existing condition*.

- The two largest government-administered health insurance programs in the United States are Medicare and Medicaid.

- The Children's Health Insurance Program (CHIP) covers many children who were previously uninsured.

- Two major supplemental insurance programs in the United States are Medigap and long-term care insurance.

- Most Americans today are covered by some form of managed care.

- The more common forms of managed care include health maintenance organizations (HMOs), preferred provider organizations (PPOs), and point-of-service (POS) options.

- The United States is the only developed country in the world without national health insurance.

- Consumer-directed health plans, including health savings accounts (HSAs), high-deductible health plans (HDHPs), health reimbursement arrangements (HRAs), and flexible spending accounts (FSAs) are becoming more popular health plan options.

- Healthcare reform in the United States has not come easily, but the Affordable Care Act has significantly increased the number of Americans who have health insurance.

- Healthcare access, costs, and quality are not as they could be in the United States; therefore, additional healthcare reform will be needed.

Scenario: Analysis and Response

1. Have you ever experienced a situation similar to the one described in the scenario? If so, briefly describe it.

2. How can this scenario be improved when considering our current United States healthcare system?

3. Please explain why or why not Mirra made the correct choice.

4. If you were Mirra, what would you have done? If your insurance paid for everything and there were no out-of-pocket costs, would it have made a difference in your choice?

5. Which of the available options to Mirra do you think are the most expensive and least expensive and why?

Review Questions

1. Why have some questioned whether the United States really has a healthcare system?

2. Describe some of the major changes that have taken place in healthcare delivery over the years.

3. What is meant by *third-party payment*?

4. Why has the cost of health care in the United States continued to grow faster than the cost of inflation?

5. What is meant by a *spectrum of health care*?

6. What are the domains of practice noted in the spectrum of health care?

7. Is there a demand for healthcare workers in the United States today? If so, why?

8. In what type of facility are most healthcare workers employed?

9. What is the difference between independent and limited (restricted) care providers?

10. What are the differences between allopathic and nonallopathic healthcare providers?

11. What is the difference between *complementary* and *alternative medicine*? Give a few examples of each.

12. What kind of education do limited (restricted) care providers have?

13. What is the difference between LPNs and RNs?

14. What are advanced practice registered nurses (APRNs)?

15. What is a physician assistant?

16. What role do public health professionals play in healthcare delivery?

17. What are the advantages of outpatient care facilities?

18. What is meant by a long-term care facility? Give two examples.

19. Why has the number of home healthcare agencies increased in recent years?

20. What is The Joint Commission? What does it do?

21. What are three major problems facing the healthcare system in the United States?

22. How is the quality of healthcare services measured?

23. Explain how each of the following types of reimbursement works: fee-for-service, packaged pricing, resource-based relative value scale, prepaid health care, capitation, and prospective reimbursement.

24. On what basic concept is insurance based?

25. Explain the following insurance policy provisions: (a) a $500 deductible, (b) 20/80 coinsurance, (c) a $4,500 fixed indemnity for a basic surgical procedure, (d) an exclusion of the pre-existing condition of lung cancer, and (e) a $10 copayment.

26. What is the difference between Medicare and Medicaid?

27. What is covered in each of the four parts of Medicare—Parts A, B, C, and D?

28. What relationship does Medigap insurance have to Medicare?

29. What is the Children's Health Insurance Program?

30. Briefly explain the differences among health maintenance organizations (HMOs), preferred provider organizations (PPOs), and a point-of-service (POS) option.

31. What are the advantages and disadvantages of managed care?

32. What is meant by the term *consumer-directed health plans*? Give some examples.

33. What is the major result of the Affordable Care Act passed in 2010?

34. Summarize the four cases about the Affordable Care Act that have been heard by the U.S. Supreme Court.

Activities

1. Using Table 13.2, identify two different healthcare facilities in your community for each of the levels of care. Briefly describe each facility and determine whether each one is private, public, or voluntary.

2. Make an appointment to interview three healthcare workers in your community who have different types of jobs. Ask them what they like and dislike about their work, what kind of education they needed, whether they are happy with their work, and whether they would recommend that others seek this line of work. Summarize your findings in a written paper.

3. Get online and look at a copy of a local newspaper (the Sunday edition is best) and look through the classified section for healthcare worker jobs. In a one-page paper, briefly describe what you have found and summarize the status of healthcare position openings in your community.

4. Create a list of all of the healthcare providers from whom your family has sought help in the past five years. Group the individuals into the six provider groups outlined in the chapter. When appropriate, identify the providers' specialties and whether they were allopathic, osteopathic, or nonallopathic providers.

5. Make an appointment to interview an administrator in the local (city or county) health department. In the interview, find out what kind of people, by profession, work in the department. Also find out what type(s) of healthcare services and clinics are offered by the department. Summarize your findings in a two-page paper.

6. Obtain a copy of the student health insurance policy available at your school. After reading the policy, summarize in writing what you have read. In your summary, indicate what type of reimbursement system is used to pay providers, list specifics about the premium costs, deductible, coinsurance, copayment, fixed indemnity, and any exclusions.

7. Visit the Healthcare.gov website and find the answers to the following: (a) When is the open enrollment period each year? (b) Who can enroll for health insurance outside of the open enrollment period during the special enrollment period? (c) What is meant by minimum essential coverage? (d) What are the special arrangements for people under the age of 30 years? and (e) What does the ACA say about same-sex spouses?

References

1. Shi, L., & Singh, D. A. (2017). *Essentials of the U.S. health care system* (4th ed.). Jones & Bartlett Learning.

2. Wilensky, S. E., & Teitelbaum, J. B. (2017). *2016 annual health reform update*. Jones & Bartlett Learning.

3. Institute of Medicine (IOM). (2003). *The future of the public's health in the 21st century*. National Academies Press.

4. Rothstein, W. G. (1972). *American physicians in the nineteenth century: From sect to science*. Johns Hopkins University Press.

5. Kongstvedt, P. R. (2007). Essentials of managed health care (5th ed.). Jones and Bartlett Publishers.

6. Sultz, H. A., & Young, K. M. (2014). *Health care USA: Understanding its organization and delivery* (8th ed.). Jones & Bartlett Learning.

7. Cambridge Research Institute. (1976). *Trends affecting the U.S. health care system* (DHEW pub. no. HRA 75-14503). U.S. Government Printing Office.

8. U.S. Department of Health, Education, and Welfare, Health Resources Administration (1974, September). *Fact sheet: The Hill-Burton program*. U.S. Government Printing Office.

9. Lokkeberg, A. R. (1988). The health care system. In E. T. Anderson & J. M. McFarlane (Eds.), *Community as client: Application of the nursing process* (pp. 3–14). Lippincott.

10. O'Connor, J. (1974). Comprehensive health planning: Dreams and realities. *Milbank Memorial Fund Quarterly, Health and Society, 52*, 391–413.

11. Koff, S. Z. (1987). *Health systems agencies: A comprehensive examination of planning and process*. Human Services Press.

12. Stockman, D. A. (1981). Premises for a medical marketplace: A neoconservative's vision of how to transform the health system. *Health Affairs, 1*(1), 5–18.

13. Wessel, D. (2006, September 7). In health care, consumer theory falls flat. *Wall Street Journal*, A2.

14. Shi, L., & Singh, D. A. (2015). *Delivering health care in America: A systems approach* (6th ed.). Jones & Bartlett Learning.

15. Zatkin, S. (1997). A health plan's view of government regulation. *Health Affairs, 16*(6), 33–35.

16. Institute of Medicine. (2001). *Crossing the quality chasm: A new health system for the 21st century*. National Academies Press.

17. World Health Organization. (2000). *World Health Organization assesses the world's health systems*. Available at http://www.who.int/whr/2000/media_centre/press_release/en/

18. Steinhauer, J. (2016, January 6). House votes to send bill to repeal health law to Obama's desk. *The New York Times*. Available at http://www.nytimes.com/2016/01/07/us/politics/house-votes-to-send-bill-to-repeal-health-law-to-obamas-desk.html

19. Centers for Disease Control and Prevention. (2016). *Hospice care*. Available at https://www.cdc.gov/nchs/fastats/hospice-care.htm

20. Centers for Medicare and Medicaid Services. (2020). *Home health compare datasets*. Available at https://data.medicare.gov/data/home-health-compare

21. Bernstein, A. B., Hing, E., Moss, A. J., Allen, K. F., Siller, A. B., & Tiggle, R. B. (2004). *Health care in America: Trends in utilization*. National Center for Health Statistics.

22. U.S. Department of Labor, Bureau of Labor Statistics. (2023 September 4). *Employment projections—2022–2023* [News release]. Available at http://www.bls.gov/news.release/pdf/ecopro.pdf

23. U.S. Department of Labor, Bureau of Labor Statistics. (2014, Spring). Health care: Millions of jobs now and in the future. *Occupational Outlook Quarterly*. Available at http://www.bls.gov/careeroutlook/2014/spring/art03.pdf

24. American Association of Colleges of Osteopathic Medicine. (2016). *A brief history of osteopathic medicine*. Available at http://www.aacom.org/become-a-doctor/about-om/history

25. National Center for Health Statistics. (2018). *Health, United States, 2017: With special feature on mortality*. NCHS.

26. American Osteopathic Association. (2016). *OMP report: Strength in primary care*. Available at https://www.osteopathic.org/inside-aoa/about/aoa-annual-statistics/Pages/strength-in-primary-care.aspx

27. American Association of Colleges of Osteopathic Medicine. (2016). *What is osteopathic medicine?* Available at https://www.aacom.org/become-a-doctor/about-osteopathic-medicine

28. Association of American Medical Colleges. (2014). *2014 physician specialty data book*. Available at https://www.aamc.org/data-reports/report/us-physician-workforce-data-dashboard

29. U.S. Department of Labor, Bureau of Labor Statistics. (2023). *Chiropractors*. Available at http://www.bls.gov/ooh/healthcare/chiropractors.htm

30. National Institutes of Health, National Center for Complementary and Alternative Medicine. (2018). *Complementary, alternative, or integrative health: What's in a name?* Available at https://www.nccih.nih.gov/health/complementary-alternative-or-integrative-health-whats-in-a-name

31. National Institutes of Health, National Center for Complementary and Alternative Medicine. (2018). *What is complementary, alternative, or integrative health?* Available at https://www.nccih.nih.gov/

32. Falci, L., Shi, Z., & Greenlee, H. (2016). Multiple chronic conditions and use of complementary and alternative medicine among US adults: Results from the 2012 National Health Interview Survey. *Preventing Chronic Disease, 13*, 150501.

33. Nahin, R. L., Barnes, P. M., Stussman, B. J., & Bloom, B. (2009). Costs of complementary and alternative medicine (CAM) and frequency of visits to CAM practitioners: United States, 2007.

National Health Statistics Reports, 18. Available at https://www.cdc.gov/nchs/data/nhsr/nhsr018.pdf

34. National Institutes of Health, National Center for Complementary and Alternative Medicine. (2016). *Paying for complementary health approaches*. Available at https://nccih.nih.gov/health/financial

35. U.S. Department of Labor, Bureau of Labor Statistics. (2019). *Occupational outlook handbook: Licensed practical and licensed vocational nurses*. Available at http://www.bls.gov/ooh/healthcare/licensed-practical-and-licensed-vocational-nurses.htm

36. U.S. Department of Labor, Bureau of Labor Statistics. (2023). *Occupational outlook handbook: Registered nurses*. Available at http://www.bls.gov /ooh/healthcare/registered-nurses.htm

37. U.S. Department of Labor, Bureau of Labor Statistics. (2020). *Occupational outlook handbook: Nursing assistants and orderlies*. Available at http://www.bls.gov/ooh/healthcare/nursing-assistants.htm

38. Stanfield, P. S., Cross, N., & Hui, Y. H. (2012). *Introduction to the health professions* (6th ed.). Jones & Bartlett Learning.

39. American Association of Nurse Practitioners. (2023). *NP fact sheet*. Available at https://www.aanp.org/all-about-nps/np-fact-sheet

40. California Health Foundation. (2019). *Expanding the role of nurse practitioners in California: Physician oversight in other states*. Available at https://www.chcf.org/wp-content/uploads/2019/05/ExpandingNP OversightStates.pdf

41. American Academy of Physician Assistants. (n.d.). *What is a PA?* Available at https://www.aapa.org/what-is-a-pa/

42. American Academy of Physician Assistants. (2020). *What is a PA?* [Infographic]. Available at https://www.aapa.org/wp-content/uploads/2020/07/WhatIsAPA-Infographic-MAY2020.pdf

43. U.S. Department of Labor, Bureau of Labor Statistics. (2022). *Occupational outlook handbook: Physician assistants*. Available at http://www.bls.gov/ooh/healthcare/physician-assistants.htm

44. American Academy of Orthopedic Surgeons. (2016). *Specialty hospitals*. Available at https://www.aaos.org/search/?q=Specialty+hospitals

45. Blumenthal, D. M., Orav, E. J., Jena, A. B., Dudzinski, D. M., Le, S. T., & Jha, A. K. (2015). Access, quality, and costs of care at physician owned hospitals in the United States: Observational study. *BMJ, 2*(351), h4466.

46. Turner, G.-M. (2015, November 6). Lift the ban on physician-owned hospitals. *Forbes*. Available at http://www.forbes.com/sites/grace marieturner/2015/11/06/lift-the-ban-on-physician-owned-hospitals/#23f664044b00

47. Griffin, D. J. (2012). *Hospitals: What they are and how they work* (4th ed.). Jones & Bartlett Learning.

48. Centers for Disease Control and Prevention. (2016). *Ambulatory care use and physician office visits*. Available at https://www.cdc.gov/nchs/data/nhsr/nhsr184.pdf

49. National Association of Community Health Centers. (2018). *Community health center chart book*. Available at http://www.nachc.org/wp-content/uploads/2018/06/Chartbook_FINAL_6.20.18.pdf

50. The Henry J. Kaiser Family Foundation. (2013). *Summary of the Affordable Care Act (#8061-02)*. Available at http://kff.org/health-reform/fact-sheet/summary-of-the-affordable-care-act/

51. Robert Wood Johnson Foundation. (2015). *Growing retail clinic industry employs, empowers nurse practitioners*. Available at https://www.rwjf.org/en/library/articles-and-news/2015/02/growing-retail-clinic-industry-employs-empowers-nurse-practitio.html

52. About Convenient Care Association. (2019). *Convenient care association*. Available at https://www.ccaclinics.org/about-us/about-cca

53. Centers for Medicare and Medicaid Services. (2021). *Home health compare datasets*. Available at https://data.medicare.gov/data/home-health-compare

54. The Joint Commission. (2023). *Joint Commission FAQ page*. Available at https://www.jointcommission.org/who-we-are/facts-about-the-joint-commission/joint-commission-faqs/

55. U.S. Department of Health and Human Services. (2020). *Affordable Care Act*. Available at https://www.hhs.gov/answers/health-insurance-reform/what-is-the-affordable-care-act/index.html

56. Turner, G.-M. (2016, January 28). *70 Changes to ObamaCare ... so far*. Galen Institute. Available at https://galen.org/2016/changes-to-obamacare-so-far-3/

57. Kissick, W. L. (1994). *Medicine's dilemmas: Infinite needs versus finite resources*. Yale University Press.

58. Obama, B. (2016). United States Health Care Reform progress to date and next steps. *Journal of American Medical Association, 316*(5), 525–532. Available at https://pubmed.ncbi.nlm.nih.gov/27400401/

59. The Henry J. Kaiser Family Foundation. (2015). *Key facts about the uninsured population*. Available at http://kff.org/uninsured/fact-sheet/key-facts-about-the-uninsured-population/

60. Martinez, M. E., Cohen, R. A., & Zammitti, E. P. (2016). *Health insurance coverage: Early release of estimates from the National Health Interview Survey, January–September 2015*. Centers for Disease Control and Prevention, National Center for Health Statistics. Available at http://www.cdc.gov/nchs/data/nhis/earlyrelease/insur201602.pdf

61. U.S. Census Bureau. (2023). *Income, poverty, and health insurance: 2023*. Available at https://www.census.gov/content/dam/Census/newsroom/press-kits/2023/iphi/presentation-iphi-overview.pdf

62. Keisler-Starkey, K., Bunch, L. N., & Lindstrom, R. A. (2023). *Health insurance coverage in the United States: 2022* (Current Population Reports). U.S. Census Bureau. https://www.census.gov/library/publications/2023/demo/p60-274.html

63. The Henry J. Kaiser Family Foundation. (2016). *Health reform FAQs*. Available at www.kff.org/medicare/issue-brief/turning-medicare-into-a-premium-support-system-frequently-asked-questions/

64. Centers for Medicare and Medicaid Services. (2016). *Overview of the SHOP marketplace*. Available at https://www.healthcare.gov/small-businesses/choose-and-enroll/shop-marketplace-overview/

65. Schneider, E., Sarnak, D., Squires, D., Shah, A., & Doty, M. (2017). *Mirror, mirror 2017 international comparison reflects flaws and opportunities for better U.S. health care*. Commonwealth Fund; 7. Available at https://www.commonwealthfund.org/publications/fund-reports/2017/jul/mirror-mirror-2017-international-comparison-reflects-flaws-and

66. Institute of Medicine. (2001). *Crossing the quality chasm: A new health care system for the 21st century*. Available at https://www.ncbi.nlm.nih.gov/pubmed/25057539

67. Institute of Medicine (US). *Committee on Quality of Health Care in America. To err is human: Building a safer health system*. Kohn LT, Corrigan JM, Donaldson MS, editors. Washington (DC): National Academies Press (US); 2000. https://pubmed.ncbi.nlm.nih.gov/25077248/

68. U.S. Department of Health and Human Services, Agency for Healthcare Research and Quality. (2015). *2014 National Healthcare quality and disparities report* (AHRQ pub. no. 15-0007). Available at https://psnet.ahrq.gov/issue/err-human-building-safer-health-system?_gl=1*1k5jbmd*_ga*MTE3MTU3ODI1MC4xNzA2NzMzNTA2*_ga_45NDTD15CJ*MTcwOTE0NTE3NC4xLjAuMTcwOTE0NTE3NC42MC4wLjA

69. National Committee for Quality Assurance. (2020). *About NCQA*. Available at http://www.ncqa.org/AboutNCQA.aspx

70. National Committee for Quality Assurance. (2020). *HEDIS® and Quality Compass®*. Available at https://www.ncqa.org/hedis/reports-and-research/

71. U.S. Department of Health and Human Services, Agency for Health care Research and Quality. (2017). *About the national quality strategy (NQS).* Available at http://www.ahrq.gov/workingforquality /about.htm

72. U.S. Department of Health and Human Services, Agency for Healthcare Research and Quality. (2015). *The national quality strategy (NQS).* Available at http://www.ahrq.gov/workingforquality /index.html

73. U.S. Department of Health and Human Services, Agency for Health care Research and Quality. (2015). *2015 annual progress report to congress: National strategy for quality improvement in health care.* Available at http://www.ahrq.gov/workingforquality/reports /annual-reports/nqs2015annlrpt.htm

74. Centers for Medicare and Medicaid Services. (2020). *Accountable care organizations (ACO).* Available at https://www.cms.gov /Medicare/Medicare-Fee-for-Service-Payment/ACO/index.html? redirect=/ACO/

75. Tu, T., Muhlestein, D., Kocot, S. L., & White, R. (2015). *The impact of accountable care: Origins and future of accountable care organizations.* Brookings Institute. Available at https://www.brookings .edu/wp-content/uploads/2016/06/Impact-of-Accountable-Care Origins-052015.pdf

76. The Henry J. Kaiser Family Foundation. (2016). *Accountable care organizations: A new paradigm for health care delivery?* Available at http://kff.org/health-costs/event/accountable-care -organizations-a-new-paradigm-for/

77. American College of Physicians. (2016). *What is the patient-centered medical home?* Available at https://www.acponline.org/running _practice/delivery_and_payment_models/pcmh/understanding /what.htm

78. Agency for Healthcare Research and Quality. (n.d.). *Defining the PCMH.* Available at https://www.pcmh.ahrq.gov/page/defining -pcmh

79. Patient-Centered Primary Care Collaborative. (2016). *About us.* Available at https://www.pcpcc.org/about

80. Centers for Medicare and Medicaid Services. (2023). *National health expenditure data.* Available at https://www.cms.gov/Research -Statistics-Data-and-Systems/Statistics-Trends-and-Reports /NationalHealth ExpendData/index.html

81. Brill, S. (2014, March 4). *Bitter pill. Time,* 16–55. Available at https:// www.ncpssm.org/entitledtoknow/bitter-pill-a-time-magazine -article-every-senior-in-medicare-should-read/

82. Centers for Medicare and Medicaid Services. (2019). *Medicare provider utilization and payment data.* Available at https:// www.cms.gov/research-statistics-data-and-systems/statistics -trends-and-reports/medicare-provider-charge-data/

83. Farell, D., Jensen, E., Kocher, B., Lovegrove, N., Melhem, F., Mendonca, L., & Parish, B. (2008, December). Accounting for the cost of US health care: A new look at why Americans spend more. *McKinsey Global Institute Report.* Available at http://www .mckinsey.com/insights/health_systems_and_services /accounting_for_the_cost_of_us_health_care

84. Bipartisan Policy Center. (2012). *What is driving U.S. health care spending: America's unsustainable health care cost growth.* Available at https://bipartisanpolicy.org/report/what-driving-us -health-care-spending-americas-unsustainable-health-care-cost -growth/

85. Martin, A. B., Hartman, M., Benson, J., Catlin, A., & The National Health Expenditure Accounts Team. (2016). National health spending in 2014: Faster growth driven by coverage expansion and prescription drug spending. *Health Affairs (Millwood), 35*(1), 150–160. doi: 10.1377/hlthaff.2015.1194

86. Congressional Budget Office. (2014). *The Budget and Economic Outlook: 2014 to 2024.* Available at https://www.cbo.gov/publication /45010

87. Centers for Medicare and Medicaid Services. (2018). *The nation's health dollar ($3.6 trillion), calendar year 2018: Where it came from.* Available at https://www.cms.gov/files/document/nations-health -dollar-where-it-came-where-it-went.pdf

88. Congressional Budget Office. (2017). *Repealing the individual health insurance mandate: An updated estimate.* Available at https://www .cbo.gov/publication/53300

89. Harrington, M. K. (2016). *Health care finance and the mechanics of insurance and reimbursement.* Jones & Bartlett Learning.

90. James, J. (2012, October 11). Health policy brief: Pay-for-performance. *Health Affairs.* Available at http://www.healthaffairs.org/health policybriefs/brief.php?brief_id=78

91. New England Journal of Medicine Catalyst. (2018). *What is pay for performance in healthcare?* Available at https://catalyst.nejm.org /doi/full/10.1056/CAT.18.0245

92. U.S. Department of Health and Human Services. (2014). *Pre-existing conditions.* Available at http://www.hhs.gov/healthcare/about-the -law/pre-existing-conditions/index.html

93. The Commonwealth Fund. (2012). *Slower growth in health insurance premiums is found—but the mystery is why.* Available at https:// www.commonwealthfund.org/publications/newsletter-article /slower-growth-health-insurance-premiums-found-mystery-why

94. Zane Benefits. (2016). *Do the majority of Americans still get health insurance through work?* Available at http://www.zanebenefits .com/blog/do-the-majority-of-americans-still-get-health-insurance -through-work

95. Kaiser Family Foundation. (2019). *The uninsured and the ACA: A primer.* [Supplemental tables]. Available at https://www.kff.org /uninsured/report/the-uninsured-and-the-aca-a-primer-key-facts -about-health-insurance-and-the-uninsured-amidst-changes-to -the-affordable-care-act/. [See Table 1: 267.5 million nonelderly people, 57.1% of whom are covered by employer-sponsored insurance.]

96. The Henry J. Kaiser Family Foundation. (2023). *Employer health benefits survey.* Available at https://www.kff.org/report-section /ehbs-2023-section-1-cost-of-health-insurance/

97. Jennings, P. (2005, December 15). Peter Jennings reporting: Breakdown—America's health insurance crisis. As cited in J. P. Rooney & D. Perrin. (2008). *America's health care crisis solved.* John Wiley & Sons.

98. The Henry J. Kaiser Family Foundation. (2016). *Health insurance premiums marketplace calculator.* Available at http://kff.org /interactive/subsidy-calculator/#state=pa&zip=17022&locale= Lancaster&income-type=dollars&income=50%2C000&employer -coverage=0&people=2&alternate-plan-family=individual &adult-count =2&adults[0][age]=36&adults[0][tobacco]=0&adults[1] [age]=38&adults[1][tobacco]=0&child-count=0&child-tobacco=0

99. Cigna. (2013, September 23). *Informed on reform.* Available at http://www.cigna.com/assets/docs/about-cigna/Webinar%20PPTs /Cigna _IoR_Sept-Web-Mtg-FAQs_10-01-13.pdf

100. U.S. Congress. (2010, March 23). *The Patient Protection and Affordable Care Act* (Public Law Numbers 111-148 and 111-152, Consolidated Print). Available at http://www.gpo.gov/fdsys/pkg /PLAW-111publ148/pdf/PLAW-111publ148.pdf

101. U.S. Department of Health and Human Services, Centers for Medicare and Medicaid Services. (2024). *Medicare costs at a glance.* Available at https://www.medicare.gov/your-medicare-costs /costs-at-a-glance/costs-at-glance.html

102. U.S. Department of Health and Human Services, Centers for Medicare and Medicaid Services. (2023). *Medicare and you 2023.* Available at https://www.medicare.gov/Pubs/pdf/10050.pdf

103. U.S. Department of Health and Human Services, Centers for Medicare and Medicaid Services. (2023). *CMS fast facts.* Available at https://www.cms.gov/fastfacts/

104. U.S. Department of Health and Human Services. (1989). *Your hospital stay under Medicare's prospective payment system* (DHHS pub. no. HCFA 02163). U.S. Government Printing Office.

105. AARP. (2014). *Is your Medicare safe?* Available at http://www.aarp.org/health/medicare-insurance/info-12-2013/medicare-and-affordable-care-act.html

106. Internal Revenue Service. (2020, February 11). *Questions and answers for the additional Medicare tax.* Available at https://www.irs.gov/businesses/small-businesses-self-employed/questions-and-answers-for-the-additional-medicare-tax

107. The Henry J. Kaiser Family Foundation. (2). *What to Know about Medicare Spending and Financing* Available at https://www.kff.org/medicare/issue-brief/what-to-know-about-medicare-spending-and-financing/

108. U.S. Department of Health and Human Services, Centers for Medicare and Medicaid Services. (2019). *Medicare trustees report shows hospital insurance trust fund will deplete in 7 years.* Available at https://www.cms.gov/newsroom/press-releases/medicare-trustees-report-shows-hospital-insurance-trust-fund-will-deplete-7-years

109. Rudowitz, R. (2013). *Financing Medicaid coverage under health reform: What is the law and the new FMAP rules.* Kaiser Commission on Medicaid and the Uninsured. Available at http://kff.org/health-reform/issue-brief/financing-medicaid-coverage-under-health-reform-the-role-of-the-federal-government-and-states/

110. Dorn, S., Teitelbaum, M., & Cortez, C. (1998). *An advocate's tool kit for the state Children's Health Insurance Program.* Children's Defense Fund.

111. U.S. Department of Health and Human Services, Centers for Medicare and Medicaid Services. (2023). *Children's Health Insurance Program (CHIP).* Available at https://www.medicaid.gov/chip/chip-program-information.html

112. National Conference of State Legislatures. (2015). *Children's Health Insurance Program overview.* Available at http://www.ncsl.org/research/health/childrens-health-insurance-program-overview.aspx

113. U.S. Department of Health and Human Services. (2023). *Biden-Harris Administration Releases New Medicaid and CHIP Renewal Data Showing the Role State Policy Choices Play in Keeping Kids Covered.* Available at https://www.hhs.gov/about/news/2023/12/18/biden-harris-administration-releases-new-medicaid-chip-renewal-data-showing-role-statepolicychoices-play-keeping-kids-covered

114. Centers for Medicare and Medicaid Services. (2020). *Choosing a Medigap policy: A guide to health insurance for people with Medicare.* Available at https://www.medicare.gov/Pubs/pdf/02110-medicare-medigap-guide.pdf

115. U.S. Department of Health and Human Services, Administration on Aging. (n.d.). *Find your path forward.* Available at https://longtermcare.acl.gov

116. Genworth Life Insurance Company. (2021). *Cost of care survey 2021: National data.* Available at https://pro.genworth.com/riiproweb/productinfo/pdf/282102.pdf

117. MCOL. (2022). *Managed care fact sheets.* Available at http://www.mcol.com/factsheetindex

118. Institute of Medicine. (1997). *Managing managed care: Quality improvement in behavioral health.* National Academies Press.

119. Kongstvedt, P. R. (2013). *Essentials of managed health care* (6th ed.). Jones & Bartlett Learning.

120. The Henry J. Kaiser Family Foundation. (2023). *Medicare advantage.* Available at https://www.kff.org/medicare/fact-sheet/medicare-advantage/

121. The Henry J. Kaiser Family Foundation. (2017). *Medicaid managed care market tracker.* Available at http://kff.org/data-collection/medicaid-managed-care-market-tracker/

122. Slee, D. A., Slee, V. N., & Schmidt, H. J. (2008). *Slee's health care terms* (5th ed.). Jones & Bartlett Learning.

123. Alliance for Health Reform. (2006, November). *HSAs and high deductible health plans: A primer.* Alliance for Health Reform.

124. IRS 26 CFR 601.602: Tax forms and instructions. (Also Part I, §§ 1, 223; Part III § 54.9831-1) Rev. Proc. (2022-2024). Available at https://www.irs.gov

125. U.S. Department of the Treasury, Internal Revenue Service. (2019). *Publication 502: medical and dental expenses (including the health coverage tax credit* (Cat. No. 15002Q). Available at https://www.irs.gov/pub/irs-pdf/p502.pdf

126. Altman, D. (2015, March 11). Health-care deductibles climbing out of reach. *The Wall Street Journal.* Available at http://blogs.wsj.com/washwire/2015/03/11/health-care-deductibles-climbing-out-of-reach/

127. The White House, United States Government. (2019). *President Trump expands access to preventive care.* Available at https://www.whitehouse.gov/articles/president-donald-j-trump-expands-access-preventive-care

128. LeTourneau, J. (2013, December). ACA changes for health reimbursement arrangements. *Broker World Magazine.* Available at https://www.wageworks.com/media/184548/WW-BW-ACA-CHANGES-FOR-HRAs.pdf

129. The White House, United States Government. (2019). *President Donald J. Trump is working to improve health insurance coverage for American workers and help small businesses.* Available at https://www.whitehouse.gov/briefings-statements/president-donald-j-trump-working-improve-health-insurance-coverage-american-workers-help-small-businesses/

130. Zane Benefits. (2016). *Flexible spending accounts (FSAs)—New 'use it or lose it' rules.* Available at http://www.zanebenefits.com/blog/bid/323382/Flexible-Spending-Accounts-FSAs-New-Use-It-Or-Lose-It-Rules

131. LeTourneau, J. (2013, November). ACA changes for flexible spending accounts. *Broker World Magazine.* https://www.wageworks.com/media/184521/ACA-Changes-LeTourneau_1113.pdf

132. Cohen, R. A., & Martinez, M. E. (2009). *Consumer-directed health care for persons under 65 years of age with private health insurance: United States, 2007* (NCHS Data Brief, No. 15). National Center for Health Statistics.

133. Cohen, R. A., & Martinez, M. E. (2018). *Health insurance coverage: Early release of estimates from the National Health Interview Survey, 2018.* Available at https://www.cdc.gov/nchs/data/nhis/earlyrelease/insur201905.pdf

134. Shaffer, E. R. (2013). The Affordable Care Act: The value of systemic disruption. *American Journal of Public Health, 103*(6), 969–972.

135. U.S. Supreme Court of the United States. (2012). *National Federation of Independent Businesses et al. versus Sebelius, Secretary of Health and Human Services, et al.* Available at http://www.supremecourt.gov/opinions/11pdf/11-393c3a2.pdf

136. U.S. Supreme Court of the United States. (2013). *Burwell, Secretary of Health and Human Services, et al. versus Hobby Lobby Stores, Inc. et al.* Available at http://www.supremecourt.gov/opinions/13pdf/13-354 _olp1.pdf

137. U.S. Department of Health and Human Services. (2016). *Birth control benefits.* Available at https://www.healthcare.gov/coverage/birth-control-benefits/

138. Liptak, A. (2014, June 30). Supreme Court rejects contraceptives mandate for some corporations. *The New York Times.* Available at http://www.nytimes.com/2014/07/01/us/hobby-lobby-case-supreme-court-contraception.html

139. Supreme Court of the United States. (2014). *King et al. versus Burwell, Secretary of Health and Human Services, et al.* Available at http://www.supremecourt.gov/opinions/14pdf/14-114_qol1.pdf

140. de Vogue, A. (2016, March 23). Supreme court hears challenge to Obamacare contraceptive mandate. *CNN Politics*. Available at http://www.cnn.com/2016/03/23/politics/supreme-court-obama care-contraceptive-mandate/

141. Rosenthal, P. (2015, October 28). Obama ACA side effects include mergers like Walgreens, Boots, Rite Aid. *Chicago Tribune*. Available at http://www.chicagotribune.com/business/ct-rosenthal-walgreens -rite-aid-1029-biz-20151028-column.html

142. Benet, L. (2014, May 21). *ACA side effects: 5 ways it may impact commercial liability insurance*. Gen Re. Available at http://www .genre.com/knowledge/blog/aca-side-effects-5-ways-it-may-impact -commercial-liability-insurance.html

143. McDonough, J., & Fletcher, M. (2015, September 18). What would Republicans do instead of the Affordable Care Act? *Health Affairs Blog*. Available at http://healthaffairs.org/blog/2015/09/18 /what-would-republicans-do-instead-of-the-affordable-care-act/

144. The White House, Office of the Press Secretary. (2009, September 9). *Excerpts of the President's address to a joint session of Congress tonight* [Press release]. Available at https://obamawhitehouse .archives.gov/the-press-office/excerpts-presidents-address -a-joint-session-congress-tonight

Environmental Health and Safety

CHAPTER 14

Community and Public Health and the Environment

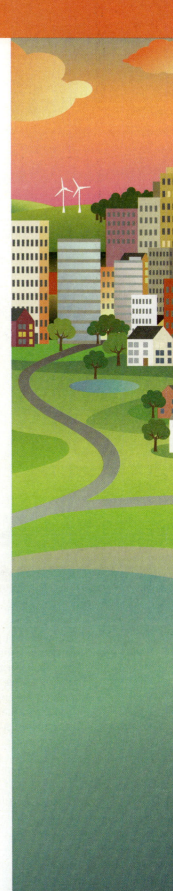

Chapter Outline

Chapter Objectives

After studying this chapter, you will be able to:

1. List the sources and types of air pollutants, including the criteria pollutants, and explain the difference between primary and secondary pollutants.

2. Describe the role of the Environmental Protection Agency in protecting the environment.

3. Outline the provisions of the Clean Air Act, and explain the purposes of the National Ambient Air Quality Standards and the Air Quality Index.

4. Recall the major types of indoor air pollutants, including radon, and describe ways to reduce exposure to them.

5. Explain the difference between point source and nonpoint source pollution.

6. Discuss the various types of pollutants that threaten the safety of our

Chapter Objectives   (continued)

drinking water and give examples of each type.

7. Define what is meant by the term *waterborne disease outbreak* and list some of the causative agents.

8. Illustrate the measures communities take to ensure the quality of drinking water and the measures communities take to manage wastewater.

9. Explain the purposes of the Clean Water Act and Safe Drinking Water Act.

10. Define the term *foodborne disease outbreak*, name some of the agents that cause these outbreaks, and describe some of the practices that increase the risk of a foodborne disease outbreak.

11. Name some of the agencies that help protect the safety of our food, and describe how they accomplish this task.

12. Define pest, pesticides, target organism, and nontarget organism. Explain some of the safety and health concerns with pesticide use.

13. Describe the composition of our municipal solid waste (MSW) and

outline acceptable MSW management strategies.

14. Define hazardous waste and give some examples.

15. Explain the purposes of the Resource Conservation and Recovery Act and the Comprehensive Environmental Response, Compensation, and Liability Act.

16. Discuss the health hazards associated with exposure to lead in our environment.

17. Define the terms *vector* and *vectorborne disease* and explain why these are community concerns.

18. Define ionizing radiation and describe the health hazards associated with it.

19. List examples of natural hazards and complex disasters and the ways they can affect the health of a community.

20. Interpret the relationships among population growth, the environment, and human health.

21. Explain the roles of the Federal Emergency Management Agency and the community partners in preparing for and providing assistance to people and communities after a disaster.

Scenario

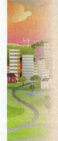

Juan and Maria had been trying to have a baby for 2 years. Their first child, Elaina, conceived before they moved to their current home and born without a problem, is now 4 and a half years old. Yesterday, Maria experienced her third miscarriage in the past 14 months. Before they moved into their current home, approximately 3 years ago, Juan and Maria had taken a sample of the well water and had it tested. At that time, the water was determined to be safe to drink.

Six months after that, however, a large-scale, rural hog farm had been built less than a half a mile away and began operations shortly afterward. At first, the smell was not noticeable, but now the stench from the huge waste lagoon is evident on most days. State inspectors had made several visits to the operation in the past year. Juan wondered whether the water in their well was still safe to drink. He decided to have their well water tested again.

Introduction

Our health is affected by the quality of our environment, including the air we breathe, the water we drink, the food we eat, and the communities in which we live. The activities of our growing population and our demand for ever-increasing amounts of energy endanger the quality of our air, the purity of our water, the safety of our food, and the health of our planet. Having recognized the implications of environmental degradation on our health and the health of our communities, we have enacted regulatory measures to address some of the most egregious environmental assaults and accept our responsibility for the stewardship of our planet.

Environmental health is the study and management of environmental conditions that affect our health and well-being. **Environmental hazards** are those factors or conditions in the environment that increase the risk of human injury, disease, or death. The aim of this chapter is to examine common environmental hazards and describe community efforts to protect our health. We begin with a discussion of environmental concerns surrounding our air, water, and food resources. Then, we discuss how communities manage solid and hazardous waste. We conclude with a discussion of natural, human-made, and environmental hazards.

The Air We Breathe

Nothing has been more important to the development of life on Earth than the composition of the air we breathe. Yet many of our everyday activities alter the quality of this essential environmental component. By polluting the air, we endanger our health and risk leaving a deteriorating environment to future generations. In some cases, we further endanger our health with unhealthy indoor air.

Outdoor Air Pollution

Air pollution is the contamination of the air by substances—gases, liquids, or solids—in amounts great enough to harm humans, the environment, or alter the climate. These contaminants or pollutants originate from natural or human sources. Natural sources include dust storms, forest fires, and volcanic eruptions. Human sources can be divided into mobile sources, such as motor vehicles, and stationary sources, such as power plants and factories.

In the United States, major sources are (1) transportation, including privately owned motor vehicles; (2) electric power plants fueled by oil and coal; and (3) industry, primarily mills and refineries. In addition to these major sources, there are many smaller sources, such as wood- and coal-burning stoves, fireplaces, dry-cleaning facilities, and waste incinerators.

Pollutants are generally divided further into primary and secondary pollutants. **Criteria or primary pollutants** include those emanating directly from the sources listed previously. They include carbon monoxide, ozone, sulfur dioxide, nitrogen dioxide, lead, and suspended particulates.[1] **Secondary pollutants** are formed when pollutants react with one another or with other atmospheric components to form new harmful chemicals. Because sunlight promotes the formation of secondary pollutants, the resulting smog is referred to as **photochemical smog** (brown smog). This term is used to contrast photochemical smog with **industrial smog** (gray smog) formed primarily by sulfur dioxide and suspended particulates.

Living in communities where air pollution reaches harmful levels can result in both acute and chronic health problems. Acute effects include irritation of the eyes, nose, and throat; wheezing or shortness of breath; coughing; and respiratory illnesses.[2] In severe pollution episodes, deaths have been reported. Chronic effects include chronic bronchitis, emphysema, and increased incidence of bronchial asthma attacks. There is even evidence of increased risk of lung cancer from air pollution (see **Figure 14.1**).[3]

Ozone (O₃), perhaps, represents the single most dangerous air pollutant. Breathing ozone can result in a variety of health problems even at low levels, including chest pain, coughing, throat irritation, congestion, bronchitis, emphysema, asthma, and reduced lung function. Repeated exposure to ground-level ozone may permanently scar lung tissue. Even healthy people can experience breathing problems if exposed to ozone at high enough levels. In many urban and suburban areas throughout the United States, concentrations of ground-level ozone can exceed air quality standards. The Environmental Protection Agency (EPA) website includes air quality data from across the United States.[4]

One cause of excessive levels of ground-level ozone is a phenomenon referred to as a **thermal inversion**. This occurs when a layer of warm air settles

Environmental health the study and management of environmental conditions that affect the health and well-being of humans

Environmental hazards factors or conditions in the environment that increase the risk of human injury, disease, or death

Air pollution contamination of the air that interferes with the comfort, safety, and health of living organisms

Primary pollutants air pollutants emanating directly from transportation, power and industrial plants, and refineries

Secondary pollutants air pollutants formed when primary air pollutants react with sunlight and other atmospheric components to form new, harmful compounds

Photochemical smog haze or fog formed when air pollutants interact with sunlight, also known as brown smog

Industrial smog haze or fog formed primarily by sulfur dioxide and suspended particles from the burning of coal, also known as gray smog

Ozone (O₃) an inorganic molecule considered to be a pollutant in the atmosphere because it harms human tissue, but considered beneficial in the stratosphere because it screens out UV radiation

Thermal inversion a condition that occurs when warm air traps cooler air at the surface of the Earth

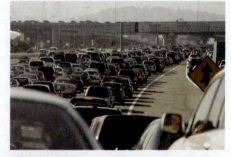

FIGURE 14.1 Air pollution from heavy traffic.

© Aaron Kohr/Shutterstock

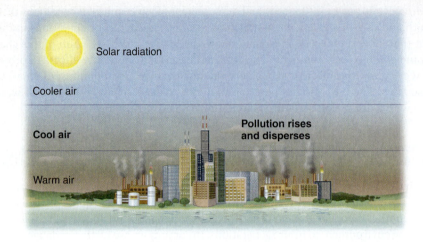

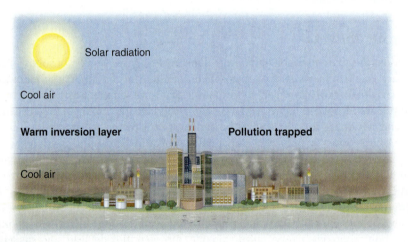

FIGURE 14.2   A thermal inversion.

Reproduced from Chiras, D.D. (2010). *Environmental Science*. 8th ed. Sudbury, MA: Jones & Bartlett Learning.

above cooler air close to the Earth's surface, preventing the cooler air from rising. The longer a thermal inversion continues, the more likely it is that pollutants, such as ozone, will reach dangerously high levels in the air we breathe (see **Figure 14.2**).[5]

Regulation of Outdoor Air Quality

Steady deterioration of air quality in the 1950s and 1960s led to the nation's first serious attempt to regulate air pollution, the **Clean Air Act (CAA)** of 1963. The CAA, which provided the federal government with the authority to address interstate air pollution problems, was amended several times prior to 1970, but much of the regulation was based on voluntary compliance.

The 1970 amendments to the CAA provided the first comprehensive approach to dealing with air pollution nationwide. Three significant components of these amendments were emission standards for automobiles, emission standards for new industries, and ambient air quality standards for urban areas.[6] The latter are known as the **National Ambient Air Quality Standards (NAAQSs)**. The 1990 amendments to the CAA set deadlines for establishing emission standards for 190 toxic chemicals that had not been previously addressed, established a tax on toxic chemical emissions, and tightened emission standards for automobiles.[7]

Clean Air Act (CAA) federal law that provides the government with authority to address interstate air pollution

National Ambient Air Quality Standards (NAAQSs) standards created by the EPA for allowable concentration levels of outdoor air pollutants

TABLE 14.1 Criteria Pollutants

Pollutants (Designation)	Form(s)	Major Sources (in order of percentage of contribution)
Carbon monoxide (CO)	Gas	Transportation, industrial processes, other solid waste, stationary fuel combustion
Lead (Pb)	Metal or aerosol	Transportation, industrial processes, stationary fuel combustion, solid waste
Nitrogen oxides (NO_2, NO)	Gas	Stationary fuel combustion, transportation, industrial processes, solid waste
Ground-level ozone (O_3)	Gas	Transportation, industrial processes, solid waste, stationary fuel combustion
Particulate matter	Solid or liquid	Industrial processes, stationary fuel combustion, transportation, solid waste
Sulfur dioxide (SO_2)	Gas	Stationary fuel combustion, industrial processes, transportation, other wastes

The U.S. **Environmental Protection Agency (EPA)** is the federal agency primarily responsible for setting, maintaining, and enforcing environmental standards. The legislation allows states to adopt and implement programs with equivalent or more stringent standards in lieu of the EPA. As such, states are empowered to regulate air quality and are authorized to levy fines against those who violate the standards. The EPA oversees these state programs or enforces standards in states where no state program exists or is inadequate.[7] The EPA sets limits on how much of a pollutant can be in the air anywhere in the United States. The air pollutants of greatest concern in the United States are called **criteria pollutants** (see **Table 14.1**). The levels of each of these six pollutants are monitored in the ambient (outdoor) air to determine if and when they exceed the NAAQSs. Between 1990 and 2022, the United States substantially reduced the ambient air concentrations of all criteria pollutants, namely, lead by 88%, particulate matter by 34%, ozone by 22%, sulfur dioxide by 90%, carbon monoxide by 81%, and nitrogen dioxide by 60%.[8] Nonetheless, in 2022, approximately 121 million people in the United States lived in counties with pollution levels above the NAAQSs.[9] This reflects a positive trend, in that 12% fewer people were living in counties exceeding the NAAQSs than in 2018.[9] This improvement is likely due to reduced travel and other economic sectors during the SARS-CoV-2 pandemic.[10] To make it easier for all of us to understand daily air quality and what it means for your health, the EPA calculates the **Air Quality Index (AQI)** for five of the criteria air pollutants. The index tells you how clean or polluted your air is and what associated health effects might be of concern for you or sensitive people in your community.

The value of the AQI on a particular day can range from 0 (good air quality) to 500 (hazardous air quality). AQI values below 100 are generally thought of as satisfactory, whereas values above 100 are considered unhealthy. Those most sensitive to air pollutants will be the first to be affected as the AQI rises above 100.[11] Weather channels and websites might use a color-coded AQI for easier understanding (see **Figure 14.3**). The AQI can be obtained for any area of the United States at http://airnow.gov.

In 2022, coal-fired power plants provided 10% of the nation's electric power.[12] Many of these plants lack essential modern pollution controls and discharge excess sulfur, mercury, and other harmful chemicals into the air and waterways. These plants are among the nation's leading sources of heat-trapping carbon dioxide (CO_2). Between 2011 and 2022, 717 coal-fired generating units were retired, leaving 510 still operational.[13,14] Replacing these units with cleaner and more efficient technology could further reduce air pollution and reduce CO_2 emissions.

Although our primary focus has been on the health benefits of air quality regulation, some mention should be made of the role of air pollution on climate change. In this regard, it should be noted that reducing the level of **greenhouse gases**, such as CO_2, chlorofluorocarbons, ozone, methane, water vapor, and nitrous oxide, will reduce heat retention in the atmosphere and slow global climate change.

Environmental Protection Agency (EPA) federal agency primarily responsible for setting, maintaining, and enforcing environmental standards or authorizing and overseeing state agencies that enforce established standards

Criteria pollutants the most pervasive air pollutants and those of greatest concern in the United States

Air Quality Index (AQI) an index that indicates the level of pollution in the air and the associated health risk

Greenhouse gases atmospheric gases, principally carbon dioxide, chlorofluorocarbons, ozone, methane, water vapor, and nitrous oxide, that are transparent to visible light but absorb infrared radiation

Air quality index levels of health concern	Numerical value	Meaning
Good (green)	0–50	Air quality is considered satisfactory, and air pollution poses little or no risk.
Moderate (yellow)	51–100	Air quality is acceptable; however, for some pollutants there may be a moderate health concern for a very small number of people who are unusually sensitive to air pollution.
Unhealthy for sensitive groups (orange)	101–150	Members of sensitive groups may experience health effects. The general public is not likely to be affected.
Unhealthy (red)	151–200	Everyone may begin to experience health effects; members of sensitive groups may experience more serious health effects.
Very unhealthy (purple)	201–300	Health alert: everyone may experience more serious health effects.
Hazardous (maroon)	>300	Health warnings of emergency conditions. The entire population is more likely to be affected.

FIGURE 14.3   Color codes for various air quality indices.

Reproduced from U.S. Environmental Protection Agency. (n.d.). *Air Quality Index (AQI) basics.* Available at https://www.airnow.gov/aqi/aqi-basics/

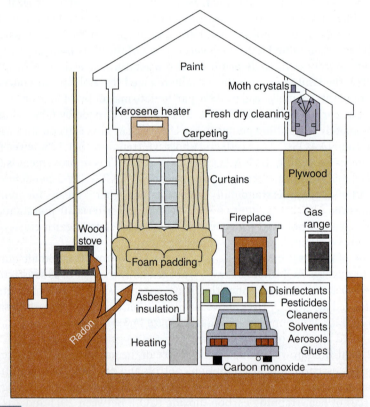

FIGURE 14.4   Air pollution sources in the home.

Data from U.S. Environmental Protection Agency & U.S. Consumer Product Safety Commission. (1995). *The inside story: A guide to indoor air quality.* Available at https://www.epa.gov/indoor-air-quality-iaq/inside-story-guide-indoor-air-quality

Indoor Air Pollutants

Asbestos a naturally occurring mineral fiber identified as a Class A carcinogen by the EPA

Sources of indoor air pollution include building and insulation materials, biogenic pollutants, combustion byproducts, home furnishings, cleaning agents, radon gas, and tobacco product smoke. These pollutants can arise from a number of sources (see **Figure 14.4**). **Asbestos** is a naturally occurring mineral fiber that was commonly used as insulation and fireproofing material. It was often used in older buildings to insulate pipes, walls, and ceilings; as a component of floor and ceiling tiles; and was sprayed in structures for fireproofing. It is harmless if intact and left alone; however, when disturbed, inhaled airborne fibers can cause serious health problems. **Biogenic pollutants** are airborne materials of biologic origin, such as living and nonliving fungi and their toxins, bacteria, viruses, molds, pollens, insect parts, and animal dander. They normally enter the human body by being inhaled. These contaminants can trigger allergic reactions, including asthma; cause infectious illnesses, such as influenza and measles; or release disease-producing toxins. Symptoms of health problems include sneezing, watery eyes, coughing, and shortness of breath, dizziness, lethargy, fever, and even digestive problems. Children, elderly people, and people with breathing problems, allergies, or lung diseases are particularly susceptible to airborne biogenic pollutants. People can minimize exposure to these pollutants by controlling the relative humidity level in a home or office; a relative humidity of 30–50% is generally recommended for homes. To reduce airborne biogenic pollutants in their homes, people should remove standing water, and any wet or water-damaged materials from around the home, and, if they suspect a problem, have the home inspected by someone knowledgeable about indoor air-pollution problems.[15] In light of the contagious nature of the SARS-CoV-2 virus (which causes COVID-19), EPA has published recommendations to minimize virus transmission in homes (see **Box 14.1**).

Combustion by-products include gases (e.g., CO, NO_2, and SO_2) and particulates (e.g., ash and soot). The major sources of these substances are fireplaces, wood stoves, kerosene heaters, secondhand tobacco smoke, and improperly maintained gas stoves and furnaces. Prolonged exposure to these substances can cause serious illness and possibly death.[17]

Volatile organic compounds (VOCs) are compounds that exist as vapors over the normal range of air pressures and temperatures. The health effects of these chemicals vary with their concentration and one's length of exposure. Acute symptoms include irritation of the eyes and respiratory tract, headaches, dizziness, and memory impairment. Some of these chemicals are known or suspected carcinogens. In any one building, one might find hundreds of different VOCs. Sources of VOCs include construction materials (e.g., insulation and paint), structural components (e.g., vinyl tile and drywall), furnishings (e.g., upholstery fabric), cleansers and solvents (e.g., liquid detergent), personal care products (e.g., deodorant), insecticides/pesticides, electrical equipment (e.g., computers), and combustion of wood and kerosene.[15] **Formaldehyde (CH2O)**, a pungent water-soluble gas, is one of the most ubiquitous VOCs. It is a widely used chemical that can be found in hundreds of products. Exposure occurs when it evaporates from wood products, such as plywood and

Biogenic pollutants airborne biological organisms or their particles or gases or other toxic materials that can produce illness

Combustion by-products gases and particulates generated by burning

Volatile organic compounds (VOCs) compounds that exist as vapor over the normal range of air pressures and temperatures

Formaldehyde (CH_2O) a water-soluble gas used in aqueous solutions in hundreds of consumer products

---

BOX 14.1   Indoor Air and Contagious Diseases

Viral diseases are commonly spread through person-to-person contact. Contagious viruses, such as SARS-CoV-2 (which causes COVID-19) may also spread by airborne particles or droplets when an infected person sneezes, coughs, or peaks. Because the airborne virus can be inhaled or contacted by a nearby person, it is the basis for social distancing recommendations. The use of masks mitigates this distance.[16] The EPA has issued best practices for reducing the potential for airborne transmission of viruses, such as SARS-CoV-2, in homes where social distancing and masks are not always practical.

- Increase outdoor ventilation by opening windows into the home.
- Use portable fans or the heating/ventilation/air conditioning (HVAC) system fan to increase indoor ventilation.
- Use the highest efficiency filter designed for your ventilation system and change it when recommended.
- Use a portable air cleaner or air purifier.

For Further Thought

Do you know which filters are best for your HVAC system? How often should you change your filters? Do you a have a room with a bathroom that you can use to isolate a sick person to minimize the potential for spread of a contagious disease to others in the home?

Data from U.S. Environmental Protection Agency. (2023). *Indoor air in homes and coronavirus (COVID-19)*. Available at https://www.epa.gov/coronavirus/indoor-air-and-coronavirus-covid-19.

particle board, in which it is a component of the glue that binds these products together. Formaldehyde can also be found in products, such as grocery bags, wallpaper, carpet, insulation, wall paneling, and wallboard.[15] Exposure to formaldehyde can cause watery eyes, burning in the eyes and throat, and difficulty in breathing. It can precipitate asthma attacks in susceptible people. Formaldehyde may also be a **carcinogen**. So, how can people protect their families and themselves? When building or renovating a residence, use exterior-grade products that emit less formaldehyde. Increase ventilation in the home, use a dehumidifier and air conditioning to control humidity, and keep temperature at moderate levels in the home to reduce formaldehyde emissions.

Radon is the number one cause of lung cancer among nonsmokers and the second-leading cause of lung cancer overall. This radioactive gas, which cannot be seen, smelled, or tasted, is responsible for about 21,000 lung cancer deaths every year.[18,19] It is a naturally occurring gas that seeps into a home from surrounding soil, rocks, and water and through openings, such as cracks, drains, and sump pumps. However, exposure to radon is preventable, and homeowners can do something about it. Every home and office building should be tested for radon, and homeowners can administer this inexpensive and easy test.

Mold is another indoor air pollutant that can be associated with allergic reactions and respiratory difficulties, such as asthma. Although eliminating mold in the indoor environment may not be possible, removing damp or wet furnishings or building materials, preventing condensation, and maintaining indoor humidity between 30–60% can reduce mold growth significantly. Venting damp air out of the home, using air conditioners, dehumidifiers, and bathroom exhaust fans, is an ideal way to control moisture in the home.[20]

Environmental tobacco smoke (ETS; secondhand smoke) includes both **mainstream smoke** (the smoke inhaled and exhaled by the smoker) and **sidestream tobacco smoke** (the smoke that comes off the end of a burning tobacco product). The involuntary inhalation of ETS by nonsmokers is referred to as **passive smoking**. Hundreds of toxic agents and more than 40 carcinogens are present in secondhand smoke. A few of these harmful agents are CO, NO_2, CO_2, hydrogen cyanide, formaldehyde, nicotine, and suspended particles.[21]

Approximately 12.5% (39 million) of adult Americans 12 years of age or older were active cigarette smokers in 2023.[22] As a result, many nonsmokers are exposed to environmental tobacco smoke. ETS is classified as a known human (group A) carcinogen and causes approximately 7,330 lung cancer deaths annually in U.S. nonsmokers.[21]

In 2014, the U.S. Public Health Service released *The Health Consequences of Smoking—50 Years of Progress: A Report of the Surgeon General*. This report discusses the progress made, efforts that have resulted in the reduction of tobacco use, and evidence of the continued burden that tobacco use imposes on the United States. It is expected that 5.6 million minors who were alive in 2014 will die prematurely due to smoking.[21] The report discusses the evidence that links ETS and adverse health effects, such as cancer, heart disease, and stroke. Additionally, such exposure has been shown to increase the risk of adverse prenatal consequences and postnatal health conditions in infants. Specifically, this exposure has been associated with intrauterine growth retardation, low birth weight, preterm delivery, orofacial clefts, respiratory tract infections, and behavioral and cognitive abnormalities.[21] Furthermore, young children are especially susceptible to secondhand smoke and are likely to suffer from coughing, wheezing, breathlessness, an increased risk of developing asthma, and disruptive behavioral disorders.[21]

Cigarette smoking among teens in 2023 had dropped to 4.8%; however, this downward trend has been countered by an increase to 28.2% of teens using a nicotine-containing tobacco product, including a 33% increase in the use of e-cigarettes since 2018. In 2023, it was estimated that 27.5% of teens were using e-cigarettes.[23] E-cigarettes result in addiction to nicotine and can cause acute onset of life-threatening illnesses. These devices contain chemicals that are toxic to cells and can cause lung disease and cardiovascular disease. E-cigarettes are not a "safe" alternative to cigarettes and likely pose a hazard due to secondhand emissions.[24] More studies and information are needed quickly to fully determine the health hazards posed by e-cigarettes.

Carcinogen agent, usually chemical, that causes cancer

Radon a naturally occurring colorless, tasteless, odorless, radioactive gas formed during the radioactive decay of uranium-238

Mold fungi that spread and reproduce by making spores; they grow best in warm, damp, and humid conditions, and can cause respiratory difficulties for sensitive people

Environmental tobacco smoke (ETS; secondhand smoke) tobacco smoke in the environment that is a mixture of mainstream and sidestream smoke that can be inhaled by nearby or transient nonsmokers

Mainstream smoke tobacco smoke inhaled and exhaled by the smoker

Sidestream tobacco smoke tobacco smoke that comes off the end of burning tobacco products

Passive smoking the inhalation of ETS by nonsmokers

Protecting Indoor Air

Because we spend up to 90% of our time indoors,[25] we need to take measures to protect the quality of our indoor air. The energy crisis of the 1970s led to a conservation movement that included reducing the ventilation rate in buildings. The accepted rate was reduced from 15 cubic feet per minute (CFM) to 5 CFM as a cost savings and energy savings measure. This reduced ventilation resulted in the creation of "tight buildings," which came to be known as "sick buildings," as reports of illness traced to such buildings increased.[26] **Sick building syndrome** refers to a situation in which the air quality in a building produces nonspecific signs and symptoms of ill health in the building occupants. Electronic controls and more efficient filtration, heating, and cooling systems have enabled the ventilation rate of 15 to 20 CFM to be reinstated.

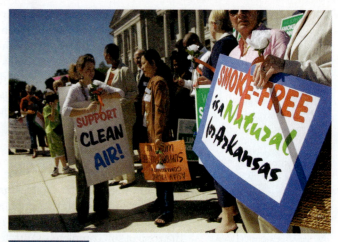

FIGURE 14.5   Nonsmokers' rights advocates sometimes take their campaign to their statehouse.

© Mike Wintroath/AP Photo

Even though indoor air pollution may be more harmful to human health than outdoor air pollution, measures to monitor and correct indoor air pollution have been limited. The U.S. government has not yet established a framework for the development of indoor air policies as it has for outdoor air. It has, however, usually supported voluntary industry standards. For example, there are safety codes for kerosene space heaters, an "action guideline" for radon, and smoking restrictions for an increasing number of public spaces. There are also requirements on the handling of asbestos during demolition and disposal and a prohibition on new uses for asbestos.

In the absence of federal indoor clean air legislation, some states, counties, and municipalities have developed their own standards. In an attempt to protect workers and citizens from heart disease, cancer, and respiratory illness and to reduce forced inhalation through passive smoking, many U.S. counties and states, as well as countries around the world, have banned or are in the process of outlawing smoking in workplaces and public areas, such as restaurants. In some areas, even outdoor smoking has been banned within a certain distance of entrances, exits, and air intakes of public and state-owned buildings. As of 2022, 28 states and the District of Columbia have met the American Lung Association's (ALA) challenge to pass comprehensive legislation prohibiting smoking in all public places and workplaces. Sixteen states and the District of Columbia have also added e-cigarettes to their smoke-free laws.[27] The ALA website includes a summary of prevention and control efforts in each state.

Some states still have preemptive laws that impede the passage and enforcement of stronger local tobacco control laws. One of the *Healthy People 2030* objectives is to eliminate state laws that preempt stronger local legislation.[28] As of 2023, legislation at the state and local level has resulted in protection for 82.3% of the U.S. population (see **Figure 14.5**).[29]

The Water We Use

Clean, uncontaminated water is essential for life and health. In many regions of the world, such as parts of Asia and Africa, the scarcity of potable water limits development and challenges health. Furthermore, lack of basic sanitation, including the inability to properly treat wastewater, has immediate and dire health consequences. Consumption of polluted water can result in outbreaks of such waterborne diseases as cholera, typhoid fever, dysentery, and other gastrointestinal diseases. Worldwide, such diseases are responsible for 1.4 million deaths every year. Most of those affected are children in developing countries. In 2022, nearly 20% of the world's population (1.5 billion people) lived without proper sanitation and 9% of the world's population (703 million people) had no access to clean drinking water.[30,31]

Sick building syndrome a situation in which the air quality in a building produces generalized signs and symptoms of ill health in the building's occupants

Sanitation the practice of establishing and maintaining healthy or hygienic conditions in the environment

Surface water precipitation that does not infiltrate the ground or return to the atmosphere by evaporation; the water in streams, rivers, and lakes

Groundwater water located under the surface of the ground

Aquifers porous, water-saturated layers of underground bedrock, sand, and gravel that can yield economically significant amounts of water

Water pollution any physical or chemical change in water that can harm living organisms or make the water unfit for other uses

Point source pollution pollution that can be traced to a single identifiable source

Here in the United States, virtually 100% of the population has access to a clean water supply and **sanitation**, the establishment and maintenance of healthy or hygienic conditions in the environment; this is among the highest reported for any world region. Nonetheless, over 100 waterborne disease outbreaks (WBDOs) linked to drinking or recreational use of water occur annually. A major source of drinking water contamination is waste produced by humans through their daily activities. Thus, both the prevention of water pollution and the treatment of polluted water are essential community activities.[32]

Sources of Water

We acquire water for our domestic, industrial, and agricultural needs from either surface water or groundwater. Water in streams, rivers, lakes, and reservoirs is called **surface water**. The water that infiltrates into the soil is referred to as subsurface water or **groundwater**. Groundwater that is not absorbed by the roots of vegetation moves slowly downward until it reaches the zone of soil completely saturated with water, referred to as an aquifer. **Aquifers** are porous, water-saturated layers of underground bedrock, sand, and gravel that can yield economically significant amounts of water.[5]

The Earth's supply of fresh water available for our use is limited. Only 0.003% of the Earth's water is available for use by humans, and much of this is hard to reach and too costly to be of practical value.[33] Thus, the continual contamination of our groundwater through the improper disposal of human waste, trash, and solid and hazardous waste should be of paramount concern to everyone.

Sources of Water Pollution

Water pollution includes any physical or chemical change in water that can harm living organisms or make it unfit for other uses, such as drinking, domestic use, recreation, fishing, industry, agriculture, or transportation. The sources of water pollution fall into two categories—point sources and nonpoint sources (see **Figure 14.6**).[5] **Point source pollution**

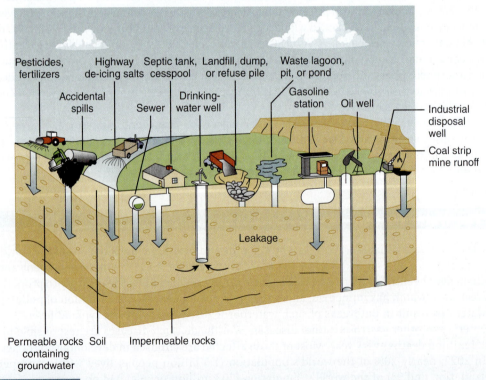

FIGURE 14.6   Sources of groundwater contamination.

refers to a single identifiable source that discharges pollutants into the water, such as a pipe, ditch, or culvert. Examples of such pollutants might include release of pollutants from a factory or sewage treatment plant. Point sources of pollution are relatively easy to identify, control, and treat.

Nonpoint source pollution includes all pollution that occurs through the runoff, seepage, or falling of pollutants into the water. Examples include the runoff of water from cities, highways, and farms, resulting from rain events (called stormwater runoff) and seepage of leachates from unlined landfills. Nonpoint source pollution is a greater problem than point source pollution is because it is often difficult to track the actual source of pollution and, therefore, to control it. Although many sanitary districts across the United States are implementing plans to capture and treat urban stormwater runoff from their streets, it is not yet a common practice. Because of increased urbanization and the growing proportion of land that is covered by impervious concrete, rainwater cannot infiltrate the land surface and is, therefore, collected by storm and sewer lines and often dumped into rivers without treatment.[34]

Types of Water Pollutants

Water pollutants can be classified as biological or nonbiological. Biological pollutants include pathogens or undesirable living organisms; nonbiological pollutants are nonliving hazardous materials, such as chemicals.

Biological Pollutants of Water

Biological pollutants are living organisms or their products that make water unsafe for human consumption. Examples include pathogens, such as parasites, bacteria, viruses, and other undesirable live micro-organisms. Waterborne viral agents and the diseases they cause include poliomyelitis virus (polio) and hepatitis A virus (hepatitis). Waterborne bacteria and the diseases they cause include *Escherichia coli* (gastroenteritis), *Legionella* spp. (legionellosis), *Salmonella typhi* (typhoid fever), *Shigella* spp. (shigellosis or bacillary dysentery), and *Vibrio cholerae* (cholera). Waterborne parasites include *Entamoeba histolytica* (amebiasis or amebic dysentery), *Giardia lamblia* (giardiasis), and *Cryptosporidium parvum* (cryptosporidiosis; see **Table 14.2**). Each of these diseases can be serious, and two in particular—typhoid fever and cholera—have killed thousands of people in single epidemics.

These pathogens enter the water mainly through human and other animal wastes that were disposed of improperly or untreated prior to disposal. Sources of such contamination include **runoff** from animal farms containing manure; failed septic systems that leach untreated or partially treated human fecal waste to groundwater and surface water; discharges of a mix of untreated storm water and human sewage overflow to rivers or streams; and stormwater runoff that carries animal and human fecal waste left on land surfaces. These biological wastes spread viruses, bacteria, and parasites into rivers, lakes, reservoirs, and drinking water supplies, where they can cause human illness. For example, people can become ill by drinking water from a groundwater well contaminated with fecal waste from a septic system or from ingesting water while swimming in a lake contaminated by runoff from nearby cities or farms.

Nonbiological Pollutants of Water

Nonbiological pollutants include heat; inorganic chemicals, such as lead, copper, and arsenic; organic chemicals; and radioactive contaminants. Among the organic chemicals are industrial solvents such as trichloroethylene (TCE); pesticides such as dichlorodiphenyltrichloroethane (DDT); herbicides such at atrazine; and the specialty chemicals, such as the polychlorinated biphenyls (PCBs), and dioxin (TCDD), a byproduct of improper incineration of chlorinated chemicals.

Historically, governmental regulation of chemical pollutants has targeted chemicals discharged by industries and municipal sewage treatment facilities. These pollutants, present in high concentrations and known to be detrimental to human health, are relatively easy to identify. Since 2002, however, two types of pollutants have been detected in U.S. waterways and are raising health concerns. These are **endocrine-disrupting chemicals (EDCs)** and **pharmaceuticals and personal care products (PPCPs)**.

Nonpoint source pollution all pollution that occurs through the runoff, seepage, or falling of pollutants into the water where the source is difficult or impossible to identify

Runoff water that flows over land surfaces (including paved surfaces), typically from precipitation

Endocrine-disrupting chemicals (EDCs) chemicals that interfere in some way with the body's endocrine (hormone) system

Pharmaceuticals and personal care products (PPCPs) synthetic chemicals found in everyday consumer healthcare products and cosmetics

TABLE 14.2 Leading Causes of Waterborne Disease Outbreaks—United States, 2020–2021

Predominant Cause of Illness	Number of Outbreaks (%)	Number of Cases (%)
Bacteria	**75 (75)**	**387 (53)**
Legionella spp.	62	237
Shigella spp.	1	4
Pseudomonas aeruginosa	4	41
Escherichia coli	3	27
Campylobacter spp.	4	75
Salmonella spp.	1	3
Other	0	0
Parasites	**5 (5)**	**79 (11)**
Cryptosporidium spp.	3	64
Giardia intestinalis	2	15
Cyclospora cayetanensis	0	0
Avian schistosomes	0	0
Cryptosporidium/Giardia spp.	0	0
Viruses	**1 (1)**	**20 (3)**
Norovirus	1	20
Hepatitis A virus	0	0
Chemicals/Toxins	**16 (16)**	**125 (17)**
Multiple	**2 (2)**	**101 (14)**
Suspected/Unidentified	**1 (1)**	**24 (3)**
Total	**100 (100)**	**736 (100)**

Data from Center for Disease Control and Prevention. (2022). *National Outbreak Reporting System (NORS)*. Available at https://wwwn.cdc.gov/norsdashboard/.

Endocrine disruptors include pesticides, commercial chemicals, and environmental contaminants that can disrupt, imitate, or block the body's normal hormonal activity, causing developmental or reproductive problems. Evidence for this has been found in certain wildlife species. Thus far, the relationship between EDCs and human disease is a complex issue; however, there is evidence of adverse reproductive outcomes and effects on the thyroid and brain.[35] The EPA has developed a two-tier process to screen and evaluate chemicals and has published a list of 109 chemicals for Tier 1 screening.[36] The EPA has completed Tier 1 screening for 52 chemicals with 20 indicating no evidence for interaction with the endocrine system, 14 with a potential interaction, and 18 with potential to interact with the estrogen pathway.[37]

PPCPs are synthetic chemicals found in everyday consumer healthcare products and cosmetics. These products include prescription and over-the-counter drugs; cosmetics, including body cleansers; fragrances; sunscreens; diagnostic agents; biopharmaceuticals; and many others. PPCPs have been detected in water supplies around the world, and their effects on human health are the subject of scientific investigations. PPCPs get into water sources when they are flushed down toilets and washed down drains and transported to wastewater treatment plants, where they are discharged, mostly unchanged, into rivers and streams. There have been a few studies conducted that have examined the effects of exposure to low-concentrations of PPCPs on humans. Screening methodologies suggest that exposure to the low concentrations measured compared with a "minimum therapeutic dose" provides a margin of safety for humans.[38] However, such an approach is unlikely to be appropriate for aquatic life and does not account for bioaccumulation through the food chain.

Although the EPA and other researchers are working to assess the effects of EDCs and PPCPs, there are no governmental regulations or guidance for the disposal of pharmaceuticals meant for personal use. Because it is important to take some personal action to reduce their presence in our environment, people should dispose of unused or unwanted medication in an environmentally sound manner. The U.S. Food and Drug Administration has developed a list of medications that can be flushed into the sewer system. For other pharmaceuticals, the options are take-back programs or disposal in household trash. Contact the local pharmacy, hospital, or law enforcement for disposal locations and times for expired or unwanted medicines.[39]

A **waterborne disease outbreak (WBDO)** is a water exposure in which at least two persons have been epidemiologically linked to recreational or drinking water by location, time, and illness. In the case of a recreational exposure, two or more persons must experience a similar illness after ingestion of drinking water or after exposure to water used for recreational purposes, and epidemiologic evidence must implicate water as the probable source of the illness.[40] In recent years, although the number of WBDOs associated with drinking water has declined, the number of WBDOs associated with recreational exposure has increased (see **Figure 14.7**). The Centers for Disease Control and Prevention (CDC) issues biennial surveillance summaries based on WBDOs reported to the Waterborne Disease and Outbreak Surveillance System. During 2020–2021, 100 waterborne disease outbreaks resulted in 736 cases of illness. In the most recent reports, 61 WBDOs associated with recreational water were reported from at least 18 states. Of these outbreaks, 61% were traced to exposure to treated water venues (swimming pools, wading pools, spas, etc.). In 66% of the outbreaks, the illnesses were described as acute respiratory illnesses, 27% as acute gastroenteritis illnesses, and 2% as skin disorders. The leading causes of WBDOs associated with recreational water was bacteria (62%) followed by chemical (26%), parasites (7%), multiples causes (3%), and viruses (2%). There were no cases where the cause was unidentified (0%).[41]

From 2020 to 2021, 124 WBDOs associated with drinking water were reported. The WBDOs associated with water intended for drinking caused illness in at least 1,429 people and resulted in 36 deaths. About 65% of the outbreaks resulted in acute respiratory illness, and 34% in acute gastrointestinal illness. In those outbreaks where the etiological agent was determined, the leading cause was bacteria (54%), followed by parasites (29%), viruses (6%), chemicals (3%), multiple causes (3%) and unidentified (5%).[41] The leading cause of WBDOs associated with drinking water is the bacterium *Legionella*.

WBDOs can usually be traced to a source either within or outside of the jurisdiction of a water utility. Outbreaks associated with municipal water systems can become quite large. The largest WBDO ever reported in the United States occurred in Milwaukee, Wisconsin, in 1993. In that outbreak, 403,000 people became ill and 4,400 were hospitalized. The disease agent was identified as the parasite *Cryptosporidium parvum*. This outbreak occurred because of a breakdown in the city's water treatment plant.[42] Public health laws that set standards for drinking water and for treated recreational water are a community's first line of defense against WBDOs. Although WBDOs occur from time to time in the United States, they occur much less frequently than they do in developing countries, where access to safe drinking water and sanitation is limited or nonexistent.

The safety of the U.S. water supply has deteriorated in many communities. Water-quality deterioration can be attributed to: (1) population growth, (2) agricultural and manufacturing activities, (3) land use practices, (4) mismanagement of hazardous materials, and (5) deteriorating water treatment and distribution infrastructure.[43] As the public's knowledge of the endangerment of water quality in the United States grows, it is hoped that greater efforts will be made to protect the water.

Ensuring the Safety of Our Water

Ensuring the safety of U.S. water supplies involves the proper treatment of water intended for drinking and a properly maintained distribution system for that water. It also requires proper construction and maintenance of water-associated recreation facilities. Safe water also depends

Waterborne disease outbreak (WBDO) a disease in which at least two persons experience a similar illness after the ingestion of drinking water or after exposure to water used for recreational purposes, and epidemiologic evidence implicates water as the probable source of the illness

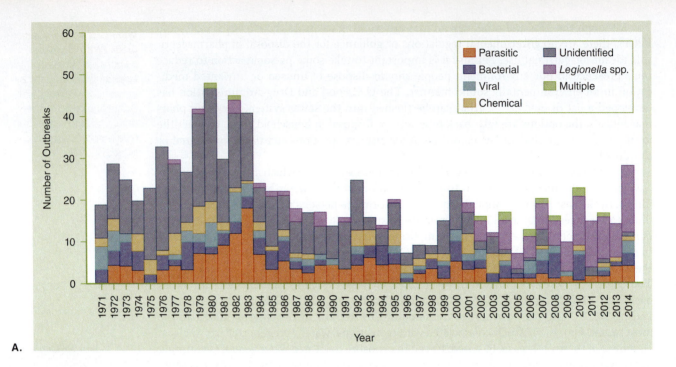

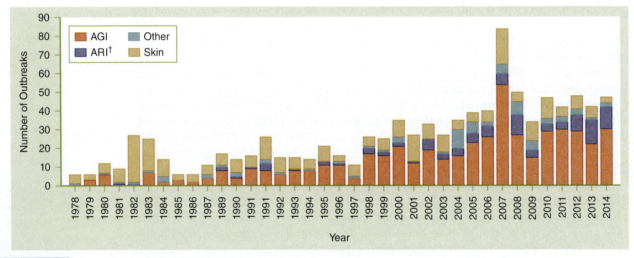

FIGURE 14.7   **A.** Number of waterborne disease outbreaks associated with drinking water (*n* = 1,212) by year and etiology—Waterborne Disease and Outbreak Surveillance System, United States, 1978–2021. **B.** Number of waterborne disease outbreaks associated with recreational water (*n* = 1,391) by predominant illness and year—Waterborne Disease and Outbreak Surveillance System, United States, 1978–2021.

*†All outbreaks of legionellosis (i.e., Legionnaires' disease and Pontiac fever) are classified as ARI.

AGI: acute gastrointestinal illness; Skin: illness, condition, or symptom related to skin; ARI: acute respiratory illness; Other: includes keratitis, conjunctivitis, otitis, bronchitis, meningitis, meningoencephalitis, hepatitis, leptospirosis, and combined illnesses.

Data from Center for Disease Control and Prevention. (2022). National Outbreak Reporting System (NORS). Available at https://wwwn.cdc.gov/norsdashboard/

on the enactment and enforcement of well-conceived water quality regulations. In addition, it requires wastewater treatment and sanitation.

Treatment of Water for Domestic Use

Water in the United States is used for many purposes, including agriculture, industry, energy generation, and domestic use. Domestic water use includes water for drinking, cooking, washing dishes and laundry, bathing, flushing toilets, and outdoor use (such as watering lawns and gardens). Although domestic use makes up only 13% of total water usage, each U.S. resident uses an average of 80 to 100 gallons of water each day, just by flushing the toilet, showering, washing laundry, and other domestic uses.[44,45]

Whereas many rural residents in the United States obtain their water from untreated private wells (groundwater), urban residents usually obtain their water from municipal water treatment plants. About two-thirds of municipalities use surface water, while one-third uses groundwater.

Virtually all surface water is polluted and needs to be treated before it can be safely consumed. The steps in the treatment of water for domestic use vary but usually include removing solids through coagulation, flocculation, and filtration. This is followed by disinfection, during which chlorine, sodium hypochlorite, ozone, or another disinfectant is added to the water to kill remaining viruses, bacteria, algae, and fungi. Disinfection is sometimes accompanied by fluoridation, which helps prevent dental decay.

Fluoridation of community drinking water has been a major factor responsible for the decline in dental caries (tooth decay) in the United States since 1950. At first, caries reduction rates of 50–70% were reported.[46] More recently, tooth decay reduction in adults and children has averaged 25%. Because fluoride has appeared in other products, such as toothpaste and mouthwashes, the difference in rates of caries between those who receive fluoridated water and those who do not has declined. By 2020, 208 million people were receiving fluoridated water, at an average cost of $0.611 to $24.38 per person per year, depending on the size of the served community. The savings from prevention of dental caries attributable to fluoridation was estimated to be $32 per person per year.[47,48]

The responsibility of municipal water treatment plants is to provide water that is chemically and bacteriologically safe for human consumption. It is also desirable that the water be aesthetically pleasing with regard to taste, odor, color, and clarity. Above all, the municipal water supply must be reliable. Reliability with regard to both quantity and quality has always been regarded as non-negotiable in operating a treatment facility.

Wastewater Treatment

Wastewater is the substance that remains after humans have used water for domestic or commercial purposes. Such water, also referred to as liquid waste or sewage, consists of approximately 99.9% water and 0.1% suspended and dissolved solids. The solids consist of human feces, soap, paper, garbage grindings (food parts), and a variety of other items that are put into wastewater systems from homes, schools, commercial buildings, hotels/motels, hospitals, industrial plants, and other facilities connected to the sanitary sewer system. The primary purpose of **wastewater treatment** is to improve the quality of wastewater to the point that it might be released into a body of water without seriously disrupting the aquatic environment, causing health problems in humans in the form of waterborne disease, or causing nuisance conditions. Most municipalities and many large companies have wastewater treatment plants that incorporate at least primary and secondary treatment processes (see **Figure 14.8**).

Primary Wastewater Treatment

Primary wastewater treatment occurs in a sedimentation tank, also called a *clarifier*, where wastewater remains in a quiescent condition for about two to four hours. Here, heavier solid particles settle to the bottom, forming a layer referred to as **sludge**. Sludge is a semisolid mixture that includes bacteria, viruses, organic matter, toxic metals, synthetic organic chemicals, and solids.[49] Above the sludge remains most of the wastewater, including many bacteria and chemicals. On top of this aqueous layer is a layer of oils and fats, also called scum. The layers of sludge and scum are removed, and the clarified wastewater enters the secondary stage of treatment.

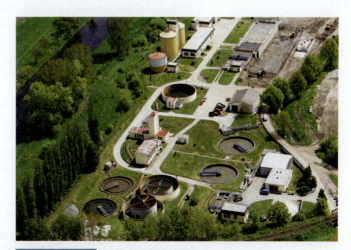

FIGURE 14.8   A wastewater treatment facility.
© Robert Malota/Dreamstime.com

Wastewater the aqueous mixture that remains after water has been used or contaminated by humans

Wastewater treatment the process of improving the quality of wastewater (sewage) to the point that it can be released into a body of water without seriously disrupting the aquatic environment, causing health problems in humans, or causing nuisance conditions

Sludge a semiliquid mixture of solid waste that includes bacteria, viruses, organic matter, toxic metals, synthetic organic chemicals, and solid chemicals

Secondary Wastewater Treatment

During secondary treatment, aerobic bacteria are added and mixed with clarified wastewater to break down the organic waste; this mixture then flows to aeration tanks. Here, oxygen is continuously added to support aerobic decomposition of organic waste into carbon dioxide, water, and minerals. When this biological process is completed (after approximately six to 10 hours), the wastewater is sent to sedimentation tanks, where solids and flocs of bacteria are separated from the treated liquid portion of wastewater in quiescent conditions. After this process, many treatment plants disinfect and discharge the treated wastewater to surface water bodies; other wastewater plants perform tertiary treatment.

Tertiary Wastewater Treatment

Tertiary wastewater treatment involves filtration through sand and carbon filters. During this process, many remaining dissolved pollutants are removed. The treated water is then disinfected and discharged. The least expensive way of disinfecting wastewater is to chlorinate it. After chlorination is completed, chlorine is removed from the water through a process called dechlorination to prevent poisoning of aquatic life in streams or rivers downstream of the discharge point. Discharges of treated wastewater are regulated by the EPA.

Septic Systems

Those who live in unsewered areas (20% of Americans) dispose of their wastewater using a septic system.[50] A septic system comprises two major components—a septic tank and a buried sand filter or absorption field (see **Figure 14.9**). The **septic tank**, which is a watertight concrete or fiberglass tank, is buried in the ground some distance from the house and is connected to it by a pipe. Sewage leaves the home via the toilets or drains and goes through the pipe to the septic tank. The wastewater is retained in quiescent conditions for one to two days, during which separation of heavier solids and lighter scum from liquid wastewater occurs in the process called sedimentation. The liquid portion of wastewater is then carried by a pipe to an **absorption field**, a system of trenches (dugout channels) where perforated pipes are surrounded by gravel. As wastewater trickles through the gravel, films of aerobic micro-organisms develop and feed on this liquid wastewater, causing decomposition of organic waste. This treated wastewater then infiltrates through the soil profile into the groundwater.

Clearly, proper installation and regular maintenance of the septic system are absolutely crucial for its optimal performance. Septic systems cannot be legally installed in most communities without a permit. Local health departments are responsible for issuing permits, inspecting the systems, and enforcing state and local regulations regarding them. The system must be (1) located in appropriate soil, (2) properly constructed and inspected prior to being buried, and (3) maintained regularly. Septic tanks need to be pumped out every three to five years to remove sludge and thus prevent overflow, sewage backup to the house, or failure of the absorption field. Failure to properly maintain the system can result in fecal contamination of both land and water sources. Improperly functioning or overflowing septic systems also provide optimal breeding sites for disease-transmitting mosquitoes, such as the northern house mosquito, *Culex pipiens*, the vector of West Nile virus (see **Figure 14.10**).

Regulating Water Quality

Surface water and drinking water are regulated by two important laws, the Clean Water Act and the Safe Drinking Water Act. Growing public concern over the pollution of surface water sources, such as rivers, lakes, estuaries, coastal waters, and wetlands, led to enactment of the Federal Water Pollution Control Act Amendments of 1972. This law, as amended, is commonly known as the **Clean Water Act (CWA)**. The goal of the CWA is to restore and maintain the chemical, physical, and biological integrity of the waters in the United States so that they can support "the protection and propagation of fish, shellfish, and wildlife and recreation in and on the water."[51] In other words, the goal is to maintain the quality of surface waters to swimmable and fishable status. To achieve this goal, the EPA employs various regulatory and nonregulatory

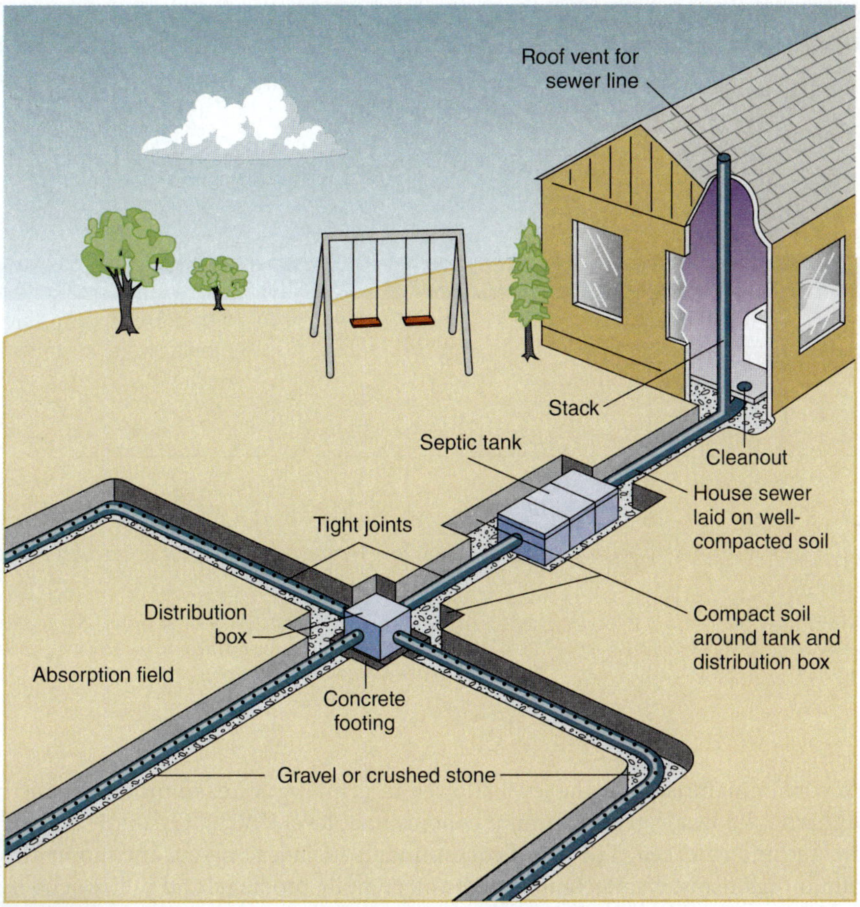

Watershed the area of land from which all of the water that is under it or drains from it goes into the same place and drains in one point; for example, the Mississippi River watershed drains and collects all of the water from the land extending from east of the Rocky Mountains to the Appalachian Mountains and from the upper Midwest all the way south to the Gulf of Mexico

Safe Drinking Water Act (SDWA) the federal law that regulates the safety of public drinking water

FIGURE 14.9 A septic system consists of a septic tank and an absorption field. This system is commonly used to treat domestic wastewater in suburban and rural areas.

programs to reduce direct pollutant discharges into waterways by industrial and wastewater treatment facilities. In addition, the agency attempts to manage polluted runoff by implementing nonregulatory programs.

In the early years of the CWA's implementation, the agency's efforts focused on regulating discharges from traditional point source facilities, such as municipal sewage plants and industrial facilities. The CWA made it unlawful for any person to discharge any pollutant from a point source into navigable waters without a permit. Since the late 1980s, however, the EPA has significantly increased its efforts to address nonpoint source pollution from urban, agricultural, and stormwater runoff, and implemented either voluntary or regulatory programs to curb this problem. In its efforts to reduce water pollution, the EPA considers land use and sources of pollution within the entire **watershed** rather than controlling and regulating only individual pollution sources or contaminants. The watershed approach emphasizes protecting healthy waters and restoring impaired ones to protect not only human but also environmental health.

The quality of drinking water is regulated by the **Safe Drinking Water Act (SDWA)** and its amendments. The SDWA implements many actions to protect drinking water and its sources (rivers, lakes, reservoirs, springs, and groundwater). Under the SDWA, the EPA sets national standards to limit the levels of contaminants in drinking water and oversees the states, localities, and water suppliers who implement those standards.[52] The national standard

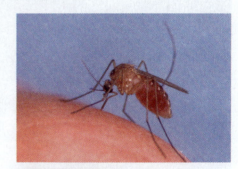

FIGURE 14.10 The northern house mosquito (*Culex pipiens*) is the most important vector of St. Louis encephalitis and West Nile virus in the eastern United States.

Courtesy of U.S. Geological Survey.

BOX 14.2   *Healthy People 2030:* **Objectives**

Objective EH-03: Increase the proportion of persons served by community water systems who receive a supply of drinking water that complies with the SDWA.
Target-setting method: Projection
Data sources: Safe Drinking Water Information System (SDWIS), EPA
Target and baseline:

Objective	2018 Baseline	2021 Data	2030 Target
EH-03 Increase the proportion of persons served by community water systems who receive a supply of drinking water that complies with the SDWA.	90.2% of persons served by community water systems	92.2% of persons	92.1% of persons served by community water systems

For Further Thought

Do you know the source of your water supply? Is it a river or underground aquifer? How do you find out if the water meets the SDWA regulations?

Data from U.S. Department of Health and Human Services, Office of Disease Prevention and Health Promotion. (2021). *Increase the proportion of people whose water supply Meets Safe Drinking Water Act regulations—EH-03.* Available at https://health.gov/healthypeople/objectives-and-data/browse-objectives /environmental-health/increase-proportion-people-whose-water-supply-meets-safe-drinking-water-act-regulations-eh-03.

for each contaminant is set at the level allowed in drinking water to protect public health; this standard is known as the maximum contaminant level (MCL). Currently, 88 MCLs are implemented and enforced. The list of contaminants includes organic and inorganic chemicals, micro-organisms, disinfectants and disinfectant by-products, and radionuclides.[53] The SDWA requires the EPA to go through a long and intensive process to identify new contaminants that may require regulation in the future. The most recent list of new contaminants to be considered for regulation includes 97 chemicals and 12 microbiological agents.[54] One of the *Healthy People 2030* objectives is to increase the number of people served by community water systems that meet the SDWA (see **Box 14.2**). As of 2021, data indicated that the objective exceeded the target.

Environmentalists and others would like to see the provisions of the SDWA strengthened and more vigorously enforced, but others point to the high administrative and enforcement costs of the SDWA and the cost burden it places on municipal and privately owned water supply systems as reasons not to strengthen the provisions. Meanwhile, the quality and safety of our drinking water remain the envy of the world (see **Figure 14.11**).

The Food We Eat

One way in which humans interact with their environment is by ingesting bits of it, which we call *food*. In a worldwide comparison, the U.S. food supply probably ranks as one of the safest. The safety of our food supply is a result of public health efforts and regulatory actions during the past century. In fact, safer and healthier foods in the United States have been designated as one of the 10 greatest achievements in public health in the twentieth century.[55]

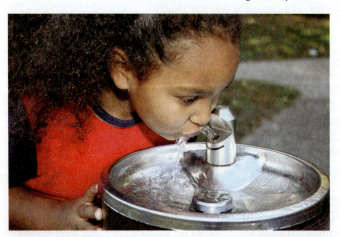

FIGURE 14.11   In the United States, virtually 100% of the population has access to clean, safe drinking water.
© Duplass/Shutterstock

Unfortunately, additional progress must be made before we completely eliminate foodborne disease. "More than 200 known diseases are transmitted through food. In these cases, food is the vehicle; and the agents can be viruses, bacteria, parasites, toxins, metals, and prions."[56] Foodborne diseases cause an estimated 48 million cases of illness, 128,000 hospitalizations, and 3,000 deaths per year in the United States.[57] A majority of these cases are never reported to the CDC. The annual economic cost of foodborne illness in the United States has been estimated to be as high as $17.6 billion.[58] Estimates vary due to the number of pathogens included in a study as well as the costs associated with illness. Healthy food can become contaminated at several points between farm or factory and the consumer. This can result in an outbreak of foodborne disease.

> **Foodborne disease outbreak (FBDO)** the occurrence of two or more cases of a similar illness resulting from the ingestion of food

Foodborne Disease Outbreaks

The CDC defines a **foodborne disease outbreak (FBDO)** as the occurrence of two or more cases of a similar illness resulting from the ingestion of a common food. During the most recent years for which data are available (2020–2021), 563 FBDOs (238 in 2020 and 335 in 2021) were reported, resulting in 11,448 cases of illness, 1,322 hospitalizations, and 15 deaths. Norovirus was the most commonly reported agent, accounting for 26% of the outbreaks, followed by *Salmonella* (24% of outbreaks). The leading causes of foodborne illness, including the number of outbreaks and cases, appear in **Table 14.3**. Common food vehicles most often implicated were fish (17%), poultry (9%), vegetable row crops (9%), dairy (8%), mollusks (6%), beef (4%), fruits (4%), and pork (2%).[41]

Leading factors that contributed to FBDOs were inadequate cooking temperatures or improper holding temperatures for foods (especially for bacterial outbreaks); unsanitary conditions or practices at the point of service, such as failure to wash hands (norovirus outbreaks); or drinking raw (nonpasteurized) milk (bacterial outbreaks).[59] State laws permitting the sale of nonpasteurized dairy products vary, but 78% of the FBDOs involving nonpasteurized dairy products were reported in states that permit their sale.[60] Other factors that often contribute to FBDOs are contaminated equipment or obtaining food from an unsafe source (such as shellfish from polluted waters).

To protect the public from foodborne diseases requires the coordinated efforts of federal, state, and local health agencies. At the federal level, the CDC, under its Emerging Infections Program, has established the Foodborne Diseases Active Surveillance Network (FoodNet) to provide better data on foodborne diseases. FoodNet tracks diseases caused by enteric pathogens transmitted through foods. The CDC coordinates these surveillance activities with officials from the U.S. Department of Agriculture's Food Safety and Inspection Service, the U.S. Food and Drug Administration's Center for Food Safety and Applied Nutrition, and respective state epidemiologists. One set of the *Healthy People 2030* objectives aims to reduce the number of outbreak-associated infections due to foodborne disease agents (see **Box 14.3**).

Growing, Processing, and Distributing Our Food Safely

Despite the surveillance efforts described earlier, much remains to be done to ensure the safety of the food supply. Greater efforts need to be made to ensure that plants and animals are free from harmful biological and chemical agents during growing, harvesting, and processing of food products before they reach retail outlets and food service establishments.

Historically, our food was supplied by independent farmers whose field crops or livestock reached the marketplace relatively free from modern chemicals. Over the past century, farming has increasingly become "big business" with more and more farmland owned by large corporations. Modern agriculture in the United States has been characterized as the process of converting petroleum into food. Although this seems like an extreme statement, it contains elements of truth. On the modern industrial farm, significant amounts of fuel are required to run the tractors, combines, and other equipment. Tractors are used to apply petroleum-based chemical fertilizers, herbicides, and insecticides, usually from plastic tanks made from petroleum. It is hard to imagine a modern farm operation without these petroleum-based materials.

TABLE 14.3   Leading Causes of Reported Foodborne Disease Outbreaks—United States, 2020-2021

Predominant Cause of Illness	Number of Outbreaks (%)	Number of Cases (%)
Bacteria	**396 (57)**	**7,558 (66)**
Salmonella spp.	170	5,469
Clostridium perfringens	2	11
Escherichia coli, Shiga toxin-producing (STEC)	51	657
Campylobacter	116	348
Bacillus	21	992
Shigella	30	52
Other bacteria	6	29
Chemical	**81 (12)**	**123 (1)**
Scombroid toxin/histamine	21	56
Ciguatoxin	60	67
Mushroom toxins	0	0
Pesticides	0	0
Other chemicals	0	0
Parasites	**26 (4)**	**1,130 (10)**
Cyclospora	25	1,1113
Giardia	2	32
Other parasites	1	4
Viruses	**187 (27)**	**2,571 (22)**
Calicivirus (*Norovirus*)	180	2,460
Hepatitis A	6	98
Other viruses	1	13
Unknown	**4 (<1)**	**38 (0)**
Multiple causes	**5 (<1)**	**28 (0)**
Total	**563 (100)**	**11,448 (100)**

Data from Centers for Disease Control and Prevention. (2022). *National Outbreak Reporting System (NORS) Dashboard.* Available at https://wwwn.cdc.gov/norsdashboard/

Two health concerns regarding the ubiquitous nature of agricultural chemicals, especially pesticides, are (1) the risk of unintentional poisonings where these chemicals are stored and used, and (2) the residues reaching food workers and consumers.

Pesticides

The term **pest** refers to any organism (plant, animal, or microbe) that has an adverse effect on human interests. Some common examples are weeds in the vegetable garden, termites in the house, and mold on the shower curtain. **Pesticides** are natural or synthetic chemicals that have been developed and manufactured for the purpose of killing pests. As of March of 2013, 18,810 products containing a total of 1,118 active ingredients held current EPA registrations. These products, produced by 1,723 companies, were being distributed by 12,777 vendors, who had arranged with the producers to sell these products under private labels.[61] In 2021, more than 900 million pounds of pesticides were applied in agricultural uses in the United States.[62] Many of these pesticides are used in agriculture, where it is estimated that pests destroy 20–25% of

Pest any organism—a multicelled animal, plant, or microbe—that has an adverse effect on human interests

Pesticides synthetic chemicals developed and manufactured for the purpose of killing pests

BOX 14.3   *Healthy People 2030:* Objectives

Objective FS-2: Reduce the number of outbreak-associated infections due to Shiga toxin-producing *E. coli* O157, or *Campylobacter*, *Listeria*, or *Salmonella* species.
Target-setting method: 10% improvement.
Data sources: Foodborne Diseases Active Surveillance Network (FoodNet), CDC, and states.
Target and baseline:

Objective	2016–2018 Baseline (infections per 100,000)	2021 Data (infections per 100,000)	2030 Target (infections per 100,000)
FS-01 *Campylobacter*	16.2	17.2	10.9
FS-02 *E. coli*	4.6	4.6	3.7
FS-03 *Listeria*	0.31	0.27	0.22
FS-04 *Salmonella*	15.3	13.3	11.5

For Further Thought

Are you aware of any foodborne outbreaks in your area? Outbreaks of *E. coli* O157:H7 have been associated with undercooked beef. How do you make sure that you are protecting yourself and your guests when you cook hamburgers at home? How do you make sure you do not contaminate fresh leafy vegetables with raw meat or poultry?

Data from U.S. Department of Health and Human Services, Office of Disease Prevention and Health Promotion. (2021). Foodborne illness. Available at https://health.gov/healthypeople/objectives-and-data/browse-objectives/foodborne-illness

the food crop before it reaches the marketplace, an estimated loss of $70 billion to consumers and producers.[63,64] Without the use of agricultural chemicals, farm production would be greatly decreased. Because of this, it seems certain that pesticides will be present in our environment for the foreseeable future.

Although chemical companies market pesticides to control a particular pest, most of them in fact kill a wide range of organisms; that is, they are broad-spectrum pesticides. The pest organism against which the pesticide is applied is referred to as the **target organism (target pest)** (see **Table 14.4**). All other organisms in the environment that may also be affected are called **nontarget organisms**. For example, most weed killers will not only kill the weeds but also (nontarget) flowers and ornamental plants. Similarly, it is not uncommon for domestic animals to be poisoned and killed by rodenticides (rat poison).

The two most widely used types of pesticides are *herbicides* (pesticides that kill plants) and *insecticides* (pesticides that kill insects). These account for 61 and 22% of the pesticides

Target organism (target pest) the organism (or pest) for which a pesticide is applied

Nontarget organisms all other susceptible organisms in the environment, for which a pesticide was not intended

TABLE 14.4 Types of Pesticides

Type of Agent	Target Pest to Be Destroyed
Acaricides/miticides	Ticks/mites
Bactericides	Bacteria
Fungicides	Fungi, molds
Herbicides	Weeds, plants
Insecticides	Insects
Larvicides/grubicides	Insect larvae
Molluscicides	Snails, slugs
Nematocides	Worms
Rodenticides	Rats, mice

applied for agriculture, respectively.[62] It is also from these two types of pesticides that most human pesticide poisonings occur. The two groups at highest risk for pesticide poisoning are young children and the workers who apply the pesticides. Many of these people live on farms or are engaged in farm work. Poisonings occur when the pesticides are consumed orally, inhaled, or when they come in contact with the skin. The majority of children poisoned by pesticides consume them orally when the pesticides are left within their reach. Most adult poisonings occur because of careless practice. Examples include eating food without washing hands after handling pesticides, mouth-siphoning to transfer pesticides from one container to another, applying pesticides while one's skin is exposed, or spilling the pesticide on one's body. In agricultural settings, poisonings often occur when agricultural workers fail to follow directions on the pesticide label. For example, workers (who may not be able to read English) may enter sprayed fields too soon after a pesticide application, even a field with posted warning signs, or employers may even tell farm workers to enter the field too soon after a pesticide application. If the workers' children are with them, the children would be at higher risk of being poisoned. In addition to occupational exposure of farm workers, consumers may be exposed to low concentrations of pesticides daily through their handling and ingestion of food.

The effects of exposure to pesticides depend on the pesticide type, dose, route and duration of exposure, and the characteristics of the person exposed. Exposures may be acute (single, high-level exposure) or chronic (repeated exposure over an extended period of time). Some signals of poisoning are headache, weakness, rash, fatigue, and dizziness. More serious effects include respiratory problems, convulsions, coma, and death. Chronic effects can include cancer, mutations, and birth defects.

Regulating Food Safety

Because of the poisonous nature of pesticides, their unregulated manufacture and sale and indiscriminate use are unthinkable. Therefore, they are regulated by a combination of federal and state authorities. The EPA regulates the registration and labeling of pesticides. Individual state agencies license those who can buy, sell, or apply pesticides within their state. The safety of our food supply at the national level is further insured by the U.S. Department of Agriculture (USDA), which inspects meat and dairy products, and the U.S. Food and Drug Administration (FDA), which is charged with ensuring the safety of the remainder of our foods (see **Figure 14.12**). In recent years, several instances have occurred that call into question the quality of food processing and its inspection process. These include scares associated with fresh spinach, romaine lettuce, tomatoes, and peanut butter products.

The task of enforcing state regulations at the local level falls on **registered environmental health specialists (REHSs; sanitarians)**. Hired by local health departments, REHSs inspect restaurants and other food-serving establishments (such as hospitals, nursing homes, churches, and schools), retail food outlets (grocery stores and supermarkets), temporary and seasonal points of food service (such as those at fairs and festivals), and food vending machines to ensure that environmental conditions favorable to the growth and development of pathogens do not exist. When unsafe or unhealthy conditions are found, establishments are cited or, in cases of eminent danger to the public, closed. By enforcing food safety laws, public health officials protect the health of the community by reducing the incidence of FBDOs.

Finally, it is important to recognize that consumers themselves can further reduce their risk for foodborne illness by following safe food-handling practices and by avoiding consumption of certain unsafe foods. Examples of foods that are often unsafe include unpasteurized milk and milk products and raw or undercooked oysters, eggs, ground beef, pork, fish, or poultry. Guidelines for preventing foodborne disease transmission at home are simple and straightforward (see **Box 14.4**).

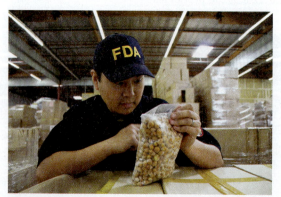

FIGURE 14.12   The U.S. Food and Drug Administration is charged with ensuring the safety of our foods, except for meat and dairy products.

Courtesy of U.S. Food and Drug Administration.

BOX 14.4   Guidelines for Preventing Foodborne Illnesses

To prevent foodborne illness, use the following strategies:

Clean: Wash Hands and Surfaces Often

- Wash your hands with warm water and soap for at least 20 seconds before and after handling food and after using the bathroom, changing diapers, and handling pets.
- Wash your cutting boards, dishes, utensils, and countertops with hot soapy water after preparing each food item and before you go on to the next food.
- Use paper towels to clean up kitchen surfaces. If you use cloth towels, wash them often in the hot cycle of your washing machine.
- Rinse fresh fruits and vegetables under running tap water, including those with skins and rinds that are not eaten.
- Rub firm-skin fruits and vegetables under running tap water or scrub with a clean vegetable brush while rinsing with running tap water.

Separate: Don't Cross-Contaminate!

- Separate raw meat, poultry, seafood, and eggs from other foods in your grocery shopping cart, grocery bags, and in your refrigerator.
- Use one cutting board for fresh produce and a separate one for raw meat, poultry, and seafood.
- Never place cooked food on a plate that previously held raw meat, poultry, seafood, or eggs.

Cook to Proper Temperature

- Use a food thermometer to measure the internal temperature and make sure that the food is cooked to a safe internal temperature (e.g., roasts and steaks to a minimum of 145°F, poultry to a minimum of 165°F in the innermost part of the thigh and wing and the thickest part of the breast). Cook ground meat to at least 160°F.
- Cook eggs until the yolk and white are firm, not runny. Don't use recipes in which eggs remain raw or only partially cooked.
- Cook fish to 145°F or until the flesh is opaque and separates easily with a fork.
- When cooking in a microwave oven, make sure there are no cold spots in food where bacteria can survive. For best results, cover food, stir, and rotate for even cooking.
- Bring sauces, soups, and gravy to a boil when reheating. Heat leftovers thoroughly to 165°F.

Chill: Refrigerate Promptly

- Refrigerate foods quickly and as soon as you get them home from the store because cold temperatures slow the growth of harmful bacteria. Keeping a constant refrigerator temperature of 40°F or below is one of the most effective ways to reduce the risk of foodborne illness.
- Never let raw meat, poultry, eggs, cooked food, or cut fresh fruits or vegetables sit at room temperature for more than 2 hours before putting them in the refrigerator or freezer.
- Never defrost food at room temperature. Food must be kept at a safe temperature during thawing, which you can achieve by defrosting your food in the refrigerator, in cold water, and in the microwave.
- Always marinate food in the refrigerator.
- Divide large amounts of leftovers into shallow containers for quicker cooling in the refrigerator.
- Use or discard refrigerated food on a regular basis.

Reproduced from Partnership for Food Safety Education. (n.d.). *The core four practices*. Available at http://www.fightbac.org/food-safety-basics/the-core-four-practices/

The Place We Live

Environmental hazards occur where we live because of our household and land management practices, including the production and mismanagement of our solid waste. The result can be environmental degradation, increased exposure to unsanitary and hazardous materials, and the amplification and transmission of vectorborne diseases.

Solid and Hazardous Waste

Solid waste is garbage, refuse, sludge, and other discarded solid materials. Most solid waste, 95–98%, can be traced to agriculture, mining, gas and oil production, and industry. The remaining 2–5%, termed **municipal solid waste (MSW)**, comprises the waste generated by households, businesses, and institutions (e.g., schools) located within municipalities.[65] In 2018, we produced a daily average of 4.91 pounds of MSW per person, up from the 2.7 pounds of waste produced per person in 1960, and up from the 4.74 pounds per person generated in 2017 (see **Figure 14.13**). There are nine major categories—paper, yard waste, food scraps, rubber and textiles, wood, metals, glass, plastics, and other. Paper makes up the largest percentage (23.1%), followed by food scraps (21.6%), yard trimmings (12.1%), and plastics (12.2%; see **Figure 14.14**).[66]

Solid waste solid refuse from households, agriculture, and businesses

Municipal solid waste (MSW) waste generated by individual households, businesses, and institutions located within municipalities

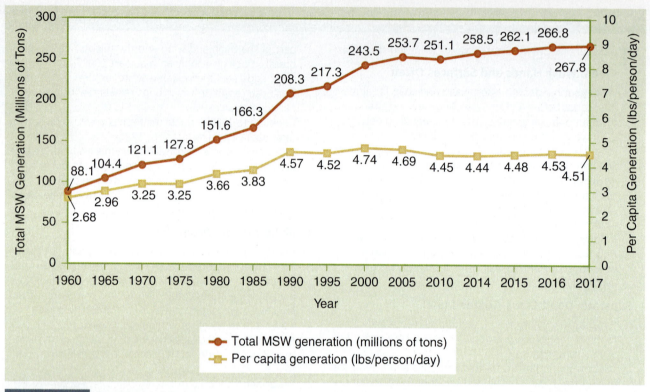

FIGURE 14.13 Municipal solid waste generation rates, 1960–2018.

Data from U.S. Environmental Protection Agency. (2020). *Advancing sustainable materials management 2018 fact sheet.* https://www.epa.gov/sites/default/files/2021-01/documents/2018_tables_and_figures_dec_2020_fnl_508.pdf

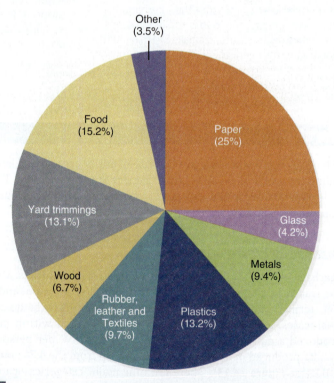

FIGURE 14.14 Total municipal solid waste generation by material.

Data from U.S. Environmental Protection Agency. (2020). Advancing sustainable materials management 2018 fact sheet. https://www.epa.gov/sites/default/files/2021-01/documents/2018_tables_and_figures_dec_2020_fnl_508.pdf

Hazardous waste is solid waste with properties that make it dangerous or potentially harmful to human health or the environment and, therefore, requires special management and disposal. A waste is hazardous if it is ignitable, corrosive, reactive, or toxic, or if it is otherwise designated hazardous by the EPA. Designated hazardous wastes can be found among the byproducts of manufacturing and industrial processes (e.g., solvents and cleaning fluids) and the byproducts of petroleum refining operations and pesticide manufacturing. Also, certain wastes, including batteries, mercury-containing instruments, and fluorescent light bulbs, fall into the category of universal (hazardous) wastes. The total amount of hazardous waste created each year in the United States is difficult to estimate but, according to the EPA's 2021 Toxic Release Inventory, 29.3 billion pounds of production-related waste were managed in 2021.[67] This statistic does not include any wastes that were discarded improperly or illegally.

Electronic waste (e-waste), not included in the preceding total, often contains hazardous components, such as polyvinylchloride, brominated flame retardants, lead, and mercury. In 2018, it was estimated that 2.7 million tons of electronics, including personal computers, displays, printers, keyboards and mice, TVs, and mobile devices (phones) were discarded (ready for end-of-life management)[68] (see **Box 14.5**).

Managing Our Solid Waste

Imagine what would happen if our local garbage and other refuse were not removed for just two or three weeks. The resulting accumulation of solid waste would produce undesirable odors and attract vermin, such as rats, flies, and other disease reservoirs and vectors; it would constitute a community-wide environmental health hazard. Although the necessity of the timely removal of MSW from community neighborhoods is evident to all, its heterogeneous makeup precludes its efficient disposal.

The **Resource Conservation and Recovery Act of 1976 (RCRA)** was an amendment to the Solid Waste Disposal Act of 1965 intended to comprehensively address the management of nonhazardous and hazardous wastes. **Solid waste management (integrated waste management)** encompasses all approaches to managing the constantly accumulating solid waste, including

Hazardous waste a solid waste or combination of solid wastes that is dangerous to human health or the environment

Resource Conservation and Recovery Act of 1976 (RCRA) the federal law that sets forth guidelines for the proper handling and disposal of hazardous wastes

Solid waste management (integrated waste management) the collection, transportation, and disposal of solid waste

---

BOX 14.5   Electronic Waste

As we become more dependent on electronic products to make our lives more convenient, we also generate a vast amount of electronic waste (e-waste) as we dispose of used and obsolete products. Electronic waste makes up about 1–2% of total municipal solid waste production. On average, a U.S. household uses 28 electronic devices, such as computers, televisions, and mobile devices.

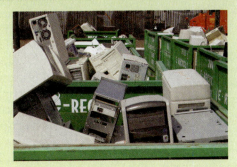
© Michael ledray/Shutterstock

Why Is e-Waste Hazardous?

e-Waste can contain toxic heavy metals, such as lead, mercury, chromium, cadmium, mercury, beryllium, nickel, and zinc, and brominated flame retardants. These toxic substances require special handling at the end of their lives. When electronics are not properly disposed of or recycled, these toxic materials can be released into the environment through landfill leachate or incinerator ash—both potential pathways to pollution that can negatively affect the health of nearby communities.

What Should I Do with Used and Obsolete Electronic Products?

Local facilities may recycle electronic products, thus promoting the safe management of hazardous components and supporting the recovery and reuse of recyclable materials. Another option is recycling electronic products by donating them for reuse by others. This extends the life of the products and keeps them out of the waste stream for a longer period of time. To learn more, visit www.epa.gov/recycle/electronics-donation-and-recycling.

Data from U.S. Environmental Protection Agency. (2023). *Basic information about electronics stewardship.* https://www.epa.gov/smm-electronics/basic-information-about-electronics-stewardship

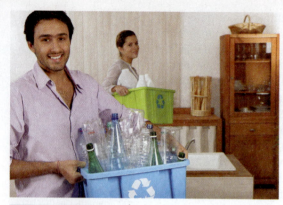

FIGURE 14.15   Recycling involves collecting, sorting, and processing materials to manufacture new products that prevent waste, pollution, and use of virgin natural resources.

© Phovoir/Shutterstock

Source reduction a waste management approach involving the reduction or elimination of the use of materials that produce an accumulation of solid waste

Recycling the collecting, sorting, and processing of materials that would otherwise be considered waste into raw materials for manufacturing new products, and the subsequent use of those new products

Composting the natural, aerobic biodegradation of organic plant and animal matter to compost

Sanitary landfills waste disposal sites on land suited for this purpose and on which waste is spread in thin layers, compacted, and covered with a fresh layer of clay or plastic foam each day

Leachates liquids created when water mixes with wastes and removes soluble constituents from them by percolation

Combustion (incineration) the burning of solid wastes

collection, source reduction, product reuse and recycling, treatment, and disposal. Of these approaches, the most desirable is **source reduction**. Examples of waste source reduction include not buying or using such throwaway products as paper towels and disposable diapers and minimizing packaging associated with groceries and carryout foods. The second-best approach to waste management is to reuse or recycle the waste. **Recycling** is the collecting, sorting, and processing of materials that would otherwise be considered waste into raw materials that can be used to manufacture new products (see **Figure 14.15**). Recycling diverts items, such as paper, glass, plastic, and metals, from the waste stream and conserves sanitary landfill space. The United States currently recycles or composts about 32.1% of its MSW.[66] Although progress has been made, the recycling rate in the United States is far below the rates of some European countries. Germany, for example, recycles or composts 68% of its household solid waste.[69] **Composting** is a form of recycling that can be done easily at home because it does not require special knowledge or equipment. In composting, yard waste and food wastes are recycled through a natural process of aerobic biodegradation during which micro-organisms convert organic plant and animal matter into compost that can be used as a mulch or fertilizer. Composting conserves precious landfill space.

Once created, MSW that cannot be reused or recycled must be disposed of. The currently acceptable methods of disposal are sanitary landfills or combustion (incineration). At present, 50% of municipal solid waste is placed in **sanitary landfills**, sites issued operating permits that are judged suitable for in-ground disposal of solid waste.[70] In 2023, there were 1,278 permitted landfills.[70] These must be located and constructed so that **leachates**, that is, liquids that drain from wastes to the bottom of a landfill, do not contaminate the underlying groundwater (see **Figure 14.16**). Despite these precautions, according to the EPA, all landfills will eventually leak.

Another concern with landfills is the accumulation of dangerous amounts of methane gas (a greenhouse gas) created by the anaerobic decomposition of refuse. In some cases, explosions have occurred when the methane gas was ignited. Although some communities have systems in place to harness the methane gas and use it as an energy source, only a small minority of landfills operating today collect gases. It has been estimated that landfills are responsible for 14.3% of all methane emissions in the United States.[71]

Nobody wants to live next to a sanitary landfill, even a properly operating one. For this reason, it is exceedingly difficult to establish new landfills in areas where they are needed most. As existing landfill space becomes more restricted, demand will drive up the cost of MSW disposal. This has led to an increased interest in combustion as an alternative to MSW waste disposal.

Combustion (incineration), or the burning of wastes, is the second major method of refuse disposal. The passage of the Clean Air Act of 1970 severely restricted the rights of individuals and municipalities to burn refuse because most could not comply with the strict emission standards. About 12% of all municipal waste is combusted.[66] Of these incinerators, 75 are waste-to-energy incinerators or energy recovery plants; that is, they are able to convert some of the heat generated from the incineration process into steam and electricity.[72] Combustion reduces the weight and volume of solid waste by as much as 75 and 85%, respectively.[72] The resulting waste, if nontoxic, will take up less sanitary landfill space, and because an incinerator can be located closer to the source of the solid waste, transportation costs may be less than for landfills. However, there are disadvantages: (1) startup costs are high because large commercial incinerators are expensive; (2) nitrogen oxides, sulfur dioxide, and other toxic air pollutants are produced; and (3) the ash may be too toxic to place in a sanitary landfill. Regular testing is required to ensure that residual ash is nonhazardous before it is placed in a landfill.

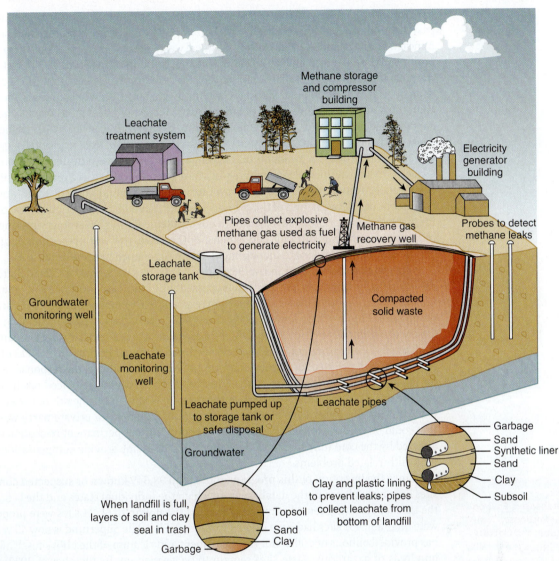

FIGURE 14.16   A state-of-the-art sanitary landfill

Data from Miller, G. T. (2008). Living in the environment: Principles, connections, and solutions (16th ed.). Brooks/Cole; Solid Waste Authority of Central Ohio. SWACO Sanitary Landfill Poster.

Managing Our Hazardous Waste

RCRA established a system for controlling hazardous waste from the time it is generated until its disposal (called cradle-to-grave regulation) and mandated strict controls over the treatment, storage, and disposal of hazardous waste. More than 400 substances are listed on the EPA's hazardous waste list. The EPA list includes neither radioactive wastes, which are controlled by the Nuclear Regulatory Commission, nor biomedical wastes, which are regulated by the individual states. The EPA Office of Solid Waste has the responsibility to oversee the management of hazardous waste, including its treatment, storage, and disposal. More than 37.5 million tons of hazardous waste were generated in United States in 2021.[73] Roughly 15 methods of hazardous waste management are overseen and regulated by the EPA. The single most common method used is deep well or underground injection, which is used for disposal of about 50% of hazardous waste.[73] Most of these wells are found in the states of Texas and Florida. The remaining 50% of hazardous waste is managed by various methods, such as special landfills, impoundment, recycling, and incineration.

Managing present and future hazardous wastes is one issue; dealing with the inappropriate past disposal of hazardous wastes is another. Leaking underground storage tanks, abandoned mine lands, and abandoned hazardous chemical waste sites all present serious threats to human health and the environment (see **Box 14.6**). An underground storage tank (UST) system includes the tank, underground connected piping, and any containment system that stores either petroleum or certain hazardous substances. Gasoline leaking from service stations is one of the most common sources of groundwater pollution. Just 1.5 cups of leaking hazardous chemicals can contaminate more than 1 million gallons of groundwater. Because nearly 102 million U.S. residents get their water from a community water system derived at least in part from groundwater, and 43 million more U.S. residents drink from private wells, groundwater pollution is a serious concern.[74] Many municipal and private wells have been shut down as a result of contamination. Additionally, fumes and vapors can travel beneath the ground and collect in areas, such as basements, utility vaults, and parking garages, where they can pose a serious threat of explosion, fire, asphyxiation, or other adverse health effects. Remediating hazardous substances released into the subsurface, is difficult and expensive; therefore, the best prevention of groundwater contamination is appropriate management and maintenance to prevent releases.

The primary participant in the cleanup of hazardous waste in the United States has been the federal government. In 1980, Congress passed the **Comprehensive Environmental Response, Compensation, and Liability Act (CERCLA)** in response to the public's demand to clean up leaking dump sites. This law, also known as the *Superfund*, created a tax on the chemical and petrochemical industries to clean up abandoned hazardous waste sites that might endanger human health and the environment. CERCLA established a National Priority List (NPL) of hazardous waste sites and provided funds for remediation. Whenever possible, the responsible parties pay for those cleanups instead of using the Superfund. These sites were placed on the list after an assessment in order of priority based on the threat posed to public health or the environment. Once on the NPL, sites were eligible for Superfund dollars if no private party was identified that could be used for remediation and for the temporary or permanent relocation of residents affected by the contaminated sites. The Superfund does not provide compensation to victims for health-related problems.

Since the inception of this program, more than 98,649 known or suspected contaminated sites have been placed in the database from which the individual states and the U.S. EPA select the sites for requiring remediation. At the end of fiscal year 2022, 24 sites were proposed, 1,334 were final, and 452 sites had been deleted from the NPL.[75] The Superfund is now 43 years old and has provided billions of dollars for the assessment and cleanup of the NPL sites. Unfortunately, hundreds of hazardous waste sites remain to be cleaned up. By October of 2022, more than $5.2 billion had been disbursed or obligated for Superfund cleanups.[75] EPA also performs 5-year reviews of remediated properties to ensure that remedies continue to protect communities.[75]

Brownfields

Another problem is the more than 450,000 abandoned industrial plants, factories, commercial worksites, junkyards, and gas stations. These so-called **brownfields** are contaminated properties where expansion, redevelopment, or reuse may be complicated by the presence or potential

Comprehensive Environmental Response, Compensation, and Liability Act (CERCLA) the federal law (known as the Superfund) created to clean up abandoned hazardous waste sites

Brownfields property where reuse is complicated by the presence of hazardous substances from prior use

---

BOX 14.6   Brownfields, Superfund Sites, and Underground Storage Tanks in Your Area

Search the EPA website (https://enviro.epa.gov/) for brownfields, Superfund sites, USTs, and abandoned mine lands and find the following maps:

- Superfund cleanup sites
- Brownfields
- Toxic release inventory (TRI explorer)

Based on the maps you found, answer the following questions:

1. What types of sites and how many have you found in your area of residence?
2. What specific contaminants of concern are at these sites?
3. Have they been cleaned up?
4. Reflect on your findings and evaluate what this means for the health of your community.

presence of a hazardous substance, pollutant, or contaminant that can pose a threat to human health.[76] Cleaning up and reinvesting in these properties take development pressures off undeveloped open land, increase local tax bases, facilitate job growth, and improve and protect both the environment and human health.

Lead and Other Heavy Metals

Among the more ubiquitous and harmful environmental hazards are heavy metals, such as lead, mercury, cadmium, chromium, and arsenic. They often contaminate well water and are ingested by unsuspecting people. Heavy metals occur naturally throughout the environment and many are also used in industrial processes or products. For example, **lead** is used in batteries, pipe, solder, paint, and plastic pigments, and, until 1986, in gasoline. EPA regulates disposal of heavy metals by industry or businesses under RCRA.

Because of its past widespread use, lead can be found in soil, household dust, air, paint, old painted toys and furniture, water pipes made of lead or soldered with lead, foods and liquids stored in lead crystal or lead-based porcelain, or contaminated private wells. In 2021, it was estimated that there were approximately 34.6 million housing units in the United States that still contain dangerous levels of lead-based paint, and that 3.3 million of these dwellings are homes to children.[77] Families living in older homes with children should have their homes tested for lead paint. Most local health departments provide this service.

The EPA has estimated that about 40 million Americans who live in homes built before 1930 (when copper began to replace lead in water pipes) are drinking water containing more than the legally permissible level of lead (15 parts per billion [ppb]). Those who are at greatest risk of lead poisoning are young children, who may inadvertently ingest lead paint, but adults can be poisoned, too. It is estimated that as much as 50% of the lead ingested by young children is absorbed, compared with only 1% in adults.[78] Absorption by the fetus in a pregnant woman is expected to be equivalent to the blood lead level (BLL) in the mother.[79]

The health problems from exposure to lead include anemia, birth defects, bone damage, depression of neurological and psychological functions, kidney damage, learning disabilities, miscarriages, and sterility.[80] Since 1976, the median BLL in children has decreased from 15 μg/dL to 0.07 μg/dL, a decrease of 95%.[81] Between 1997 and 2018, the percentage of children under 6 years of age with elevated blood lead levels (≥10 μg/dL) declined from 7.61% to 0.4% of those tested.[82] Unfortunately, disparities remain among racial and ethnic groups. The children with the highest blood lead levels are non-Hispanic Black children.[77] The major source of lead exposure for these children is dust and chips of lead paint in their homes (see **Figure 14.17**). However, increased attention is being given to exposure to high lead levels in household water due to older infrastructure or inadequate water treatment (see **Box 14.7**). Unlike children, the major source of lead intake for adults is occupational exposure through inhalation.

The solution to preventing lead poisoning includes education, regulation, and prudent behavior. Educational efforts to inform people of the dangers of lead in paint have been in effect for a number of years, and for the most part they seem to have been well received, although significant effort is required to reach the *Healthy People 2030* objective to reduce BLLs in the general population to 1.74 μg/dL.[83] Over 500,000 children under 5 years of age are estimated to have BLLs greater than the action level of 3.5 μg/dL. In 2021, CDC lowered the action level.[84]

Controlling Vectorborne Diseases

Standing water, including runoff water from overflowing septic systems or overloaded sewer systems, and improperly handled solid waste are more than unsavory sights. They provide

Lead a naturally occurring mineral element found throughout the environment and used in large quantities for industrial products, including batteries, pipes, solder, paints, and pigments

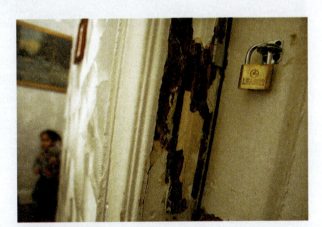

FIGURE 14.17   Lead poisoning from paint dust continues to be a problem in the United States.

© Spencer Platt/Getty Images News/Getty Images

BOX 14.7 Lead in Drinking Water in Flint, Michigan

Lead piping that was installed in the early twentieth century can pose a health threat due to mismanagement of water supplies by municipal governments that may result in harmful consequences, not only in terms of lead exposure to children but to the infrastructure that provides drinking water to a community.

In 2014, the water supply for Flint, Michigan, was changed from Lake Huron to a less expensive option: the Flint River. This change would likely not have been noticeable except for the fact that a corrosion inhibitor, which cost $80 to $100 per day, was not added to the Flint River water as part of the required treatment to ensure that the water was safe to distribute to the community. This oversight resulted in water that was corrosive to the iron and lead pipes of the distribution system. As a result, household water in Flint became discolored, foul-smelling, and distasteful, and contained high levels of lead. Unbelievably, local and state officials reassured the public often that the water was safe to drink.

From 1998 to 2014, BLLs ≥5 μg/dL for children in Flint decreased from greater than 40% to 2.2%. In 2015, a preliminary study concluded that BLLs in Flint increased by approximately 2% for all children. In one area, however, lead levels exceeded 13,000 ppb in some homes, and BLLs increased by approximately 6.6%. Although the water supply no longer comes from the Flint River, the damage to the piping will continue to contaminate the water, even properly treated water, until it is replaced. In this case, the lead exposure and damage to infrastructure was entirely preventable. The BLLs for children in Flint peaked in 2015 at 3.7% and has continued to decrease.

Data from Hanna-Attisha, M., LaChance, J., Sadler, R. C., & Schnepp, A. C. (2016). Elevated blood lead levels in children associated with the flint drinking water crisis: A spatial analysis of risk and public health response. American Journal of Public Health, 106(2), 283–290. Doi: 10.2105/AJPH.2015.303003; Sanburn, J. (2016, February 1). The toxic tap: How a disastrous chain of events corroded Flint's water system—and the public trust. Time, 14 (online); Gómez, H., Borgialli, D., Sharman, M., Shah, K., Scolpino, A., Oleske, J., & Bogden, J. (2018). Blood lead levels of children in Flint, Michigan: 2006–2016. The Journal of Pediatrics, 197, 158–164.

Vector a living organism, usually an insect or other arthropod that can transmit a communicable disease agent to a susceptible host (e.g., a mosquito or tick)

Vectorborne disease outbreak (VBDO) an occurrence of an unexpectedly large number of cases of disease caused by an agent transmitted by insects or other arthropods

a habitat for, and support the proliferation of, disease vectors. As discussed earlier, a **vector** is a living organism, usually an insect or other arthropod, which transmits microscopic disease agents to susceptible hosts. Examples of vectors and the diseases they transmit include mosquitoes, fleas, lice, and ticks (see **Table 14.5**).

Mosquito larvae require standing water in which to complete their development. The improper handling of wastewater or inadequate drainage of rainwater provides an ideal habitat for mosquitoes and increases the risk for a **vectorborne disease outbreak (VBDO)**. Of particular concern in this regard is the northern house mosquito, *Culex pipiens* (see Figure 14.10). *Culex pipiens* is the most important vector of St. Louis encephalitis (SLE) in the eastern United States. In California, SLE virus is transmitted by another mosquito species, *Culex tarsalis*, which proliferates in mismanaged irrigation water. SLE is a disease to which the elderly are particularly susceptible. Those at greatest risk live in unscreened houses without air conditioning.

TABLE 14.5 Vectorborne Biological Hazards

Hazard	Agent	Vector	Disease
Virus	SLE virus	Mosquito	St. Louis encephalitis
	LaCrosse	Mosquito	LaCrosse encephalitis
	Chikungunya virus	Mosquito	Chikungunya virus
	West Nile virus	Mosquito	West Nile fever, encephalitis, or meningitis
	Zika virus	Mosquito	Zika virus
Rickettsiae	*Rickettsia typhi*	Flea	Murine typhus
	Rickettsia rickettsii	Tick	Rocky Mountain spotted fever
	Ehrlichia chaffeensis	Tick	Ehrlichiosis
Bacteria	*Yersinia pestis*	Flea	Bubonic plague
	Borrelia burgdorferi	Tick	Lyme disease
Protozoa	*Plasmodium* spp.	Mosquito	Malaria

Data from Heymann, D. L. (Ed.). (2015). *Control of communicable diseases manual* (20th ed.). American Public Health Association; Centers for Disease Control and Prevention, Division of Vector-Borne Diseases (2015). West Nile virus. Available at http://www.cdc.gov/westnile/

Culex pipiens also transmits West Nile virus (WNV), which causes West Nile fever, West Nile encephalitis, and West Nile meningitis. The latter two are severe forms of the disease that affect the nervous system. *Encephalitis* refers to an inflammation of the brain; *meningitis* is an inflammation of the membrane surrounding the brain and spinal cord. WNV first appeared in New York in 1999, where it caused 62 human cases of disease, including seven deaths.[85] The virus quickly spread westward until it became established throughout the country. The occurrence of West Nile cases varies from year to year. Since 1999, an average number of 2,357 cases and 116 deaths have occurred annually.[86] The lowest incidence of cases and deaths occurred in 2000 with 21 and 2, respectively. However, the highest incidences occurred in different years, with 9,862 cases in 2003 and with 286 deaths in 2012.[87]

Another species of mosquito that thrives on environmental mismanagement in the north-central and eastern United States is the eastern tree-hole mosquito, *Aedes triseriatus*. Whereas the natural habitat for this mosquito is tree holes, it flourishes in water held in discarded automobile and truck tires. It is estimated that 264 million used tires are generated annually in the United States, of which 90.8% are consumed for beneficial use or disposed of in legal landfills. However, this results in 24 million tires being illegally dumped or added to the environment each year.[88] In the eastern United States, *A. triseriatus* transmits LaCrosse encephalitis, an arbovirus that produces a serious and sometimes fatal disease in children.

C. pipiens and *A. triseriatus* are only two of several hundred species of mosquitoes that are present in the United States. Because we have become a global economy, new exotic pest species are constantly being introduced into our country. Two of these are the Asian tiger mosquito, *Aedes albopictus*, first discovered in Texas in 1985[88] and *Aedes japonicus*, first detected in 1998.[89] Although no human cases of disease have been traced directly to either of these vectors in the United States, laboratory studies indicate that both can transmit pathogenic viruses.

Aedes aegypti and *Aedes albopictus* are commonly involved in the transmission of the Chikungunya virus and Zika virus. Chikungunya infections were initially identified in the United States in 2006. Between 2006 and 2013, an average of 28 persons per year were identified as infected.[90] In 2014, a peak occurred in the incidence of the disease as 7,521 cases were reported from U.S. states and territories.[90] Post-2014, the incidence of disease has declined to 81 cases reported in 2022, with an average of 278 cases from 2015 through 2022.[90] The Zika virus, a nationally notifiable disease, typically results in mild symptoms. However, reports from South America in 2016 potentially linked the virus to incidents of Guillain-Barré syndrome and birth defects in babies born to women who contracted the disease while pregnant.[91]

Federal, state, and local governments all have units whose primary responsibility is the prevention and control of vectorborne diseases. At the federal level, the lead agency is the CDC's Division of Vector-Borne Diseases (DVBD), a unit of the National Center for Emerging and Zoonotic Infectious Diseases (NCEZID). The DVBD conducts and funds research on vectorborne diseases, maintains surveillance of vectorborne diseases, assists states in investigating vectorborne disease outbreaks, and, in some cases, assists other countries with vectorborne problems. Most state departments of health also have offices or labs that maintain vectorborne disease surveillance programs and provide expertise to local health departments, which have the primary task of reducing mosquito populations and preventing disease transmission. Most of us have seen county or district mosquito abatement workers inspecting or treating standing water or driving through our neighborhood with a mosquito sprayer or fogger. Although most of us appreciate these efforts to protect our health and our comfort, it is discouraging to think that despite the millions of dollars spent on mosquito control in communities across the country, many cases of mosquito-borne diseases are reported annually. Proper land, solid waste, and wastewater management; mosquito control efforts; the promotion of personal protection against mosquito bites; and active surveillance for vectorborne diseases are all important defenses against mosquito-borne disease outbreaks.

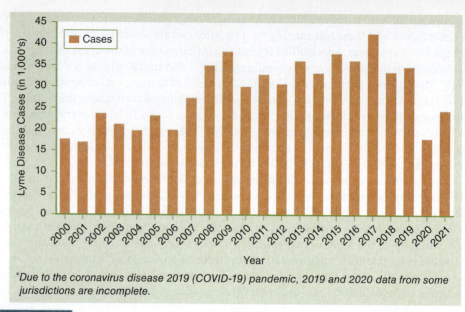

*Due to the coronavirus disease 2019 (COVID-19) pandemic, 2019 and 2020 data from some jurisdictions are incomplete.

FIGURE 14.18 Number of reported cases of Lyme disease in the United States from 2000 to 2021.

Data from Centers for Disease Control and Prevention. (2022). *Lyme disease Surveillance data.* Available at https://www.cdc.gov/lyme/data-research/facts-stats/surveillance-data-1.html

The number one vectorborne disease in the United States is not a mosquito-borne disease, but a tick-borne disease, Lyme disease. In 2021, more than 24,610 confirmed and probable cases of Lyme disease were reported to the CDC (see **Figure 14.18**).[92] Lyme disease is transmitted by the black-legged tick, *Ixodes scapularis*, a species of tick that flourishes when deer are abundant. During the latter half of the twentieth century, deer populations rapidly increased in the United States through conservation efforts. This resulted in an explosion of populations of the black-legged tick, sometimes called "deer tick." The tick transmits the bacterial spirochete *Borrelia burgdorferi*, the cause of Lyme disease. It is important to note that Lyme disease is a bigger problem in some regions of the country. For example, of the 10 states reporting the highest incidences of Lyme disease in 2021, seven were in the east. Listed in order, beginning with the highest incidence, the 10 states were: New Jersey, New York, Pennsylvania, Wisconsin, Minnesota, West Virginia, Maine, Rhode Island, Maryland, and Michigan.[93]

Because there is no vaccine for Lyme disease, and community tick control is virtually nonexistent, personal protection is the best defense. Health departments often remind citizens to take the following precautions: (1) avoid entering tick-infested areas when possible; these are usually wooded and bushy areas with high grass and a lot of leaf litter; (2) if entering an area possibly infested with ticks, dress appropriately—wear long pants and tuck them into your socks and wear a long-sleeved shirt; (3) apply a tick repellent; (4) examine yourself and family members for ticks after leaving the area; and (5) carefully remove any ticks found with a pair of tweezers. Tick control efforts include using landscaping techniques that discourage ticks—reduce leaf litter and tall grass, and establish a litter-free (and tick-free) border around the perimeter of the yard. Keep the lawn short and, if using acaricides, do so in accordance with instructions on the label.

Improper management of waste—such as occurs at open dumps, ill-managed landfills, and urban slums—fosters the expansion of rat and mouse populations. These rodents are hosts for fleas that transmit murine typhus, a rickettsial disease characterized by headache, fever, and rash. The closing of most of the open dumps has relegated murine typhus to the status of an uncommon disease in the United States, but improper MSW management could provide an environment conducive to murine typhus transmission.

Natural Hazards

A **natural hazard** is a naturally occurring phenomenon or event that produces/releases energy in amounts that exceed human endurance, causing injury, disease, or death. Examples include naturally occurring radiation, geologic activity (earthquakes and volcanoes), and severe weather-driven events (tornados, hurricanes, and floods). When a natural hazard involves human injuries and deaths, it is often termed a **natural disaster**.

Radiation

Radiation is the process in which energy is emitted as particles or waves. Heat, sound, and visible light are examples of long-wavelength, low-energy radiation. High-energy (ionizing) radiation is radiation with shorter wavelengths, such as ultraviolet (UV) light, X-rays, and gamma rays, or particles, such as alpha or beta particles (see **Box 14.8**). High-energy **ionizing radiation** is released when atoms are split or naturally decay from a less-stable to a more-stable form. This type of radiation has enough energy to knock electrons out of orbit and break chemical bonds among molecules in living cells and tissues. Mild tissue damage may be able to be repaired, but if the damage is too severe or widespread, it cannot be repaired and is manifested as radiation burns, radiation sickness, or both. Radiation sickness includes nausea, weakness, hair loss, skin burns, diminished organ function, premature aging, cancer, or even death. The amount of radiation and the duration of exposure affect the severity of the injury or illness.

Radiation from Natural Sources

Radiation arises from both natural and human-made sources. Sources of natural radiation are extraterrestrial (outer space and the Sun) or terrestrial (radioactive minerals emanating from the Earth). The radiation we receive from the Sun is considerable. Sunshine comprises energy in many wavelengths, including visible light, heat, and **ultraviolet (UV) radiation**. UV radiation includes energy at wavelengths between 10 and 400 nanometers (nm). UV radiation between 290 and 330 nanometers, called UV-B, causes the most harm to humans.

> **Natural hazard** a naturally occurring phenomenon or event that produces or releases energy in amounts that exceed human endurance, causing injury, disease, or death (such as radiation, earthquakes, tsunamis, volcanic eruptions, hurricanes, tornados, and floods)
>
> **Natural disaster** a natural hazard that results in substantial loss of life or property
>
> **Radiation** a process in which energy is emitted as particles or waves
>
> **Ionizing radiation** high-energy radiation that can knock an electron out of orbit, creating an ion, and can thereby damage living cells and tissues (includes UV radiation, gamma rays, X-rays, alpha and beta particles)
>
> **Ultraviolet (UV) radiation** radiant energy with wavelengths of 10 to 400 nanometers

---

BOX 14.8   About the Electromagnetic Spectrum

Electromagnetic radiation emitted from different sources has characteristic wavelengths. Taken together, these types of radiation make up the electromagnetic spectrum, which ranges from the very-long-wavelength radiation of power lines (thousands of meters) to the very-short-wavelength cosmic radiation that originates in outer space (less than one-trillionth of a meter).

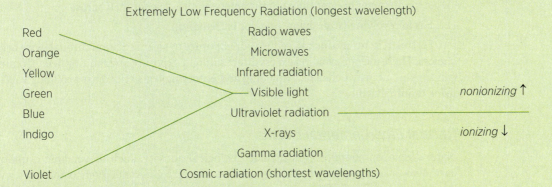

Extremely Low Frequency Radiation (longest wavelength)

Red	Radio waves
Orange	Microwaves
Yellow	Infrared radiation
Green	Visible light — *nonionizing* ↑
Blue	Ultraviolet radiation
Indigo	X-rays — *ionizing* ↓
	Gamma radiation
Violet	Cosmic radiation (shortest wavelengths)

In the middle of the electromagnetic spectrum, infrared and ultraviolet radiation bracket the familiar spectrum of visible light. Sunlight is made up of infrared radiation, visible light, and ultraviolet radiation. Infrared radiation is simply heat; any object that is warmer than its surroundings gives off infrared radiation.

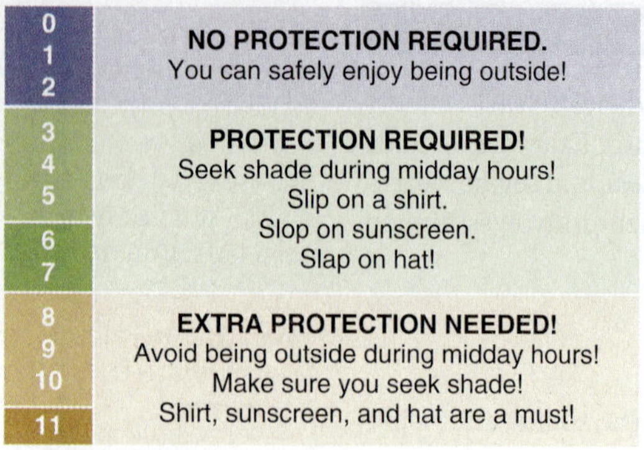

FIGURE 14.19 UV index scale.

Reproduced with permission of World Health Organization. (2023). "UV Index." Available at https://www.who.int/news-room /questions-and-answers/item/radiation-the-ultraviolet-(uv)-index

Much of the UV radiation emanating from the Sun is screened out by the layer of ozone in the stratosphere. In recent years, with the erosion of the ozone layer, the quantity of UV-B radiation reaching the Earth has been increasing.[94] Each year, more than 1 million new cases of skin cancer are reported in the United States. The incidence rate of skin cancer in 2023 was reported to be stabilizing for those before 50 years of age, but increasing by 1% per year for those over 50 years of age.[95] The vast majority of these cases are the highly curable basal cell and squamous cell carcinomas, the most common forms of cancer. The most serious and least common skin cancer is malignant melanoma. The American Cancer Society estimated that more than 186,680 cases of melanoma would be diagnosed and about 7,990 patients died from this disease in 2023. This type of skin cancer is the most dangerous because of its ability to grow and spread quickly. However, like the other skin cancers, melanoma is curable if discovered and treated early.[95]

Skin cancer morbidity and mortality rates can be lowered by reducing one's exposure to UV radiation and by early detection and treatment. One can reduce the risk of exposure by staying out of direct sunlight or by covering the skin with clothing or commercial sunscreens. Sunscreens work by absorbing, reflecting, or scattering ultraviolet light, thereby reducing the amount that reaches the skin. To reduce exposure to UV radiation, individuals can also find out the UV index for a specific day through the weather forecast on the Internet or visit EPA's Sun Safety website.[96] The UV index is reported on a scale of 1 (low danger) to 11 (extreme danger; see **Figure 14.19**). The EPA also issues UV alerts, which are warnings when the level of solar radiation in a particular area is predicted to be unusually high. Obtaining information about the strength of UV radiation is the most important step people can take in protecting their health.

The second way people can protect their health is through early diagnosis and prompt treatment. The key to discovering whether treatment is warranted is to practice monthly skin self-examination. Basal and squamous cell carcinomas often appear as a pale, waxlike, peely nodule or a red, scaly, sharply outlined patch. A physician should check either of these abnormalities or the sudden change in a mole's appearance. Melanomas often appear first as small mole-like growths. The simple ABCDE rule from the American Cancer Society outlines warning signs of melanoma.[97]

A. is for asymmetry (half of the mole does not match the other half).

B. is for border irregularity (the edges are ragged, notched, or blurred).

C. is for color (the pigmentation is not uniform).

D. is for diameter greater than 6 millimeters or one-quarter inch across.

E. E is for evolving (size, shape, or color is changing).

Fortunately, most of us can reduce our exposure to solar radiation through wise behavioral choices. These include avoiding excess direct sunlight exposure and tanning beds. Communities can support healthy behavior by passing and enforcing legislation that prohibits youths from using tanning facilities.

Natural Environmental Events

Natural environmental events include geological activity, such as volcanic eruptions and earthquakes (and resulting tsunamis), and weather-driven events, such as tornados, cyclones, hurricanes, and floods. These events can result in serious physical and psychological health consequences for humans. Examples of recent natural disasters include the geological activity resulting in the 2004 tsunami that struck Southeast Asia, including Thailand and Indonesia, and the earthquakes that struck Haiti and Chile in 2010; and the weather-driven events, such as tornados like the one that struck Joplin, Missouri, in 2012 and hurricanes, such as Hurricane Katrina (2005) and Hurricane Maria (2017; see **Figure 14.20**).

In each of these natural disasters, health concerns included not only the immediate loss of life and destruction of homes and businesses but also the unavailability of clean water, food, and sanitation. Also, the loss of loved ones left many survivors feeling sad, depressed, and in need of social services.

Longer-term consequences from such events usually continue for days or months afterward. For example, volcanic eruptions that release large quantities of ash into the atmosphere are responsible for the acute respiratory symptoms commonly reported by people during and after ash falls, including nasal irritation and discharge (runny noses), throat irritation and sore throat, coughing, and uncomfortable breathing. People with pre-existing conditions can develop severe bronchitis, shortness of breath, wheezing, and coughing. Similarly, flooded homes can become contaminated with high levels of mold, which may lead to respiratory problems. Flooding can also produce prodigious numbers of mosquitoes, resulting in outbreaks of vectorborne diseases, including encephalitis and malaria.

After a natural disaster, because of the remaining physical, biological, sociological, and psychological conditions, a variety of needs may exist, including clean water, food, shelter, health care, and clothing. Failure of a community, state, or nation to provide for these needs in an efficient and effective manner can exacerbate the extent of human suffering.

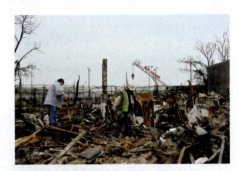

FIGURE 14.20 Natural disasters, such as earthquakes, tsunamis, hurricanes, tornadoes, and floods, can result in substantial loss of life and property.

© FashionStock.com/Shutterstock

Complex Disasters or Emergency

A **complex disaster** or emergency can result when a natural disaster further escalates an ongoing crisis, such as a civil war, or causes a technological disaster. A complex disaster can result from several different hazards and include a combination of natural and human-made causes.[98] An example of a complex disaster was the Tohoku earthquake in 2011, which caused the tsunami that resulted in the destruction of the Fukushima Daiichi Nuclear Power Plant. The damage to the Fukushima Daiichi facility resulted in widespread radioactive contamination and displacement of the nearby populations. Hazardous materials, such as radioactive substances, not only cause physical damage and add to the needs resulting from the natural disaster but they also result in psychological, sociological, and economic consequences that are not easily overcome.

Radiation from Human-Made Sources

Sources of human-made radiation are those associated with medical and dental procedures, such as X-rays, nuclear medicine diagnoses, and radiation therapy; consumer products, such as smoke detectors, television and computer screens; and nuclear energy and weaponry. Most would agree that most of radiation used for medical and dental purposes is beneficially justifiable.

However, there is less agreement about the cost–benefit question in the case of nuclear power plants. The advantages and disadvantages of nuclear power are often discussed. As of 2020, 94 operating nuclear power stations currently generate about 20% of our nation's total electricity and fit comfortably into the nation's electricity grid.[99] They do this while producing very little air pollution. However, these facilities produce radioactive waste, pose significant environmental and human health risks should failure occur, and are costly to build, operate, and decommission. The contamination of the environment caused by a release of nuclear materials due to an accident is long lasting because the half-life of uranium is measured in the billions of years and necessitates expensive remediation or abandonment of the contaminated areas.

The health effects that have resulted from the 1986 meltdown of the nuclear facility at Chernobyl, in Ukraine, are staggering. Hundreds of thousands of people, including many children, were exposed to high levels of radiation. A large increase in the incidence of thyroid

Complex disaster a natural disaster that further escalates an ongoing crisis or causes a technological disaster, resulting in communities being affected by the consequences of a combination of natural and human-made hazards

cancer has occurred among people who were young children or adolescents at the time of the disaster. The incidence of leukemia doubled in those who experienced high doses of radiation, and there have been an estimated 4,000 additional cancer deaths in the highest exposed groups. Other concerns are cataracts, cardiovascular disease, mental health effects, and reproductive and hereditary effects.[100] In 2011, an earthquake and tsunami led to a release of radioactive material from the Fukushima Daiichi nuclear power station. Review of data available in 2013 by the United Nations Scientific Committee on the Effects of Atomic Radiation estimated that compared with baseline risk, a general radiation-related increase in the incidence of cancer of those exposed in the Fukushima accident is not expected to be discernible.[101] A contributing factor may be the prompt evacuation of residents resulting in a lower exposure. It will take many years to establish the totality of health issues that result from this exposure, including those impacts on psychological and social well-being.

Psychological and Sociological Hazards

Living around other people exposes us to psychological and sociological hazards that can affect our health. Among these are overpopulation and crowding, hate crimes, wars, and acts of terrorism. Many of these hazards can be related directly or indirectly to population growth.

Population Growth

Population growth can be attributed to three factors—birth rate, death rate, and migration. In considering world population growth, migration is not a factor, so that when the birth rate and death rate are equal, population growth is zero. When the birth rate exceeds the death rate, the population size increases. Increases in population size and per capita consumption result in an ever-increasing environmental impact. The maximum population that can be supported by available resources (air, water, shelter, etc.) is referred to as the **carrying capacity** of the environment.[102]

The world's population now exceeds 8 billion. During the past three decades, the rate of world population growth has begun to decline (see **Figure 14.21**). Although the population growth rate is projected to continue to decline, the world population is forecast to grow to 10 billion by the end of the twenty-first century[103] (see **Figure 14.22**).

Approximately 80% of the world's population lives in the world's less-developed countries (LDCs), and virtually all of the world's population increase between now and 2050 will occur in these countries.[103,104] The largest percentage of growth during the next 40 years (2010–2050) is expected to occur in Africa and Asia. Whereas the growth rate remains high for LDCs as a whole, fertility rates are decreasing in these regions, and the growth rate for more-developed countries (MDCs) has fallen. In fact, in many MDCs, fertility rates are below replacement levels (the level at which children born would just replace those persons lost to mortality). In 2020, the rate of population growth fell below 1% per year. This is the first time since 1950, and is expected to continue to slow throughout this century.[103]

Although exponential world population growth is no longer occurring in absolute terms, world population growth continues to be substantial, and the world's population is growing at a rate that is unsustainable if we wish to maintain the quality of life and health we enjoy today. The ramifications of overpopulation include the prospects of climate change, acid rain, vast waste landfills, increasing crime rates, increasing vulnerability to epidemics and pandemics, smog, exhaustion of usable water supplies, contamination of soils and groundwater, degradation of arable land, and growing international tensions, and complex emergencies. Each year, humans degrade millions of acres of arable land.[105] Also, there will be a dwindling of natural resources available for energy, housing, and living space. Since 1950, the urban population has more than tripled. It is estimated that 55% of the current population is located in urban areas.[106] In 1975, there were only five megacities (cities of more than 10 million residents) in the world; now there are 33.[106,107] By 2030, there will be 43 megacities accounting for 9% of the

Carrying capacity the maximum population of a particular species that a given habitat can support over a given period of time

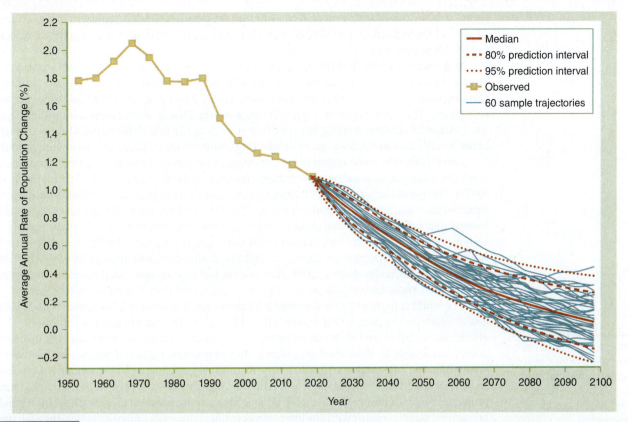

FIGURE 14.21   World population growth rate between 1950 and 2100.

Data from United Nations, Department of Economic and Social Affairs. (2022). Probabilistic projection of average annual rate of population change by country or area, 2022-2100 (percentage). Available at https://population.un.org/wpp/Download/Files/2_Indicators%20(Probabilistic)/EXCEL_FILES/2_Population/UN_PPP2022_Output_PopGrowthRate.xlsx

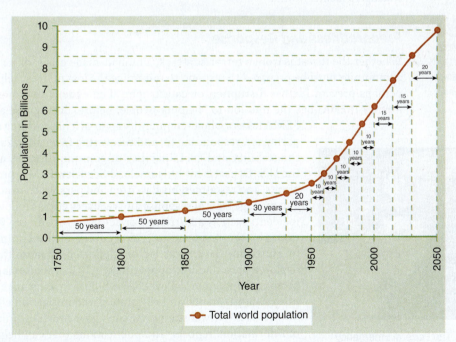

FIGURE 14.22   World population growth in historical perspective between 1800 and 2050, a typical J-shaped curve.

Data from United Nations, Department of Economic and Social Affairs, Population Division. The World at Six Billion. Retrieved November 21, 2023 from https://www.un.org/development /desa/pd/sites/www.un.org.development.desa.pd/files/files/documents/2020/Jan/un_1999_6billion.pdf; United Nations, Department of Economic and Social Affairs. "World Population Prospects, the 2022 Revision. Total population (both sexes combined) by major area, region and country, annually for 1950-2100 (thousands)." Available at November 21, 2023 from https://population.un.org/wpp/Download/Files/1_Indicators%20(Standard)/EXCEL_FILES/2_Population/WPP2022_POP_F01_1_POPULATION_SINGLE_AGE_BOTH_SEXES.xlsx

global urban population or more than 400 million persons.[107] Such rapid growth and large density of humans in one area results in pollution and degradation that negatively affects the health of everyone.

Most experts agree that the world population is approaching the maximum sustainable limit. However, no one knows what the ultimate population size will be, what the ultimate carrying capacity of the Earth is, and how many people it can support. There are some encouraging signs. The world population growth rate was over 2% just 50 years ago; it is now less than 1%.[103] Although there are still great concerns regarding the population growth rates in parts of the Middle East and Africa, some developing countries have succeeded in slowing growth.

The so-called humane means of limiting population growth include (1) various methods of conception control, such as the oral contraceptive pill, physical or chemical barrier methods, or sterilization (tubal ligation and vasectomy); (2) birth control methods, such as intrauterine devices, legalized abortion, and morning-after pills; and (3) social policies, such as financial incentives and societal disincentives for having children. Although some of these methods are unacceptable to certain people, all are proactive solutions to the mounting population problem. The alternative is to allow exponential population growth to continue until it declines naturally, by way of famine, epidemic diseases, and perhaps warfare. Nature's way will require a good deal more environmental deterioration, social disintegration, poverty, and human suffering. The choice is still ours.

The world is more of a global community than ever. The terms *global economy* and *global health* illustrate the notion that we are "all in it together," that we are one big community. Yet ethnic, racial, tribal, and religious differences remain. Whereas some celebrate this diversity, others are unable to shed their prejudices, suspicions, and hatred of peoples unlike themselves. **Bias and hate crimes** are crimes that occur "when offenders choose a victim because of some characteristic—for example, race, ethnicity, or religion—and provide evidence that hate prompted them to commit the crime."[108] When these acts are committed, not against individuals but against populations or with the intention of influencing government or policy, they fall into the realm of terrorism.[109] Terrorism is a sociological hazard because it not only affects entire societies, but it is also a psychological hazard because it produces fear, stress, and hysteria and endangers mental health.

Preparedness and Response

Whether the threat is from a terrorist attack, a human-made crisis, or a natural disaster, a community must be prepared to respond to minimize the loss of lives, help the injured, and perhaps prevent further disruption or catastrophe. The **Federal Emergency Management Agency (FEMA)** has the mission to "helping people, before, during and after disasters."[110]

FEMA takes a whole-community approach in providing resources for preparing for, responding to, and recovering from all hazards that threaten the stability and sustainability of communities. As an agency within the U.S. Department of Homeland Security, FEMA provides programs, grants, and resources, both written and personnel, to achieve its mission and manage federal response and recovery efforts following any national incident, such as a hurricane or act of terrorism (see **Figure 14.23**). For example, the response to and recovery of the communities affected by Hurricane Sandy was led or supported by more than 7,500 FEMA-deployed personnel and approximately 10,000 additional deployed federal personnel and provided over $25.5 billion in assistance to victims, flood insurance payments, and restoration and mitigation efforts.[111,112]

The FEMA website (www.fema.gov) provides links to a vast array of information, reports, and publications that can help individuals and communities prepare for emergencies. FEMA works in partnership with other organizations that are part of the nation's emergency management system, including state and local emergency management agencies, other federal agencies, and numerous nongovernmental organizations, such as the **American Red Cross**.

Bias and hate crimes criminal offenses against a person or property by offenders who are motivated in whole or in part by bias against a race, religion, disability, sexual orientation, ethnicity, gender, or gender identity

Federal Emergency Management Agency (FEMA) the nation's official emergency response agency

American Red Cross a nonprofit, humanitarian organization led by volunteers and guided by its congressional charter that provides relief to victims of disasters

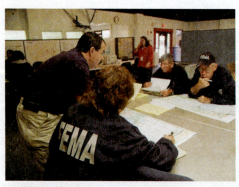

FIGURE 14.23   The Federal Emergency Management Agency (FEMA) helps communities prepare for disasters and manages federal response and recovery efforts following a national incident.

Courtesy of Patsy Lynch/FEMA.

Natural disasters can occur at any place and at any time. Although a variety of federal and state agencies and other non-governmental organizations (NGOs) have as all or part of their mission to respond to such disasters, recent experiences should have taught us that local communities, especially those located in high-risk areas, also need to prepare. Only through careful planning and preparation can communities hope to minimize loss of human health and life if a disaster should occur. It is also important to involve all community resources in response to complex emergencies. Research has identified that most disease outbreaks resulting from complex emergencies involve vaccine-preventable diseases, especially if populations from developing countries are involved. The lack of vaccination can result in displaced populations' exposure to diseases for which they have no immunity or introduce diseases into new areas.[113]

Community preparedness begins at home. Families need to be familiar with the types of emergencies and disasters that can occur in the area and plan. FEMA provides online information on how to prepare at www.ready.gov and in the mobile app. The information is free and includes forms for planning to ensure family members stay safe and can find each other if they are separated during an emergency. Planning must include stocking medicine, food, and water; backing up critical documents in cloud-based storage or another secure location; planning for pets; understanding alerts and warnings when they are issued by local authorities and establishing a communication plan.[114] Even though preparedness begins at home, government and NGO partnerships are essential to community resilience and recovery. For example, local health departments found that well-established partnerships strengthened the local health department's ability to engage the community in public health preparedness. Surveys of partnerships that existed before and after disasters found that those that developed in response to a disaster were less durable than those that were established during non-disaster time.[115] An additional benefit is that these partnerships not only benefit the community during recovery but also enable local health departments to deliver services more effectively during non-disaster periods or during an influx of displaced populations.

Although disease surveillance via wastewater is not new, the relationship between the CDC, local public health and public works, and analytical laboratories to track community disease outbreaks became a priority during the SARS-CoV-2 outbreak. Wastewater collection and treatment systems can be used for detecting disease outbreaks and can trigger an appropriate community response to minimize an outbreak. To affect this process, the CDC needs to establish standards for a national wastewater surveillance system, and the local community partners work together to develop procedures for implementing detection methods, data interpretation, and criteria for response.[116]

Chapter Summary

- Environmental health is the study and management of environmental conditions that affect our health and well-being. Environmental hazards increase our risk of injury, disease, or death.

- Air pollution is the contamination of the air by gases, liquids, or solids in amounts that harm humans, other living organisms, or the ecosystem, or that change the climate. Sources of primary air pollutants are stationary or mobile. Secondary air pollutants arise from the interaction of primary air pollutants and sunlight.

- Efforts to regulate air quality include the Clean Air Act of 1963 and its amendments, which resulted in the establishment of the National Ambient Air Quality Standards. The U.S. Environmental Protection Agency calculates the Air Quality Index to help people relate air quality to their health.

- Indoor air pollutants include asbestos, biogenic materials, combustion byproducts, and volatile organic compounds. Radon gas and environmental tobacco smoke pose additional indoor air threats to health.

- The United States has the safest water in the world. Nonetheless, both point source and nonpoint source pollution threaten the safety of our water supply.

- Waterborne disease outbreaks caused by biological and nonbiological pollutants are reported each year, with an increasing proportion of outbreaks being associated with recreational water use.

- Population growth, chemical manufacturing, and reckless land use practices contribute to the deterioration of our water quality.

- Municipal water treatment plants provide water for domestic use, and wastewater treatment plants remove much of the waste before used water is returned to the environment.

- Water quality is regulated by two important laws: the Clean Water Act and the Safe Drinking Water Act.

- More than 200 known diseases are transmitted through the food we eat. Foodborne disease outbreaks occur each year and are reported to the Centers for Disease Control and Prevention (CDC).

- The U.S. Department of Agriculture and the U.S. Food and Drug Administration inspect food-processing plants and enforce health and safety standards. Registered environmental health specialists inspect local restaurants and retail food outlets to enforce food preparation and food-handling laws, thereby protecting consumers.

- The Resource Conservation and Recovery Act (RCRA) governs the management of both municipal solid waste and hazardous solid waste, and the Comprehensive Environmental Response, Compensation, and Liability Act (CERCLA) governs the cleanup of existing hazardous waste sites.

- Of special concern are the many toxic chemicals and heavy metals, such as lead, that can leach into sources of our drinking water.

- Vectorborne diseases, such as West Nile fever, St. Louis encephalitis, LaCrosse encephalitis, Lyme disease, murine typhus, and Zika virus represent another group of environmental health concerns. These diseases affect thousands of people each year and are difficult to predict or control.

- Natural hazards include high-energy radiation and natural environmental events, such as earthquakes, tsunamis, volcanic eruptions, and weather-driven events, such as tornados, hurricanes, and floods. Natural disasters occur when these events involve human injuries and/or deaths.

- Avoiding exposure to ionizing radiation can reduce one's risk for skin cancer and other health problems.

- A complex disaster or emergency is a humanitarian crisis that often results when a natural disaster further escalates an ongoing crisis, such as a civil war, or causes a technological disaster.

- Uncontrolled population growth can contribute to psychological and sociological hazards.

- The Federal Emergency Management Agency (FEMA) and the American Red Cross are two agencies that prepare for and respond to natural disasters. Affected communities can improve their resilience to disasters by developing strong partnerships with nongovernmental agencies and services and preparation by individual households.

Scenario: Analysis and Response

Please take a moment to reread the scenario at the beginning of this chapter. Then, reflect on the questions that follow.

1. Many people like Juan and Maria live where industrial poultry or livestock operations have become established. What additional precautions could Juan and Maria have taken before moving into their current home to protect their health?

2. Suppose the well water is found to contain high levels of nitrates. Assuming that Juan and Maria cannot move, what steps could they take to improve their chances of a successful pregnancy? What might they do to restore the safety of their well water? What local, state, or federal agencies might be able to help them? Environmental injustice is a term used to describe situations in which undesirable industries or waste disposal sites are preferentially located in racial and ethnic minority areas. Is there anything about this situation that might suggest that this is a case of environmental injustice?

Review Questions

1. What are the major sources of air pollutants? What are criteria pollutants? What is the difference between primary and secondary pollutants?

2. What role does the Environmental Protection Agency (EPA) play in protecting the environment?

3. What is the Clean Air Act? What are the National Ambient Air Quality Standards? What is the Air Quality Index? Why were air pollution levels reduced during the SARS-CoV-2 pandemic?

4. What are some major kinds of indoor air pollutants? How can we reduce our exposure to them? What is radon and why is it dangerous? What recommendations were made by the CDC to minimize transmission of viruses in indoor spaces?

5. What is the difference between point source and non-point source pollution? Which is the bigger problem?

6. What types of pollutants threaten our water supply? Give an example of each type. Did the local community where you live track SARS-CoV-2 outbreak through wastewater surveillance?

7. What are waterborne disease outbreaks? Name some waterborne disease agents.

8. What are pharmaceuticals and personal care products, and why should we be concerned with their disposal?

9. How do communities ensure the quality of drinking water, and what steps do communities take to reduce the likelihood that their wastewater harms the environment?

10. What are the purposes of the Clean Water Act and the Safe Drinking Water Act?

11. What is a foodborne disease outbreak? What factors contribute to foodborne disease outbreaks? Name some common foodborne disease causative agents.

12. What are some of the local, state, and federal agencies that help protect our food? How do they accomplish this task?

13. What is a pest? Explain the difference between target organisms and nontarget organisms and give examples. Explain some safety and health concerns associated with the use of pesticides.

14. What types of refuse make up our municipal solid waste (MSW)? How much MSW do we generate per person per year? What options do communities have for managing MSW?

15. What is hazardous waste? Can you give some examples?

16. What are the purposes of the Resource Conservation and Recovery Act (RCRA) and the Comprehensive Environmental Response, Compensation, and Liability Act (CERCLA)?

17. How does lead get into our environment? How is lead harmful to our health? Which segment of our population is at highest risk for lead poisoning?

18. What is a vector? What is a vectorborne disease? Give some examples of each.

19. What is ionizing radiation? Why is it a health hazard? How can individuals lower their health risk?

20. What is a natural disaster, and what is a complex disaster or emergency? How do disasters affect the health of a community? What planning activities can a community engage in to minimize the impact of disasters? How can an influx of displaced populations result in a public health crisis in a community?

21. How would you interpret the relationships among population growth, the environment, and human health?

22. How do local partnerships between public health agencies and non-governmental agencies and service increase resilience and contribute in preparing for and responding to catastrophic events?

Activities

1. For two weeks, monitor a weather program that mentions the Air Quality Index (AQI). During that two-week period, chart the AQI in graph form and identify the major pollutant for each day.

2. During the next week, create a list of at least 10 things you could have done to conserve the water you use.

3. Write a one-page paper describing either your support for or opposition to (a) nuclear power plants or (b) strengthening the Safe Drinking Water Act.

4. In a one-page paper, identify what you believe to be the number one waste or pollution problem faced by the United States, and explain why.

5. Call your local health department and find out what kind of efforts have been made to eliminate lead poisoning. Ask about education programs and possible state or local laws. Also, find out if the health department will test for lead in the water and paint. If they

will, ask about the procedures they use to do so. Write the results of your findings in a two-page paper.

6. For all of us to be better stewards of our environment, we need to be aware of how our community handles various important environmental issues. Find the answers to the following about your community and state:

a. How does your community dispose of solid waste?

b. How far do you live from a secured landfill? What is the closest community to it?

c. Where does your community get its water? If you personally get your water from a well, when was the last time the water was evaluated?

d. Where is the closest nuclear power plant to your home? What are you supposed to do in case of an accident?

e. Does your state have legislation to protect communities and individuals from factory farm operations that might pollute aquifers or surface water?

7. Make arrangements to interview a director of environmental health in a local health department. Find answers to the following questions and summarize these answers in a two-page paper.

   a. What are all the tasks this division of the health department carries out?

   b. What is the primary environmental health problem in your community? Why is it a problem? How is it being dealt with?

c. If they inspect restaurants, which ones have the best sanitation practices?

d. What is an average day like for a health department sanitarian?

8. Monitor the Internet or reporting service, such as www.gdacs.org, for two weeks and record in a table the number, type, and location of disasters reported.

   a. How many are due to natural hazards? How many are complex disasters or human made? What are the possible health consequences?

   b. Go to www.ready.gov and develop a plan for a natural hazard based on where you live.

References

1. U.S. Environmental Protection Agency. (2023). *NAAQS table.* Available at https://www.epa.gov/criteria-air-pollutants/naaqs-table.

2. U.S. Environmental Protection Agency. (n.d.). *AirNow: Your health.* https://www.airnow.gov/air-quality-and-health/your-health/

3. National Institute of Environmental Health Sciences. (n.d.). *Air Pollution and Your Health.* Available at https://www.niehs.nih.gov/health/materials/air_pollution_and_your_health_508.pdf

4. U.S. Environmental Protection Agency. (2023). *Air databasic information.* https://www.epa.gov/outdoor-air-quality-data/air-data-basic-information

5. Miller, G. T. (1979). *Living in the Environment (2nd ed.).* Wadsworth Publishing Co.

6. U.S. Environmental Protection Agency. (2023). *EPA history: Clean Air Act of 1970/1977.* Available at https://www.epa.gov/history/epa-history-clean-air-act-19701977

7. U.S. Environmental Protection Agency. (2023). *1990 Clean air act amendment summary.* Available at https://www.epa.gov/clean-air-act-overview

8. U.S. Environmental Protection Agency. (2022). *Our nation's air: Status and trends through 2022.* Available at https://gispub.epa.gov/air/trendsreport/2023/#welcome

9. U.S. Environmental Protection Agency. (2023). *Summary nonattainment area population exposure report.* Available at https://www3.epa.gov/airquality/greenbook/popexp.html

10. National Aeronautics and Space Administration. (2021). *Emission reductions from Pandemic Had Unexpected Effects on Atmosphere.* Available at https://climate.nasa.gov/news/3129/emission-reductions-from-pandemic-had-unexpected-effects-on-atmosphere/

11. U.S. Environmental Protection Agency. (n.d.). *What is the U.S. Air Quality Index.* Available at https://www.airnow.gov/aqi/aqi-basics/

12. U.S. Energy Information Administration. (2022). *U.S. energy facts explained.* Available at https://www.eia.gov/energyexplained/us-energy-facts/

13. U.S. Energy Information Administration. (2022). *Electric power annual.* Table 4.3. *Existing Capacity by Energy Source, 2022. (Megawatts).* Available at https://www.eia.gov/electricity/annual/html/epa_04_03.html

14. U.S. Energy Information Administration. (2017). *Coal-fired electric power plants. Detailed EIA-860.* Available at https://www.eia.gov/coal/data.php

15. U.S. Environmental Protection Agency. (2008). Indoor Air Quality (IAQ) *EPA 402/F-08/008, Care for your air: A guide to indoor air quality.* Available at https://www.epa.gov/sites/default/files/2014-08/documents/careforyourair.pdf

16. U.S. Centers for Disease Control and Prevention. (2023). *COVID-19 Overview and Infection Prevention and Control Priorities in non-U.S. Healthcare Settings.* Available at https://www.cdc.gov/coronavirus/2019-ncov/hcp/non-us-settings/overview/index.html

17. U.S. Environmental Protection Agency. (2023). *Sources of combustion products: An introduction to indoor air quality.* Available at https://www.epa.gov/indoor-air-quality-iaq/sources-combustion-products

18. Lantz, P. M., Mendez, D., & Philbert, M. A. (2013). Radon, smoking, and lung cancer: The need to refocus radon control policy. *American Journal of Public Health, 103*(3), 443–447.

19. U.S. Environmental Protection Agency. (2024). *Health risk of radon.* Available at https://www.epa.gov/radon/health-risk-radon

20. U.S. Environmental Protection Agency. (2024). *Ten things you should know about mold.* Available at https://www.epa.gov/mold/ten-things-you-should-know-about-mold

21. U.S. Department of Health and Human Services. (2014). *The health consequences of smoking—50 years of progress: A report of the Surgeon General.* Available at https://www.ncbi.nlm.nih.gov/books/NBK179276/

22. American Lung Association. (2024). *State of tobacco control 2024.* Available at https://www.lung.org/research/sotc

23. American Lung Association. (2023). *Overall tobacco trends.* Available at https://www.lung.org/research/trends-in-lung-disease/tobacco-trends-brief/overall-tobacco-trends

24. American Lung Association. (2023). *E-cigarettes & vaping.* Available at https://www.lung.org/quit-smoking/e-cigarettes-vaping

25. U.S. Environmental Protection Agency. (2023). Report on the environment—indoor air quality. Available at https://www.epa.gov/report-environment/indoor-air-quality

26. U.S. Environmental Protection Agency. (1991). *Indoor air facts no. 4, sick building syndrome.* Available at https://www.epa.gov/sites/production/files/2014-08/documents/sick_building_factsheet.pdf

27. American Lung Association. (2022). *Smokefree air laws.* Available at https://www.lung.org/policy-advocacy/tobacco/smokefree-environments/smokefree-air-laws

28. U.S. Department of Health and Human Services, Healthy People 2030. (2020). *Eliminate policies in states, territories, and DC that preempt local tobacco control policies—TU-20.* Available at https://health.gov/healthypeople/objectives-and-data/browse-objectives/tobacco-use/eliminate-policies-states-territories-and-dc-preempt-local-tobacco-control-policies-tu-20

29. American Nonsmokers' Rights Foundation. (2023). *Overview list – number of smokefree and other tobacco-related laws.* Available at https://no-smoke.org/wp-content/uploads/pdf/mediaordlist.pdf

30. World Health Organization. (2022). *Water, sanitation and hygiene (WASH).* Available at https://www.who.int/health-topics/water-sanitation-and-hygiene-wash#tab=tab_1

31. World Health Organization. (2023). Unsafe water, sanitation and hygiene: a persistent health burden. Available at https://pubmed.ncbi.nlm.nih.gov/37663869/

32. Centers for Disease Control and Prevention. (2021). *2021 Waterborne Disease Outbreaks Annual Surveillance Report.* Available at https://www.cdc.gov/healthywater/surveillance/2021-waterborne-outbreaks-annual-report.html

33. U.S. Geological Survey. (2019). *How much water is there on earth?* Available at https://www.usgs.gov/special-topics/water-science-school/science/how-much-water-there-earth

34. U.S. Environmental Protection Agency. (2018). *Basic information about nonpoint source (NPS pollution).* Available at https://www.epa.gov/nps/basic-information-about-nonpoint-source-nps-pollution

35. U.S. Environmental Protection Agency. (2024). *Endocrine disruptor screening program (EDSP).* Available at https://www.epa.gov/endocrine-disruption

36. U.S. Environmental Protection Agency. (2013). Endocrine disruptor screening program: Final second list of chemicals and substances for tier 1 screening. *Federal Register, 78*(115), 35922–35928. Available at https://www.federalregister.gov/documents/2013/06/14/2013-14232/endocrine-disruptor-screening-program-final-second-list-of-chemicals-and-substances-for-tier-1

37. U.S. Environmental Protection Agency. (2023). *Endocrine disruptor screening program (EDSP) tier 1 assessments.* Available at https://www.epa.gov/endocrine-disruption/endocrine-disruptor-screening-program-edsp-tier-1-assessments

38. U. S. Geological Survey. (2018). *Pharmaceuticals in water.* Available at https://www.usgs.gov/special-topics/water-science-school/science/pharmaceuticals-water

39. U.S. Food and Drug Administration. (2019). *Where and how to dispose of unused medicines.* Available at https://www.fda.gov/consumers/consumer-updates/where-and-how-dispose-unused-medicines

40. Centers for Disease Control and Prevention. (2019). *Waterborne disease outbreak surveillance reporting detecting and investigating waterborne diseases and outbreaks.* Available at https://www.cdc.gov/healthywater/surveillance/detecting-investigating.html

41. Centers for Disease Control and Prevention. (2022). *National Outbreak Reporting System (NORS).* Available at https://wwwn.cdc.gov/norsdashboard/

42. Centers for Disease Control and Prevention. (1996). Surveillance for waterborne disease outbreaks—United States, 1993–1994. *Morbidity and Mortality Weekly Report, 45*(SS-1), 1–33. Available at https://www.cdc.gov/mmwr/PDF/ss/ss4501.pdf

43. United Nations, Environmental Programme. (2010). *Clearing the waters: A focus on water quality solutions.* Nairobi: United Nations at Nairobi. Available at https://wedocs.unep.org/handle/20.500.11822/7906

44. Maupin, M. A. (2015). *Summary of estimated water use in the United States in 2015.* U.S. Geological Survey Fact Sheet 2018-3035. Available at https://pubs.er.usgs.gov/publication/fs20183035

45. U.S. Geological Survey. (2015). *Water Q&A: How much water do I use at home each day?* Available at https://www.usgs.gov/special-topics/water-science-school/science/water-qa-how-much-water-do-i-use-home-each-day

46. Centers for Disease Control and Prevention. (1999). Achievements in public health, 1900-1999: Fluoridation of drinking water to prevent dental caries. *Morbidity and Mortality Weekly Report, 48*(41), 933–940. Available at https://www.cdc.gov/mmwr/preview/mmwrhtml/mm4841a1.htm

47. Centers for Disease Control and Prevention. (2023). *Over 75 years of community water fluoridation.* Available at *https://www.cdc.gov/fluoridation/basics/anniversary.htm*

48. Centers for Disease Control and Prevention. (2023). *Cost savings of community water fluoridation.* Available at https://www.cdc.gov/fluoridation/basics/cost.htm

49. Roychoudhury, A., & Das, N. (2022). *Sewage Sludge Treatment and Involvement of Microbes.* In: Rajput, V. D., Yadav, A. N., Jatav, H. S., Singh, S. K., & Minkina, T. (eds) Sustainable Management and Utilization of Sewage Sludge. Springer, Cham. Available at https://doi.org/10.1007/978-3-030-85226-9_8

50. U.S. Environmental Protection Agency. (2023). *About septic systems.* Available at https://www.epa.gov/septic/about-septic-systems

51. U.S. Environmental Protection Agency. (20116). *EPA history: Water- The challenge of the environment: A primer on EPA's statutory authority.* Available at https://www.epa.gov/archive/epa/aboutepa/epa-history-water-challenge-environment-primer-epas-statutory-authority.html

52. U.S. Environmental Protection Agency. (2023). *Overview of the Safe Drinking Water Act.* Available at https://www.epa.gov/sdwa/overview-safe-drinking-water-act

53. U.S. Environmental Protection Agency. (2024). *National primary drinking water regulations.* Available at https://www.epa.gov/ground-water-and-drinking-water/national-primary-drinking-water-regulations

54. U.S. Environmental Protection Agency. (2023). *CCL 4 frequent questions.* Available at https://www.epa.gov/ccl/ccl-4-frequent-questions

55. Centers for Disease Control and Prevention. (1999). Achievements in public health, 1900–1999: Safer and healthier foods. *Morbidity and Mortality Weekly Report, 48*(4), 905–913.

56. Centers for Disease Control and Prevention. (1999). Food-related illness and death in the United States. *Emerging Infectious Diseases, 5*(5), 607–625. Available at https://doi.org/10.3201/eid0505.990502

57. Centers for Disease Control and Prevention. (2018). *Burden of foodborne illness: Findings.* Available at https://www.cdc.gov/foodborneburden/2011-foodborne-estimates.html

58. U.S. Department of Agriculture. (2023). *Cost estimates of foodborne illnesses.* Available at https://www.ers.usda.gov/data-products/cost-estimates-of-foodborne-illnesses.aspx

59. Centers for Disease Control and Prevention. (2023). *Four steps to food safety: clean, separate, cook, chill.* Available at https://www.cdc.gov/foodsafety/keep-food-safe.html

60. Centers for Disease Control and Prevention. (2023). *Raw milk questions and answers.* Available at https://www.cdc.gov/foodsafety/rawmilk/raw-milk-questions-and-answers.html

61. National Pesticide Information Retrieval Systems. (n.d.). *PPIS.* Purdue University. http://ppis.ceris.purdue.edu/

62. Food and Agriculture Organization of the United Nations. (2021). *Pesticides use.* Available at https://www.fao.org/faostat/en/#data/RP

63. Food and Agriculture Organization of the United Nations. (2019). *New standards to curb the global spread of plant pests and diseases.* Available at https://www.fao.org/newsroom/detail/New-standards-to-curb-the-global-spread-of-plant-pests-and-diseases/en

64. World Economic Forum. (2021). *40% of global crop production is lost to pests. And it's getting worse.* Available at https://www.weforum.org/agenda/2021/06/climate-change-insects-pests-crops-agriculture/

65. Bradford, A., Broude, S., & Truelove, A. (2018). *Trash in America moving from destructive consumption to a zero-waste system.* Available at https://uspirg.org/sites/pirg/files/reports/US%20-%20Trash%20in%20America%20-%20Final.pdf

66. U.S. Environmental Protection Agency. (2020). *Advancing sustainable materials management 2018 fact sheet.* Available at https://www.epa.gov/sites/default/files/2021-01/documents/2018_ff_fact_sheet_dec_2020_fnl_508.pdf

67. U.S. Environmental Protection Agency. (2021). *Introduction to the 2021 TRI National Analysis.* Available at https://www.epa.gov/trinationalanalysis/introduction-2021-tri-national-analysis

68. U.S. Environmental Protection Agency. (2023). *Basic information about electronics stewardship.* Available at https://www.epa.gov/smm-electronics/basic-information-about-electronics-stewardship

69. European Environment Agency. (2023). *Municipal waste recycling rates in Europe by country* Available at https://www.eea.europa.eu/data-and-maps/daviz/municipal-waste-recycled-and-composted-7#tab-chart_7

70. University of Michigan. (2023). U.S. *municipal solid waste.* Available at https://css.umich.edu/sites/default/files/2023-10/U.S.%20MSW_CSS04-15.pdf

71. U.S. Environmental Protection Agency. (2023). *Basic Information about landfill gas.* Available at https://www.epa.gov/lmop/basic-information-about-landfill-gas

72. U.S. Environmental Protection Agency. (2023). *Energy recovery from the combustion of municipal solid waste (MSW).* Available at https://www.epa.gov/smm/energy-recovery-combustion-municipal-solid-waste-msw#EnergyRecovery

73. U.S. Environmental Protection Agency. (2021). *Management methods.* Available at https://rcrapublic.epa.gov/rcrainfoweb/action/modules/br/management/view

74. Centers for Disease Control and Prevention. (2019). *Ground water awareness week.* Available at https://www.cdc.gov/healthywater/drinking/groundwater-awareness-week.html

75. U.S. Environmental Protection Agency. (2023). *Superfund remedial annual accomplishment metrics.* Available at https://www.epa.gov/superfund/superfund-remedial-annual-accomplishments-metrics

76. U.S. Environmental Protection Agency. (2024). *Brownfields.* Available at https://www.epa.gov/brownfields/about

77. U.S. Department of Housing and Urban Development. (2021). *American healthy homes survey II lead findings.* Available at https://www.hud.gov/sites/dfiles/HH/documents/AHHS%20II_Lead_Findings_Report_Final_29oct21.pdf

78. MAYO Clinic Health System. (2023). *Reducing lead exposure in children.* Available at https://www.mayoclinichealthsystem.org/hometown-health/speaking-of-health/reducing-lead-exposure-in-children

79. Loyola University. (2024). *Effects of lead poisoning during pregnancy.* WHO Document Production Services. Available at https://www.luc.edu/healthyhomes/leadsafeillinois/familysafety/effectsofleadpoisoningduringpregnancy/

80. Centers for Disease Control and Prevention, The National Institute for Occupational Safety and Health. (2023). *Lead: Information for workers.* Available at https://www.cdc.gov/niosh/topics/lead/workerinfo.html

81. President's Task Force on Environmental Health Risks and Safety Risks to Children. (2018). *Federal action plan to reduce childhood lead exposures and associated health impacts.* Available at https://www.epa.gov/sites/default/files/2018-12/documents/fedactionplan_lead_final.pdf

82. Centers for Disease Control and Prevention, National Center for Environmental Health. (2018). *Blood lead levels (µg/dL) among U.S. children <72 months old, by age, by state, year, and blood lead level (BLL) group.* Available at https://www.cdc.gov/nceh/lead/docs/cbls-national-data-table-508.pdf

83. U.S. Department of Health and Human Services, Healthy People 2030. (2020). *Reduce exposure to lead—EH-08.* Available at https://health.gov/healthypeople/objectives-and-data/browse-objectives/environmental-health/reduce-exposure-lead-eh-08/data

84. Centers for Disease Control and Prevention. (2023). *Overview of childhood lead poisoning prevention.* Available at https://www.cdc.gov/nceh/lead/overview.html#print

85. Centers for Disease Control and Prevention. (1999). Outbreak of West Nile–like viral encephalitis—New York, 1999. *Morbidity and Mortality Weekly Report, 48*(38), 845–849.

86. Centers for Disease Control and Prevention, Division of Vector- Borne Infectious Diseases. (2024). *West Nile Historic data (1999-2022).* Available at https://www.cdc.gov/westnile/statsmaps/historic-data.html

87. U.S Tire Manufacturers Association. (2020). *2019 U.S. scrap tire management summary.* Available at https://www.ustires.org/sites/default/files/2019%20USTMA%20Scrap%20Tire%20Management%20Summary%20Report.pdf

88. Moore, C. G., & Mitchell, C. J. (1997). *Aedes albopictus* in the United States: Ten-year presence and public health implications. *Emerging Infectious Diseases, 3*(3), 329–334. Available at https://dx.doi.org/10.3201/eid0303.970309

89. European Centre for Disease Prevention and Control. (2014). *Aedes japonicus: Factsheet for experts.* Available at https://www.ecdc.europa.eu/en/disease-vectors/facts/mosquito-factsheets/aedes-japonicus

90. Centers for Disease Control and Prevention. (2019). *Chikungunya virus in the US.* Available at https://www.cdc.gov/chikungunya/geo/chikungunya-in-the-us.html

91. Centers for Disease Control and Prevention. (2024). *Zika.* Available at https://wwwnc.cdc.gov/eid/spotlight/zika

92. Centers for Disease Control and Prevention. (2019). *Lyme disease surveillance data.* Available at https://www.cdc.gov/lyme/datasurveillance/surveillance-data.html

93. Centers for Disease Control and Prevention. (2021). *Lyme disease surveillance data, top ten states by year.* Available at https://www.cdc.gov/lyme/datasurveillance/surveillance-data.html.

94. U.S. Environmental Protection Agency. (2023). *Health and environmental effects of ozone layer depletion.* Available at https://www.epa.gov/ozone-layer-protection/health-and-environmental-effects-ozone-layer-depletion

95. American Cancer Society. (2019). *Cancer facts & figures 2023.* Available at https://www.cancer.org/content/dam/cancer-org/research/cancer-facts-and-statistics/annual-cancer-facts-and-figures/2023/2023-cancer-facts-and-figures.pdf

96. U.S. Environmental Protection Agency. (2023). *UV index.* Available at https://www.epa.gov/sunsafety/uv-index-1

97. American Cancer Society. (2020). *How to spot skin cancer.* Available at https://www.cancer.org/latest-news/how-to-spot-skin-cancer.html

98. Culver, A., Rochat, R., & Cookson, S. T. (2017). Public health implications of complex emergencies and natural disasters. *Confl Health, 11*(32). Available at https://doi.org/10.1186/s13031-017-0135-8

99. U.S. Energy Information Administration. (2023). *Monthly energy review.* Available at https://www.eia.gov/totalenergy/data/monthly/pdf/sec8.pdf

100. World Health Organization. (2005). *Chernobyl: The true scale of the accident.* Available at https://www.who.int/news/item/05-09-2005-chernobyl-the-true-scale-of-the-accident

101. United Nations Scientific Committee on the Effects of Atomic Radiation. (2022). *Scientific Reports UNSCEAR 2020/2021 Report.* Available at https://www.unscear.org/unscear/en/publications/scientific-reports.html

102. Pulselli, F., & Coscieme, L. (2014). Earth's Carrying Capacity. In: Michalos, A.C. (eds) Encyclopedia of Quality of Life and Well-Being Research. Springer, Dordrecht. Available at https://doi.org/10.1007/978-94-007-0753-5_800

103. United Nations, Economic and Social Affairs. (2022). *World population prospects: 2022: Summary of results.* Available at https://www.un.org/development/desa/pd/sites/www.un.org.development.desa.pd/files/wpp2022_summary_of_results.pdf

104. United Nations Conference on Trade and Development. (2022). *Now 8 billion and counting: Where the world's population has grown most and why that matters.* Available at *https://unctad.org/data-visualization/now-8-billion-and-counting-where-worlds-population-has-grown-most-and-why*

105. Hinrichsen, D., & Robey, B. (2000). *Population and the environment: The global challenge* (Population Reports, Series M, no. 15). Johns Hopkins University School of Public Health, Population Information Program.

106. United Nations, Department of Economic and Social Affairs, Population Division. (2022). *World's cities report 2022.* Available at https://unhabitat.org/sites/default/files/2022/06/wcr_2022.pdf

107. United Nations, Department of Economic and Social Affairs, Population Division. (2018). *The world's cities in 2018.* Available at https://www.un.org/development/desa/pd/content/worlds-cities-2018-data-booklet

108. U.S. Department of Justice, Federal Bureau of Investigation. (2022). *Hate crimes.* Available at https://www.fbi.gov/news/podcasts/inside-the-fbi-hate-crimes-031122

109. U.S. Department of Justice, Federal Bureau of Investigation. (2020). *Domestic terrorism: definitions, terminology, and methodology.* Available at file:///C:/Users/Jamie3/Downloads/ndaa-report-dt-definitions-terminology-methodology-111220.pdf

110. Federal Emergency Management Agency. (n.d.). *About us.* Available at https://www.fema.gov/about

111. Federal Emergency Management Agency. (2013). *Hurricane Sandy FEMA after-action report.* Available at https://www.scarsdaleschools.k12.ny.us/cms/lib5/NY01001205/Centricity/Domain/182/Hurricane%20Sandy%20FEMA%20After-Action%20Report.pdf

112. Federal Emergency Management Agency. (2017). *Remembering Sandy five years later.* Available at https://www.fema.gov/press-release/20210318/remembering-sandy-five-years-later

113. Culver, A., Rochat, R., & Cookson, S. T. (2017). Public health implications of complex emergencies and natural disasters. *Conflict and Health. 11*(32). doi: 10.1186/s13031-017-0135-8. PMID: 29209410; PMCID: PMC5706345.

114. Federal Emergency Management Agency. (2024). *Ready.* Available at https://www.ready.gov/

115. Acosta, J. D., Burgette, L., Chandra, A., Eisenman, D. P., Gonzalez, I., Varda, D., & Xenakis, L. (2018). How community and public health partnerships contribute to disaster recovery and resilience. *Disaster Medicine and Public Health Preparedness, 12*(5), 635–643. doi: 10.1017/dmp.2017.130. Epub 2018 Feb 1. PMID: 29388518.

116. National Academies of Sciences, Engineering, and Medicine. (2023). *Wastewater-based Disease Surveillance for Public Health Action.* Washington, DC: The National Academies Press. Available at https://doi.org/10.17226/26767.

CHAPTER 15

Injuries as a Community and Public Health Problem

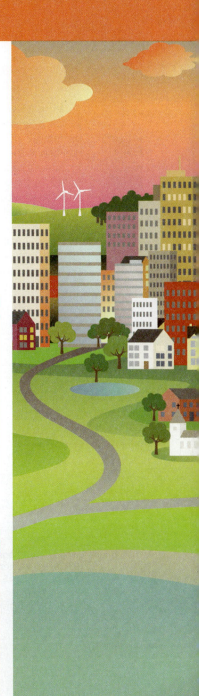

Chapter Outline

Chapter Objectives

After studying this chapter, you will be able to:

1. Describe the importance of injuries as a community and public health problem.

2. Explain why the terms *accidents* and *safety* have been replaced by the currently more acceptable terms *unintentional injuries, injury prevention,* and *injury control* when dealing with such occurrences.

3. Briefly discuss the difference between intentional and unintentional injuries and provide examples of each.

4. Summarize the epidemiology of unintentional injuries, that is, when, where, and to whom injuries occur.

5. List strategies for the prevention and control of unintentional injuries.

6. Explain how education, regulation, automatic protection, and litigation can reduce the number and seriousness of unintentional injuries.

7. Define the term *intentional injuries*, and provide examples of behaviors that result in intentional injuries.

8. Describe the significance of intentional injuries as a community and public health problem in the United States.

9. Discuss risk factors for intimate partner violence.

10. List some contributing factors to domestic violence and some strategies for reducing it.

11. Define the term *youth gang*. Explain why some young people join these gangs.

12. Discuss local, state, and national resources available to communities for reducing the number and severity of intentional injuries resulting from violence in the community.

13. Give examples of ways communities can reduce firearm violence.

Scenario

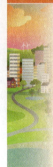

Sam is 15 years old and a high school sophomore. On a Sunday afternoon, he volunteered to clean his family's garage. While reorganizing a cabinet, he reached to the top shelf and felt a metal object. It was his father's handgun. Sam's parents owned a gun safe, but there the gun was, unlocked and loaded. He had never touched a firearm before. However, he thought about the escalating tension between his friends and another group of students at school, which had recently turned to threats of fighting. Sam had felt increasingly worried about what might happen. He decided to take the gun and hide it in his backpack just in case. He figured he could return it to the cabinet before his parents noticed.

In the parking lot after school on Monday, Sam saw the rival group getting ready to confront his friends. He reached into his backpack to move the gun to his waistband. He hoped those students would see it and avoid picking a fight with him. As he rummaged around his bag, Sam heard a pop and felt a sharp pain in his foot. The gun had discharged, striking Sam. Sam's friends and the other students in the parking lot scattered. A few moments later, a school security officer arrived to detain Sam and wait for an ambulance.

Injury damage that results when a human body is suddenly or briefly subjected to intolerable levels of energy

Unintentional injury an injury that occurs without anyone intending that harm be done

Intentional injury an injury that is purposely inflicted, either by the victim or by another

Fatal injury an injury that results in one or more deaths

Introduction

This chapter first defines and then examines the scope, causes, and significance of both unintentional and intentional injuries in community and public health. Approaches to the prevention and control of injuries and injury deaths also are reviewed.

Definitions

The word **injury** is derived from the Latin word for "not right."[1] Injury is defined as "physical damage that results when a human body is suddenly or briefly subjected to intolerable levels of energy."[2] An injury may occur after exposure to mechanical, radiant, thermal, electrical, or chemical energy. The term can also refer to a critical impairment in function that occurs because of a lack of at least one vital element, like oxygen or heat (e.g., drowning is the lack of oxygen).[2] In this chapter, we discuss both **unintentional injury**, an injury judged to have occurred without anyone intending that harm be done (such as those that result from car crashes, falls, drowning, and fires), and **intentional injury**, an injury judged to have been purposely inflicted, either by another or oneself (such as assaults, intentional shootings and stabbings, and suicides).

Cost of Injuries to Society

Injuries are costly to society in terms of both human suffering and economic loss. Injuries are a leading cause of death and disability in the world. Globally, over 4 million people die from injuries each year, accounting for 8% of the world's deaths.[3]

Each year in the United States, more than 300,000 people die from a **fatal injury**.[4] Injuries, from all causes—unintentional and intentional—account for 53% of all deaths among people aged 1 to 44 years in the United States. Of all injury deaths, 224,935 (73%) were classified as unintentional injury deaths, 48,183 (16%) as suicides, and 26,031 (9%) as homicides. Of the remaining deaths, 6,259 (2%) were of undetermined intent and 669 (less than 1%) were the result of legal intervention (see **Figure 15.1**).[4]

Deaths are only a small part of the total cost of injuries. Worldwide, just over 10% of the human burden of disease can be attributed to injuries.[5] Each year in the United States, there are millions of **medically consulted injuries** (person consults with a healthcare professional for medical treatment or advice). In 2022, 26,564,105 people in the United States visited an emergency

Undetermined
6,259
(2%)

Legal
intervention
616 (<0.2%)

Homicide
26,031
(9%)

Suicide
48,183
(16%)

Unintentional
224,935
(73%)

Total injury deaths: 306,024

FIGURE 15.1   Injury deaths: United States, 2021.

Modified from Centers for Disease Control and Prevention. (2023). *Fatal injury reports.* National Center for Injury Prevention and Control (WISQARS™). Available at https://wisqars.cdc.gov/reports

TABLE 15.1 Years of Potential Life Lost (YPLL) and Percentage of Deaths for Selected Leading Causes of Death—United States, 2021

Disease or Condition	Age-Adjusted YPLL Before Age 75 (per 100,000 population)	Percentage of Deaths
Injury	1,842.9	19.1%
Cancer	1,080.8	14.2%
Heart disease	1,002.0	12.7%
COVID-19	1,015.5	12.2%
Suicide	471.7	4.9%
Homicide	363.9	3.7%
Liver disease	275.6	3.1%
Diabetes mellitus	222.5	2.8%
Chronic lower respiratory diseases	141.3	2.0%
Septicemia	81.6	1.0%
Influenza and pneumonia	65.7	0.8%

Modified from Centers for Disease Control and Prevention, National Center for Injury Prevention and Control. (2023). *Years of potential life lost before age 75* (WISQARS™). Available at https://wisqars.cdc.gov/lcd

Medically consulted injury an injury for which a healthcare professional is consulted for medical treatment or advice, either by phone or in person

Injury prevention (control) an organized effort to prevent injuries or to minimize their severity

department because of an injury or poisoning. Of these visits, 3.8 million (14.5%) required hospitalization or transfer to another medical facility.[6] In addition to the physical and emotional harm caused by these injuries and poisonings, there are significant associated economic costs. For example, in 2021, the National Safety Council estimated the total cost of all injuries at more than $1,255 billion, including $665 billion in wage and productivity losses, $255 billion in medical expenses, $195 billion in administrative costs, $89 billion in motor vehicle damage, $35 billion in employer uninsured costs, and $16 billion in fire losses.[7] The true economic burden of injuries is much greater than this estimate because it does not include the value of life lost to premature mortality, loss of patient and caregiver time, and nonmedical expenditures, such as insurance costs, property damage, litigation, decreased quality of life, and disability.

Injuries are a major contributor to premature deaths (deaths that occur before reaching the age of one's life expectancy) in the United States. Leading causes of years of potential life lost before 75 years of age (YPLL-75) and percentage of deaths for selected leading causes of death are shown in **Table 15.1**.[8] Unintentional injuries are the leading cause of YPLL-75.

Unintentional Injuries

Unintentional injuries are the cause of nearly three-fourths of all injury-related deaths in the United States and were ranked as the fourth leading cause of death in 2021. There were 223,610 unintentional injury deaths in 2021.[9] Accounting for those deaths were unintentional poisonings; 101,965 (46.7%); followed by motor vehicle crashes, 45,294 (20.7%); and falls 46,677 (20.5%), along with other causes.[9] In addition to the human death toll were the economic costs, mentioned earlier. Clearly, unintentional injuries constitute one of the United States' major public health problems.

The term *accident* has fallen into disfavor and disuse with many public health officials whose goal is to reduce the number and seriousness of all injuries. The word "accident" suggests a chance occurrence or an unpreventable mishap. Yet we know that many, if not most, accidents are preventable. The term *unintentional injury* is now used in its place. Similarly, the rather vague term *safety* has largely been replaced by **injury prevention (control)**. These terms are inclusive of all measures to prevent injuries, both unintentional and intentional, or to minimize their severity.

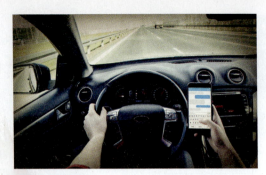

FIGURE 15.2   An unsafe act is a behavior that increases the probability of an injury.

© guteksk7/Shutterstock

Four significant features characterize unintentional injuries: (1) They are unplanned events; (2) they usually are preceded by an unsafe act or condition (hazard); (3) they often are accompanied by economic loss; and (4) they interrupt the efficient completion of a task.

An **unsafe act** is any behavior that would increase the probability of an unintentional injury. For example, driving an automobile while impaired by alcohol or operating a power saw without eye protection is an unsafe act (see **Figure 15.2**). An **unsafe condition** is any environmental factor (physical or social) that would increase the probability of an unintentional injury. Icy streets are an example of an unsafe condition. An unsafe act or unsafe condition is a **hazard**. Whereas hazards do not actually cause unintentional injuries (an alcohol-impaired person may reach home uninjured, even over icy streets), they do increase the probability that an unintentional injury will occur.

Unsafe act any behavior that would increase the probability of an injury occurring

Unsafe condition any environmental factor or set of factors (physical or social) that would increase the probability of an injury occurring

Hazard an unsafe act or condition

Types of Unintentional Injuries

There are many types of unintentional injuries. The majority occur as a result of unintentional poisonings, motor vehicle crashes, falls, suffocation, drowning, fires and burns, and firearms. These are discussed briefly here.

Poisonings

Poisonings were the leading cause of unintentional deaths in 2021 when unintentional poisoning deaths numbered 101,965.[9] These deaths resulted from unintentional ingestion of fatal doses of narcotics, prescription medicines, alcohol and other drugs; exposure to gases and vapors; and from exposure to chemical and toxic substances. More than 90% of all poisonings happen at home.[10] Contributing to poisoning death totals is the current epidemic of opioid pain reliever–related deaths. More information on this epidemic is available elsewhere in this text.

Motor Vehicle Crashes

Road traffic crash victims can be found throughout the world. Worldwide, 1.19 million people are killed (3,200 each day) and tens of millions are injured or disabled in road traffic crashes annually. Road traffic injuries are the leading cause of death for children and young adults aged five to 29 years and the twelfth leading cause of death for people of all ages with low-income countries experiencing road traffic deaths at a three times higher rate than high-income countries. Pedestrians, cyclists, and motorcyclists account for more than half of global road traffic deaths, demonstrating a global neglect in road traffic system design in many countries.[11]

In the United States, motor vehicle–related deaths are the second leading cause of unintentional injury deaths with 42,939 people killed in motor vehicle traffic crashes on U.S. roadways in 2021, a 10% increase over the previous year and a 16-year high.[12] The increase in traffic fatalities may be attributed to an increase in unsafe behaviors, such as speeding, driving while impaired by alcohol, and failure to use a seatbelt.[12] A majority of those killed were drivers (51%), followed by pedestrians (17%), passengers (15%), motorcyclists (14%), and pedal cyclists (2%).[13]

Because of its public health importance, motor vehicle fatality rates were included in the *Healthy People 2030 (HP2030)* set of objectives. Targets were set to focus the nation's attention on reducing deaths from motor vehicle crashes per 100,000 population. Unfortunately, the fatal injury rate increased between 2019 and 2021, and the fatality rate per 100,000 population is moving away from the HP2030 target rate. Improving motor vehicle safety continues to be a priority (see **Box 15.1**).[14]

Falls

The third leading cause of unintentional fatal injuries is falls, which resulted in 46,677 deaths (20.5% of deaths from unintentional injuries) in 2021.[9] Falls account for nearly one-third of all nonfatal injuries in the United States and disproportionately affect older adults (65 and older), with approximately one in four older people falling each year.[6,15]

with a BAC of 0.08 g/dL or higher. Although 31% represents a significant decline from the 55% reported in 1982, it is still too high. There has also been a decline in the percentage of those killed in crashes who had a BAC of 0.15+ g/dL—from 48% in 1982 to 21% in 2021.[17]

The rate of alcohol impairment among drivers involved in a fatal crash is 2.8 times higher at night than during the day and is almost two times higher on weekends than during the week. Motorcycle drivers have the highest rates of fatal crashes among all drivers with a BAC of 0.08 g/dL or higher, accounting for 28% of fatal crashes compared with 24% of car drivers. The 21- to 24-year-old and 25- to 34-year-old age groups are involved in the greatest number of fatal crashes with a BAC of 0.08 g/dL, accounting for a total of 54% of drivers in fatal crashes.[17] Drivers with BACs of 0.08 g/dL or higher involved in fatal crashes were almost four times more likely to have prior driving while intoxicated (DWI) convictions.[17]

Tragically, drivers are not the only persons killed in alcohol-related motor vehicle crashes. Motor vehicle crashes are the leading cause of death among those aged 5 to 24 years in the United States.[9] When drivers involved in fatal crashes are unrestrained, 69% of children were also unrestrained. The combination of being unrestrained and a passenger of a driver under the influence is deadly, as 25% of children killed in traffic crashes were killed in alcohol-related driving crashes.[18]

Passage of primary enforcement safety belt laws (laws that allow police to stop and ticket a driver or passenger solely because an occupant is unbelted) exists in only 34 states, the District of Columbia, and Puerto Rico.[19] Child restraint laws exist in all 50 states but vary from state to state. Passage of primary enforcement safety belt laws in the remaining states, and stricter enforcement of both laws in all states, could reduce passenger deaths among both adults and children.[19]

Alcohol has also been determined to be an important factor in other types of unintentional injuries and deaths, including water-related deaths, accounting for upwards of 70% of adolescent and adult deaths associated with water recreation.[20] Alcohol continues to be the primary contributing factor in fatal boating accidents, accounting for 16% of total fatalities.[21] According to a U.S. Coast Guard study, where the cause of death is known, 75% of boating accident victims drowned, and of those who drowned, 85% were not wearing a lifejacket, reinforcing that alcohol consumption lowers a person's chance of survival should that person end up in the water (see **Figure 15.7**).[21] Clearly, alcohol consumption and water-related recreation are a dangerous combination.

Prevention Through Epidemiology

Sometimes it has been society's nature to wait until after a tragedy before correcting an existing hazard or dangerous situation. Most implementation of prevention activities related to injuries occurs only after costly disasters.

Early Contributors to Injury Prevention and Control

The first important efforts toward injury prevention and control began early in the twentieth century. Four of the most important contributors to early efforts at injury control were Hugh DeHaven, John E. Gordon, James Gibson, and William Haddon, Jr. Hugh DeHaven was a World War I combat pilot, who, after surviving a plane crash, dedicated his professional life to studying victims of falls in an effort to design ways to reduce the force of impact on a body. Many of his ideas have led to better design concepts, including structural adaptations to protect drivers and other occupants of moving vehicles. For example, today we have at our disposal the protection of safety belts, air bags, collapsible steering assemblies, and padded dashboards. Many of these safety devices were built on the early work of Hugh DeHaven.[22]

In 1949, John E. Gordon proposed that the tools of epidemiology be used to analyze injuries. Because of Gordon's work, a great deal was learned about risk factors, susceptible populations, and the distribution of injuries in populations.

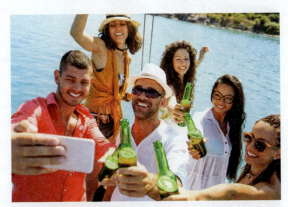

FIGURE 15.7 Alcohol consumption while boating lowers your chances of survival should you end up in the water.

© Valentinrussanov/Getty Images

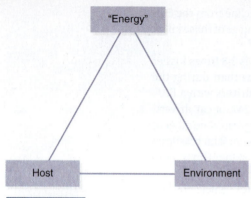

FIGURE 15.8 The public health model for unintentional injuries.

In 1961, James Gibson proposed the idea that injury harm was caused by "energy interchange." Although this definition did not fit well with certain injury deaths, such as drowning and freezing, William Haddon, Jr., realized that in these cases, injury occurred because of the lack of necessary energy elements. Thus, the definition of injury supported by the National Center for Injury Prevention and Control (NCIPC) is "any intentional or unintentional damage to the body resulting from acute exposure to thermal, mechanical, electrical, or chemical energy or from the absence of such essentials as heat or oxygen."[22]

William Haddon, Jr. was both an engineer and a physician, and he is often considered the founding father of modern injury prevention research.[22] He was an unrelenting proponent of the epidemiologic approach to injury control and insisted that the results of this work be used in the development of public policy. He was the foremost expert on highway safety in the 1960s and developed many successful countermeasures to reduce the number of unintentional highway injuries.

A Model for Unintentional Injuries

Model for unintentional injuries the public health triangle (host, agent, and environment) modified to indicate energy as the causative agent of injuries

Until the 1950s, little progress occurred in the reduction of unintentional injuries and deaths. One reason for this was the failure to identify the causative agent associated with unintentional injuries. The public health model describes communicable diseases in terms of the host, agent, and environment, arranged in a triangle; this was discussed in detail elsewhere in the text. A similar **model for unintentional injuries** has been proposed. In this model, the injury-producing agent is energy (see **Figure 15.8**).

Examples of injury-producing energy are plentiful. A moving car, a falling object (or person), and a speeding bullet all have kinetic energy. When one of these moving objects strikes another object, energy is released, often resulting in injury or trauma. Similarly, a hot stove or pan contains energy in the form of heat. Contact with one of these objects results in the rapid transfer of heat. If the skin is unprotected, tissue damage (a burn) occurs. Electrical energy is all around us and represents a potential source of unintentional injuries. Even accidental poisonings fit nicely into the model that incorporates energy as the causative agent of injury. Cleansers, drugs, and medicines represent stored chemical energy, which, when released inappropriately, can cause serious injury or death.

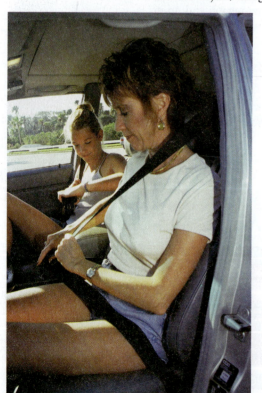

FIGURE 15.9 Safety belts reduce injuries caused by motor vehicle crashes and save lives.
© Yuri Arcurs/Shutterstock

Prevention and Control Tactics Based on the Model

Based on the epidemiologic model just described, four types of actions can be taken to prevent or reduce the number and seriousness of unintentional injuries and deaths.[22] These four tactics are modified from those of Haddon. The first is to prevent the accumulation of the injury-producing agent, energy. Examples of implementing this principle include reducing speed limits to decrease motor vehicle injuries, lowering the height of children's high chairs and diving boards to reduce fall injuries, and lowering the settings on water heaters to reduce the number and seriousness of burns. In our electrical example, circuit breakers in the home prevent the accumulation of excess electrical energy.

The second type of action is to prevent the inappropriate release of excess energy or to modify its release in some way. Flame-resistant fabric that will not ignite is an example of this type of prevention. Currently, federal regulations require that such a fabric be used in the manufacture of children's pajamas. The use of automobile safety belts is another example. In this case, excess energy (movement of a human body) is released into the safety belt instead of into the car's windshield (see **Figure 15.9**). In the prevention of fall injuries, handrails, walkers, and nonslip surfaces in bathtubs prevent the inappropriate release of kinetic energy resulting from falls.

The third tactic involves placing a barrier between the host and agent. The insulation around electrical wires and the use of potholders and insulated handles on cookware are examples of this preventive strategy. The use of sunscreen lotion and the wearing of a hat in the summer place a barrier between the sun's energy and a person's skin. Another example is the cable barriers now visible between opposing traffic lanes on many interstate highways. These installations not only serve as a barrier to protect oncoming traffic but also modify the release of energy and provide drivers and occupants with a relatively soft landing.

Finally, it is sometimes necessary or useful to completely separate the host from potentially dangerous sources of energy. Examples include the locked gates and high fences around electrical substations and swimming pools. At home, locking up guns and poisons provides protection against the likelihood of unintentional injury of young children.

Other Tactics

By viewing energy as the cause of unintentional injuries and deaths, it is possible to take positive steps in their prevention and control. There are still other actions that a community can take. First, injury-control education in schools and other public forums can be helpful. Second, improvements in the community's ability to respond to emergencies, such as encouraging the public to enroll in first aid and cardiopulmonary resuscitation (CPR) classes and expanding 911 telephone services, can limit disability and save lives. Third, communities can ensure that they have superior emergency and paramedic personnel by instituting the best possible training programs. The result will be improved emergency medical care and rehabilitation for the injured. Finally, communities can strengthen ordinances against high-risk behaviors, such as driving while impaired by alcohol, and then support their enforcement.

Community Approaches to the Prevention of Unintentional Injuries

An estimated 39% of unintentional injury deaths could be prevented by correcting the following hazards: lack of vehicle restraint use, lack of motorcycle helmet use, unsafe consumer products, and drug and alcohol use (including prescription drug misuse, exposure to occupational hazards, and unsafe home and community environments).[23] There are four broad strategies for preventing unintentional injuries—education, regulation, automatic protection, and litigation.

Education

Injury prevention education is the process of changing people's health-directed behavior in such a way as to reduce unintentional injuries. Education certainly has a place in injury prevention. Many of us remember the school fire drill, lessons on bicycle safety, and the school crossing guard. Undoubtedly, millions of injuries were prevented in these ways. However, injury prevention education has its limitations. **Figure 15.10** illustrates both the inefficiency of public education and the difficulties of measuring a successful outcome.

Regulation

The former 55-mile-per-hour national speed limit is an example of the power of **regulation**—the enactment and enforcement of laws to control conduct—as a means of reducing the number and seriousness of unintentional injuries. For years, motorists were advised to drive more responsibly. Public service announcements in the 1960s and 1970s informed audiences that "speed kills," and advised motorists not to "drink and drive." However, the highway death toll continued to mount until 1974, when then-President Gerald Ford issued the national 55-mile-per-hour speed limit. Although the primary purpose of the slower speed limit was to conserve gasoline during the oil embargo by the Organization of the Petroleum Exporting Countries (OPEC), more than 9,000 lives were saved as the number of motor vehicle deaths dropped from 55,511 in 1973 to 46,200 in 1974 because of the slower speeds.

State laws requiring child safety seats and safety belt use are another example of regulation to reduce injuries. Beginning in the 1980s, automobile child restraint and safety belt legislation spread across the United States. All states now have occupant restraint requirements (seatbelt

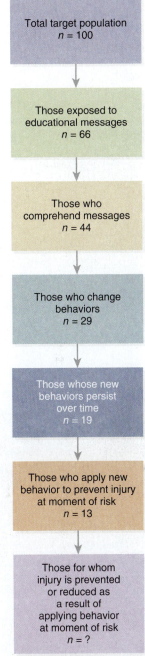

FIGURE 15.10

Attenuation of the effect of a public health education program.

Modified from McLoughlin, E., Vince, C. J., Lee, A. M., & Crawford, J. D. (1982). Project burn prevention: Outcome and implications. *American Journal of Public Health, 72*(3), 241–247. As presented in U.S. Congress, Office of Technology Assessment (February 1988). *Healthy Children: Investing in the Future* (pub no. OTA-H-345). U.S. Government Printing Office.

Injury prevention education the process of changing people's health-directed behavior to reduce unintentional injuries

Regulation the enactment and enforcement of laws to control conduct

laws) for children, and all states except for New Hampshire have occupant restraint laws for adults.[24] State laws vary with regard to enforcement, level of fines, seats of the vehicle covered (front seat or all seats), and type of vehicle covered. Passage and vigorous enforcement of safety belt regulations is one reason why motor vehicle fatalities have declined in recent decades. Enforcement laws can be primary (allowing police to stop drivers and issue citations solely because occupants were unbelted) or secondary (allowing police to issue a seatbelt citation after stopping the motorist for another reason). Research supports the implementation of primary enforcement laws as the rate of seatbelt use is consistently higher in states with primary enforcement laws.[24] Regulation is often aimed not at the consumer, but at the industry. For example, beginning with the 1990 models, car makers were required to equip all passenger cars with safety belts or air bags.

Distracted driving is now recognized as a major roadway hazard for everyone. In 2021, distracted driving claimed 3,522 lives, although many instances may go unreported.[25] Since the first workshop on distracted driving research was held by the National Highway Traffic Safety Administration (NHTSA) in 2000, the number of personal electronic devices in use has increased dramatically. Examples are mobile phones, smartwatches, laptops, electronic notebooks, iPods, iPads, and global positioning devices (GPSs). Furthermore, beyond texting, a variety of social media available on these devices—TikTok, Instagram, Facebook, Snapchat, and a variety of music applications—vie for the driver's attention. In addition, the availability of in-car entertainment as a result of constant Internet access is more widespread than ever. Drivers who use mobile phones up to 10 minutes before a crash are associated with a fourfold increased likelihood of a crash.[26] Researchers also report that high school students who text while driving (nearly half of all U.S. high school students who drive) are more likely to engage in additional risky motor vehicle behaviors, such as not always wearing seatbelts, riding with a driver who had been drinking alcohol, and drinking alcohol and driving.[27]

Use of electronic devices is only part of the problem. Drivers also become distracted when eating or drinking, putting on makeup, tending to children, talking to a passenger, looking for something in the car or a bag, and fidgeting with controls. But add to these all of the technological devices now in widespread use, and the impact of distracted driving on highway safety becomes significant. In 2021, 3,522 people died in distraction-affected crashes, which shows a 12% decrease from 2017.[25] Drivers aged 25 to 34 years have the highest proportion of fatal crashes in which the driver was reported as being distracted at the time of the crash (25%).[25]

States are taking a comprehensive approach to reducing distracted driving, including education, legislation, and enforcement. To date, 34 states have passed primary enforcement laws banning the use of handheld cell phones while driving, thus an officer may cite a driver for using a handheld cell phone without any other traffic offense. Additionally, 49 states and the District of Columbia have banned text messaging for all drivers. Legislation is in place in 25 states that bans all cell phone use by school bus drivers and in 36 states for novice drivers.[19]

In a "free society," such as the one in which Americans live, there is a limit to how much can be accomplished through legislation. For example, it has been very difficult to reduce the number of firearm injuries in the United States through legislation because the National Rifle Association (NRA), gun and ammunition manufacturers, and other interests have been able to lobby successfully against restrictions on gun ownership.

Another example of the difficulty of achieving a balance between personal freedoms and society's legitimate health interests is motorcycle helmet legislation. Current research indicates that helmets reduce motorcycle fatalities by 37% for riders and 41% for passengers and reduce the risk of brain injury by 41%.[28] In 1975, all but two states required motorcyclists to use helmets. Beginning in 1976, states began to repeal these laws. Currently, only 18 states, Puerto Rico, and the District of Columbia require a helmet for all motorcyclists.[19]

The strategy of prevention through regulation can be difficult to implement. The idea of regulating health behavior grates against the individual freedom that Americans have come to expect. Why should someone be required to wear a safety belt? The answer to that is: for the good of the total public—to protect the resources, including human life, of the greater public. Others say, "It's my life, and if I choose to take the risk of dying by not wearing a safety belt, who should care?" That response is all well and good, but when life is lost, it affects many others, such as family members, friends, and coworkers, not just the deceased. This scenario would become worse if the person not wearing a safety belt does not die but becomes a paraplegic and a ward of the state. Many public resources would then be required.

At what point is some legislation enough? It is known that safety belts and air bags are good and effective, but so are helmets—at least they think so at the Indianapolis 500. So, should people now work to pass a law that requires all automobile and truck drivers to wear helmets? How much legislated health behavior is enough?

Automatic Protection

When engineered changes are combined with regulatory efforts, remarkable results can sometimes be achieved. The technique of improving product or environmental design to reduce unintentional injuries is termed **automatic (passive) protection**.[22] A good example is childproof safety caps (see **Figure 15.11**). Childproof safety caps on aspirin and other medicines were introduced in 1972. By 1977, deaths attributed to ingestion of analgesics and antipyretics had decreased by 41%.[29] We are all familiar with automatic protection devices. Common examples include automatic shutoff mechanisms on power tools (such as lawn mowers), safety caps on toxic products, and the warning lights and sounds that remind us to buckle our safety belts, warn us that a nearby vehicle is backing up, or, in some newer cars, let us know if we are too close to another vehicle. NHTSA released a rule requiring that, as of 2018, all vehicles under 10,000 pounds be equipped with rear visibility technology.[30]

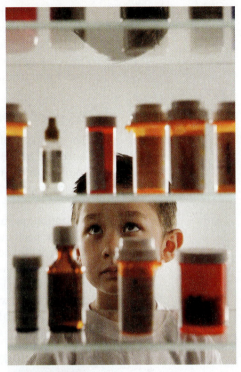

FIGURE 15.11 Child safety caps are an example of automatic or passive protection.
© Chris Stein/Stone/Getty Images

Litigation

When other methods fail, behavioral changes can sometimes come about through the courts. **Litigation**—lawsuits filed on behalf of injured victims or their families—has been successful in removing dangerous products from store shelves or otherwise influencing changes in dangerous behavior. Litigation against a manufacturer of unsafe automobile airbags, for example, might result in safer airbags. Sometimes these lawsuits can be very large. In 2014, the National Highway Traffic Safety Administration initiated what would become the largest safety recall in United States history for faulty airbags, affecting more than 70 million cars. In these cases, airbags manufactured by the automotive parts supplier, Takata, contained defective propellant. As a result, there was an increased risk that the airbags would deploy with explosive force and even eject metal shards. More than 400 people were injured and 26 died in the United States. The company agreed to a $1 billion settlement over their handling of the recall, and, as of 2024, automobiles continue to be recalled because of the airbags.[31] In these ways, litigation can encourage companies to provide safer products.

Lawsuits against bartenders and bar owners for serving alcohol to alcohol-impaired customers, who have then injured other people, have produced more responsible server behavior at public bars. Alcohol-related deaths and injuries on college campuses have caused insurance companies to re-examine their liability insurance policies with fraternities and sororities. This has forced some of these organizations and the universities themselves to restrict the way alcohol is used. The outcome may be a drop in unintentional injuries on these campuses.

Automatic (passive) protection the modification of a product or environment to reduce unintentional injuries

Litigation the process of seeking justice for injury through courts

Intentional Injuries

Intentional injuries, the outcome of self-directed and interpersonal violence, are a staggering community health problem in the United States. More than 74,800 people die, and millions of others receive nonfatal injuries, each year as a result of self-directed or interpersonal violence.

In 2021, an estimated 1.6 million persons were treated for nonfatal physical assault-related injuries, and over 340,000 were hospitalized.[32] Although the physical assault rate is higher for males than for females, the rate of ED visits for sexual assault–related injuries is eight times higher for females. The highest injury rates for both males and females that resulted in ED visits were for individuals aged 20 to 29 years.[32]

Types of Intentional Injuries

The spectrum of violence includes assaults, rapes, suicides, and homicides. These acts of violence can be perpetrated against family members (children, elders, and intimate partners), community members, or complete strangers. In 2022, 3.5 million U.S. residents aged 12 years or older reported being victims of a violent crime, resulting in 6.2 million incidents. Although this represents an increase in violent crime incidents over the previous year, the overall victimization rate has declined since 1993.[33]

Interpersonal violence is a costly community and public health problem, not only because of the loss of life and productivity but also because of the economic cost. Consider the community, state, and national resources expended because of interpersonal violence. There are numerous costs for the police, the legal system, the penal system, emergency healthcare services, medical services, social workers, and many others. Clearly, this is a problem for which prevention is the most economical approach.

Epidemiology of Intentional Injuries

To better understand the problem of intentional injuries, it is instructive to look more closely at both the victims and the perpetrators of violence. Interpersonal violence disproportionately affects those who are frustrated and hopeless, those who are jobless and live in poverty, and those with low self-esteem. More violent acts, whether self-directed or directed at others, are committed by males. Firearms are increasingly involved in violent acts, with ever-increasing fatal consequences. Abuse of drugs, especially alcohol, also contributes to the number of intentional injuries. Additionally, perpetrators of violent acts are more likely to have been abused or neglected as children or exposed to violence and aggression earlier in their lives.

Homicide, Assault, and Rape

In 2022, 21,156 murders (6.3 per 100,000 population) were reported to the Federal Bureau of Investigation (FBI).[34] Although the U.S. homicide rate has declined from 9.3 per 100,000 inhabitants in 1992, the COVID-19 pandemic marked a dramatic turning point in the trends. Between 2019 and 2020, the murder rate increased by 30% from 5.2 per 100,000 population to 6.8, the largest single-year increase since 1905. It remains unclear which factors drove the increase in murders; however, the societal and economic impacts of the pandemic, an increase in gun ownership, and changes in police-community relationships are likely culprits.[35,36] Homicide and legal intervention were ranked as the 16th leading cause of death for the overall population in the United States in 2021.[9] In the 15 to 24 age group, homicide ranked as the second leading cause of death and the third leading cause among the 1 to 4, 5 to 9, and 25 to 34 age groups.[9] Firearms accounted for 81% of all homicides reported in the United States in 2021, the highest proportion ever recorded by the CDC since it began tracking such data in 1968.[37]

Males, Black people, and people aged 18 to 24 experienced the highest rates of violent victimization in 2022.[33] Married and widowed people experience lower than average violent victimization rates. In 2022, males experienced violent victimization at a rate of 17.5 per 1,000 population compared with 15.5 per 1,000 for females. In comparison, victimization rates per 1,000 were 18.5 for Black people; 16.1 for White people; 15.9 for Hispanics; 9.9 for Asians, Native Hawaiians, and Pacific Islanders; and 45.1 for those of other races. Overall, it is estimated that only 41.5% of all violent crimes committed in 2022 were reported to police. In the case of rapes or sexual assaults, even fewer (21.4%) were reported to police.[33] This makes the acquisition of accurate statistics on rape and attempted rape difficult. If the perpetrator is a stranger, the incident is more likely to be reported to the police. However, eight out of 10 sexual violence incidents involve an offender who was a family member, intimate partner, friend, or acquaintance.[38]

Suicide and Attempted Suicide

As previously indicated, more than 48,000 suicides are reported each year in the United States, accounting for one-sixth of all injury mortality. In 2021, 48,183 suicide deaths were reported, making this the 11th leading cause of death.[9] Firearms were the most common method of suicide (54.6%). Other methods of suicide included suffocation (25.8%) and poisoning (11.6%).[39] Although data on suicide attempts is incomplete, research suggests that 1.7 million adults attempted suicide. Adult women attempt suicide 1.3 times more often than men, but men die by suicide 3.9 times more than women.[40] The age-adjusted suicide rate for men (22.8 per 100,000) was nearly four times that for women (5.7 per 100,000) in 2017.[41]

Suicide is the second-leading cause of death for the 10 to 14, and 25 to 34 age groups and the third-leading cause of death for the 15 to 24 age group.[9] The rate of suicide among women is highest in the 45 to 64 age group (8.2 per 100,000). For men 25 to 44 years old, the suicide rates are highest (30 per 100,000). The suicide rate for men aged 75 years and older is the highest for any population subgroup (42.2 per 100,000) and 10 times higher than the rate for elderly women (4.4 per 100,000).[41] When suicide rates are reported by race, American Indian/Alaskan Natives have the highest rates for both men (42.6 per 100,000) and women (13.8 per 100,000).[41] These data present suicide as a challenging public health issue with differences consistently reported by method, sex, age, and method, as well as occupation, geographic location, sexual minority status, and disability status.[42]

Firearm Injuries and Injury Deaths

Statistics on fatal and nonfatal firearm injuries include data covering both intentional and unintentional incidents. When one considers all firearm deaths—those that result from both intentional and unintentional acts—firearms were the second leading cause of injury deaths after poisoning in 2021 (see **Figure 15.12**).[4] In 2021, there were 48,830 firearm injury deaths.

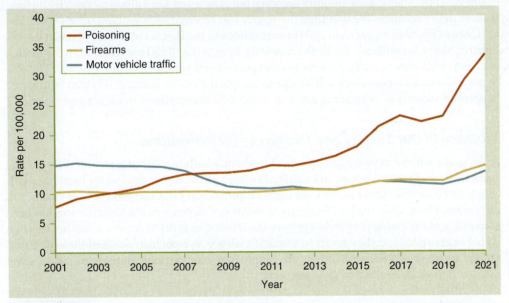

FIGURE 15.12 Leading causes of injury deaths, 1979 to 2021. By 2008, poisonings had superseded motor vehicle crashes as the leading cause of injury death in the United States.

Data from Centers for Disease Control and Prevention. (2023). *Fatal injury data.* Injury Prevention & Control (WISQARS™). Available at https://wisqars.cdc.gov/reports

Of these, 26,328 (54%) were classified as suicides, 21,495 (44%) as homicides and legal interventions, 549 (1%) as unintentional, and 458 (<1%) of undetermined intent.[4] In 2021, as in most years, males were six times more likely to die or be treated in an emergency department for a gunshot wound than females.[4]

In recent years, the proportion of homicides and suicides in which a firearm was used has reached historic highs. The firearm homicide rate increased by 34.6% between 2019 and 2020 and increased another 8.3% between 2020 and 2021. As previously discussed, 81% of homicides were attributed to firearm injuries in 2021.[43] The firearm suicide rate increased by 1.5% between 2019 and 2020 and increased another 5.9% between 2020 and 2021. Although this was a smaller increase compared with firearm homicide data, as of 2021, 55% of suicides were attributed to firearm injuries; this was the highest percentage since 2001.[43,44] The increase of firearm injuries in the United States throughout 2020 and 2021 occurred against the backdrop of the COVID-19 pandemic and protests against the use of lethal force by law enforcement. Although researchers have not established a causal relationship between these events and the increase in firearm injury, it is possible that interruptions to health, social, and emergency services and the worsening of social and economic conditions increased the risk of homicide and suicide.[43,44]

At highest risk for homicide involving firearms are teenage boys and young men, aged 15 to 39.[4] As is reported in the Youth Risk Behavior Surveillance System (YRBSS) 2021 report, 5.0% of high school males had carried a gun on at least one occasion during the 12 months before the survey.[45] Gun-carrying behavior increases the risk of deadly violence against others as well as oneself; over 22% of high school students indicated that they had seriously considered suicide at least once in the 12 months before the survey.[45]

One barrier to preventing firearm injuries and deaths is the absence of a detailed, federally supported reporting system. Unlike the highly developed reporting system for motor vehicle crashes and crash injuries, there is no such system for firearm-related injuries. Each year since 1996, at the bequest of the national gun lobby, the U.S. Congress has approved the Dickey Amendment, a provision added to the national spending bill that prevents the CDC from using federal funds to advocate or promote gun control. CDC officials have historically understood the language to prohibit any research on firearms whatsoever.[46] However, in 2018, Congress approved a softening of the provision's language to allow the CDC to research the causal factors of gun violence. Additionally, the 2018 spending bill earmarked $25 million for the CDC to fund firearm injury research, the first time the agency had received such funding since 1996.[47] The CDC began distributing funds in 2020 to nine states and the District of Columbia under its new Firearm Injury Surveillance Through Emergency Rooms (FASTER) program. With the money, recipients can create surveillance systems that provide real-time data on gun violence. The ultimate goal is that communities will be able to use the data to understand why gun injuries are happening, identify priority areas, and improve public health efforts to reduce gun violence.[47]

Violence in Our Society and Resources for Prevention

A 6th-grade student brings a gun to school to shoot a bully, a mother is run off the road and injured by an aggressive driver, and a child dies from physical punishment for breaking a rule at home. These newspaper reports are signs of unnecessary but common acts of violence in our communities. Over the past few years, it seems as if violence in the United States has been increasing. Many young people do not have the interest or skills to resolve a conflict through verbal negotiation, and they resort to physical violence to resolve it. Some of these confrontations are gang-related, while others are simply individual actions. In the next sections, we discuss individual, family, and gang violence.

Individuals and Violence

A significant number of violent acts committed in the United States each year are committed by individuals who lack basic communication and problem-solving skills. Many of these people are not interested in resolving an argument through discussion, compromise, and understanding. Instead, they are intent on "winning" their argument, by physical force, if necessary. (After all, isn't that the way arguments are won on television, in computer games, and in the movies?)

The availability and proliferation of firearms make this approach particularly deadly. In 2021 among Black American people, homicide and legal intervention were the number one cause of death in the 15 to 24 year age group and the second-leading cause of death in the 1 to 14 year and 25 to 34 year age groups.[9] Among the entire American population, homicide and legal intervention accounted for approximately 1 in 10 deaths.[4] Because of the level of violence, many schools and community organizations offer conflict resolution programs that teach youths alternative ways to resolve disagreements. These programs are designed for various grade levels and teach about the nature of conflicts, the harmful effects of violence, alternatives to violent behavior, and how to make safe decisions. Some of these programs can be found by searching the Violence Prevention website of the Centers for Disease Control and Prevention, where programs are listed by social setting (youth, intimate partner, elder). An example of one such program is the STRYVE: Striving to Reduce Youth Violence Everywhere program.[48]

Family Violence and Abuse

Family violence includes the maltreatment of children, intimate partner violence, sibling violence, and violence directed toward older family members. Because children are our most important resources, and because being abused or neglected as a child increases one's risk for violent behavior as an adult, it is of paramount importance that society increases its efforts to intervene in cases of family violence. In recent years, there has been increased attention paid to family violence, including violence against children and intimate partners. The victimization rates for intimate partners and children steadily declined between 1993 and 2014 but have fluctuated since then. Although the rates began to decline again in 2019 and 2020, they increased in 2021 and 2022.[33] Some of the decline in the 1990s can be attributed to improved efforts by social service agencies that are tasked with intervening and preventing family violence. But some can be attributed to economic conditions—lower unemployment rates mean less domestic violence. Beginning in 2001, as the economy weakened, the decline in intimate partner violence rate slowed while the overall violent crime rate continued to decline. During the COVID-19 pandemic, the risk of family violence increased again as many households experienced economic hardship. Households that reported experiencing income loss were twice as likely to experience abuse with greater frequency. Females were more likely to experience verbal abuse than males, and sexual minorities were more likely to experience family violence than their heterosexual peers.[49]

Child Maltreatment

Child maltreatment is an act or failure to act by a parent, caretaker, or other person as defined under state law that results in physical abuse, neglect, medical neglect, sexual abuse, emotional abuse, or an act or failure to act that presents an imminent risk of serious harm to a child. Also included are other forms of child maltreatment, such as child abandonment and congenital drug addiction. **Child abuse** can be physical, emotional, verbal, or sexual. Physical abuse is the intentional (nonaccidental) inflicting of injury on another person by shaking, throwing, beating, burning, or other means. Emotional abuse can take many forms, including showing no emotion and the failure to provide warmth, attention, supervision, or normal living experiences. Verbal abuse is the demeaning or teasing of another verbally. Sexual abuse includes the physical acts of fondling or intercourse, nonphysical acts, such as indecent exposure or obscene phone calls, or violent physical acts, such as rape and battery. **Child neglect** is a type of maltreatment that refers to the failure by the parent or legal caretaker to provide necessary, age-appropriate care when financially able to do so, or when offered financial or other means to do so. Neglect may be physical, such as the failure to provide food, clothing, medical care, shelter, or cleanliness. It also may be emotional, such as the failure to provide attention, supervision, or other support necessary for a child's well-being. In addition, it may be educational, such as the failure to ensure

Family violence the use of physical force by one family member against another, with the intent to hurt, injure, or cause death

Child maltreatment an act or failure to act by a parent, caretaker, or other person as defined under state law that results in physical abuse, neglect, medical neglect, sexual abuse, emotional abuse, or an act or failure to act that presents an imminent risk of serious harm to a child

Child abuse the intentional physical, emotional, verbal, or sexual mistreatment of a minor

Child neglect the failure of a parent or guardian to care for or otherwise provide the necessary subsistence for a child

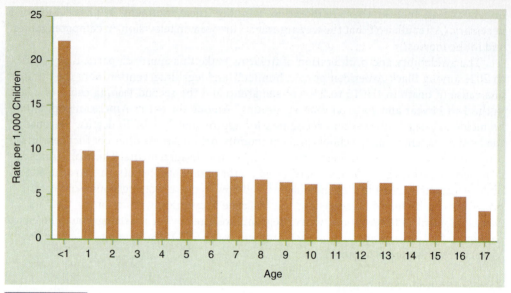

FIGURE 15.13   Victimization rates per 1,000 children by age, 2022.

Modified from U.S. Department of Health and Human Services, Administration for Children & Families, Administration on Children, Youth and Families, Children's Bureau. (2024). *Child maltreatment 2022*. Available at https://www.acf.hhs.gov/sites/default/files/documents/cb/cm2022.pdf

that a child attends school regularly. Educational neglect is one of the most common categories of neglect, followed by physical, and then emotional neglect.

In 2022, 558,899 children under the age of 18 years were victims of abuse or neglect nationwide at a rate of 7.7 per 1,000 children. Seventy-six percent of the perpetrators were parents.[50] Although it marked a 20.0% decrease from the number of victims reported in 2018, some states reported an increase between 2021 and 2022. This was due, in part, to the end of COVID-19 restrictions, allowing children to return to in-person learning and be observed by educational personnel. Of the 558,899 children who were maltreated in 2022, three-fourths (74.3%) suffered neglect, 17.0% suffered physical abuse, 10.6% were sexually abused, and 6.8% were psychologically maltreated. Many children suffered more than one kind of maltreatment, with the most common combination being neglect and physical abuse.[50] The highest victimization rates were for infants (22.2 maltreatments per 1,000 children) and children 1 year of age (9.9 per 1,000 children), and these rates decline with age (see **Figure 15.13**). Victimization rates vary by race and ethnicity. In 2022, the lowest rates were for Asian children (1.3 per 1,000 children), and the highest rates were for American Indian and Alaska Native children (14.3 per 1,000 children), followed by Black children (12.1 per 1,000 children), and Pacific Islander children (9.3 per 1,000 children), Hispanic children (7.0 per 1,000 children), and White children (6.6 per 1,000 children). Multiracial children experienced abuse at a rate of 9.4 per 1,000 children.[50]

An estimated 1,990 children died of abuse or neglect in 2022, at a rate of approximately 2.7 deaths per 100,000 children. Sixty-six percent of all child fatalities were under the age of three years. The highest child maltreatment fatality rate (24.3 per 100,000 children) was among those younger than 1 year of age (see **Figure 15.14**). One or both parents caused 81.8% of all child fatalities.[50]

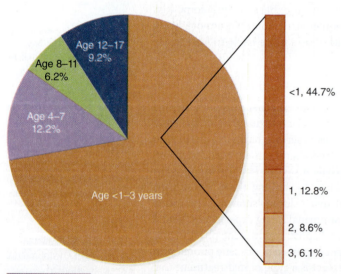

FIGURE 15.14   Percentage of child fatalities resulting from maltreatment by age, 2022.

Modified from U.S. Department of Health and Human Services, Administration for Children & Families, Administration on Children, Youth and Families, Children's Bureau. (2024). *Child maltreatment 2022*. Available at https://www.acf.hhs.gov/sites/default/files/documents/cb/cm2022.pdf

Maltreatment deaths were more often associated with neglect than with abuse. Parental drug and alcohol use is a significant factor in reported child maltreatment and fatality cases, as is being the perpetrator or victim of domestic violence.[50]

Children who physically survive maltreatment may be scarred emotionally. What happens to abused and neglected children after they grow up? Do the victims of violence and neglect later become criminals or violent offenders? Research suggests adolescent and early adulthood risky behavior may be more likely for young children who experienced physical abuse.[51]

Prevention of Child Maltreatment

One of the keys to protecting children from maltreatment is a system of timely reporting and referral to one of the many state and local child protective service (CPS) agencies. Anyone may make such a report (e.g., a relative, neighbor, or teacher). In 2022, 70% of child abuse and neglect reports were received from professional law enforcement personnel (21.2%), educational personnel (20.7%), and medical personnel (11.2%). Nonprofessionals—friends, neighbors, and relatives—were responsible for 15.2% of reports.[50] Signs of neglect include extremes in behavior, an uncared-for appearance, evidence of a lack of supervision at home, or the lack of medical care.

CPS agencies provide services to prevent future instances of child abuse or neglect and to remedy harm that has occurred as a result of child maltreatment. These services are designed to increase the parents' child-rearing competence and knowledge of the developmental stages of childhood. There may be an assessment of the family's strengths and weaknesses, development of a plan based on the family's needs, and post-investigative follow-up services. Services might include respite care, parenting education, housing assistance, substance-use treatment, daycare, home visits, counseling, and other services. The goal is to ensure the safety of the child or children.[50]

There are many useful sources of information and support for those interested in preventing child abuse and neglect. The Child Welfare Information Gateway, sponsored by the Children's Bureau of the U.S. Department of Health and Human Services Administration for Children and Families, provides information, products, and technical assistance services to help professionals locate information related to child abuse and neglect and related child welfare issues (www.childwelfare.gov). Another source of information is the Committee for Children. Its mission is to promote the safety, well-being, and social development of children (www.cfchildren.org). The Centers for Disease Control and Prevention, Injury Prevention and Control Division of Violence Prevention has valuable information on child maltreatment prevention (www.cdc.gov/violenceprevention/childmaltreatment/index.html).

Elder Maltreatment

The maltreatment of elders (persons 65 years of age and older) is a problem worldwide, where it is estimated that one in six people aged 60 years and older experienced some form of abuse in community settings during the past year.[52] Globally, maltreatment of elders is expected to increase as populations age; the number of those 60 years of age and older is predicted to double from 900 million in 2015 to 2 billion in 2050.[52] In the U.S. population, the proportion of the population made up of elders is growing. Elders living in the United States numbered 57.8 million in 2022 but is expected to increase to 82.1 million by 2050.[53,54] Although elders experience violent crime at a lower rate than people of other ages, approximately one in six to one in 13 elders experienced maltreatment within the past year.[6,55] Women tend to be more vulnerable to elder abuse as are those with low social support, cognitive deficits, functional impairment, and poor health.[56]

Abuse can be physical, sexual, psychological, emotional, or financial, or it may involve abandonment, neglect, or self-neglect. Elders may be kicked, hit, denied food and medical care, or have their Social Security checks or other financial resources stolen or otherwise misappropriated. Most cases of elder abuse are not reported or only become apparent following other

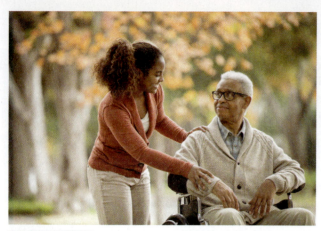

FIGURE 15.15   Listening to the needs and concerns of elders and their caregivers can help prevent abuse.

© Terry Vine/DigitalVision/Getty Images

legal or medical proceedings; thus, accurate statistics on the incidence of elder abuse are unavailable. As the American population ages, elder maltreatment is likely to become a community health problem of increasing importance.

Prevention of Elder Maltreatment

Prevention of elder maltreatment begins with learning the signs of elder abuse, listening to elders and their caregivers, learning how to report maltreatment, and reporting maltreatment to Adult Protective Services (see **Figure 15.15**).[57] One could also learn the risk and protective factors for perpetration. Perpetrators of elder abuse and neglect may have mental illness or misuse substances, they may have high levels of stress or inadequate coping skills, or they may have been abused as a child.[57] Finally, one may wish to seek assistance by calling the Eldercare Locator hotline at 1-800-677-1116. More information is available from the National Center on Elder Abuse (www.ncea.acl.gov).

Intimate Partner Violence

The term **intimate partner violence (IPV)** refers to physical or sexual violence, emotional, economic, or technological abuse, stalking, or psychological aggression that occurs in a romantic relationship. It can be perpetrated by a current or former spouse or dating partner in opposite-sex and same-sex relationships.[58,59] Each year, countless women and men are victimized by their intimate partners with nearly one in three women and one in four men reporting severe physical violence from an intimate partner in their lifetime.[58] For IPV survivors, approximately 75% of female and 48% of male survivors experience some sort of physical injury. United States crime reports suggest that one in five homicide victims are killed by an intimate partner.[58]

Injuries from intimate partner violence are under-reported, with thousands of individuals injured as a result of IPV requiring medical treatment each year. In addition to physical injuries, survivors of IPV may experience depression and post-traumatic stress disorder (PTSD) symptoms. The health care, time away from work, and criminal justice costs of intimate partner violence exceed $3.6 trillion.[58]

Each year, thousands of American children witness IPV within their families as more than 15 million children live in homes in which domestic violence has happened at least once. Witnessing such violence is a risk factor for developing long-term physical and mental health problems, including becoming a victim of abuse and perpetrating IPV.[60]

Risk factors for IPV perpetration include experiencing economic stress, a belief in strict gender roles, and a history of abuse during childhood and aggressive behavior during adolescence.[61] In a dysfunctional relationship, the perpetrator may seek to exert power and control over the victim, resulting in a cycle in which violence recurs (see **Figure 15.16**).[59] The cycle of violence depicts the progression of steps leading up to an attack or episode of violence and the restoration of calm. A violent episode may result from the loss of a job, a divorce, illness, death of a family member, or misbehavior (actual or perceived)

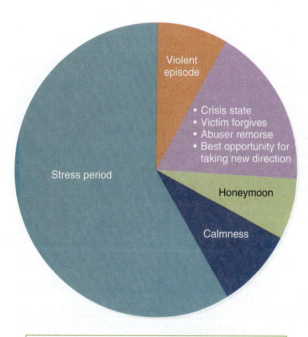

Stress factors	Characteristics of abuser
• Isolation—pregnancy	• Possessive—jealous
• Economics	• Low impulse control
• Alcohol/drugs	• Substance abuse
• Death—role change	• Rigid role expectations
• Change in family structure	• Controlling—dictatorial
• Sexual dysfunction	
• Medical problem	

FIGURE 15.16   Cycle of violence.

Domestic Abuse Intervention Project in Duluth, Minnesota, as reported in *AHEC News*, a publication of the Area Health Education Centers of Oklahoma (February 1994). *AHEC News*, *2*(1), 9. Used with permission.

of children or an intimate partner. The likelihood that abuse will occur is greatly increased if alcohol has been consumed. While selected interventions aimed at one factor (for example, the abuser) might mitigate against family violence, community efforts to reduce violence should be both comprehensive, involving a variety of approaches, and coordinated among all agencies involved in order to be effective.

Prevention of Intimate Partner Violence

Prevention of IPV involves improvements in identifying and documenting cases of IPV and increasing access to services for victims and perpetrators of IPV and their children. Coordinating community initiatives strengthens the safety networks for high-risk individuals and families. Some communities have established a "Violence Coordinating Council" that holds monthly meetings to set an agenda and action plans for the community and to determine and clarify the roles and responsibilities of agencies and individuals. It is important for communities to develop and implement a coordinated response with strong advocates from criminal justice, victim services, children's services, and allied professions. Healthcare providers make up a particularly important group in this regard. Educational materials and programs on IPV and sexual assault are available at the National Center for Injury Prevention and Control website (www.cdc.gov/injury/).

> **Intimate partner violence (IPV)** describes physical or sexual violence, emotional, economic, or technological abuse, stalking, or psychological aggression by a current or former spouse or dating partner, including opposite-sex and same-sex couples

Violence in Schools

Although schools are one of the safest places for children to spend their time (see **Figure 15.17**), even rare acts of violence in schools strike terror into parents, teachers, and the children themselves. Highly publicized incidents of fatal shootings on school grounds have focused the nation's attention on the question of just how safe (or unsafe) our nation's schools are.

Our nation's schools should be safe havens for teaching and learning, free of crime and violence. Any instance of crime or violence at school not only affects the individuals involved but also may disrupt the educational process and affect bystanders, the school itself, and the surrounding community.

The National Center for Educational Statistics (NCES), in the U.S. Department of Education (DoE), and the Bureau of Justice Statistics (BJS) in the U.S. Department of Justice jointly collect and publish data annually on the frequency, seriousness, and incidence of violence in elementary and secondary schools.[62] During the 2019 to 2020 school year, 25 student, staff, and nonstudent school-associated violent deaths were recorded, which included 23 homicides, one suicide, and one legal intervention. In 2021, among students aged 12 to 18 years, there were about 170,600 nonfatal victimizations at school (i.e., theft and nonfatal violent victimization). In 2021, the rate of violent victimization in school (7 per 1,000 students) was lower than the rate away from school (20 per 1,000), which represents a decline in total victimization rates since 2019 (30 per 1,000 students). However, these data were collected when many states suspended in-person classes due to the COVID-19 pandemic. Thus, these figures may only represent that students were not in the school setting as much as in previous years, as opposed to a true decline in school violence. For reference, the 2019 nonfatal victimization rate was not statistically different from the 2010 rate.[62]

Fighting and weapon carrying are also concerns. In 2021, nearly one-fifth (18.3%) of students in grades 9 to 12 reported they had been in a fight during the previous year, 5.8% on school property. Nationwide, 3.1% of students had carried a weapon (for example, a gun, knife, or a club) on school property on at least one day in the 30 days prior to the survey. As stated previously, 7.7% of males in grades 9 to 12 reported carrying a gun in the past 30 days in 2017.[45]

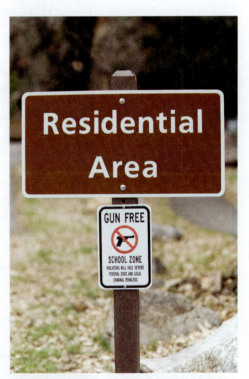

FIGURE 15.17   Despite several highly publicized tragic events, schools are one of the safest places for students to spend time.

© Simon Balson/Alamy Stock Photo

Most schools try to deal with violence problems by instituting zero-tolerance policies toward serious student offenses. These policies, defined as school or district policy mandating predetermined consequences for various student offenses, have come under fire because administering such policies sometimes leads to somewhat extreme outcomes. In 2020, almost all schools utilized some type of security measure, such as controlling access to school buildings (97%), using security cameras (91%), and requiring faculty to wear badges or picture IDs (77%). Most schools (65%) also report having at least one security staff on school grounds at least once a week.[63] Some schools have established electronic notification systems for schoolwide emergencies and/or implemented, structured anonymous threat systems.

Bullying and being bullied at school are increasingly being recognized as associated with violence-related behavior (such as carrying a weapon to school, fighting, or becoming injured in a fight). Bullying includes being made fun of; being made the subject of rumors; being threatened with harm; being pushed, shoved, tripped, or spat on; being pressured to do something one does not want to do; being excluded, or having one's property destroyed. In 2019, 22% of 12- to 18-year-olds reported having been bullied at school during the school year and 16% reported having been electronically bullied.[62]

Safe Schools/Healthy Students Initiative

The Safe Schools/Healthy Students Initiative is a unique grant program jointly administered by the U.S. Departments of Education, Health and Human Services (Mental Health Services), and Justice. The program promotes a comprehensive, integrated problem-solving process for use by communities in addressing school violence. The Safe Schools/Healthy Students framework integrates strategic approaches (i.e., collaboration and partnerships, policy change and development, and capacity building) with core components (i.e., promoting mental, emotional, and behavioral health or creating safe schools) and guiding principles (cultural competency, resource leveraging, and sustainability) to guide grantees in developing evidence-based approaches to mental health promotion and youth violence prevention.[63]

Youth Violence After School

Although violence in schools has grabbed the headlines, the real problem area is violence committed after school. Fewer and fewer children have a parent waiting for them at home after school. Whereas many youths are able to supervise themselves and their younger siblings responsibly after school or are engaged in sports or other after-school activities, some are not. Statistics show that serious violent crime committed by juveniles peaks in the hours immediately after school (see **Figure 15.18**). Also, during these after-school hours, juveniles are most likely to become victims of crime, including violent crimes, such as robberies and aggravated assaults.[64]

For individuals and communities that want to engage in youth violence prevention, a variety of federal and state government agencies and private organizations offering leadership and support can be found by searching the Internet. The Centers for Disease Control and Prevention has an excellent website that lists information and resources for youth violence and youth violence prevention.[65]

Violence in Our Communities

Youth gangs, human trafficking, and firearm violence contribute to the overall level of violence in the community and are a drain on community resources.

Youth Gang Violence

Whereas most young people in the United States grow up subscribing to such American ideals as democracy, individualism, equality, and education, others do not. Many of those who do not are economically disadvantaged and have lost faith in society's capacity to work on their behalf. Some of these seek refuge and reward in organized subculture groups of peers who feel similarly disenfranchised.

One popular subculture structure is the **youth gang**, a self-formed association of peers bound together by mutual interests, with identifiable leadership and well-defined lines of authority. Youth gangs act in concert to achieve a specific purpose, and their acts generally

Youth gang an association of peers, bound by mutual interests and identifiable lines of authority, whose acts generally include illegal activity and control over a territory or an enterprise

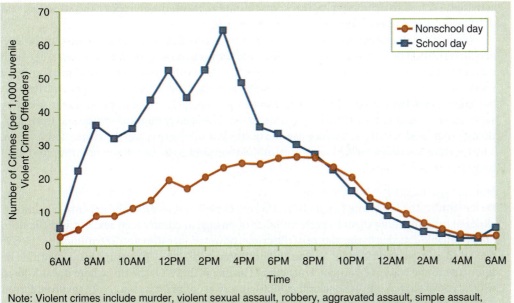

Note: Violent crimes include murder, violent sexual assault, robbery, aggravated assault, simple assault, and kidnapping. Data are from law enforcement agencies in 45 states and the District of Columbia.

FIGURE 15.18   Serious violent crime committed by juveniles peaks in the hours immediately after school.

Modified from U.S. Department of Justice, Office of Juvenile Justice and Delinquency Prevention. (2022). *Offending by juveniles: Time of day.* Available at https://ojjdp.ojp.gov/statistical-briefing-book/offending-by-youth/faqs/qa03301

include illegal activities and the control over a particular territory or enterprise. Types of illegal activities in which gang members participate include larceny/theft, aggravated assault, burglary/breaking and entering, and street drug sales.

In 2019, 9% of students aged 12 to 18 years reported gang presence at their school. This was a decline since 2009 when 20% of students reported gang presence.[62] An estimated 8% of all youth have joined a gang by the time they reach adolescence. The social status and excitement of gang membership may entice many young people, but others may join a gang because they believe it will offer them protection from neighborhood violence or because they fear for their safety if they do not join. The good news is that most gang membership is short-term, with fewer than one in 10 gang members remaining involved for four or more years. However, gang membership inherently increases the risk of perpetrating or being the victim of violence. Even after leaving a gang, former members are at long-term risk of substance use and mental health disorders.[66]

Youth gangs and youth gang–related violence present an enormous drain on the law enforcement resources of a community beyond the injuries and injury deaths that result from their activities. Pressured to "do something," field officers may be pulled from other duties and not replaced. If additional police are hired, it can cost the community $75,000 per year per officer. In short, the suppression of gangs by law enforcement is costly for communities, often depleting resources for other needed community improvements.

Youth Gang Prevention

Many communities have responded effectively to the increased violence resulting from gang-related activity. Perhaps the best approach is a multifaceted effort involving law enforcement, education, diversion activities, and social services support. Suppression of gang activity by law enforcement is justified because many gang-related activities—such as selling illicit drugs, carrying and discharging weapons, and defacing property—are illegal. Education of children, teachers, parents, and community leaders is another facet of gang-related violence prevention. Just as there are drug abuse prevention curricula in schools, there are now anti-gang awareness programs in some schools. Diversion activities, including job opportunities and after-school

Human trafficking a crime in which traffickers exploit and profit at the expense of adults or children by compelling them to perform labor or engage in commercial sex

activities, such as enrichment programs, sports, and recreation, can reduce the attractiveness of less wholesome uses of free time.

Most, if not all, states have agencies with programs aimed at preventing or reducing the level of injuries caused by intentional violence. Many of the agencies or programs are concerned with both unintentional and intentional injury prevention. Funding sources for these programs are variable. Some are funded as line items on state budgets; other programs are grant-driven. At the federal level, the Office of Justice Programs (www.ojp.gov) aims to improve public safety by supporting law enforcement and the justice system. The agency monitors crime and victimization, gang-related activity, substance use and crime, juvenile justice, and the corrections system. Their Crime Solutions website (www.crimesolutions.ojp.gov) lists many community-based programs under "topics."

Human Trafficking

Human trafficking is a crime in which "traffickers exploit and profit at the expense of adults or children by compelling them to perform labor or engage in commercial sex."[67] It is difficult to obtain reliable data due to the nature of the crime; however, an estimated 27.6 million people are trafficked each year worldwide.[67] In the United States in 2021, 16,710 victims were identified by tips made to the National Human Trafficking Hotline in 2021. Of the tips where it was known which type of trafficking was occurring, 83.6% involved commercial sex, 11.9% involved forced labor, and 4.5% involved both.[68] Although any person can be victimized by human trafficking, members of marginalized communities, such as runaway youth and youth who are homeless, undocumented immigrants, people of racial and sexual minority groups, and people with disabilities, are more at risk of being targeted by criminals. It is also important to note that human traffickers can be of any age, race, and occupation group, and trafficking occurs both in the shadows of illegal labor industries and in plain view of the public.[69] The U.S. Department of Health and Human Services Office on Trafficking in Person's (OTIP) National Human Trafficking Training and Technical Assistance Center (NHTTAC) (www.nhttac.acf.hhs.gov/) provides training and technical assistance to community stakeholders who may come into contact with human trafficking victims or those who are at risk. NHTTAC has a trauma-informed and person-centered framework and focuses on education, prevention, response, and intervention.[70]

Firearm Violence

As described earlier, firearm violence is a significant problem for many communities in the United States. Historically, most legislative attempts aimed at making it more difficult for certain persons to acquire handguns and/or automatic weapons have failed to reduce the level of firearm injuries and deaths. Some local governments have banned guns in their jurisdictions in an effort to reduce the frequency of firearm injuries. However, many of these bans are now in jeopardy. In a 6-to-3 ruling in June of 2022, the U.S. Supreme Court struck down New York's concealed carry law, ruling that American citizens have the right to carry a handgun in public for self-defense. The decision has potentially paved the way for challenges to gun control measures in other states.[71] However, that same week, President Joe Biden signed a landmark gun violence bill, the first of its kind to pass Congress in 30 years. Among its provisions were more stringent background checks for people aged 18 to 21 years attempting to purchase a gun and new language that prevents dating partners, in addition to current and former spouses, convicted of domestic abuse from owning a gun.[72]

Firearm injuries can be prevented through collaboration among experts (both those within and outside of public health) addressing the risk factors for gun violence (see **Box 15.2**). Requiring households with minor children to securely store unattended firearms can reduce the risk of unintentional shootings and suicides. Initiatives like hospital-based violence intervention programs can provide at-risk individuals with crucial mental health and social services that may prevent the cycle of violence from continuing.[73,74] The CDC's VetoViolence website (www.vetoviolence.cdc.gov/) lists evidence-based, violence-prevention strategies and training based on the best available evidence. Many of the topics presented on the website can complement firearm injury prevention efforts, including resources for preventing suicide, youth violence, and intimate partner violence.

BOX 15.2   The Public Health Approach to Violence Prevention

The public health approach to community violence prevention focuses on understanding and addressing the root causes. The approach involves a systematic four-step process, and stakeholders from various sectors (such as healthcare, law enforcement, and education) collaborate on one or more of these steps to develop and implement a prevention strategy.

Steps	Guiding Questions	Resource Examples
Define the problem	• What problem do I want to prevent? • How many people are affected? Who are they? • When and where is the problem occurring?	• Web-based Injury Statistics Query and Reporting System (WISQARS) (https://wisqars.cdc.gov/) • Kids Count Data Center (www.datacenter.aecf.org) • State and local vital records, hospital records, or police reports
Identify risk and protective factors	• What are the risk and protective factors for the problem identified in Step 1?	• CDC's Division of Violence Prevention (www.cdc.gov/ViolencePrevention)
Develop and test prevention strategies	• Are there effective strategies based on best available evidence? If no strategies exist, what resources do I need to develop based on Steps 1 and 2? • Where can I find research partners to help evaluate the selected strategy? • Was the strategy effective?	• Blueprints for Healthy Youth Development (www.blueprintsprograms.org) • The Community Guide to Preventive Services (www.thecommunityguide.org) • VetoViolence (www.vetoviolence.cdc.gov/)
Assure widespread adoption	• Who would benefit from this strategy (e.g., parents, educators, policymakers, etc.)? • How do I get this strategy to them? • Where can I get help for implementing an effective strategy? For ongoing monitoring and evaluation?	• EvaluACTION (wwwvetoviolence.cdc.gov/apps/evaluaction) • University of Kansas Community Toolbox (www.ctb.ku.edu)

Modified from Centers for Disease Control. (2018). The Public Health Approach to Violence Prevention (CS221239B). National Center for Injury Prevention and Control. Available at https://www.govinfo.gov/app/details/GOVPUB-HE20-PURL-gpo89860

In conclusion, intentional injuries resulting from interpersonal violence remain a national as well as a community concern. Significant resources are available at the federal level (from the U.S. Departments of Health and Human Services and Justice) to help states and local communities reduce the number and seriousness of violence-related injuries. It is up to each concerned citizen to make sure that their community is taking advantage of these resources.

Chapter Summary

- Injuries are the second-leading cause of death in the United States and the leading cause of premature deaths and years of potential life lost (YPLL).
- Unintentional and intentional injuries represent a major community and public health problem, not only because of the loss of life but also because of lost productivity, medical costs, and the increase in the number of Americans who are disabled.
- Unintentional injuries are unplanned events that are usually preceded by an unsafe act or condition. They are often accompanied by economic loss, and they interrupt the efficient completion of a task.

- Unintentional injuries occur across all age groups; however, they are the leading cause of death for younger Americans, aged 1 to 44 years.
- Poisonings are the leading cause of unintentional injury deaths, followed by motor vehicle crashes.
- Males and certain minority groups suffer proportionately more unintentional injuries.
- Measures to prevent or reduce the number and severity of unintentional injuries and injury fatalities can be successful when based on a familiar public health model in which energy is the causative agent for injuries.
- Four broad strategies can prevent unintentional injuries—education, regulation, automatic protection, and litigation. Together, these strategies may be used to reduce the number and seriousness of unintentional injuries in the community.
- Intentional injuries are the outcome of self-directed or interpersonal violence.
- The spectrum of violence includes suicides, assaults, rapes, robberies, and homicides in our communities, and the maltreatment of children, older adults, and intimate partners in our homes.
- Minorities and young adults are at the highest risk for injury or death from an intentional violent act.
- Family violence, including child and elder maltreatment and intimate partner violence, is a serious and pervasive community and public health problem.
- Widely publicized fatal shootings in schools have once again focused national attention on violence in our schools. However, schools remain a relatively safe place for the nation's youth.
- Gangs and human traffickers pose a danger to at-risk youth and public health. Community members can work together to reduce the risk factors and help survivors.
- Significant resources are available at the state and federal levels (from the U.S. Departments of Health and Human Services and Justice) to assist local communities in reducing the number and seriousness of violence-related injuries.

Scenario: Analysis and Response

Please take a moment to reread the scenario at the beginning of this chapter. Then, reflect on the questions that follow.

1. Should the incident described in the scenario be classified as an unintentional injury or intentional injury? Defend your response.

2. Identify and explain the unsafe acts and unsafe conditions that influenced the events in the scenario. Give two examples of each.

3. What can be done at the individual level to prevent similar incidents from happening in the future? At the school level? At the community level? Give at least one example for each.

Review Questions

1. List the ways in which injuries are costly to society, and quantify the costs in terms of the United States.

2. Identify the leading types of unintentional injury deaths and the risk factors associated with each type of death.

3. Why have the terms *accident* and *safety* lost favor with injury prevention professionals?

4. What is a hazard? Do hazards cause accidents? Explain your answer.

5. How does alcohol consumption contribute to unintentional injuries?

6. Describe the epidemiologic model for injuries, and provide three examples of how energy causes injuries.

7. For each of your examples from Question 6, explain how the injury could have been prevented using prevention and control tactics.

8. Identify the different types of violent behavior that result in intentional injuries.

9. Describe the cost of intentional injuries to society.

10. Define family violence, and give some examples.

11. Explain the difference between child abuse and child neglect. List some contributing factors to these phenomena.

12. What is intimate partner violence? List the types of behaviors included in the definition.

13. How safe are our schools for children? For teachers and staff? How are schools responding to safety concerns?

14. What resources are available at the state and federal levels to help communities reduce the number and seriousness of injuries resulting from violence?

Activities

1. Visit the webpage of a local news station and find three stories dealing with unintentional injuries. Provide a two- or three-sentence summary of each article and then provide your best guess of (a) what the unsafe act or condition that preceded the event was, (b) what the resulting economic loss or injury was, and (c) what task was not completed.

2. Make an appointment and interview the director of safety on your campus. Find out what the most prevalent unintentional injuries are on campus, what strategies have been used to deal with them, and what could be done to eliminate them.

3. With guidance from your course instructor, conduct a random survey of a safety topic, such as texting and driving or safety belt use at your campus. Collect the data in such a manner that you can compare the results between school employees and students. Then, analyze your results and draw some conclusions.

4. Survey your home, apartment, or residence hall and create a room-by-room list of the unsafe conditions that may exist. Then, create a strategy for changing each condition.

5. Using an Internet search engine, locate three news articles that deal with violence. For each article, (a) provide a two-sentence summary, (b) identify and describe the victim and the perpetrator, (c) identify what you feel was the underlying cause of the violence, and (d) offer a suggestion as to how the violence could have been avoided or prevented.

6. Make an appointment with an officer of the local police department to interview them about violent crime in your hometown. Write a two-page summary of your interview and include answers to the following questions: (a) What is the number one violent crime? (b) What is the law enforcement department doing to control violent crime? (c) Does the city have a comprehensive program against crime? (d) How does the police department work with other professionals (e.g., those working in medicine, public health, education, community organizations) to reduce crime? (e) What can the typical citizen do to help reduce violence?

7. Using Box 15.2, choose an intentional injury topic and follow the four-step public health approach:

   a. How many people are affected and what are their demographic characteristics? Where is the problem occurring (city, county, state)? The CDC's *Fatal Injury Explore* and *Nonfatal Injury Explore* tools (https://wisqars.cdc.gov) can help you locate this information.

   b. Use the Internet to research any risk and protective factors for this problem.

   c. Identify or brainstorm a strategy that could be effective. Review this chapter for ideas.

   d. With whom could you share this strategy? For example, youth, parents, educators, policymakers, medical professionals, or law enforcement officials.

References

1. Baker, S. P. (1989). Injury science comes of age. *Journal of the American Medical Association*, 262(16), 2284–2285.

2. World Health Organization. (2001). *Injury surveillance guidelines*. Available at https://iris.who.int/bitstream/handle/10665/42451/9241591331.pdf?sequence=1

3. World Health Organization. (2022). *Preventing injuries and violence: An overview*. Available at https://iris.who.int/bitstream/handle/10665/361331/9789240047136-eng.pdf?sequence=1

4. Centers for Disease Control and Prevention. (2023). *Fatal and nonfatal injury reports*. National Center for Injury Prevention and Control (WISQARS™). Available at https://wisqars.cdc.gov/reports

5. Roser, M., Ritchie, H., & Spooner, F. (2021). *Burden of disease*. Global Change Data Lab. Available at https://ourworldindata.org/burden-of-disease

6. Centers for Disease Control and Prevention. (2024). *Fatal and nonfatal injury reports*. National Center for Injury Prevention and Control (WISQARS™). Available at https://wisqars.cdc.gov/reports

7. National Safety Council. (2024). *Injury facts*. Available at https://injuryfacts.nsc.org

8. Centers for Disease Control and Prevention, National Center for Injury Prevention and Control. (2023). *Leading causes of death* (WISQARS™). Available at https://wisqars.cdc.gov/lcd

9. Centers for Disease Control and Prevention, National Center for Injury Prevention and Control. (2023). *Leading causes of death* (WISQARS™). Available at https://wisqars.cdc.gov/lcd

10. National Safety Council. (2024). *Prevent poisoning and drug overdose*. Available at https://www.nsc.org/community-safety/safety-topics/other-poisons/poison-prevention-home

11. World Health Organization. (2023). *Global status report on road safety 2023*. Available at https://iris.who.int/bitstream/handle/10665/375016/9789240086517-eng.pdf

12. Stewart, T. (2023). *Overview of motor vehicle traffic crashes in 2021* (Report No. DOT HS 813 435). National Highway Traffic Safety Administration. Available at https://crashstats.nhtsa.dot.gov/Api/Public/ViewPublication/813435

13. National Center for Statistics and Analysis. (2023). *Traffic safety facts 2021: A compilation of motor vehicle traffic crash data* (Report No. DOT HS 813 527. National Highway Traffic Safety Administration. Available at https://crashstats.nhtsa.dot.gov/Api/Public/ViewPublication/813527

14. U.S. Department of Health and Human Services. (2024). *Health People 2030 objectives and data*. Available at https://health.gov/healthypeople/objectives-and-data

15. Kakara, R., Bergen, G., Burns, E., & Stevens, M. (2023). Nonfatal and fatal falls among adults aged ≥65 Years — United States, 2020–2021.

Morbidity and Mortality Weekly Report, 72, 938–943. Available at https://www.cdc.gov/mmwr/volumes/72/wr/mm7235a1.htm

16. Centers for Disease Control and Prevention. (2022). *Teen drivers and passengers: Get the facts.* Available at https://www.cdc.gov/transportationsafety/teen_drivers/teendrivers_factsheet.html

17. National Highway Traffic Safety Administration. (2023). *Traffic safety facts 2021 data: Alcohol-impaired driving.* (DOT HS 813 450, June 2023). U.S. Department of Transportation. Available at https://crashstats.nhtsa.dot.gov/Api/Public/ViewPublication/813450

18. National Highway Traffic Safety Administration. (2023). *Traffic safety facts 2021 data: Children.* (DOT HS 813 456). Washington, DC: U.S. Department of Transportation. Available at https://crashstats.nhtsa.dot.gov/Api/Public/ViewPublication/813456

19. Governors Highway Safety Association. (2023). *State laws.* Available at https://www.ghsa.org/state-laws

20. Centers for Disease Control and Prevention. (2024). *Drowning facts.* Available at https://www.cdc.gov/drowning/facts/index.html

21. U.S. Department of Homeland Security, U.S. Coast Guard. (2023). *2022 recreational boating statistics* (COMDTPUB P16754.36). Available at https://www.uscgboating.org/library/accident-statistics/Recreational-Boating-Statistics-2022.pdf

22. Christoffel, T., & Gallagher, S. S. (2006). *Injury Prevention and public health: Practical knowledge, skills, and strategies* (2nd ed.). Jones & Bartlett Learning.

23. Centers for Disease Control and Prevention. (2014). Potentially preventable deaths from the five leading causes of death—United States, 2008–2010. *Morbidity and Mortality Weekly Report, 63*(17), 369–374. Available at http://www.cdc.gov/mmwr/pdf/wk/mm6317.pdf

24. National Highway Traffic Safety Administration. (2019). *Traffic safety facts 2017 data: Occupant protection in passenger vehicles* (DOT HS 812 691). National Center for Statistics and Analysis US Dept of Transportation. Available at https://crashstats.nhtsa.dot.gov/Api/Public/ViewPublication/812691

25. National Highway Traffic Safety Administration. (2021). *Traffic safety facts: Distracted driving in 2021* (DOT HS 813 443). National Center for Statistics and Analysis US Dept of Transportation. Available at https://crashstats.nhtsa.dot.gov/Api/Public/ViewPublication/813443

26. McEvoy, S. P., Stevenson, M. R., McCartt, A. T., Woodward, M., Haworth, C., Palmara, P., & Cercarelli, R. (2005). Role of mobile phones in motor vehicle crashes resulting in hospital attendance: A case-crossover study. *British Medical Journal, 331*(7514), 428–430.

27. Olsen, E. O., Shults, R. A., & Eaton, D. K. (2013). Texting while driving and other risky motor vehicle behaviors among U.S. high school students. *Pediatrics, 131*(6), e1798–e1715. Available at http://pediatrics.aappublications.org/content/early/2013/05/08/peds.2012-3462

28. Centers for Disease Control and Prevention. (2022). *Motorcycle safety.* Available at https://www.cdc.gov/transportationsafety/mc/index.html

29. Centers for Disease Control and Prevention. (1982). Unintentional and intentional injuries—United States. *Morbidity and Mortality Weekly Report, 31*(18), 240–248.

30. National Highway Traffic Safety Administration. (2020). *NHTSA announces final rule requiring rear visibility technology* [Press Release]. Available at https://www.ishn.com/articles/98349-nhtsa-announces-final-rule-requiring-rear-visibility-technology

31. Consumer Reports. (2024). *Takata airbag recall: Everything you need to know.* Available at https://www.consumerreports.org/cars/car-recalls-defects/takata-airbag-recall-everything-you-need-to-know-a1060713669/

32. Centers for Disease Control and Prevention. (2023). *Injury prevention & control: Data and statistics.* Available at https://wisqars.cdc.gov/

33. Thompson, A., & Tapp, S. N. (2023). *Criminal victimization, 2022* (NCJ 307089). Washington, DC: U.S. Department of Justice, Bureau of Justice Statistics. Available at https://bjs.ojp.gov/document/cv22.pdf

34. Federal Bureau of Investigation. (2023). *Crime data explorer: 2022 CIUS estimations.* Available at https://cde.ucr.cjis.gov/

35. Gramlich, J. (2021). *What we know about the increase in U.S. murders in 2020.* Pew Research Center. Available at https://www.pewresearch.org/short-reads/2021/10/27/what-we-know-about-the-increase-in-u-s-murders-in-2020

36. Anderson, M. (2023). *4 key takeaways from the FBI's annual crime report.* NPR. Available at https://www.npr.org/2023/10/20/1207276234/fbi-crime-report-takeaways

37. Gramlich, J. (2023). *What the data says about gun deaths in the U.S.* Pew Research Center. Available at https://www.pewresearch.org/short-reads/2023/04/26/what-the-data-says-about-gun-deaths-in-the-u-s/

38. RAINN (Rape, Abuse & Incest National Network). (2024*). Perpetrators of sexual violence: Statistics.* Available at https://www.rainn.org/statistics/perpetrators-sexual-violence

39. Centers for Disease Control and Prevention. (2023). *Suicide data and statistics.* Available at https://www.cdc.gov/suicide/suicide-data-statistics.html

40. American Foundation for Suicide Prevention. (2024). *Suicide statistics.* Available at https://afsp.org/suicide-statistics/

41. Garnett, M. F., & Curtin, S. C. (2023). Suicide mortality in the United States, 2001-2021. *NCHS Data Brief, 464*, 1-8. Available at https://dx.doi.org/10.15620/cdc:125705

42. Centers for Disease Control and Prevention. (2023). *Disparities in suicide.* Available at https://www.cdc.gov/suicide/facts/disparities-in-suicide.html

43. Kegler, S. R., Simon, T. R., Zwarl, M. L., et al. (2022). Vital signs: Changes in firearm homicide and suicide rates — United States, 2019–2020. *Morbidity and Mortality Weekly Report, 71*, 656–663. Available at http://dx.doi.org/10.15585/mmwr.mm7119e1

44. Simon, T. R. (2022). Notes from the field: Increases in firearm homicide and suicide rates — United States, 2020-2021. *Morbidity and Mortality Weekly Report, 71*, 1286–1287. http://dx.doi.org/10.15585/mmwr.mm7140a4

45. Centers for Disease Control and Prevention, Adolescent and School Health. (2023). *YRBSS results.* Available at https://www.cdc.gov/healthyyouth/data/yrbs/results.htm

46. Rostron, A. (2018). The Dickey Amendment on federal funding for research on gun violence: A legal dissection. *American Journal of Public Health, 108*(7), 865–867.

47. Neuman, S. (2023). *The CDC is helping states address gun injuries after years of political roadblocks.* NPR. Available at https://www.npr.org/2023/07/07/1184739094/cdc-gun-violence-research-dickey-amendment-faster-grants

48. Centers for Disease Control and Prevention, Violence Prevention. (2021). *Striving to reduce youth violence everywhere (STRYVE).* Available at https://www.cdc.gov/violenceprevention/youthviolence/stryve/index.html

49. Drotning, K. J., Doan, L., Sayer, L. C., Fish, J. N., & Rinderknecht, R. G. (2023). Not all homes are safe: Family violence following the onset of the Covid-19 pandemic. *Journal of Family Violence, 38*, 189–201. https://doi.org/10.1007/s10896-022-00372-y

50. U.S. Department of Health and Human Services, Administration for Children & Families, Administration on Children, Youth and Families, Children's Bureau. (2024). *Child maltreatment 2022.* Available at https://www.acf.hhs.gov/sites/default/files/documents/cb/cm2022.pdf

51. Lansford, J. E., Miller-Johnson, S., Berlin, L., Dodge, K., Bates, J., & Pettit, G. (2007). Early physical abuse and later violence delinquency:

A prospective longitudinal study. *Child Maltreatment, 12*(3): 233–245.

52. World Health Organization. (2020). *Abuse of older people.* Geneva, Switzerland: Author. Available at https://www.who.int/news-room/fact-sheets/detail/abuse-of-older-people

53. U.S. Census Bureau. (2023). *Data Profiles: United States of America.* Available at https://data.census.gov/table/ACSDP1Y2022.DP05?

54. U.S. Census Bureau. (2023). *2023 National Population Projections Tables: Main Series.* Available at https://www.census.gov/data/tables/2023/demo/popproj/2023-summary-tables.html

55. National Center on Elder Abuse, for Community Living. (2024). *Prevalence of Elder Mistreatment.* Available at https://ncea.acl.gov/prevalenceofeldermistreatment

56. National Center on Elder Abuse, for Community Living. (2024). *Risk factors & protective factors.* Available at https://ncea.acl.gov/riskfactorsandprotectivefactors

57. Centers for Disease Control and Prevention, National Center for Injury Prevention & Control, Division of Violence Prevention. (2021). *Fast facts: Preventing elder abuse.* Available at https://www.cdc.gov/violenceprevention/elderabuse/fastfact.html

58. Centers for Disease Control and Prevention. (2022). *Fast facts: Preventing intimate partner violence.* Available at https://www.cdc.gov/violenceprevention/intimatepartnerviolence/fastfact.html

59. Office on Violence Against Women, U.S. Department of Justice. (2023). *Domestic violence.* Available at https://www.justice.gov/ovw/domestic-violence

60. U.S. Department of Health and Human Services, Office of Women's Health. (2021). *Effects of domestic violence on children.* Available at https://www.womenshealth.gov/relationships-and-safety/domestic-violence/effects-domestic-violence-children

61. Centers for Disease Control and Prevention. (2021). *Risk and protective factors for perpetration.* Available at https://www.cdc.gov/violenceprevention/intimatepartnerviolence/riskprotectivefactors.html

62. Irwin, V., Wang, K., Cui, J., & Thompson, A. (2023). *Report on indicators of school crime and safety: 2022* (NCES 2023-092/NCJ 307328). National Center for Education Statistics, U.S. Department of Education, and Bureau of Justice Statistics, Office of Justice Programs, U.S. Department of Justice. Available at https://bjs.ojp.gov/document/iscs22.pdf

63. National Center for Healthy Safe Children. (2024). *Safe Schools/Healthy Students.* Available at https://healthysafechildren.org/grantee/safe-schools-healthy-students

64. U.S. Department of Justice, Office of Juvenile Justice and Delinquency Prevention. (2022). *Violent crime by youth time of day (per 1,000 youth who committed a violent crime).* Available at https://ojjdp.ojp.gov/statistical-briefing-book/offending-by-youth/faqs/qa03301

65. Centers for Disease Control and Prevention, National Center for Injury Prevention & Control. (2022). *Youth violence.* Available at https://www.cdc.gov/violenceprevention/youthviolence/index.html

66. National Gang Center. (n.d.). *Frequently asked questions about gangs.* U.S. Department of Justice, Office of Justice Programs. Available at https://nationalgangcenter.ojp.gov/about/faq

67. U.S. Department of State. (n.d.). *About human trafficking.* Available at https://www.state.gov/humantrafficking-about-human-trafficking/

68. National Human Trafficking Hotline. (2024). *National statistics.* Available at https://humantraffickinghotline.org/en/statistics

69. U.S. Department of Justice. (2023). *What is human trafficking?* Available at https://www.justice.gov/humantrafficking/what-is-human-trafficking

70. National Human Trafficking Training and Technical Assistance Center. (2024). *About NHTTAC.* U.S. Department of Health & Human Services, Administration for Children & Families. Available at https://nhttac.acf.hhs.gov/about-nhttac

71. Totenberg, N. (2022). *Supreme Court strikes down N.Y. law that restricts concealed carrying of guns.* NPR. Available at https://www.npr.org/2022/06/23/1102995474/supreme-court-opinion-guns

72. Clyde, D., & Miranda, S. (2022). *Biden signs gun safety bill into law.* NPR. Available at https://www.npr.org/2022/06/25/1107626030/biden-signs-gun-safety-law

73. Centers for Disease Control and Prevention. (2023). *Fast facts: Firearm violence and injury prevention.* Available at https://www.cdc.gov/violenceprevention/firearms/fastfact.html

74. Johns Hopkins Bloomberg School of Public Health. (2023). *The public health approach to prevent gun violence.* Available at https://publichealth.jhu.edu/center-for-gun-violence-solutions/research-reports/the-public-health-approach-to-prevent-gun-violence

CHAPTER 16

Safety and Health in the Workplace

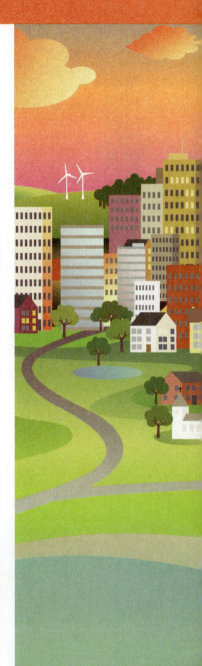

Chapter Outline

Chapter Objectives

After studying this chapter, you will be able to:

1. Describe the scope of the occupational safety and health problem in the United States and its importance to the community.
2. Identify some pioneers in the prevention of occupational injuries and disease.
3. Provide a short history of state and federal legislation on occupational safety and health.
4. Explain the difference between occupational injuries and occupational illnesses and give several examples of each.
5. Discuss the types of injuries that frequently occur in the workplace and describe their occurrence with regard to person, place, and time.
6. Briefly describe broad strategies for preventing injuries in the workplace.
7. Outline the causes of, and risk factors for, violence in the workplace and describe prevention strategies.
8. Name the different types of occupational illnesses and diseases, and list some of the causative agents.
9. Outline some general strategies for preventing and controlling these diseases and illnesses.
10. List several occupational safety and health professions and describe what the professionals in each of these do.
11. List and describe several kinds of workplace safety and health programs.
12. Explain the purpose of worksite health and wellness promotion programs and describe some of their features.
13. Discuss the concept behind Total Worker Health.

Scenario

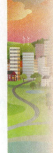

Nguyen Thi Linh had been working at her summer job in a nail salon business for six weeks. With the money she earned as a manicurist, Linh planned to eventually continue her college education. Linh worked quickly and accurately and enjoyed her work. Now, though, she had begun to worry about the safety of the chemicals in the various nail products used in the salon—products, such as polishes, strengtheners, removers, and artificial nail liquids. Sometimes, after a long day in the salon, Linh would experience headaches. Once, when she was there alone, she read the list of contents of some of the products: acetone, acetonitrile, butyl acetate, dibutyl phthalate, ethyl acetate, ethyl methacrylate, formaldehyde, isopropyl acetate, methacrylic acid, methyl methacrylate, quaternary ammonium compounds, toluene . . . Linh wrote down the names of some of the chemicals. When she returned home, she searched the Internet to learn whether any of them could be responsible for her headaches. She learned that some of these chemicals irritate the skin and nose and cause asthma. Others cause headaches, dizziness, and irritated eyes, nose, and throat; still others can damage liver and kidneys and can even pose harm to a fetus. Linh began to wonder whether she should continue to work as a nail technician.

Introduction

The global workforce exceeds 3.6 billion workers and is continually growing.[1] Approximately 30% of these workers are in the least developed countries, where working conditions are more hazardous than in more developed countries.[2] Each year, as many as 395 million workers experience nonfatal occupational injuries, and 330,000 workers are fatally injured. This amounts to more than 1 million workplace injuries and almost 1,000 injury deaths every day. Also, each year, an estimated 2.678 million workers die from diseases acquired in the workplace. Therefore, more than 7,000 workers die each day from workplace exposure.[3] The human cost of these occupational injuries and diseases is estimated to be nearly 5.4% of the global gross domestic product each year.[4]

The number of civilian Americans employed in the labor force, as of April of 2024, was approximately 161 million.[5] After home, Americans spend the next largest portion of their time at work; thus, safe and healthy workplaces are essential if the United States is to reach its future health objectives. It is not always easy to distinguish between the terms *occupational injury* and *occupational illness* or *disease*. However, it is generally accepted that an **occupational illness** is any abnormal condition or disorder, other than one resulting from an occupational injury, caused by factors associated with employment. It includes acute or chronic illnesses or disease that may be caused by inhalation, absorption, ingestion, or direct contact. An **occupational injury** is any injury, such as a cut, fracture, sprain, or amputation, that results from a work-related event or from a single, instantaneous exposure in the work environment.[6]

Scope of the Problem

Each day in the United States, on average, approximately 15 workers die from an injury sustained at work. Although even one worker death is one too many, it is instructive to note that the work-related fatality rates in the United States have declined significantly over the past 90 years. In 1933, an estimated 14,500 work-related injury deaths occurred, a death rate of 37 per 100,000 workers.[7] In 2022, there were 5,486 such deaths, and the death rate for occupational injury deaths had fallen to 2.7 per 100,000 workers.[8]

Nearly 2.8 million nonfatal injuries and illnesses were reported in private industry workplaces during 2022, resulting in a rate of 2.7 cases per 100 equivalent full-time workers. Over 2021 and 2022, nearly two-thirds of the 2.2 million injury or illness cases in private industry required recuperation away from work beyond the day of the incident or transfer or restriction of job duties.[9]

Occupational injuries and illnesses are an economic issue. In the United States, in 2022, it has been estimated that workplace injuries and illnesses cost $167 billion annually, including

Occupational illness an abnormal condition or disorder, other than an occupational injury, caused by an exposure to environmental factors associated with employment

Occupational injury an injury that results from exposure to a single incident in the work environment

$50.7 billion in lost wages and productivity, $37.6 billion in medical costs, and $54.4 billion in administrative costs. It also includes employers' uninsured costs of lost time of workers other than those with disabling injuries ($15.0 billion), investigation costs, vehicle damage losses, and fire losses. Each worker in the United States must produce $1,040 in goods and services just to offset the cost of work-related injuries and illnesses.[10]

Importance of Occupational Safety and Health to the Community

Due to the worrisome statistics previously stated, it is important to recognize how occupational and community health problems are linked. The population of those working in industry is a subset of the population of the larger community in which the industry is located. Workers, usually the healthiest people in the community, are exposed in the course of their jobs to specific hazardous materials at the highest concentrations. It is in the factory that the most accurate exposure and health data are available for extrapolation to the general community. Most pollutants with stated safe exposure levels were first studied and measured in the workplace for investigation into occupational exposure of workers.

Hazardous agents in the workplace not only affect workers but also those outside the worksite. This can occur through soil and groundwater contamination with solids and liquids or air pollution with industrial gasses and dusts. It can also occur through clothing and vehicle contamination, as in the case of asbestos workers whose wives and children became exposed to asbestos from these sources or, more recently, electronic waste recyclers who unknowingly exposed their families to lead dust from their workplace. It is important to note that the general population, which includes children, older adults, and pregnant women, is more sensitive to exposure to pollutants than the workforce, generally, because of their developing or compromised immune system.

Another way that industries and their communities share health problems is in the instance of an industrial disaster. Examples include the Three Mile Island (Pennsylvania) nuclear reactor near-meltdown in the United States in 1979, the Bhopal tragedy in India in 1984, and the Chernobyl nuclear catastrophe in the Ukraine in 1986. In these cases, the risk of exposure to a chemical or nuclear energy source, which was originally limited to the workplace, became a community-wide risk.

Finally, it is important to recognize the workers themselves as a community, with common social problems and environmental risks. The failure to recognize the community nature of occupational groups and to monitor chronic conditions, such as dermatitis, headaches, blood pressure, or blood chemistries has been a major weakness in our conventional approach to occupational health problems.

History of Occupational Safety and Health Problems

Occupational risks undoubtedly occurred even in prehistoric times, not only during hunting and warfare but also in more peaceful activities, such as the preparation of flint by knapping. The discovery of flint heaps suggests that even these earliest workers may have been at risk for silicosis (dust in the lungs).

An extensive historic review of occupational safety and health problems from early Egyptian times to late in the twentieth century has been published.[11] Among the early milestones was George Agricola's treatise on mining in 1561, *De Re Metallica*, which emphasized the need for the ventilation of mines. In 1567, the work of Philippus Aureolus Theophrastus Bombastus von Hohenheim, also known as Paracelsus, was published under the title, *On the Miners' Sickness and Other Miners' Diseases*. These were the first significant works describing specific occupational diseases. The first work on occupational diseases in general was Ramazzini's *Discourse on the Diseases of Workers*, which appeared in 1700.[12,13] In this chapter, we concentrate only on recent events in the United States and make only brief references to earlier milestones.

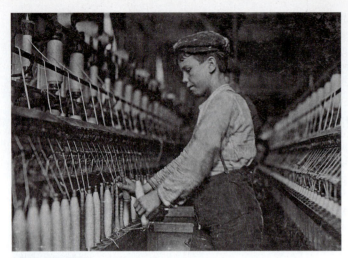

FIGURE 16.1   Cotton mills in the late nineteenth century offered little protection from injuries.

Courtesy of Library of Congress, Prints & Photographs Division, National Child Labor Committee Collection [reproduction number LC-DIG-nclc-01640].

Occupational Safety and Health in the United States Before 1970

The Industrial Revolution, which began in Britain in the eighteenth century, soon spread to continental Europe and then to the United States. Factors creating and driving the Industrial Revolution were the substitution of steam and coal for animal power, the substitution of machines for human skills, and other advances in industrial technology. These changes resulted in the rise of mass manufacturing, the organization of large work units, such as mills and factories, and eventually, the exposure of masses of workers to new hazards. Although mining remained the most dangerous form of work, there were soon other unsafe occupations, such as iron smelting and working in cotton mills and textile factories (see **Figure 16.1**).

The recognition of the need to reduce workplace injuries began long before any attention was paid to workplace diseases. The earliest efforts of those responsible for inspecting workplaces were aimed primarily at the sanitation and cleanliness of workplaces. They soon became concerned with equipment safeguards and tending to those who had become injured or ill at work.[13] These efforts, while much needed and appreciated, did little to improve the overall health of the workforce.

State Legislation

The first official responses to new hazards in the workplace did not occur until 1835, when Massachusetts passed the first Child Labor Law, and later in 1867, when it created a Department of Factory Inspection to enforce it (see **Figure 16.2**). Under this law, factories were prohibited from hiring children younger than 10 years of age.[14] At this time, the federal government was concerned only with working conditions of federal employees. In 1877, Massachusetts passed the first worker safety law, aimed at protecting textile workers from hazardous spinning machinery.[15]

In 1902, Maryland became the first state to pass any kind of workers' compensation legislation. In 1908, the U.S. Congress, at the insistence of President Theodore Roosevelt, finally enacted the first of several **workers' compensation laws**; this first law covered certain federal employees. Over the next 40 years, all states and territories eventually enacted some type of workers' compensation legislation, beginning with New York in 1910 and ending with Mississippi in 1948.[11] So ended the first wave of reform in occupational safety and health. With the exception of several other legislative efforts, little progress was achieved during the first half of the twentieth century in protecting workers from injuries in the workplace, and almost nothing was done about occupational illnesses.

There was one exception. Alice Hamilton (1869–1970) was a strong proponent of occupational health and a true pioneer in this field (see **Figure 16.3**). Over her 40-year career in occupational health, she led crusades to reduce poisonings from heavy metals, such as lead and mercury. She investigated silicosis in Arizona copper mines, carbon disulfide poisoning in the viscose rayon industry, and many other industrial health problems.[14]

> **Workers' compensation laws** a set of federal laws designed to compensate those workers and their families who suffer injuries, disease, or death from workplace exposure

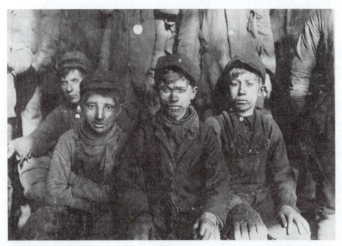

FIGURE 16.2   Before child labor laws were passed, many children worked long hours at dangerous jobs, such as mining.

Courtesy of Library of Congress, Prints & Photographs Division, National Child Labor Committee Collection [reproduction number LC-DIG-nclc-01137].

In spite of Hamilton's efforts, progress in occupational health legislation was slow in the first half of the twentieth century. Occupational diseases were by and large ignored. There was some safety legislation, such as the Coal Mine Safety Act of 1952. Beginning in the 1960s, some people began to take a closer look at the various state workers' safety and workers' compensation laws. It was discovered that in most states, legislation was a fragmentary patchwork of laws; some states had good laws, but many had inadequate legislation. Many of the laws had failed to keep up with new technology or with inflation. Some groups of workers, including agricultural workers, were not covered at all by legislation. Other problems were the division of authority among various departments within state governments, fragmented record keeping, and inadequate administrative personnel.[16]

Federal Legislation

In 1884, the federal government created a Bureau of Labor; in 1910, the Federal Bureau of Mines; and in 1914, the Office of Industrial Hygiene and Sanitation in the Public Health Service. In 1916, Congress passed the Federal Employees' Compensation Act, which provided federal employees compensation if injured while on the job.[15] Quite a few important laws were passed between 1908 and 1970 (see **Table 16.1**), but the two most comprehensive laws were the Coal Mine Health and Safety Act of 1969 and the **Occupational Safety and Health Act of 1970 (OSH Act)**, also known as the Williams-Steiger Act in honor of Senator Harrison A. Williams, Jr., and Congressman William A. Steiger, who worked for passage of the Act. At the time the Act was passed, 14,000 workers died each year on the job. Since its passage, the Act has served to raise the consciousness of both management and labor to the problems of health and safety in the workplace.

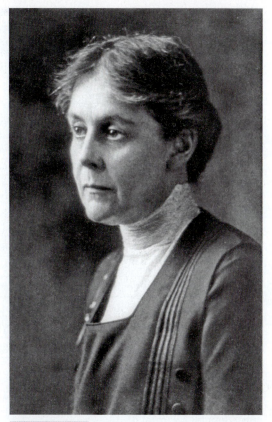

FIGURE 16.3   Alice Hamilton (1869–1970) was a pioneer in occupational safety and health in the United States.
© National Library of Medicine

Occupational Safety and Health Act of 1970

The purpose of the Occupational Safety and Health Act of 1970 is to ensure that employers in the private sector furnish each employee "employment and a place of employment which are free from recognized hazards that are causing or likely to cause death or serious physical harm."[15] Furthermore, employers were henceforth required to comply with all occupational safety and health standards promulgated and enforced under the Act by the **Occupational Safety and Health Administration (OSHA)**, which was established by the legislation.

Also established by the OSH Act was the **National Institute for Occupational Safety and Health (NIOSH)**, a research body now located in the Centers for Disease Control and Prevention of the U.S. Department of Health and Human Services. NIOSH is responsible for recommending occupational safety and health standards to OSHA, which is located in the U.S. Department of Labor (DOL).

The OSH Act contains several noteworthy provisions. Perhaps the most important is the employee's right to request an OSHA inspection. Under this right, any employee or any employee representative may notify OSHA of violations of standards or of the general duty obligation (to provide a safe and healthy workplace) by the employer. Under the Act, the employee's name must be withheld if desired, and the employee or a representative may accompany the OSHA inspectors in their inspection. By another provision of the OSH Act, individual states can regain local authority over occupational health and safety by submitting state laws that are and will continue to be as effective as the federal programs.[15]

Occupational Safety and Health Act of 1970 (OSH Act) comprehensive federal legislation aimed at ensuring safe and healthful working conditions for working men and women

Occupational Safety and Health Administration (OSHA) the federal agency located within the U.S. Department of Labor and created by the OSH Act, which is charged with the responsibility of administering the provisions of the OSH Act

National Institute for Occupational Safety and Health (NIOSH) a research body within the U.S. Department of Health and Human Services, which is responsible for developing and recommending occupational safety and health standards

TABLE 16.1   Highlights of Federal Occupational Safety and Health Legislation

Year	Legislation
1908	Federal Workmen's Compensation Act—limited coverage
1916	Federal Highway Aid Act
1926	Federal Workmen's Compensation Act—amended to include all workers
1927	Federal Longshoremen's and Harbor Workers' Compensation Act
1936	Walsh-Healey Public Contracts Act
1952	Coal Mine Safety Act
1958	Federal Longshoremen's and Harbor Workers' Compensation Act—amended to include rigid safety precautions
1959	Radiation Standards Act
1960	Federal Hazardous Substances Labeling Act
1966	National Traffic and Motor Vehicle Safety Act
1966	Child Protection Act—banned hazardous household substances
1967	National Commission on Product Safety created
1968	Natural Gas Pipeline Safety Act
1969	Construction Safety Act
1969	Child Protection Act—amended to broaden the coverage
1969	**Coal Mine Health and Safety Act**
1970	**Occupational Safety and Health Act**

Data from U.S. Department of Labor, Bureau of Labor Statistics. (2015). *Labor law highlights, 1915–2015.* Available at https://www.bls.gov/opub/mlr/2015/article/labor-law-highlights-1915-2015.htm

Prevalence of Occupational Injuries, Diseases, and Deaths

In this section, a brief overview of current trends in workplace injuries and illness is followed by a discussion of the occurrence and prevalence of work-related injuries and work-related diseases.

Overview of Recent Trends in Workplace Injuries and Illnesses

Since 1992, there has been a decline in the number of workplace injuries and illnesses reported in private industry. There were 2.8 million injuries and illnesses reported in 2022, resulting in a rate of 2.7 cases per 100 equivalent full-time workers per year. Approximately 1.86 million of these injuries and illnesses were cases with days away from work.[9]

In the private sector in 2022, the estimated rate of occupational injuries and illnesses ranged from 4.1 cases per 100 full-time workers in agriculture, forestry, fishing, and hunting to 0.3 cases in finance and insurance. The healthcare and social assistance industry accounts for the highest number of injuries and illnesses, resulting in nearly 1 in 4 cases of injury and illness (see **Figure 16.4**).[9]

Unintentional Injuries in the Workplace

Unintentional injuries in the workplace include minor injuries (such as bruises, cuts, abrasions, and minor burns), and major injuries (such as amputations, fractures, severe lacerations, eye losses, acute poisonings, and severe burns). Statistics on injuries and injury deaths are available from several sources, including the National Center for Health Statistics (NCHS), the National Safety Council (NSC), the Bureau of Labor Statistics (BLS), and NIOSH. For this reason, estimates of the number of occupational injuries and injury deaths vary. However, beginning in 1992, the NSC adopted the figures published by BLS reports, including its

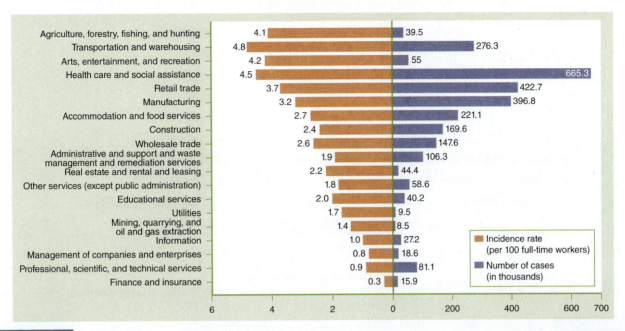

FIGURE 16.4   Incidence rates and numbers of nonfatal occupational injuries and illnesses by private industry sector, 2022.

Data from U.S. Department of Labor, Bureau of Labor Statistics. (2023). Employer-reported workplace injuries and illnesses—2021–2022. https://www.bls.gov/charts/injuries-and-illnesses/number-and-rate-of-nonfatal-work-injuries-and-illnesses-by-industry.htm

Census of Fatal Occupational Injuries (CFOI) and its annual report on workplace injuries and illnesses. The BLS reports are the source of figures used in this text.[9,17]

Fatal Work-Related Injuries

In 2022, there were 5,486 fatal work-related injuries, or 15 per day. The fatal occupational injury rate for 2022 was 3.7 per 100,000 full-time equivalent workers.[17] Overall, the 2022 total of fatal occupational injuries increased slightly from the previous years. While the overall trend of workplace fatalities is down, there are still several industries with significant increases in workplace fatality rates. The death rate in the mining industry increased by 11%, while death rates increased in the information and leisure and hospitality industries by 14% and 20%, respectively.[18]

Transportation incidents (2066) accounted for two out of every five fatal workplace injuries. Roadway incidents continued to lead the way, with 1,369 deaths (25% of the total); followed by falls, with 865 deaths (16%); violence, with 849 deaths (15%); exposure to harmful substances or environments, with 839 deaths (15%); being struck by an object or equipment, with 484 deaths (9%); and fire and explosions, with 107 deaths (2%) (**Figure 16.5**).[17]

The industries with the highest rates of fatal occupational injuries per 100,000 employees in 2022 were agriculture, forestry, fishing, and hunting (23.5), construction and extraction (13.0), and transportation and material moving (14.6). Industries with the lowest fatality rates were leisure and hospitality (2.8), manufacturing (2.6), retail trade (2.19), and educational and health services (0.8) (see **Figure 16.6**).[19]

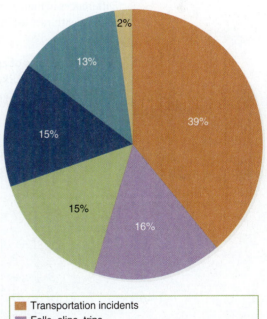

- Transportation incidents
- Falls, slips, trips
- Violence and other injuries by persons or animals
- Exposure to harmful substances or environments
- Contact with objects and equipment
- Fires and explosions

FIGURE 16.5   Fatal occupational injuries by major event, 2022.

Data from U.S. Department of Labor, Bureau of Labor Statistics. (2023). Census of fatal occupational injuries summary, 2022. Available at https://www.bls.gov/charts/census-of-fatal-occupational-injuries/fatal-occupational-injuries-by-event-drilldown.htm

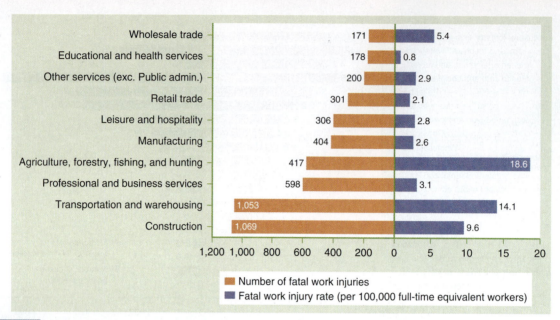

FIGURE 16.6 Number and rate of fatal occupational injuries, by industry sector, 2022.

Data from U.S. Department of Labor, Bureau of Labor Statistics. (2023). Census of fatal occupational injuries summary, 2022. Available at https://www.bls.gov/charts/census-of-fatal
-occupational-injuries/number-and-rate-of-fatal-work-injuries-by-industry.htm

Characteristics of Workers Involved in Fatal Work-Related Injuries

Differences in injury and injury death rates are often related to the age and gender of the worker. Injury death rate differences may vary according to minority racial or ethnic status.

Age

Workers (17 years of age or younger) had the lowest rates of fatal workplace injuries in 2022. The rate of fatal workplace injuries grew with each age group, with those aged 65 and older experiencing significantly more fatal work injuries than younger members of the workforce (see **Figure 16.7**).[19]

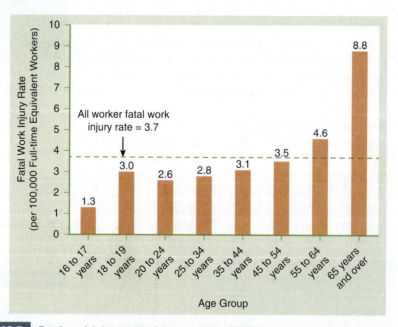

FIGURE 16.7 Fatal work injury rates, by age group, 2022.

Data from U.S. Department of Labor, Bureau of Labor Statistics. (2023). Census of fatal occupational injuries summary, 2022. Available at https://
www.bls.gov/news.release/cfoi.nr0.htm

Gender

Women die of work-related injuries at much lower rates than men. In 2022, only 8.1% of those who died of an injury in the workplace were women, even though historic data suggest that women work between 40–45% of all worked hours.[17] A significant portion of the difference results from men being employed in more dangerous jobs. Both men and women experience the highest percentage of fatal injuries due to roadway incidents. While the number of homicides due to fatal occupational injuries is higher among men, proportionally, homicides are greater for women, accounting for nearly one in five of women's job-related fatalities.[17]

Minority Status

In 2022, fatality rates for Hispanic or Latino workers were the highest among worker groups (4.6 fatalities per 100,000 full-time workers). Black or African-American (non-Hispanic) workers had workplace fatality rates above the national average at (4.2), while White (non-Hispanic) workers were just below the national average, at (3.5). Asian (non-Hispanic) workers had the lowest workplace fatality rates (1.7 fatalities per 100,000 full-time workers).[20]

Nonfatal Work-Related Injuries

Nonfatal work-related injuries diminish productivity and jeopardize both employee wages and employer profits. In 2022, 2.8 million nonfatal injuries and illnesses were reported in private industry, up 7.5% from 2021. Almost 1.2 million cases resulted in days away from work in private industry, with a median number of days off of 10.9.[21] The economic burden of worker injuries and illnesses has been estimated at more than $167 billion annually.[10]

Disabling injuries or illnesses are those in which the injured worker remains away from work because of injury beyond the day on which the injury occurred. In 2022, the incidence rate of disabling injuries or illnesses was 2.3 per 100 full-time workers.[9] Police officers and sheriff's patrol officers, nursing assistants, laborers, and heavy tractor-trailer truck drivers are among the occupations that account for the greatest number of the days away from work cases. Overexertion and bodily reaction made up 52.1% (521,350 cases) of all cases that required days away from work, with an incidence rate of 26.2 cases per 10,000 full-time equivalent workers, with a median of 14 days away from work. Between 2021 and 2022, 96.3% of the total exposure to harmful substances or environments cases required at least one day away from work. This high percentage can be attributed to COVID-19's inclusion in this category; however, it is only the fourth most common event or exposure type.[9,22]

Healthy People 2030 has set objectives to help make work conditions safer for employees through reducing work-related injuries and through health promotion efforts (see **Box 16.1**).[23]

Characteristics of Workers Involved in Work-Related Injuries

Age

Workers aged 55 to 64 years had the highest incidence of workplace injuries and illnesses (113.4 cases per 10,000 full-time workers). Workers aged 45 to 54 years had the next highest rate (104.5 cases per 10,000 full-time workers).[21] Younger workers typically experience a lower rate of fatal workplace injuries, but a higher rate of nonfatal injuries than workers 25 years of age and older. Younger workers typically spend fewer days away from work for each disabling injury.[21] Younger workers spent the lowest median number of days away from work (five days) for each disabling injury or illness of any age group. The fewer days away from work per disabling injury or illness and the lower fatality rates experienced by younger workers may reflect the types of employment of today's young people—fewer hold manufacturing jobs, and more are employed in service-providing industries. Generally, as people age, the rates of injury and the amount of time spent away from work for a disabling injury increase.[21]

One group of workers that is of special concern is children. An estimated 36.8% of 16 to 19-year olds work for pay.[24] Although some level of employment may be desirable, studies show that teens who work more than 20 hours per week do worse academically and are more likely to abuse drugs and alcohol. The five most dangerous jobs for teens in 2015 were (1) tobacco harvesting, (2) harvesting crops and using machinery, (3) traveling youth sales crews,

---

BOX 16.1   *Healthy People 2030*: Objectives Related to Workplace Safety

Data sources: U.S. Department of Health and Human Services, Office of Disease Prevention and Health Promotion, Healthy People 2030.

Target and baseline:

Objective	Status (year)	2030 Target
	Injuries per 10,000 Full-time Equivalent Workers	
OSH-2 Reduce employer-reported nonfatal work-related injuries resulting one or more days away from work.	73.2 (2021)	63.8
ECBP-D03 Increase the proportion of worksites that offer an employee health promotion program.		Developmental (no reliable baseline data available)

For Further Thought

What are the consequences of employees missing one or more days of work due to work-related injuries? What strategies might workplaces implement in order to improve workplace safety? What role do employee health promotion programs play in improving workplace safety?

Data from U.S. Department of Health and Human Services, Office of Disease Prevention and Health Promotion. (2024). *Healthy People 2030*. Available at https://health.gov/healthypeople/objectives-and-data/browse-objectives/workplace

---

(4) construction and height work, and (5) landscaping, groundskeeping, and lawn service.[25] Agriculture is usually ranked as the most dangerous industry by the National Safety Council.[26]

At particular risk are those youth who are employed in violation of child labor laws. An estimated 148,000 youth are illegally employed during an average week in the United States. This figure does not include the roughly 300,000 to 500,000 youth aged 6 to 17 years old who are working as migrant and seasonal farmworkers.[25] Violations of child labor regulations are all too common and not always rigorously enforced. Youth employment peaks during the summer, when an estimated 2.1 million youths find jobs.[27] Young workers are at particular risk for injury because (1) they may not be trained to perform the assigned task, (2) they may not be adequately supervised, (3) they lack experience and maturity needed to perform assigned tasks and to recognize hazards, and (4) they may be unaware of child labor laws aimed at protecting them. **Box 16.2** provides recommendations for protecting the safety and health of young workers.[28]

Gender

Nearly 81 million women are part of the American labor force. Since 1950, the labor force participation rate for women has nearly doubled, so that today, more than half of all adult women work. In 2023, females made up nearly 47% of the American workforce.[29] In 2017, on the days they worked, employed men worked 52 minutes more than employed women.[30] Because men work more hours and because there are still some dangerous jobs filled predominantly by males, in 2022, males accounted for 54% of all the injury and illness cases involving days away from work; males also account for 92% of all fatal occupational injuries.[26,8]

Working women are more likely than nonworking women to receive certain health benefits, such as workplace prenatal education, weight control programs, and cancer education. Women in the workforce are more likely to be covered by health insurance than nonworking women and are more likely to have preventive health tests.

Poverty and Minority Status

Nonfatal injury and illness rates for those of minority status and income levels are not available from the BLS because the numbers of workers within these characteristics are not known. In 2022, White workers accounted for 30% of cases with days away from work, and Hispanic

BOX 16.2   Hazardous Work for Adolescents and Practical Steps for Protecting Their Safety and Health

Work Too Hazardous for Adolescents

- Working in or around motor vehicles
- Operating tractors and other heavy equipment
- Working in retail and service industries where there is a risk of robbery-related homicide
- Working on ladders, scaffolds, roofs, or construction sites
- Continuous manual lifting or lifting of heavy objects

Recommendations

Young Workers

Young workers should take the following steps to protect themselves:

1. *Know about and follow safe work practices.*
   - Recognize the potential for injury at work.
   - Follow safe work practices.
   - Seek information about safe work practices from employers, school counselors, parents, state labor departments, and the Department of Labor (DOL). Visit www.youthrules.gov, or call 1-866-4-USWAGE.
2. *Ask about training.* Participate in training programs offered by your employer, or request training if none is offered.
3. *Ask about hazards.* Don't be afraid to ask questions if you are not sure about the task you are asked to do. Discuss your concerns with your supervisor or employer first.
4. *Know your rights.* Be aware that you have the right to work in a safe and healthful work environment free of recognized hazards. Visit www.osha.gov/youngworkers/index.html
   - You have the right to refuse unsafe work tasks and conditions.
   - You have the right to file complaints with the DOL when you feel your rights have been violated or your safety has been jeopardized.
   - You are entitled to workers' compensation for a work-related injury or illness.
5. *Know the laws.* Before you start work, learn what jobs young workers are prohibited from doing. State child labor laws may be more restrictive than federal laws, and they vary considerably from state to state. Visit www.youthrules.gov or call 1-866-4-USWAGE

Employers

Employers should take the following steps to protect young workers:

1. *Recognize the hazards.*
   - Reduce the potential for injury or illness in young workers by assessing and eliminating hazards in the workplace.
   - Make sure equipment used by young workers is safe and legal. Visit www.dol.gov/general/topic/youthlabor or call 1-866-4-USADOL.
2. *Supervise young workers.*
   - Make sure that young workers are appropriately supervised.
   - Make sure that supervisors and adult coworkers are aware of tasks young workers may or may not perform.
   - Label equipment that young workers cannot use, or color-code uniforms of young workers so that others will know they are not permitted to perform certain jobs.
3. *Provide training.*
   - Provide training in hazard recognition and safe work practices.
   - Have young workers demonstrate that they can perform assigned tasks safely and correctly.
   - Ask young workers for feedback about the training.
4. *Know and comply with the laws.* Know and comply with child labor laws and occupational safety and health regulations that apply to your business. State laws may be more restrictive than federal laws, and they vary considerably from state to state. Post these regulations for workers to read. For information about federal child labor laws, visit www.dol.gov/general/topic/youthlabor or call 1-866-4-USADOL. Links to state labor offices are also available at this site. Information about OSHA regulations that apply to workers of all ages is available at www.osha.gov
5. *Develop an injury and illness prevention program.* Involve supervisors and experienced workers in developing a comprehensive safety program that includes an injury and illness prevention program and a process for identifying and solving safety and health problems. OSHA consultation programs are available in every state to help employers identify hazards and improve their safety and health management programs.

(continues)

BOX 16.2   Hazardous Work for Adolescents and Practical Steps for Protecting Their Safety and Health   *(continued)*

Educators

Educators should take the following steps to protect young workers:

1. *Talk to students about work.* Talk to students about safety and health hazards in the workplace and students' rights and responsibilities as workers.
2. *Ensure the safety of school-based work experience programs.* Ensure that vocational education programs, school-to-work, or Workforce Investment Act partnerships offer students work that is allowed by law and is in safe and healthful environments free of recognized hazards. All such programs should include safety and health training.
3. *Include worker safety and health in the school curriculum.* Incorporate occupational safety and health topics into high school and junior high curricula (e.g., safety and health regulations, how to recognize hazards, how to communicate safety concerns, where to go for help). For more information, call 1-800-321-OSHA or visit https://www.osha.gov/young-workers/parents-educators
4. *Know the laws.* If you are responsible for signing work permits or certificates, know the child labor laws. State laws may be more restrictive than federal laws, and they vary considerably from state to state. Visit www.youthrules.gov (or call 1-866-4-USWAGE).

Parents

Parents should take the following steps to protect young workers:

1. *Take an active role in your child's employment.*
   - Know the name of your child's employer and your child's work address and phone number.
   - Ask your child about the types of work involved, work tasks, and equipment they use at work.
   - Ask your child about training and supervision provided by the employer.
   - Be alert for signs of fatigue or stress as your child tries to balance demands of work, school, home, and extracurricular activities.
2. *Know the laws.* Be familiar with child labor laws. State laws may be more restrictive than federal laws, and they vary considerably from state to state. Do not assume that your child's employer knows about these laws. Visit www.youth-rules.gov (or call 1-866-4-USWAGE).
3. *Be aware of young workers' rights.* Report unsafe working conditions or employment in violation of child labor laws to DOL. Young workers are eligible for workers' compensation benefits if injured on the job.
4. *Share information with other parents.* Studies have shown that most young workers and parents are not aware of the laws and rights of young workers.

Reproduced from U.S. Department of Health and Human Services, Centers for Disease Control and Prevention, National Institute for Occupational Safety and Health. (2003). *NIOSH alert: Preventing deaths, injuries, and illnesses of young workers.* (DHHS [NIOSH] Pub. No. 2003-128). Available at http://www.cdc.gov/niosh/docs/2003-128/pdfs/2003128.pdf

or Latino workers accounted for almost 12% of injuries and illnesses involving days away from work. However, race and ethnicity were unreported in 48% of all cases, so a true picture is not known.[26]

Geographic Differences in Workplace Injuries

For 2022, occupational injury and illness rates were highest in the following states: Maine, Vermont, Washington, Oregon, California, Montana, and Alaska.[22] In all, 18 states reported private injury and illness rates above the national average of 2.7 cases per 100 full-time workers, while 15 states and the District of Columbia reported rates below the average. Nine states were not significantly different from the national average. Eight states did not report a rate (see **Figure 16.8**).[22]

Workplace Injuries by Industry and Occupation

Fatal and nonfatal occupational injury rates vary according to type of industry and type of occupation.

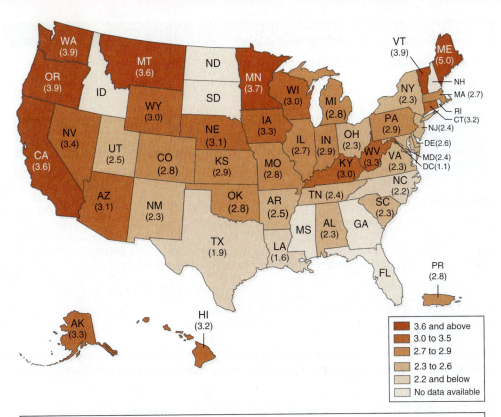

• State rate not available (8 states) (Idaho, North Dakota, South Dakota, Florida, New Hampshire, Rhode Island, Georgia, Mississippi)
• State rate statistically greater than national rate (18 states)
• State rate not statistically different from national rate (9 states)
• State rate statistically less than national rate (15 states and DC)
• Average Total recordable cases (per 100 full-time workers): 2.7

FIGURE 16.8 State nonfatal occupational injury and illness incidence rates compared with the national rate, private industry, 2022. (Total recordable cases [TRC] incidence rate per 100,000 full-time workers.)

Reproduced from U.S. Department of Labor, Bureau of Labor Statistics. (2024). Survey of occupational injuries and illnesses data. Available at https://www.bls.gov/charts/injuries-and-illnesses/rate-of-total-recordable-cases-by-state.htm

Fatal Occupational Injuries by Industry

Some jobs are more dangerous than others. Injury death rates are one indication of the risk associated with employment in an industry or in a particular job within an industry (see **Box 16.3**). Although the total number of deaths is highest in the construction industry, workers in agriculture, forestry, fishing, and hunting have the highest workplace fatality rates (18.6 deaths per 100,000 full-time workers; see Figure 16.6).[19] Within this industry category, logging and commercial fishing and hunting were the most dangerous occupations in 2022, with death rates of 100.7 and 50.9 deaths per 100,000 workers, respectively. (Remember the overall fatality rate for American workers is less than four deaths per 100,000 workers.) Aircraft pilots and flight engineers have the fifth highest fatality rates (35.9 deaths per 100,000 workers; see **Table 16.2**).[19]

Nonfatal Occupational Injuries and Illnesses by Industry

A total of 2.8 million nonfatal injuries and illnesses were reported in public and private industry workplaces during 2022, resulting in a rate of 2.7 cases per 100 equivalent full-time workers.[29] Among goods-producing industries, agriculture, forestry, fishing, and hunting had the highest incidence rate in 2022 (4.1 cases per 100 full-time workers). In the service-producing industries,

BOX 16.3 *Healthy People 2030*: Objectives

Objective OSH-01: Reduce deaths from work-related injuries.
Data sources: Census of Fatal Occupational Injuries (CFOI), Department of Labor/BLS.
Target and baseline:

Objective	2017 Baseline	2022	2030 Target
	Deaths per 100,000 Full-time Workers		
OSH-01	3.5	3.7	2.9

For Further Thought

Targets call for continued reduction in deaths from work-related injuries. Previously, this target was reported by industry (e.g., mining, construction, agriculture). Why might the objective have been revised to eliminate the separate industries? How might workplaces use the tools for action and evidence-based resources to develop individualized interventions?

Data from U.S. Department of Health and Human Services, Office of Disease Prevention and Health Promotion. (2020). *Healthy People 2030.* Available at https://health.gov/healthypeople

transportation and warehousing had the highest incidence rate (4.8 per 100 full-time workers), followed by health care and social assistance (4.5 cases per 100 full-time workers; see Figure 16.4).[9]

Agricultural Safety and Health

One particularly hazardous occupation is farming. Those working on farms are at considerable risk not just for injuries, but for lung diseases, noise-induced hearing loss, skin diseases, and certain cancers associated with chemical use and sun exposure. In 2023, there were approximately 2.3 million full-time workers involved in production agriculture. In addition, 1.4 to 2.1 million seasonal crop workers are hired annually.[31] More than 890,000 youth lived on farms in 2014 and nearly half worked on their farm. Also, more than 260,000 youth were hired to work on U.S. farms that year. Every day, approximately 33 children are injured, and about every three days, a child dies in an agriculture-related incident.[32] In 2017, 416 farm-related deaths were reported, and farming and ranching alone ranked seventh among the top 10 most dangerous jobs in 2018 (see Table 16.2).[19,31]

TABLE 16.2 Top 10 Deadliest Jobs in 2018

Rank	Occupation	Death Rate per 100,000	Total Deaths
1	Logging workers	100.7	54
2	Roofers	57.5	105
3	Fishers and hunting workers	50.9	16
4	Helpers, construction trades	38.5	20
5	Aircraft pilots and flight engineers	35.9	72
6	Driver/sales workers and truck drivers	30.4	1,115
7	Refuse and recyclable material collectors	22.6	22
8	Structural iron and steel workers	21.3	14
9	Underground mining machine operators	20.1	8
10	Miscellaneous agricultural workers	20.0	146

Data from U.S. Department of Labor, Bureau of Labor Statistics. (2024). Census of fatal occupational injuries (CFOI)—current and revised data. Available at https://www.bls.gov/charts/census-of-fatal-occupational-injuries/civilian-occupations-with-high-fatal-work-injury-rates.htm

A major contribution to farm-related fatalities is farm machinery, particularly farm tractors. For more than two out of five farm worker deaths, the source of the fatal injury was a tractor, and more than half of these deaths resulted from tractor rollovers. Rollover incidents are those in which the tractor tips sideways or backward (especially when the tractor is improperly hitched), crushing the operator. Although all tractors manufactured since 1985 are fitted with seat belts and **rollover protective structures (ROPS)**, many tractors in use in the United States lack this equipment. Although today's tractors are the safest ever, transportation incidents remain the leading cause of farm deaths.[31]

Farming is one of the few industries in which the families of workers are also exposed to many of the same risks. It is not unusual for farm boys under the age of 12 to be seen driving tractors (see **Figure 16.9**). Additionally, according to the U.S. Department of Labor, agricultural work classified as 'particularly hazardous' may be performed by children as young 16, or at any age if the farm is owned or operated by their parents.[32] Today, approximately one in three agriculture related emergency room visits are child injuries.[33]

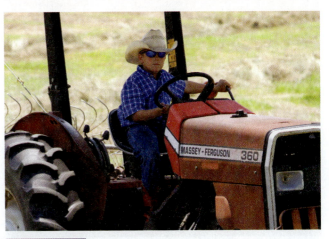

FIGURE 16.9   It is not unusual for farm children under the age of 12 to be seen driving tractors.
© David R. Frazier Photolibrary, Inc./Alamy Stock Photo

Another group of workers who are exposed to health and safety risks in agricultural settings are members of the migrant workforce, where children as young as 12, 10, 8, and even 4 years of age can be found working in the fields. Testimony before the U.S. Senate Committee on Labor and Human Resources by Fernando Cuevas, Jr., paints a grim picture of migrant children (see **Box 16.4**).[34]

The United States relies heavily on migrant workers during the peak harvest season. These migrant workers experience poverty, frequent mobility, low literacy, and language and cultural barriers, all of which impede access to social services and cost-effective primary care.[34] In many cases, working conditions are hazardous, and water shortages require workers to drink water from irrigation ditches. Not only is such water unpurified, it is usually laden with agricultural chemicals and biologic wastes. Migrant workers are also exposed to long hours in the sun, wildfire smoke, other unsanitary conditions, and numerous harmful pesticides from crop-dusting airplanes.

It is an unfortunate fact that little progress has been made in addressing the plight of migrant farm workers. In 2000, Human Rights Watch (HRW) documented the exploitative and dangerous conditions under which these workers and their children labor in a report titled, *Fingers to the Bone: United States Failure to Protect Child Farmworkers*. Nearly 10 years later, when HRW re-examined the situation, they discovered that conditions for child farmworkers were essentially unchanged.[35] Although some farming industries have established policies to protect young children from hazardous child labor, many of the risks remain.[36] Children often work 10 or more hours per day and, during peak harvest times, may

Rollover protective structures (ROPS) factory-installed or retrofitted reinforced framework on a cab to protect the operator of a tractor in case of a rollover

---

BOX 16.4   Comments of a Young Farm Worker

"When I was younger it was all a game to me. But as I started getting older it became a job, and at the age of about 7 and 8, I was competing with my parents and my older sisters. . . . I was able to get out of the fields permanently at the age of 15 to try and get a decent education. I also became an organizer for the Farm Labor Organizing Committee at the age of 16, and I continue to see many, many young children working out in the fields at the same age that I was—4-, 5-, 6-, 7-, and 8-year-olds. They are still working out in the fields. I see it every year, up in Ohio, I see it down in Texas, I see it in Florida, I see it anywhere that we go and organize."

Data from Committee on Labor and Human Resources. (1991, March 19). Prepared Statement of Fernando Cuevas, Jr. *Childhood Labor Amendments of 1991* (S. HRG. 102-201, S. 600). U.S. Government Printing Office.

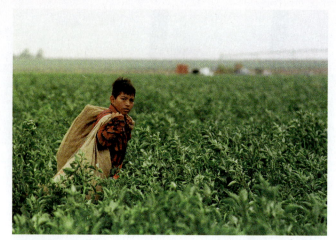

FIGURE 16.10 Children of migrant farm workers often work 10 or more hours per day and tend to drop out of school at a rate four times the national average.

© Pat Sullivan/AP Images

work from dawn to dusk (see **Figure 16.10**). They typically earn less than the minimum wage and are often forced to spend their own money on tools, gloves, and even drinking water. They may be exposed to agricultural chemicals that make them sick. Because of missed days at school, farm-working youth drop out of school at a rate four times higher than the national average.

Even these lax labor laws are not enforced diligently. Between 2001 and 2009, enforcement of child labor laws overall by the U.S. Department of Agriculture declined dramatically. Despite the hazardous conditions and frequent injuries and illnesses suffered by farmworkers, relatively few complain for fear of being fired or even deported. Even though many of the children may be U.S. citizens, the entire family may fear being deported.

Despite breaches of international child labor conventions, both in legislation and practice, the U.S. has spent tens of millions of dollars to eliminate child labor in other parts of the world.[32] Legislation aimed at eliminating the double standard in child labor laws is introduced during each session of Congress. So far, none of these bills has reached a vote. The Children's Act for Responsible Employment in Agriculture, or the CARE Act of 2024, was introduced to the U.S. Senate and might be voted on later in the year.

Prevention and Control of Unintentional Injuries in the Workplace

Reducing the number and seriousness of injuries and illnesses in the workplace involves four fundamental tasks: anticipation, recognition, evaluation, and control.[37] Anticipation involves the foresight to envision future adverse events and take action to prevent them. A hazard inventory should be conducted to detect and record physical, ergonomic, chemical, biological, and psychological hazards in the workplace. Recognition involves surveillance and monitoring of the workforce for injuries and illnesses, including near misses. It includes inspections of the workplace for hazards, monitoring it for toxins, recording injuries, and conducting employee health screenings.

All of the aforementioned activities include data collection. Evaluation is the assessment of the data that were collected during the recognition and monitoring activities. This step includes toxicological, exposure, and clinical assessment as well as risk assessment. Epidemiology is part of the evaluation process. Risk assessment enables the translation of scientific information about hazards into decisions and policies that can improve workplace safety and health. Upon establishing the need for intervention, a decision concerning control can be made. The control may involve changes in the production process to make it safer, changes in the work environment to make it safer, or improvements in the use of personal protective equipment or apparel to protect individual workers. Finally, the education and training of workers can help to reduce workplace injuries and illnesses.[37]

National leadership in reducing the number and seriousness of workplace injuries and illnesses resides with OHSA and NIOSH. In 1996, in collaboration with more than 500 public and private outside organizations and individuals, NIOSH established the National Occupational Research Agenda (NORA) to establish priorities and a plan for research on workplace safety and health problems. Partners include stakeholders from universities, large and small businesses, professional societies, government agencies, and worker organizations. Partners work together to develop research goals and objectives for resolving the most critical workplace issues based upon (1) the numbers of workers at risk, (2) the seriousness of the hazard or issue, and (3) the probability that new information and approaches will make a difference. The various councils within NORA are based upon sectors in the North American Industry Classification System (NAICS). Examples include the following: agriculture, forestry, and fishing; construction; health care and social assistance; manufacturing; mining; and so on.[38] Some of the ongoing projects coming out of NORA include projects on paid leave connected with self-reported depression and anxiety, protecting and promoting employee mental health, noise-related health risks, and creating inclusive workplaces.[39]

Workplace Violence: Intentional Workplace Injuries

Although only a small number of the incidents of workplace interpersonal violence that occur each day make the news, over 57,000 Americans report having been victims of workplace violence between 2021 and 2022.[40] In 2022, there were 525 workplace homicide victims reported, making homicide the fifth leading cause of workplace fatalities behind transportation and roadway incidents, contact with objects and equipment, falls, and exposure to harmful substances or environments.[17]

There are many reasons for workplace homicides and violence. Researchers have divided workplace violence into four categories[41]:

- *Criminal intent (Type I).* The perpetrator has no legitimate relationship to the business or its employees and is usually committing a crime, such as robbery, shoplifting, and trespassing.
- *Customer/client (Type II).* The perpetrator has a legitimate relationship with the business and becomes violent while being served. This type of violence, often referred to as client-on-worker violence, occurs most frequently in emergency or psychiatric treatment settings, waiting rooms, and geriatric settings.
- *Worker-on-worker (Type III).* The perpetrator is an employee or past employee of the business who attacks or threatens another employee or past employee of the workplace. Bullying, verbal and emotional abuse, or humiliating are some of the behaviors observed in this type of violence.
- *Personal relationship (Type IV).* The perpetrator usually does not have a relationship with the business but has a personal relationship with the intended victim. This category includes victims of domestic violence who are assaulted or threatened at work.

Risk Factors

Risk factors for encountering violence at work are listed in **Box 16.5**. They include working with the public, working around money or valuables, working alone, and working late at night. Additionally, certain industries and occupations put workers at particular risk. Healthcare workers, service providers, and education workers are more prone to workplace violence than others. For example, taxi drivers are more than 20 times more likely to be murdered on the job than other workers.[40]

BOX 16.5   Know the Warning Signs - Behaviors that Might Signal Future Violence

- Excessive use of alcohol or drugs
- Unexplained absenteeism, change in behavior, or decline in job performance
- Depression, withdrawal or suicidal comments
- Resistance to changes at work or persistent complaining about unfair treatment
- Violation of company policies
- Emotional responses to criticism, mood swings
- Paranoia

Reproduced from National Security Council. (2024). Assault Fifth Leading Cause of Workplace Deaths. Available at https://www.nsc.org/work-safety/safety-topics/workplace-violence

Prevention Strategies

Prevention strategies for workplace violence can be grouped into three categories: environmental designs, administrative controls, and behavior strategies. Before these strategies can be implemented, a workplace violence prevention policy should be in place. Such a policy should clearly indicate a zero tolerance of violence at work. Just as workplaces have mechanisms for reporting and dealing with sexual harassment, they must also have a policy in place to deal with violence. Such a policy must spell out how such incidents are to be reported, to whom, and how they are to be addressed.

Environmental designs to limit the risk of workplace violence might include implementing safer cash handling procedures, physically separating workers from customers, improving lighting, and installing better security systems at entrances and exits. Administrative controls include staffing policies (having more staff is generally safer than having fewer staff), procedures for opening and closing the workplace, and reviewing employee duties (such as handling money) that may be especially risky. Behavior strategies include training employees in non-violent response and conflict resolution and educating employees about risks associated with specific duties and about the importance of reporting incidents and adhering to administrative controls. Training should also include instruction on the appropriate use and maintenance of any protective equipment that may be provided.[40]

Occupational Illnesses

Precise data on the number of cases of occupational illnesses are more difficult to acquire than data on injuries. It is more difficult to link illnesses to occupational exposure. Some illnesses that can result from occupational exposure (e.g., tuberculosis, cancer, and asthma) appear no different from those that result from exposure elsewhere. Also, there is usually a lengthy period of time between exposure and the appearance of disease, unlike injuries, which are usually evident immediately. Since the outbreak of COVID-19, the landscape of workplace illnesses has changed significantly. Reported cases of illnesses in the workplace in 2022 accounted for 16.5% of the approximately 2.8 million injury and illness cases compared with 4.5% of total cases in 2018. In private industry, 460,700 new cases of occupational illness were reported, a rate of 45.2 cases per 10,000 full-time workers in all employment settings. Respiratory illness had the highest incidence, 35.8 cases per 10,000 full-time workers, compared with skin diseases and disorders, which, before COVID-19, had the highest incidence, 1.9 cases per 10,000 full-time workers, followed by hearing loss, 1.5 cases per 10,000 full-time workers.[8] Some conditions, such as various cancers, are slow to develop and are difficult to associate with the workplace. These diseases and conditions are often unrecognized and under-reported in annual reports of injuries and illnesses.

Types of Occupational Illnesses

Occupational diseases can be categorized by cause and by the organ or organ system affected. For example, exposure to asbestos is a cause of illness; the respiratory system, especially the lung, is the system affected.

Skin Diseases

Reported skin disorders include allergic and irritant dermatitis, eczema, rash, oil acne, chrome ulcers, and chemical burns. The natural resources and mining industry has one of the highest incidences of occupational skin disorders. The skin may serve as the target organ for disease, or it may be the route through which toxic chemicals enter the worker's body.

Noise-Induced Hearing Loss

Noise-induced hearing loss is another form of repeated trauma. Approximately 22 million Americans are exposed to hazardous noise on the job.[42] Cases include workers with permanent noise-induced hearing loss or with a standard threshold shift. Most of the cases were reported within manufacturing.

Respiratory Conditions

Occupational respiratory conditions are the result of the inhalation of toxic substances present in the workplace. The lungs, like the skin, can be both the target organ of disease and a portal of entry for toxic substances. Occupational lung diseases are chronic and early recognition is difficult (the latent period for such diseases may be 15 to 30 years). Also, there is the problem of multiple or mixed exposures in the home and the workplace.

Work-related asthma (WRA) is one of the most commonly reported occupational respiratory diseases, even though estimates suggest that most cases are not recognized or reported as being work related. There is no estimate on how many cases of WRA occur nationwide. It is important for physicians and other healthcare providers to ask adult-onset asthma patients about work-related exposure. Unfortunately, sometimes complete exposure cessation is the only intervention for a worker who has become sensitized to the agent or agents causing asthma.[42]

One of the most important categories of lung diseases is **pneumoconiosis**, a fibrotic (scarring) lung disease caused by the inhalation of dusts, especially mineral dusts. During the period 1999 to 2018, pneumoconiosis was either the underlying or contributing cause in 43,366 deaths of U.S. workers.[43]

Types of pneumoconiosis include coal workers' pneumoconiosis, asbestosis, silicosis, and byssinosis. The largest number of pneumoconiosis deaths was from coal workers' pneumoconiosis (CWP). **Coal workers' pneumoconiosis** (also called black lung disease) is an acute or chronic lung disease that is caused by inhaling coal dust (see **Figure 16.11**).

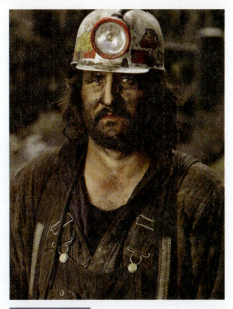

Historically, deaths from CWP clearly outnumber all other types of pneumoconiosis deaths. During the period from 1999 to 2018, there were 43,366 deaths attributed to CWP, making up more than 50% of all reported pneumoconiosis deaths for that period. However, deaths from CWP have declined during the last 40 years, from a high of 2,910 in 1972 to 363 in 2014.[43] The human cost of CWP can be measured another way, through analysis of years of potential life lost (YPLL). During the period 1968 to 2014, a total of 915,196 YPLL were attributed to CWP, an average of 11.7 years per fatality.[43] This means that workers who developed CWP during this period died, on average, 11.7 years sooner than expected. Most troubling is the finding that, after a period of decline, the number of YPLL has been increasing, from a low of 9.9 years in 2002 to 13.6 years in 2014.[43]

NIOSH has been monitoring trends in CWP, including progressive massive fibrosis (PMF), an advanced debilitating and lethal form of CWP. The incidence of PMF, which results solely from the inhalation of coal dust, has increased dramatically among miners in the Appalachian states (see **Figure 16.12**).[44] This increase could be caused by the changing nature of the coal dust inhaled, to inadequate enforcement of standards and unrepresentative dust sample measurements, or to miners working longer hours. With the widest coal seams already mined, modern day miners must work narrower seams surrounded in some cases by rock containing silica. Also, machinery used now creates finer dust particles. So miners inhale both coal dust and silica dust.[45] No effective medical treatment is available for pneumoconiosis; therefore, primary prevention is essential.

Asbestos workers suffer from diseases that include **asbestosis** (an acute or chronic lung disease), lung cancer, and malignant mesothelioma (cancer of the epithelial linings of the heart and other internal organs). In contrast to CWP, asbestosis deaths increased from 78 in 1968 to 1,221 in 2014. During the same period (1968 to 2014), the YPLL for each death for which asbestosis was either the underlying cause or a contributing case was 11.5 years. During the period from 1999 to 2014, 42,662 mesothelioma deaths were reported. A total of 2,785 mesothelioma deaths were reported in 2014.[43] The average number of YPLL for these deaths was 13.5 years.[43] The number of deaths from lung cancer to which asbestosis may have contributed has not been determined. The negative impact of asbestos is likely to start falling off as ongoing uses

Pneumoconiosis a fibrotic lung disease caused by the inhalation of dusts, especially mineral dusts

Coal workers' pneumoconiosis (CWP) an acute and chronic lung disease caused by the inhalation of coal dust (black lung disease)

Asbestosis an acute or chronic lung disease caused by the deposition of asbestos fibers on lungs

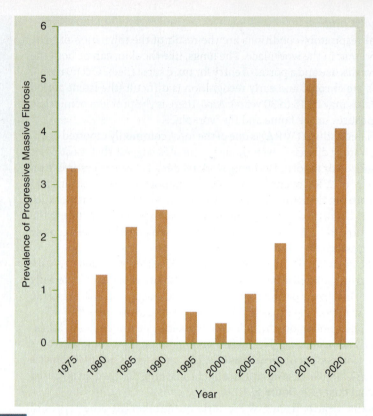

FIGURE 16.12   Prevalence of progressive massive fibrosis among working underground coal miners with 25 or more years of underground mining tenure (1974–2018) in Kentucky, West Virginia, and Virginia.

of asbestos were just banned in March of 2024 by the Environmental Protection Agency (EPA) under the new Toxic Substance Control Act.[46]

Other agents that can affect the lungs include metallic dusts, gasses and fumes, and aerosols of biologic agents (viruses, bacteria, and fungi). Health conditions that can result from exposure to these agents include occupational asthma, asphyxiation, pulmonary edema, histoplasmosis, and lung cancer.

Other Work-Related Illnesses

Other types of work-related illnesses are those that arise from poisonings and infections. Poisoning agents include heavy metals (including lead), toxic gasses, organic solvents, pesticides, and other substances. Pesticides, when used properly, offer benefits to society, increasing crop production, preserving produce, and combating insect infestations. However, pesticides do represent a health risk, especially for agricultural workers. Approximately 1.1 billion pounds of pesticide active ingredients are used annually in the United States, where 20,000 separate pesticide products are marketed. Each year, 10,000 to 20,000 physician-diagnosed pesticide poisonings occur among the approximately 2 million agricultural workers.[47]

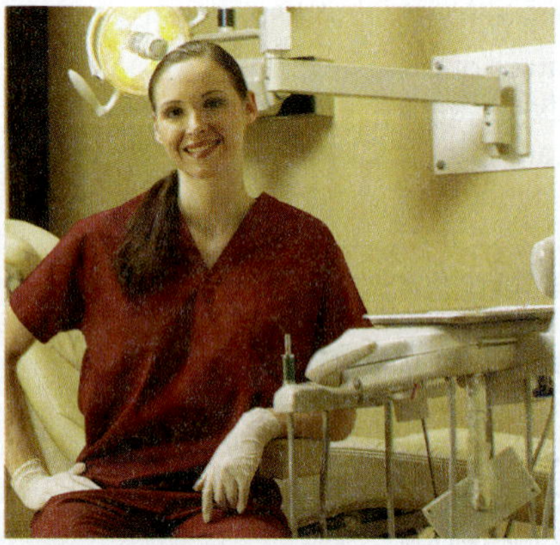

In 2022, 14.7 million people were employed in the healthcare industry in the United States, making up nearly 9.3% of the employed workforce.[48] Many of these workers are exposed to a variety of hazardous conditions, including infectious disease agents (see **Figure 16.13**). Among the agents of concern are viruses, such as COVID-19, hepatitis B, and human immunodeficiency virus (HIV). Healthcare workers are at risk if they become exposed to the blood or bodily fluids of patients or coworkers. The major route of exposure to these agents is

FIGURE 16.13   Healthcare workers are exposed to a variety of workplace hazards, including infectious diseases.

© Photos.com

percutaneous exposure (injuries through the skin) via contaminated sharp instruments, such as needles and scalpels. Exposure also occurs through contact with the mucous membranes of the eyes, nose, or mouth, exposure to broken or abraded skin, and through human bites. While healthcare workers are at an increased risk for acquiring various infectious diseases, practicing universal precautions and workplace safety initiatives have significantly reduced the risk in recent years. The COVID-19 outbreak highlighted both workplace exposure risk and the impact of proper workplace and personal safety precautions, in general, but specifically in the healthcare industry.

One positive impact of pandemic COVID-19 is a cultural shift in the workplace away from the stigma associated with health related time off. This transition toward prioritizing both individual and organizational health is still ongoing and has a ways to go before work policies and culture reflect optimal health policies across the country.

As stated previously, many of our most prevalent chronic health problems may arise from multiple exposures, both within the workplace and at home. Among these are cardiovascular diseases, cancers, and reproductive disorders. Perhaps a million or more workers are exposed to agents that can produce cancer, for example. However, there are no reliable estimates on the actual number of cancer deaths that can be traced directly to occupational exposure. Thus, we have only discussed conditions generally accepted to be solely or predominantly related to work.

Prevention and Control of Occupational Diseases and Disorders

Preventing and controlling occupational diseases requires the vigilance of employer and employee alike and the assistance of governmental agencies. The agent-host-environment disease model is applicable to the preventive strategies outlined here. Specific activities that should be employed to control occupational diseases include identification and evaluation of agents, standard setting for the handling of and exposure to causative agents, elimination or substitution of causative factors, engineering controls to provide for a safer work area, environmental monitoring, medical screenings, personal protective devices, health promotion, disease surveillance, therapeutic medical care and rehabilitation, and compliance activities. In this regard, prevention and control of occupational diseases and disorders is similar to the prevention of occupational injuries.[37] Coordinated programs to monitor and reduce occupational hazards require professionally trained personnel who work with employers and employees to reduce the number and seriousness of workplace injuries and illnesses.

Resources for Preventing Workplace Injuries and Illnesses

Prevention of workplace injuries and illnesses requires professional expertise as well as effective prevention and intervention programs.

Occupational Safety and Health Protection Professionals

The need for safety and health protection professionals in the workplace is substantial. Among those with specialized training in their fields are safety engineers and certified safety professionals, health physicists, industrial hygienists, occupational physicians, and occupational health nurses.

Safety Engineers and Certified Safety Professionals

A number of academic institutions offer accredited programs that train occupational safety professionals. Many of these professionals will join the professional organization called the American Society of Safety Professionals (ASSP). Founded in 1911, ASSP is the longest-running professional safety organization. It has more than 35,000 members dedicated to making their workplaces safer and healthier.[49]

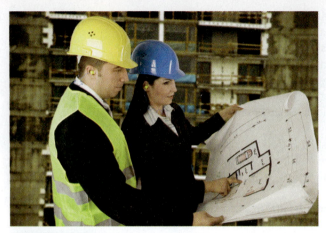

FIGURE 16.14 Safety engineers prevent workplace injuries by detecting hazards.

Another recognizable group of trained professionals in this field is the Board of Certified Safety Professionals (BCSP). This group, founded in 1969, was organized as a peer certification board with the purpose of certifying practitioners in the safety profession.[50] Certification usually requires a bachelor's degree in engineering or in another scientific curriculum and the passing of an associated examination.

Safety engineers and **certified safety professionals (CSPs)** design safety education programs, detect hazards in the workplace, and try to correct them (see **Figure 16.14**). Increased federal regulations have made the workload heavier for these occupational health professionals.

Health Physicists

Health physicists are concerned with radiation safety in the workplace. They monitor radiation within the work environment and develop plans for decontamination and coping with accidents involving radiation. Many of these belong to the Health Physics Society, an international scientific organization of professionals that traces its beginning to 1956. Health physicists are dedicated to promoting the practice of radiation safety.[51]

Industrial Hygienists

Whereas the safety engineer or certified safety professional is primarily concerned with hazards in the workplace and injury control, the **industrial hygienist** is concerned with environmental factors that might cause illness. Examples of such factors might include poor ventilation, excessive noise, poor lighting, and the presence of hazardous substances.

Many industrial hygienists choose to hold the title of certified industrial hygienist (CIH), which requires an academic degree with specific coursework along with professional experience to be eligible to take the certification exam.[52]

Occupational Medicine Physicians

The **occupational medical practitioner (OMP)** is a medical practitioner whose primary concern is preventive medicine in the workplace. Many OMPs belong to the American College of Occupational and Environmental Medicine (ACOEM), which represents physicians and other healthcare professionals specializing in the field of occupational and environmental medicine (OEM). The American Board of Preventive Medicine (ABPM) recognizes and certifies qualified physicians in the medical specialty of occupational medicine.[53]

Because physicians are highly skilled and highly salaried occupational health professionals, only the largest companies maintain full-time OMPs. Smaller companies may hire OMPs on a part-time basis or as consultants.

Occupational Health Nurses

The role of the **occupational health nurse (OHN)** has changed over the years from running the company's medical department and first aid station to one of greater emphasis on health promotion and illness prevention. It is likely that the OHN is the only health professional employed in smaller plants, so if injury prevention and health promotion programs are to be offered, the job will fall to this individual.

The OHN must be a registered nurse (RN) in the state in which they practice. It is unlikely that these persons will have had much formal training in occupational health nursing prior to receiving their baccalaureate degrees because most nursing curricula do not provide much training in this area. However, the American Board of Occupational Health Nurses, Inc.

Safety engineers safety professionals employed by a company for the purpose of reducing unintentional injuries in the workplace

Certified safety professionals (CSPs) health and safety professionals, trained in industrial and workplace safety, who have met specific requirements for board certification

Health physicists safety professionals with responsibility for developing plans for coping with radiation accidents

Industrial hygienist health professional concerned with health hazards in the workplace and with recommending plans for improving the healthiness of workplace environments

Occupational medical practitioner (OMP) a practitioner (physician) whose primary concern is preventive medicine in the workplace

Occupational health nurse (OHN) a registered nurse (RN) whose primary responsibilities include prevention of illness and promotion of health in the workplace

(ABOHN), established in 1972, now offers certifications. Requirements include many hours of continuing-education credits and five years of experience in the field of occupational health nursing. ABOHN is the only certifying body for occupational health nurses in the United States. An estimated 3,500 active, certified occupational health nurses are working today.[54] Many OHNs belong to the American Association of Occupational Health Nurses (AAOHN), which was founded in 1942 and includes over 3,200 members.[55]

Worksite Safety, Health, and Wellness Promotion Programs

A number of programs can be put in place in occupational settings to reduce injuries and diseases. These include preplacement examinations, health maintenance programs, safety awareness programs, health promotion programs, investigation of accidents, stress management programs, employee assistance programs, and rehabilitation programs.

Preplacement Examinations

The purpose of **preplacement examinations** is to make sure that the worker fits the job. By selecting the employee who is the best physically and mentally qualified for a specific job, probabilities of job-related injuries or illnesses are minimized. Periodic evaluations are necessary to ensure that the selected individual continues to be physically and mentally qualified to carry out the job assignment. Examinations are also recommended for transferred and return-to-work employees. Sometimes, a phasing in of these employees is desirable.

Occupational Disease Prevention Programs and Safety Programs

Occupational health services that facilitate preventive activities in the workplace include disease prevention programs and safety programs.

Disease Prevention Programs

Originally, occupational disease programs focused on controlling occupational diseases that one might succumb to from exposure in the work environment. Agents of concern were chemicals, radiation, and perhaps even psychological and social factors that could lead to sickness or disability. Gradually, these disease prevention efforts broadened into health maintenance programs and included the early detection and treatment of such diseases as hypertension, diabetes, obesity, and heart disease to keep employees healthier and on the job longer.

Safety Programs

Safety programs are those portions of the workplace health and safety program aimed at reducing the number and seriousness of unintentional injuries on the job. Each company needs to have a policy statement, safe operating procedures, a disaster plan, policies for hazard control, and policies for the investigation of injuries in the workplace. Provisions must be made for regular safety inspections of the workplace and for the maintenance of accurate records for each injury and for analysis of such records. Each safety program should include safety orientation and training programs and programs on first aid and cardiopulmonary resuscitation.

Worksite Health and Wellness Promotion Programs

Worksite health and wellness promotion (WHWP) programs are workplace-based programs aimed at improving the health and wellness of employees through changes in behavior and lifestyle. The goals for the employer include reduction of absenteeism, lowering health insurance premiums, increasing productivity, and improving employee morale. Other reasons why employers might support WHWP programs include reducing workers' compensation costs, increasing employee retention, and enhancing the company's image.[56]

In the United States, historically, health insurance has come through one's employment. In 1965, the employers' share of the nation's health care bill was 18%; today, it is approximately

Preplacement examination a physical examination of a newly hired or transferred worker to determine medical suitability for placement in a specific position

Safety programs those parts of the workplace safety and health program aimed at reducing unintentional injuries on the job

Worksite health and wellness promotion (WHWP) programs workplace-based programs aimed at improving the health and wellness of employees by identifying and acting on existing health conditions and by encouraging employees to optimize their health by improving health behaviors and lifestyle choices

40%. In some companies, the cost of providing health insurance for employees is equal to about 50% of the companies' profits.[56] Obviously, this upward trend in the cost of health insurance for employers cannot continue much longer. Until this system changes, however, employers are making serious efforts to reduce healthcare costs, and one effective way to do this is worksite health and wellness promotion.

WHWP programs go by various names, such as "Working Well," "Worksite Health and Family Services," "Work-Life Balance," or "Wellness and Work/Life." Generally, the objectives of these programs are to facilitate changes in behavior or lifestyle to prevent disease and to promote employee health and wellness. WHWP programs range in size from modest programs that might include only a wellness assessment, and, perhaps, hypertension screening, to more comprehensive programs that offer cancer risk screening, nutrition and weight management, fitness classes, smoking cessation, stress management programs, telephone health coaching to help manage chronic conditions, and medication therapy management. Physical activity is an important component of any wellness program and linkages to or agreements with recreation facilities is essential. But the goals of these programs have evolved from simply improving the physical health of employees to improving the quality of life, especially as it relates to work/life balance. Many include incentives, such as a free fitness tracker, or even monetary rewards, for participation by employees.

All indications are that WHWP programs will continue to grow. Corporations, colleges, and universities not only see them as a means to control healthcare costs and show a concern for the employees but also as a means by which to retain current employees and recruit new ones. Undergraduate and graduate programs now exist to specifically train people to staff these programs; these professionals go by such titles as worksite wellness coordinator, worksite wellness manager, or wellness instructor.

Located in the Centers for Disease Control and Prevention, NIOSH supports and promotes worksite wellness programs through its **Total Worker Health (TWH)** program. TWH is defined as policies, programs, and practices that integrate protection from work-related safety and health hazards with promotion of injury and illness prevention efforts to advance worker well-being.[57] The TWH approach advocates for a holistic understanding of the factors that contribute to worker well-being. Scientific evidence now supports what many safety and health professionals, as well as workers themselves, have long suspected—that risk factors in the workplace can contribute to health problems previously considered unrelated to work. The TWH website provides resources for those wishing to start or enhance existing workplace programs and policies for improving worker health and well-being.[57]

Employee Assistance Programs

Employee assistance programs (EAPs) are programs that assist employees who have substance use, family, psychological, or social problems that interfere with their work performance. These programs, which arrived at many workplaces before WHWP programs, originally arose in response to occupational alcohol problems. EAPs provide help to employees with a variety of problems that affect their work performance. EAPs may be administered separately from WHWP programs or even through a contract with a third party. The goal of EAPs is intervention when an employee has a behavioral or other problem that interferes with their work before such problems become costly for both the employer and employee. During the intervention, EAP personnel, together with the employee, try to identify and resolve the problem so that the employee's work performance can return to normal.

While statistics are incredibly powerful and informative metrics to understand a complicated landscape, no one statistical measure can explain an entire situation and might even be misleading. For example, comparing the global deaths from work-related factors in 2019, 2.93 million, to the global deaths from work-related factors in 2000, 2.62 million, sees a 12% increase. This comparison shows a significant increase in global work-related deaths, leading to the conclusion that working conditions are worsening. However, this increase can be explained by a 26% increase in the global workforce from 2000 to 2019 and drastic improvements to diagnostic tools, increasing the number of cases detected. A

Total Worker Health (TWH) policies, programs, and practices that integrate protection from work-related safety and health hazards with promotion of injury and illness prevention efforts to advance worker well-being (CDC/NIOSH)

Employee assistance programs (EAPs) workplace-based programs that assist employees who have substance use, domestic, psychological, or social problems that interfere with their work performance

more accurate statistical comparison would be between incidence rates from 2000 to 2019. In 2000, the incidence of global deaths from work-related factors was 95.27 per 100,000, and in 2019 it was 84.68 per 100,000 workers, showing an 11% decrease. This comparison would indicate improvement in workplace health and safety. Be mindful of what exactly the statistic is telling you and question if there are any statistics that represent the situation more completely or alternative explanations to the conclusions that you have made or that was presented.

Chapter Summary

- After time spent at home, Americans spend the next largest portion of their time at work; thus, safe and healthy workplaces are essential if the United States is to reach its health potential.

- Every day, approximately 15 people die from work-related injuries, and many more people die of work-related diseases.

- Occupational health issues affect the quality of life economically as well as medically in communities in which workers live. Although occupational injuries and illnesses have been a long-standing concern of workers in the United States, rapid progress in reducing the number and seriousness of workplace injuries and illnesses became possible only after the passage of the Occupational Safety and Health Act (OSH Act) of 1970.

- The OSH Act established the Occupational Safety and Health Administration (OSHA) and the National Institute of Occupational Safety and Health (NIOSH) and required private industry to provide safe jobs and workplaces.

- The number and type of workplace injuries vary by person, place, time, and type of industry. Construction, transportation, agriculture, forestry, fishing, and hunting industries have the largest numbers of workplace fatalities each year.

- Nonfatal work-related injuries diminish productivity and jeopardize both employee wages and employer profits.

- Workplace violence affects tens of thousands of workers in the United States each year, and homicide is the fifth leading cause of workplace fatalities.

- Work-related injuries can be controlled by applying a variety of injury prevention strategies, including eliminating a dangerous job, improving the work environment, using safer machinery, and improving the selection and training of workers.

- Work-related illnesses and disorders kill thousands of workers and former workers each year.

- The types of illnesses and diseases that can be attributed to workplace exposure are many, including dermatological conditions, lung diseases, and cancers, among many others.

- There are numerous resources to aid in the prevention of occupational injuries and diseases, including occupational health professionals, workplace injury and illness prevention programs, and worksite health promotion programs.

- Worksite health and wellness promotion (WHWP) programs are workplace-based programs aimed at improving the health and wellness of employees through changes in behavior and lifestyle.

- Total Worker Health is defined as policies, programs, and practices that integrate protection from work-related safety and health hazards with promotion of injury and illness prevention efforts to advance worker well-being.

Scenario: Analysis and Response

Please take a moment to reread the scenario at the beginning of this chapter. Here is some additional information on the nail salon industry from the CDC/NIOSH website:

Nearly 200,000 people are employed as manicurists and pedicurists in the United States according to the U.S. Bureau of Labor Statistics. These estimates indicate the workforce is largely female with the industry employing a large number of minority workers. Nail salon employees are potentially exposed to dozens of chemicals, including acrylates, solvents, and biocides as dusts or vapors.[58]

Then, reflect on the questions that follow.

1. If you were Linh, what would you do?

2. What federal agencies, mentioned in this chapter (or elsewhere in the text), provide information, advice, or assistance? Does your state regulate nail salon operations in a way that protects nail technicians?

3. This scenario raises concerns about workplace exposure to environmental hazards that occur in nail salons, but environmental hazards can occur anywhere. What types of environmental hazards might be present where you work?

4. Suppose you suspected that you were being exposed to a toxic agent where you worked. What would you do? Who would you contact? How could OSHA be of assistance?

Review Questions

1. Provide definitions of the terms *occupational injury* and *occupational illness*, and give three examples of each.

2. In what ways are health problems in the workplace related to health problems in the general community?

3. How did the Industrial Revolution contribute to an increase in occupational health problems?

4. Who was Alice Hamilton? What did she do?

5. What were the deficiencies in state occupational safety and health laws in the early 1960s?

6. Briefly discuss the purpose of the Occupational Safety and Health Act of 1970 and outline its major provisions.

7. What is OSHA and what does it do? What is NIOSH and what does it do?

8. What are some of the most frequently reported workplace injuries? Which are the leading causes of workplace injury deaths?

9. Which age group and gender of workers suffer the most occupational injuries? Which have the most fatal injuries?

10. Why is farming a particularly hazardous occupation? Describe some of the workplace hazards experienced by migrant farmworkers and their children.

11. What are the risk factors for encountering violence in the workplace? Which occupation is at greatest risk for workplace homicides?

12. Outline some general control strategies that can reduce the number and seriousness of workplace injuries.

13. What is the most frequently reported occupational disease?

14. List two well-documented lung conditions that are related to occupational exposure. Name the occupations whose workers are at high risk for each of these conditions.

15. Why is it often difficult to prove that a disease or condition resulted from workplace exposure?

16. Outline some features of a workplace program to prevent or control occupational diseases. For each activity, indicate whether it is aimed at the agent, host, or environment aspect of the disease model.

17. List five health occupations that deal with worker safety and health. Describe their training and job assignments.

18. Name and describe four occupational safety and health programs.

19. What are some of the benefits of worksite health and wellness promotion programs for employers and employees?

Activities

1. Examine your local news online every day for a week for articles dealing with occupational injury or illness. Find three articles and, after reading them, provide the following: a brief summary, the resulting injury or disease, the cause of the injury or disease, and a brief plan for how the organization could eliminate the cause.

2. Interview someone who works in the profession you wish to enter after graduation. Ask about prevalent injuries and illnesses connected with their job. Also ask about specific preservice and in-service education the interviewee has had to protect against these problems. Finally, ask them to propose measures to prevent future injuries or illnesses. Summarize your interview on paper in a two-page report.

3. If you have ever become injured or ill as a result of a job, explain what happened to you. In a two-page paper, identify the causative agent, how the injury could have been prevented, and what kind of training you had to prepare you for a safe working environment.

4. Research the injuries and diseases connected with your future profession. Create a public service announcement to describe the major problems and

what employers and employees should do about them and express concerns that you have about working in the profession because of these problems.

5. Visit any job site related to your future profession. At that site, find 10 things that employers and employees are doing to make it a safe work environment. List these 10 things briefly and explain the benefits of each one.

6. Visit any job site related to your future profession. At that site, interview a manager or executive on the challenges of injuries and illnesses on the side of the company or organization. List the responses of the manager and add any additional challenges you think are relevant. For each challenge listed, explain one strategy that could help mitigate it.

References

1. The World Bank. (2023). Labor force, total. Available at https://data.worldbank.org/indicator/SL.TLF.TOTL.IN?end=2023&start=1991&view=chart

2. International Labour Organization. (2022). Present and future of work in the Least Developed Countries. Available at https://www.ilo.org/wcmsp5/groups/public/---dgreports/---integration/documents/publication/wcms_844025.pdf

3. International Labour Organization. (2023). A call for safer and healthier working environments. Available at https://www.ilo.org/publications/call-safer-and-healthier-working-environments

4. International Labour Organization. (2022). Safety and health at work. Available at https://webapps.ilo.org/wcmsp5/groups/public/---europe/---ro-geneva/---ilo-brussels/documents/publication/wcms_849789.pdf

5. U.S. Department of Labor, Bureau of Labor Statistics. (2024). The Employment Situation — April 2024. Available at https://www.bls.gov/news.release/pdf/empsit.pdf

6. U.S. Department of Labor, Bureau of Labor Statistics. (2024). BLS glossary. Available at http://www.bls.gov/bls/glossary.htm

7. Center for Disease Control. (1999). Achievements in Public Health, 1900-1999. Available at https://www.cdc.gov/mmwr/preview/mmwrhtml/mm4822a1.htm

8. U.S. Department of Labor, Bureau of Labor Statistics. (2024). Injuries, Illnesses, and Fatalities. Available at https://www.bls.gov/iif/home.htm

9. U.S. Department of Labor, Bureau of Labor Statistics. (2023). *Employer-reported workplace injuries and illnesses—2021-2022.* Available at http://www.bls.gov/news.release/pdf/osh.pdf

10. National Safety Council. (2024). *Costs.* Available at https://injuryfacts.nsc.org/work/costs/work-injury-costs/

11. Felton, J. S. (1986). History of occupational health and safety. In J. LaDou (Ed.). *Introduction to occupational health and safety.* National Safety Council.

12. Rosen, G. (1993). *A history of public health.* Johns Hopkins University Press.

13. LaDou, J., Olishifski, J., & Zenz, C. (1986). Occupational health and safety today. In J. LaDou (Ed.), *Introduction to occupational health and safety.* National Safety Council.

14. Schilling, R. S. F. (1989). Developments in occupational health. In H. A. Waldron (Ed.), *Occupational health practice.* Butterworth-Heinemann.

15. Ashford, N. A. (1976). *Crisis in the workplace: Occupational disease and injury—A report to the Ford Foundation.* MIT Press.

16. Page, J. A., & O'Brien, M. W. (1973). *Bitter wages.* Grossman Publishers.

17. U.S. Department of Labor, Bureau of Labor Statistics. (2024). *Census of fatal occupational injuries summary, 2022.* Available at https://www.bls.gov/news.release/cfoi.htm

18. National Safety Council. (2024). Work-related Fatality Trends. Available at https://injuryfacts.nsc.org/work/work-overview/work-related-fatality-trends/data-details/

19. U.S. Department of Labor, Bureau of Labor Statistics. (2024). *Census of fatal occupational injuries (CFOI)—current and revised data.* Available at https://www.bls.gov/iif/oshcfoi1.htm#2022

20. National Security Council. (2024). Work Injuries and Illnesses by Race or Ethnic Origin. Available at https://injuryfacts.nsc.org/work/industry-incidence-rates/work-injuries-and-illnesses-by-race-or-ethnic-origin/

21. U.S. Department of Labor, Bureau of Labor Statistics. (2024). Employer-reported Workplace Injuries and Illnesses. Available at https://www.bls.gov/charts/injuries-and-illnesses/

22. U.S. Department of Labor, Bureau of Labor Statistics. (2024). *Survey of occupational injuries and illnesses data.* Available at https://www.bls.gov/iif/nonfatal-injuries-and-illnesses-tables.htm

23. U.S. Department of Health and Human Services, Office of Disease Prevention and Health Promotion. (2024). Goal: Promote the health and safety of people at work. Available at https://health.gov/healthypeople/objectives-and-data/browse-objectives/workplace

24. U.S. Department of Labor, Bureau of Labor Statistics. (2024). Civilian labor force participation rate by age, sex, race, and ethnicity. Available at https://www.bls.gov/emp/tables/civilian-labor-force-participation-rate.htm

25. Child Labor Coalition. (2013). *The CLC's open letter to President Obama on his next secretary of labor.* Available at http://stopchildlabor.org/?p=3381

26. National SafetyCouncil. (2024). Work Safety Introduction. Available at https://injuryfacts.nsc.org/work/work-overview/work-safety-introduction/

27. U.S. Department of Labor, Bureau of Labor Statistics. (2022). Employment and Unemployment Among Youth — Summer 2022. Available at https://www.bls.gov/news.release/archives/youth_08172022.pdf

28. U.S. Department of Health and Human Services, Centers for Disease Control and Prevention, National Institute for Occupational Safety and Health. (2024). *Young worker safety and health.* Available at http://www.cdc.gov/niosh/topics/youth/

29. U.S. Department of Labor, Bureau of Labor Statistics. (2024). *Labor force statistics from the current population survey.* Available at https://www.bls.gov/cps/

30. Fry, R., & Stepler, R. (2017). *Women may never make up half of the U.S. workforce.* Pew Research Center. Available at https://www.pewresearch.org/fact-tank/2017/01/31/women-may-never-make-up-half-of-the-u-s-workforce

31. Centers for Disease Control and Prevention, National Institute for Occupational Safety and Health, Division of Safety Research. (2024). Agriculture Worker Safety and Health. Available at https://www.cdc.gov/niosh/agriculture/about/index.html

32. Human Rights Watch. (2010). Fields of peril: Child labor in U.S. agriculture. Available at http://www.hrw.org/node/90126

33. National Children's Center for Rural and Agricultural Health and Safety. (2022). 2022 Fact Sheet – Childhood Agricultural Injuries. Available at https://doi.org/10.21636/nfmc.nccrahs.injuryfactsheet.r.2022

34. Committee on Labor and Human Resources. (1991, March 19). *Prepared statement of Fernando Cuevas, Jr.: Childhood labor amendments of 1991.* (S. HRG. 102-201. S 600). U.S. Government Printing Office.

35. National Center for Farmworker Health, Inc. (2022). *Facts about agricultural workers.* Available at https://www.ncfh.org/uploads/3/8/6/8/38685499/facts_about_farmworkers_fact_sheet_1.10.23.pdf

36. Human Rights Watch. (2015). *Teens of the tobacco fields: Child labor in United States tobacco farming.* Available at https://www.hrw.org/world-report/2016/photo-essay-tobacco-fields-united-states

37. Weeks, J. L., Wagner, G. R., Rest, K. M., & Levy, B. S. (2005). A public health approach to preventing occupational diseases and injuries. In B. S. Levy, G. R. Wagner, K. M. Rest, & J. L. Weeks (Eds.), *Preventing occupational disease and injury* (2nd ed.). American Public Health Association.

38. Centers for Disease Control and Prevention, National Institute of Occupational Safety and Health. (2024). *The national occupational research agenda (NORA).* Available at https://www.cdc.gov/nora/

39. Centers for Disease Control and Prevention, National Institute of Occupational Safety and Health. (2024). *eNews*, 22(1). Available at https://www.cdc.gov/niosh/enews/enewsv22n1.html

40. National Safety Council. (2024). Assault Fifth Leading Cause of Workplace Deaths. Available at https://www.nsc.org/work-safety/safety-topics/workplace-violence

41. Centers for Disease Control and Prevention, National Institute for Occupational Safety and Health. (2022). Workplace *violence: A Report to the Nation.* Available at https://www.cdc.gov/niosh/learning/safetyculturehc/module-2/10.html

42. United States Department of Labor, Occupational Safety and Health Administration. (2024). Occupational Noise Exposure. Available at https://www.osha.gov/noise

43. Centers for Disease Control and Prevention, National Institute for Occupational Safety and Health. (2024). About *Work-related asthma.* Available at https://www.cdc.gov/niosh/work-related-asthma/about/index.html

44. Centers for Disease Control and Prevention, Morbidity and Mortality Weekly Report. (2020). Trends in Pneumoconiosis Deaths — United States, 1999–2018. Available at https://www.cdc.gov/mmwr/volumes/69/wr/mm6923a1.htm

45. Hall, N. B., Blackley, D. J., Halldin, C. N., & Laney, A. S. (2019). Current Review of Pneumoconiosis Among US Coal Miners. *Current Environmental Health Report*, 6(3), 137–147.

46. U.S. Environmental Protection Agency. (2024). Biden-Harris Administration finalizes ban on ongoing uses of asbestos to protect people from cancer. Available at https://www.epa.gov/newsreleases/biden-harris-administration-finalizes-ban-ongoing-uses-asbestos-protect-people-cancer

47. U.S. Department of Health and Human Services, Centers for Disease Control and Prevention, National Institute for Occupational Safety and Health. (2012). *NIOSH pesticide poisoning monitoring program protects farmworkers.* (DHHS [NIOSH] Pub. No. 2012-108). Available at http://www.cdc.gov/niosh/docs/2012-108/

48. U.S. Bureau of Labor Statistics. (2024). Spotlight on Statistics. Available at https://www.bls.gov/spotlight/2023/healthcare-occupations-in-2022/home.htm

49. American Society of Safety Professionals. (2024). *Website*. Available at https://www.assp.org

50. Board of Certified Safety Professionals. (2024). *Website*. Available at http://www.bcsp.org

51. Health Physics Society. (2024). *Website*. Available at https://www.aahp-abhp.org

52. American Board of Industrial Hygiene. (2024). *Website*. Available at http://www.abih.org

53. American College of Occupational and Environmental Medicine. (2024). *About ACOEM.* Available at http://www.acoem.org

54. American Board for Occupational Health Nurses, Inc. (2024). About Us. Available at https://www.abohn.org/about-abohn/about-us

55. American Association of Occupational Health Nurses, Inc. (2024). *About AAOHN.* Available at http://www.aaohn.org

56. Chenoweth, D. H. (2007). *Worksite health promotion* (2nd ed.). Human Kinetics.

57. Centers for Disease Control and Prevention, National Institute for Occupational Safety and Health. (2024). Total Worker Health Program. Available at https://www.cdc.gov/niosh/twh/programs/index.html

58. Estill, C. F. (May 13, 2015). *Protecting nail salon workers. Centers for Disease Control and Prevention.* Available at https://blogs.cdc.gov/niosh-science-blog/2015/05/13/nail-salon/#:~:text=Nail%20salon%20employees%20are%20potentially,well%20as%20other%20health%20conditions

GLOSSARY

absorption field The element of a septic system in which the liquid portion of waste is distributed.

accreditation The process by which an agency or organization evaluates and recognizes an institution as meeting certain predetermined standards.

acculturation One cultural group learns and adopts elements of another cultural group, integrating them into their original culture

accountable care organization (ACO) Group of doctors, hospitals, and other healthcare providers, who come together voluntarily as a legal entity to give coordinated high-quality care to their Medicare patients.

active immunity Occurs when exposure to a disease-causing organism prompts the immune system to develop antibodies against that disease.

activities of daily living (ADLs) Tasks such as eating, toileting, dressing, bathing, walking, getting in and out of a bed or chair, and getting outside.

acute disease A disease with a brief duration of days to a few weeks.

Administration for Children and Families (ACF) An operating division of the U.S. Department of Health and Human Services that coordinates programs that promote the economic and social well-being of families, children, individuals, and communities.

Administration on Aging An operating division of the U.S. Department of Health and Human Services designated to carry out the provisions of the Older Americans Act of 1965.

adolescents and young adults Those people who fall into the 10- to 24-year-old age range.

adult daycare programs Daytime care provided to older adults who are unable to be left alone.

aftercare The continuing care provided to the recovering former drug abuser.

age-adjusted rates Rates used to make comparisons across groups and over time when groups differ by age structure.

ageism A form of prejudice and discrimination resulting from ignorance, misconceptions, and half-truths about aging and older adults.

Agency for Healthcare Research and Quality (AHRQ) An operating division of the U.S. Department of Health and Human Services that has the responsibility of overseeing healthcare research.

Agency for Toxic Substances and Disease Registry (ATSDR) An operating division of the U.S. Department of Health and Human Services created by Superfund legislation to prevent or mitigate adverse health effects and diminished quality of life resulting from exposure to hazardous substances in the environment.

agent (pathogenic agent) The cause of the disease or health problem.

age pyramid A conceptual model that illustrates the age distribution of a population.

airborne disease A communicable disease that is transmitted through the air (e.g., influenza).

air pollution Contamination of the air that interferes with the comfort, safety, and health of living organisms.

Air Quality Index (AQI) An index that indicates the level of pollution in the air and associated health risk.

Alcoholics Anonymous (AA) A fellowship of recovering alcoholics who offer support to anyone who desires to stop drinking.

Alcohol use disorder (AUD) A medical condition characterized by an impaired ability to stop or control alcohol use despite adverse social, occupational, or health consequences.

alcoholism A disease characterized by impaired control over drinking, preoccupation with drinking, and continued use of alcohol despite adverse consequences.

alien A person born in and owing allegiance to a country other than the one in which they live.

allied healthcare professional Healthcare worker who provides services that assist, facilitate, and complement the work of physicians and other healthcare specialists.

allopathic provider Independent provider whose remedies for illnesses produce effects different from those of the disease.

American Cancer Society A voluntary health agency dedicated to fighting cancer and educating the public about cancer.

American Health Security Act of 1993 The comprehensive healthcare reform introduced by then President Bill Clinton, but never enacted.

American Red Cross A nonprofit, humanitarian organization led by volunteers and guided by its Congressional Charter that provides relief to victims of disasters.

amotivational syndrome A pattern of behavior characterized by apathy, loss of effectiveness, and a more passive, introverted personality.

amphetamines A group of synthetic drugs that act as stimulants.

anabolic drugs Compounds, structurally similar to the male hormone testosterone, that increase protein synthesis and thus muscle building.

analytic study An epidemiological study aimed at testing hypotheses.

anthroponosis A disease that infects only humans.

aquifers Porous, water-saturated layers of underground bedrock, sand, and gravel that can yield economically significant amounts of water.

asbestos A naturally occurring mineral fiber that has been identified as a class A carcinogen by the Environmental Protection Agency.

asbestosis Acute or chronic lung disease caused by the deposition of asbestos fibers on lungs.

Asian American 20 million people living in the United States who trace their roots to more than 20 countries in East Asia, Southeast Asia, and the Indian subcontinent.

assertive community treatment (ACT) Service that uses active outreach by a team of providers over an indefinite period of time to deliver intensive, individualized services.

Assimilation   The complete adoption of the ways of life of the new cultural group, resulting in the assimilated group losing nearly all of its original or native culture. A potential outcome of acculturation.

assisted-living facility   "A system of housing and limited care that is designed for senior citizens who need some assistance with daily activities but do not require care in a nursing home." (Merriam-Webster Online Dictionary. (n.d.). *Assisted living*. http://www.merriam-webster.com /dictionary/assisted%20living.)

assisted outpatient treatment (AOT)   Laws mandating involuntary psychiatric treatment for individuals who do not understand their illness, to protect the individual from harm and safeguard the public.

attack rate   An incidence rate calculated for a particular population for a single disease outbreak and expressed as a percentage.

automatic (passive) protection   The modification of a product or the environment to reduce unintentional injuries.

bacteriological period of public health   The period of 1875 to 1900, during which the causes of many bacterial diseases were discovered.

barbiturates   Depressant drugs based on the structure of barbituric acid.

behavioral healthcare services   The managed care term for mental health and substance abuse/dependence care services.

Baylor Plan   Established in 1929 by Baylor administrators during the Great Depression to help area citizens afford hospital care. It is the first prepaid hospital insurance plan in the United States and the predecessor of Blue Cross.

benzodiazepines   Nonbarbiturate depressant drugs.

best experience   Intervention strategies used in prior or existing programs that have not gone through the critical research and evaluation studies and thus fall short of best practice criteria.

best practices   "Recommendations for interventions based on critical review of multiple research and evaluation studies that substantiate the efficacy of the intervention." (Green, L. W., & Kreuter, M. W. (2005). *Health program planning: An educational and ecological approach* (4th ed.). McGraw-Hill.)

best processes   Original intervention strategies that the planners create based on their knowledge and skills of good planning processes, including the involvement of those in the priority population and the theories and models.

bias   A prejudice in favor of or against one thing, person, or group compared with another usually in a way that is considered to be unfair.

bias and hate crimes   Criminal offenses against a person or property by offenders who are motivated in whole or in part by bias against a race, religion, disability, sexual orientation, ethnicity, gender, or gender identity.

binge drinking   Consuming five or more alcoholic drinks in a row for males and four or more for females in a 2-hour period.

biogenic pollutants   Airborne biological organisms or their particles or gases or other toxic materials that can produce illness.

biological hazards   Living organisms (and viruses), or their products, that increase the risk of disease or death in humans.

bioterrorism   The deliberate use of viruses, bacteria, or toxins or other agents to cause illness or death in people, animal, or plants.

bipolar disorder   An affective disorder characterized by distinct periods of elevated mood alternating with periods of depression.

birth rate   See *natality (birth) rate*.

blood alcohol concentration (BAC)   The percentage of concentration of alcohol in the blood.

bloodborne pathogens   Disease agents, such as HIV, that are transmissible in blood and other body fluids.

Bloodborne Pathogen Standard   A set of regulations promulgated by the Occupational Safety and Health Administration that sets forth the responsibilities of employers and employees with regard to precautions to be taken concerning bloodborne pathogens in the workplace.

body mass index (BMI)   The ratio of weight (in kilograms) to height (in meters, squared).

bottom-up community organization   Organization efforts that begin with those who live within the community affected.

brownfield   Property where reuse is complicated by the presence of hazardous substances from prior use.

built environment   "The design, construction, management, and land use of human-made surroundings as an interrelated whole, as well as their relationship to human activities over time." (Coupland, K., Rikhy, S., Hill, K., & McNeil, D. (2011). *State of evidence: The Built environment and health 2011–2015*. Public Health Innovation and Decision Support, Population, & Public Health, Alberta Health Services.)

Bureau of Alcohol, Tobacco, Firearms, and Explosives (ATF)   The federal agency in the U.S. Department of Justice that regulates alcohol, tobacco, firearms, and explosives.

Bureau of Indian Affairs (BIA)   The original federal government agency charged with the responsibility for the welfare of American Indians.

byssinosis   Acute or chronic lung disease caused by the inhalation of cotton, flax, or hemp dusts; those affected include workers in cotton textile plants (sometimes called brown lung disease).

capitation   A method of paying for covered healthcare services on a per-person premium basis for a specific time period prior to the service being rendered.

carcinogen   Agent, usually chemical, that causes cancer.

care manager   One who helps identify the healthcare needs of an individual but does not actually provide the healthcare services.

care provider   One who helps identify the healthcare needs of an individual and also personally performs the caregiving service.

carrier   A person or animal that harbors a specific communicable agent in the absence of discernible clinical disease and serves as a potential source of infection to others.

carrying capacity   The maximum population of a particular species that a given habitat can support over a given period of time.

case   A person who is sick with a disease.

categorical programs   Programs available only to people who can be categorized into a group based on specific variables.

census   See *U.S. Census.*

Center for Mental Health Services (CMHS)   The federal agency, housed within the U.S. Department of Health and Human Service's Substance Abuse and Mental Health Services Administration, whose mission it is to conduct research on the causes and treatments for mental disorders.

Centers for Disease Control and Prevention (CDC)   One of the operating divisions of the U.S. Public Health Service; charged with the responsibility for surveillance and control of diseases and other health problems in the United States.

Centers for Medicare and Medicaid Services (CMS)   The federal agency responsible for overseeing Medicare, Medicaid, and the related quality assurance activities.

cerebrovascular disease (stroke)   A chronic disease characterized by damage to blood vessels of the brain, resulting in disruption of circulation to the brain.

certified safety professional (CSP)   A health and safety professional, trained in industrial and workplace safety, who has met specific requirements for board certification.

chain of infection   A model to conceptualize the transmission of a communicable disease from its source to a susceptible host.

chemical hazard   Hazard caused by the mismanagement of chemicals.

chemical straitjacket   A drug that subdues a psychiatric patient's behavior.

child abuse   The intentional physical, emotional, verbal, or sexual mistreatment of a minor.

childhood diseases   Infectious diseases that normally affect people in their childhood (e.g., measles, mumps, rubella, and pertussis).

child maltreatment   The act or failure to act by a parent, caretaker, or other person as defined under state law that results in physical abuse, neglect, medical neglect, sexual abuse, or emotional abuse, or an act or failure to act that presents an imminent risk of serious harm to the child.

child neglect   The failure of a parent or guardian to care for or otherwise provide the necessary subsistence for a child.

children   Persons between one and nine years of age.

Children's Health Insurance Program (CHIP)   A title insurance program under the Social Security Act that provides health insurance to uninsured children.

chiropractor   A nonallopathic, independent healthcare provider who treats health problems by adjusting the spinal column.

chlorpromazine   The first and most famous antipsychotic drug, introduced in 1954 under the brand name Thorazine.

chronic disease   A disease or health condition that lasts longer than 3 months.

citizen-initiated community organization   See *bottom-up community organization.*

Clean Air Act (CAA)   The federal law that provides the government with authority to address interstate air pollution.

Clean Water Act (CWA)   The federal law aimed at ensuring that all rivers are swimmable and fishable and that limits the discharge of pollutants in U.S. waters to zero.

closed-panel HMO   An organization in which private physicians are contracted on an exclusive basis for services at a health maintenance organization.

club drugs   A general term for those illicit drugs, primarily synthetic, that are most commonly encountered at night clubs and "raves." Examples include MDMA, LSD, GHB, GBL, PCP, ketamine, Rohypnol, and methamphetamines.

coalition   "A formal alliance of organizations that come together to work for a common goal." (Butterfoss, F. D. (2007). *Coalitions and partnerships in community health.* Jossey-Bass.)

coal workers' pneumoconiosis (CWP)   Acute and chronic lung disease caused by the inhalation of coal dust (sometimes called black lung disease).

cocaine   The psychoactive ingredient in the leaves of the coca plant, *Erythroxylum coca*, which, when refined, is a powerful stimulant/euphoriant.

cognitive-behavioral therapy   Treatment based on learning new thought patterns and adaptive skills, with regular practice between therapy sessions.

coinsurance   The portion of insurance company's approved amounts for covered services that the beneficiary is responsible for paying.

combustion by-products   Gases and other particulates generated by burning.

combustion (incineration)   The burning of solid wastes.

common source epidemic curve   A graphic display of a disease where each case can be traced to a single source of exposure.

communicable disease model   The minimal requirements for the occurrence and spread of communicable diseases in a population—agent, host, and environment.

communicable (infectious) disease   An illness caused by some specific biological agent or its toxic products that can be transmitted from an infected person, animal, or inanimate reservoir to a susceptible host.

community   A collective body of individuals identified by common characteristics such as geography, interests, experiences, concerns, values, race, ethnicity, or culture.

community analysis   A process by which community needs are identified.

community building   An orientation to practice focused on community, rather than a strategic framework or approach, and on building capacities, not fixing problems.

community capacity   "The characteristics of communities that affect their ability to identify, mobilize, and address social and public health problems." (Minkler, M., & Wallerstein, N. (2012). Improving health through community organization and community building: perspectives from health education and social work. In M. Minkler (Ed.), *Community organizing and community building for health and welfare* (3rd ed., pp. 37–58). Rutgers University Press.)

community diagnosis   See *community analysis*.

community health   The health status of a defined group of people and the actions and conditions to promote, protect, and preserve their health.

community mental health center (CMHC)   A fully staffed center originally funded by the federal government that provides comprehensive mental health services to local populations.

community organizing   "The process by which community groups are helped to identify common problems or change targets, mobilize resources, and develop and implement strategies for reaching their collective goals." (Minkler, M., & Wallerstein, N. (2012). Improving health through community organization and community building: Perspectives from health education and social work. In M. Minkler (Ed.), *Community organizing and community building for health and welfare* (3rd ed., pp. 37–58). Rutgers University Press.

Community Support Program   A federal program that offers financial incentives to communities to develop a social support system for the mentally ill.

complementary/alternative medicine (CAM)   "A group of diverse medical and health care systems, practices, and products that are not presently considered to be a part of conventional medicine." (National Institutes of Health, National Center for Complementary and Alternative Medicine. (2012). *CAM basics: What is complementary and alternative medicine?* https://nccih.nih.gov/sites/nccam.nih.gov/files/D347_05-25-2012.pdf)

complex disaster   A natural disaster that further escalates an ongoing crisis or causes a technological disaster resulting in communities being affected by the consequences of a combination of natural and human-made hazards.

composting   The natural, aerobic biodegradation of organic plant and animal matter to compost.

Comprehensive Environmental Response, Compensation, and Liability Act (CERCLA)   The federal law (known as Superfund) created to clean up abandoned hazardous waste sites.

congregate meal programs   Community-sponsored nutrition programs that provide meals at a central site, such as a senior center.

consumer-directed health plan (CDHP)   Healthcare plan that combines a pretax payment account to pay for out-of-pocket medical expenses with a high-deductible health plan (HDHP).

continuing care   Long-term care for chronic health problems, usually including personal care.

continuing care retirement communities (CCRCs)   Planned communities for older adults that guarantee a lifelong residence and health care.

continuous source epidemic   A type of epidemic where cases are exposed to a common source over time.

controlled substances   Drugs regulated by the Comprehensive Drug Abuse Control Act of 1970, including all illegal drugs and prescription drugs that are subject to abuse and can produce dependence.

Controlled Substances Act of 1970 (Comprehensive Drug Abuse Control Act of 1970)   The central piece of federal drug legislation that regulates illegal drugs and legal drugs that have a high potential for abuse.

coordinated school health (CSH)   An organized set of policies, procedures, and activities designed to protect, promote, and improve the health and well-being of pre-K through 12th grade students and staff, thus improving a student's ability to learn. It includes, but is not limited to, health education; school health services; a healthy school environment; school counseling, psychological, and social services; physical education; school nutrition services; family and community involvement in school health; and school-site health promotion for staff.

copayment   A negotiated set amount a patient pays for certain services.

core functions of public health   Health assessment, policy development, and health assurance.

coronary heart disease (CHD)   A chronic disease characterized by damage to the coronary arteries in the heart.

Crisis Intervention Team   Specially trained police, in direct collaboration with mental health authorities, to remove barriers to mental health care for people with mental illness involved in the justice system.

criteria of causation   Aspects of the association between two variables that should be considered before deciding that the association is one of causation.

criteria pollutants   The most pervasive air pollutants and those of greatest concern in the United States.

cross-cultural communication   Communication with members across cultures from different nations.

cross-sectional study   An observational study where information about exposure and disease are collected at the same time.

crude rate   A rate in which the denominator includes the total population.

cultural and linguistic competence   A set of congruent behaviors, attitudes, and policies that come together in a system, agency, or among professionals that enables effective work in cross-cultural situations.

cultural communication   A process that helps to serve as a sense-making function to better understand the meaning people ascribe to the verbal and nonverbal messages and behaviors of others.

cultural competence   Service provider's degree of compatibility with the specific culture of the population served, for example, proficiency in language(s) other than English, familiarity with cultural idioms of distress or body language, folk beliefs, and expectations regarding treatment procedures (such as medication or psychotherapy) and likely outcomes.

culturally sensitive   Having respect for cultures other than one's own.

culture shock   The degree to which a person feels trauma related to being exposed to a new culture.

curriculum   A written plan for instruction.

cycles per second (cps)   A measure of sound frequency.

death rate   See *mortality (fatality) rate.*

deductible   The amount of expense that the beneficiary must incur before the insurance company begins to pay for covered services.

deinstitutionalization   The process of discharging, on a large scale, patients from state mental hospitals to less restrictive community settings.

demography   The study of a population and those variables bringing about change in that population.

Department of Health and Human Services (HHS)   The largest federal department in the United States government, formed in 1980 and headed by a secretary who is a member of the president's cabinet.

dependency ratio   A ratio that compares the number of individuals whom society considers economically unproductive to the number it considers economically productive.

depressant   A psychoactive drug that slows down the central nervous system.

descriptive study   An epidemiological study that describes a disease with respect to person, place, and time.

designer drugs   Drugs synthesized illegally that are similar to, but structurally different from, known controlled substances.

diagnosis-related groups (DRGs)   A procedure used to classify the health problems of all Medicare patients when they are admitted to a hospital.

direct transmission   The immediate transfer of an infectious agent by direct contact between infected and susceptible individuals.

disability-adjusted life years (DALYs)   A measure for the burden of disease that takes into account premature death and loss of healthy life resulting from disability.

disinfection   The killing of communicable disease agents outside of the host, on countertops, for example.

diversity   An appreciation and respect for differences and similarities in the workplace (and beyond), including the varied perspectives, approaches, and competencies of coworkers and populations served.

Dobbs v. Jackson Women's Health Organization   Supreme Court decision that overturned Roe v. Wade, eliminating the federal constitutional right to abortion and leaving the legality of abortion to individual states

dose   The number of program units delivered as part of the intervention.

drug   A substance other than food or vitamins that, when taken in small quantities, alters one's physical, mental, or emotional state.

drug abuse   Use of a drug when it is detrimental to one's health or well-being.

drug abuse education   Provides information about drugs and the dangers of drug abuse, changing attitudes and beliefs about drugs, and provides skills necessary to abstain from drugs, ultimately changing drug abuse behavior.

drug (chemical) dependence   A psychological and sometimes physical state characterized by a craving for a drug.

Drug Enforcement Administration (DEA)   The federal government's lead agency with the primary responsibility for enforcing the nation's drug laws, including the Controlled Substances Act of 1970.

drug misuse   Inappropriate use of prescription or nonprescription drugs.

drug use   A nonevaluative term referring to drug-taking behavior in general; any drug-taking behavior.

drug abuse education   Instruction that includes information about drugs and the dangers of drug abuse, changing attitudes and beliefs about drugs, and provides skills necessary to abstain from drugs, ultimately changing drug abuse behavior.

Earth Day   Annual public observance for concerns about the environment; the first was held April 22, 1970.

electroconvulsive therapy (ECT)   A method of treatment for mental disorders involving the administration of electric current to the scalp to induce convulsions and unconsciousness.

employee assistance program (EAP)   Workplace-based program that assists employees who have substance abuse, domestic, psychological, or social problems that interfere with their work performance.

empowerment   "Social action process for people to gain mastery over their lives and the lives of their communities." (Minkler, M., & Wallerstein, N. (2012). Improving health through community organization and community building: Perspectives from health education and social work. In M. Minkler (Ed.), *Community organizing and community building for health and welfare* (3rd ed., pp. 37–58). Rutgers University Press.)

endocrine-disrupting chemical (EDC)   A chemical that interferes in some way with the body's endocrine (hormone) system.

endemic disease   A disease that occurs at an expected level in a population or in a certain location.

end-of-life practice   Healthcare services provided to individuals shortly before death.

environmental hazard   Factor or condition in the environment that increases the risk of human injury, disease, or death.

environmental health   The study and management of environmental conditions that affect the health and well-being of humans.

Environmental Protection Agency (EPA)   The federal agency primarily responsible for setting, maintaining, and enforcing environmental standards.

environmental sanitation   The practice of establishing and maintaining healthy or hygienic conditions in the environment.

environmental tobacco smoke (ETS; secondhand smoke)   Tobacco smoke in the environment that is a mixture of mainstream and sidestream smoke, and that can be inhaled by nearby or transient nonsmokers.

epidemic   An unexpectedly large number of cases of an illness, specific health-related behavior, or other health-related event in a particular population.

epidemic curve   A graphic display of the cases of disease according to the time or date of onset of symptoms.

epidemiologist   One who practices epidemiology.

epidemiology   The study of the distribution and determinants of health-related states or events in specific populations, and the application of this study to control health problems.

eradication   The complete elimination or uprooting of a disease (e.g., smallpox eradication).

ethnicity   A subcultural group within a multicultural society.

ethnocentrism   When an individual believes the customs and practices of one's own culture are superior to those of others.

etiology   The cause of a disease.

evaluation   Determining the value or worth of the objective of interest.

evidence   The body of data that can be used to make decisions.

evidence-based   Way of delivering services to people using scientific evidence that shows that the services actually work.

evidence-based interventions (evidence-based programs)   Programs or practices that are peer-reviewed and based on empirical evidence of effectiveness.

evidence-based practice   Systematically finding, appraising, and using evidence as the basis for decision making.

exclusion   A health condition written into a health insurance policy indicating what is not covered by the policy.

experimental (interventional) study   An analytic study in which investigators allocate exposure or intervention and follow development of disease.

Family and Medical Leave Act (FMLA)   Federal law that provides up to a 12-week unpaid leave to men and women after the birth of a child, an adoption, or an event of illness in the immediate family.

family planning   Determining the preferred number and spacing of children and choosing the appropriate means to accomplish it.

family violence   The use of physical force by one family member against another, with the intent to hurt, injure, or cause death.

fatal injury   An injury that results in one or more deaths.

fatality rate   See *mortality (fatality) rate*.

Federal Emergency Management Agency (FEMA)   The nation's official emergency response agency.

Federal Water Pollution Control Act Amendments   See *Clean Water Act (CWA)*.

Federally Qualified Health Centers (FQHCs)   Those community health centers that receive funding under Section 330 of the Public Health Service (PHS) Act.

fee-for-service   A method of paying for health care in which after the service is rendered, a fee is paid.

fertility rate   The number of live births per 1,000 women of childbearing age (15–44 years).

fetal alcohol spectrum disorder (FASD)   A range of disorders caused by prenatal exposure to alcohol. FASD refers to conditions such as fetal alcohol syndrome (FAS), fetal alcohol effects (FAE), alcohol-related neuro-developmental disorder (ARND), and alcohol-related birth defects (ARBD).

fetal alcohol syndrome (FAS)   A condition in babies born to mothers who have consumed heavy amounts of alcohol during their pregnancies; affected babies may experience abnormal facial features, growth problems, central nervous system problems, and have problems with learning, memory, attention span, communication, vision, or hearing.

fetal death   Death in utero with a gestational age of at least 20 weeks.

fight-or-flight response   The body's natural psychological response to a stressful, frightening, or dangerous situation.

fixed indemnity   The maximum amount an insurer will pay for a certain service.

flunitrazepam   See *Rohypnol*.

Food and Drug Administration (FDA)   A federal agency in the U.S. Department of Health and Human Services charged with ensuring the safety and efficacy of all prescription and nonprescription drugs.

foodborne disease   A disease transmitted through the contamination of food.

foodborne disease outbreak (FBDO)   The occurrence of two or more cases of a similar illness resulting from the ingestion of food.

formaldehyde (CH_2O)   A water-soluble gas used in aqueous solutions in hundreds of consumer products.

formative evaluation   The evaluation that is conducted during the planning and implementing processes to improve or refine a program.

full-service hospital   A hospital that offers services in all or most of the levels of care defined by the spectrum of health-care delivery.

functional limitation   Difficulty in performing personal care and home management tasks.

gag rule   Regulations that barred physicians and nurses in clinics receiving federal funds from counseling clients about abortions.

gatekeeper   One who controls, both formally and informally, the political climate of the community.

gender   A multidimensional social and cultural construct that includes gender roles, expressions, behaviors, activities, power dynamics, and/or attributes that a given society associates with being a woman, man, girl, or boy, as well as relationships with each other. As a social construct, gender varies from society to society and can change over time.

gender expression How one chooses to convey one's gender identity through behavior, clothing, and other external characteristics.

gender identity An individual's innermost concept of self as male, female, a blend of both, or neither; this identity is not necessarily visible to others.

global health Describes health problems, issues, and concerns that transcend national boundaries, may be influenced by circumstances or experiences in other countries, and are best addressed by cooperative actions and solutions.

governmental health agency Health agency that is part of the governmental structure (federal, state, or local) and that is funded primarily by tax dollars.

government hospital A hospital that is supported and managed by governmental jurisdictions.

grassroots A process that begins with those affected by the problem/concern.

grassroots participation "Bottom-up efforts of people taking collective actions on their own behalf; they involve the use of a sophisticated blend of confrontation and cooperation in order to achieve their ends." (Perlman, J. (1978). Grassroots participation from neighborhood to nation. In S. Langton (Ed.), *Citizen participation in America* (pp. 65–79). Lexington Books.)

greenhouse gases Atmospheric gases, principally carbon dioxide, chlorofluorocarbons, ozone, methane, water vapor, and nitrous oxide, that are transparent to visible light but absorb infrared radiation.

groundwater Water located under the surface of the ground.

group model HMO An HMO that contracts with a multispecialty group practice.

hallucinogen Drug that produces profound distortions of the senses.

hard-to-reach population Those in a priority population that are not easily reached by normal programming efforts.

hate crimes See *bias and hate crimes.*

hazard An unsafe act or condition.

hazardous waste A solid waste or combination of solid wastes that is dangerous to human health or the environment.

health A dynamic state or condition of the human organism that is multidimensional in nature, a resource for living, and results from a person's interactions with and adaptations to their environment; therefore, it can exist in varying degrees and is specific to each individual and their situation.

health-adjusted life expectancy (HALE) The number of years of healthy life expected, on average, in a given population.

health disparities The higher burden of illness, injury, disability, and/or mortality that is experienced by one group of people relative to another due to current or historic disadvantage, oppression, or racism, which is manifested through inequitable social, economic, and environmental systems.

health education "Any combination of planned learning experiences using evidence-based practices and/or sound theories that provide the opportunity to acquire knowledge, attitudes, and skills needed to adopt and maintain health behaviors." (Joint Committee on Health Education and Promotion Terminology. (2012). *Report of the 2011 Joint Committee on Health Education and Promotion Terminology.* American Association of Health Education, 43(2), 1–19.)

Health Insurance Marketplace Organization established to create more organized and competitive markets for purchasing health insurance.

health insurance policy A contract between an insurer and the insured that outlines what health services are covered and how they will be paid for.

health maintenance organization (HMO) Group that supplies prepaid comprehensive health care with an emphasis on prevention.

health physicist A safety professional with responsibility for monitoring radiation within a plant environment, developing instrumentation for that purpose, and developing plans for coping with radiation accidents.

health promotion "Any planned combination of educational, political, environmental, regulatory, or organizational mechanisms that support actions and conditions of living conducive to the health of individuals, groups, and communities." (Joint Committee on Health Education and Promotion Terminology. (2012). *Report of the 2011 Joint Committee on Health Education and Promotion Terminology.* American Association of Health Education, 43(2), 1–19.)

Health Resources and Services Administration (HRSA) An operating division of the U.S. Department of Health and Human Services established in 1982 to improve the nation's health resources and services and their distribution to underserved populations.

health resources development period The years 1900 to 1960; a time of great growth in healthcare facilities and providers.

Healthy People 2030 The fifth set of health goals and objectives for the United States that defines the nation's health agenda and guides its health policy.

healthy school environment The promotion, maintenance, and utilization of safe and wholesome surroundings in a school.

herbicide A pesticide designed specifically to kill plants.

herd immunity The resistance of a population to the spread of an infectious agent based on the immunity of a high proportion of individuals.

Hispanic A term introduced by the Office of Management and Budget in 1977 that included persons of Mexican, Puerto Rican, Cuban, Central American, South American, or some other Spanish origin regardless of race.

homebound A person unable to leave home for normal activities.

home health care   Care that is provided in the patient's residence for the purpose of promoting, maintaining, or restoring health.

hospice care   "A cluster of special services for the dying which blends medical, spiritual, legal, financial, and family support services. The venue can vary from a specialized facility, to a nursing home, to the patient's own home." (Shi, L., & Singh, D. A. (2015). *Delivering health care in America: A systems approach* (6th ed.). Jones & Bartlett Learning.)

Hospital Survey and Construction Act of 1946 (Hill-Burton Act)   Federal legislation that provided substantial funds for hospital construction.

host   A person or other living organism that affords subsistence or lodgment to a communicable agent under natural conditions.

human trafficking   A crime in which traffickers exploit and profit at the expense of adults or children by compelling them to perform labor or engage in commercial sex.

hypercholesterolemia   High levels of cholesterol in the blood.

hypertension stage one   A systolic pressure equal to or greater than 130 mm Hg and/or diastolic pressure equal to or greater than 80 mm Hg for extended periods of time.

illicit (illegal) drugs   Drugs that cannot be legally manufactured, distributed, bought, or sold and that usually lack recognized medical value. Drugs that have been placed under Schedule I of the Controlled Substances Act of 1970.

immigrant   Individual who migrates from one country to another for the purpose of seeking permanent residence.

impact evaluation   The evaluation that focuses on immediate observable effects of a program.

impairments   Defects in the functioning of one's sense organs or limitations in one's mobility or range of motion.

implementation   Putting a planned program into action.

incidence rate   The number of new health-related events or cases of a disease divided by the total number in the population at risk.

incubation period   The period of time between exposure to a disease and the onset of symptoms.

independent practice association (IPA)   Legal entity separate from the HMO that is a physician organization composed of community-based independent physicians in solo or group practices that provide services to HMO members.

independent provider   Healthcare professional with the education and legal authority to treat any health problem.

Indian Health Service (IHS)   An operating division of the U.S. Department of Health and Human Services whose goal is to raise the health status of the American Indians and Alaska Natives to the highest possible level by providing a comprehensive health services delivery system.

indirect transmission   Communicable disease transmission involving an intermediate step.

individual placement and support (IPS)   An evidence-based model of employment services emphasizing real work opportunities, integrated mental health services, and individualized job supports.

industrial hygienist   Health professional concerned with health hazards in the workplace and with recommending plans for improving the healthiness of workplace environments.

industrial smog   Haze or fog formed primarily by sulfur dioxide and suspended particles from the burning of coal, also known as gray smog.

infant death (infant mortality)   Death of a child under one year of age.

infant mortality rate   The number of deaths of children under one year of age per 1,000 live births.

infection   The lodgment and growth of a virus or microorganism in a host organism.

infectious disease   See *communicable disease.*

infectivity   The ability of a biological agent to enter and grow in a host.

informal caregiver   One who provides unpaid care or assistance to one who has some physical, mental, emotional, or financial need that limits their independence.

inhalant   Breathable substance that produces mind altering effects.

injury   Damage that results when a human body is suddenly or briefly subjected to intolerable levels of energy.

injury prevention (control)   An organized effort to prevent injuries or to minimize their severity.

injury prevention education   The process of changing people's health-directed behavior to reduce unintentional injuries.

inpatient care facilities   Any facility in which a patient stays overnight, such as a hospital.

insecticide   Pesticide designed specifically to kill insects.

instrumental activities of daily living (IADLs)   More complex tasks such as handling personal finances, preparing meals, shopping, doing housework, traveling, using the telephone, and taking medications.

integrated surveillance information systems   Health information systems for the National Notifiable Diseases Surveillance System (NNDSS) that are based on the National Electronic Disease Surveillance System (NEDSS) architectural standards.

integrative care   Care a patient receives from a team of primary healthcare and behavioral health clinicians, working together with patients and families, using shared, cost-effective care plans that incorporate patient goals.

integrative medicine   Combines evidence-based conventional medicine and evidence-based complementary therapies to achieve appropriate care.

intensity   Cardiovascular workload measured by heart rate.

intentional injury   An injury that is purposely inflicted, either by the victim or another.

intern   A first-year resident.

intersectionality   A description of how race, class, gender, and other individual characteristics "intersect" with one another and overlap.

intervention   (1) Efforts to control a disease in progress. (2) An activity or activities designed to create change in people.

intimate partner violence (IPV)   Describes physical violence or sexual violence, emotional, economic, or technological abuse, stalking, or psychological aggression by a current or former spouse or dating partner, including opposite-sex and same-sex couples.

intracultural communication   Communication with members of the same culture or subculture.

intercultural communication   Communication with members of different cultures or subcultures.

ionizing radiation   High-energy radiation (e.g., UV radiation, gamma rays, X-rays, alpha and beta particles) that can knock an electron out of orbit, creating an ion, and can thereby damage living cells and tissues.

isolation   The separation of infected persons from those who are susceptible.

labor-force ratio   A ratio of the total number of those individuals who are not working (regardless of age) to the number of those who are.

law enforcement   The application of federal, state, and local laws to arrest, jail, bring to trial, and sentence those who break drug laws or break laws because of drug use.

leachate   Liquid created when water mixes with wastes and removes soluble constituents from them by percolation.

lead   A naturally occurring mineral element found throughout the environment and used in large quantities for industrial products, including batteries, pipes, solder, paints, and pigments.

legal leverage   Service providers controlling the disability income or other benefits received by a person with mental illness to enforce participation in treatment in return for suspending a criminal sentence imposed by a court of law.

licensed practical nurse (LPN)   Those prepared in one- to two-year programs to provide nontechnical bedside nursing care under the supervision of physicians or registered nurses.

life expectancy   The average number of years a person from a specific cohort is projected to live from a given point in time.

limited (restricted) care provider   Healthcare provider who provides care for a specific part of the body.

limited-service hospital   A hospital that offers only the specific services needed by the population served.

litigation   The process of seeking justice for injury through the courts.

lobotomy   Surgical severance of nerve fibers of the brain by incision.

long-term care   Different kinds of help that people with chronic illnesses, disabilities, or other conditions that limit them physically or mentally need.

low birth weight infant   One that weighs less than 2,500 grams, or 5.5 pounds, at birth.

Lyme disease   A systemic bacterial tickborne disease with symptoms that include dermatological, arthritic, neurological, and cardiac abnormalities.

macro practice   The methods of professional change that deal with issues beyond the individual, family, and small group level.

mainstream smoke   Tobacco smoke inhaled and exhaled by the smoker.

major depressive disorder   An affective disorder characterized by a dysphoric mood and/or loss of interest or pleasure in almost all usual activities or pastimes.

majority   Those with characteristics that are found in more than 50% of a population.

malignant neoplasm   Uncontrolled new tissue growth resulting from cells that have lost control over their growth and division.

managed care   "A system that integrates the functions of financing, insurance, delivery, and payment and uses mechanisms to control costs and utilization of services." (Shi, L., & Singh, D. A. (2015). *Delivering health care in America: A systems approach* (6th ed.). Jones & Bartlett Learning.)

mapping community capacity   A process of identifying community assets.

marijuana   Dried plant parts of the hemp plant, *Cannabis sativa*.

maternal, infant, and child health   The health of women of childbearing age and that of the child up to adolescence.

maternal mortality   The death of a woman while pregnant or within 42 days of termination of pregnancy, irrespective of the duration and the site of the pregnancy, from any cause related to or aggravated by the pregnancy or its management but not from accidental or incidental causes.

maternal mortality rate   Number of mothers dying per 100,000 live births in a given year.

Meals on Wheels program   A community-supported nutrition program in which prepared meals are delivered to individuals in their homes, usually by volunteers.

median age   The age at which half of the population is older and half is younger.

Medicaid   A jointly funded federal–state health insurance program for low-income Americans.

medically indigent   Those lacking the financial ability to pay for their own medical care.

medically consulted injury   Injury for which a healthcare professional is consulted for medical treatment or advice, either by phone or in person.

medical preparedness   "The ability of the health care system to prevent, protect against, quickly respond to, and recover from health emergencies, particularly those whose scale, timing, or unpredictability threatens to overwhelm routine capabilities." (Centers for Disease Control and Prevention. (2014). The community guide: Emergency preparedness and response. Available from http://www.thecommunityguide.org /emergencypreparedness/index.html)

Medicare   A national health insurance program for people 65 years of age and older, certain younger disabled people, and people with permanent kidney failure.

Medigap   Private health insurance that supplements Medicare benefits.

mental disorders   Health conditions characterized by alterations in thinking, mood, or behavior (or some combination thereof) associated with distress and/or impaired functioning.

mental health   Emotional and social well-being, including one's psychological resources for dealing with the day-to-day problems of life.

mental health court Court where the judges have special training and use nonadversarial procedures that mandate treatment and rehabilitation rather than incarceration if a person with mental illness is found guilty of a crime.

mental illness A collective term for all diagnosable mental disorders.

Mental Retardation Facilities and Community Mental Health Centers Act A law that made the federal government responsible for assisting in the funding of mental health facilities and services.

metastasis The spread of cancer cells to distant parts of the body by the circulatory or lymphatic system.

methamphetamine The amphetamine drug most widely abused.

methaqualone An illicit depressant drug.

methcathinone (cat) An illicit, synthetic drug, similar to the amphetamines, that first appeared in the United States in 1991.

microaggressions The everyday slights, insults, put downs, invalidations, and offensive behaviors that people experience in daily interactions with generally well-intentioned individuals who may be unaware that they have engaged in demeaning ways.

middle old Those 75 to 84 years of age.

migration Movement of people from one country to another.

minority groups Subgroups of the population that consist of less than 50% of the population.

minority health The distinctive health characteristics and attributes of racial and/or ethnic minority populations who are socially disadvantaged due in part to being subject to racist or discriminatory acts and are underserved in health care.

mixed model HMO A hybrid form of a health maintenance organization.

model for unintentional injuries The public health triangle (host, agent, and environment) modified to indicate energy as the causative agent of injuries.

modern era of public health The era of public health that began in 1850 and continues today.

modifiable risk factor Contributor of a noncommunicable disease that can be altered by modifying one's behavior or environment.

mold Fungi that spread and reproduce by making spores; grow best in warm, damp, and humid conditions; and can cause respiratory difficulties for sensitive people.

moral treatment A nineteenth century treatment in which people with mental illness were removed from the everyday life stressors of their home environments and given "asylum" in a rural setting, including rest, exercise, fresh air, and amusements.

morbidity (sickness) rate The number of people who are sick divided by the total population at risk.

mortality (fatality) rate The number of deaths in a population divided by the total population.

multicausation disease model A visual representation of the host, together with various internal and external factors that promote and protect against disease.

multiplicity The number of components or activities that make up the intervention.

municipal solid waste (MSW) Waste generated by individual households, businesses, and institutions located within municipalities.

narcotic Drug derived from or chemically related to opium that reduces pain and induces stupor, such as morphine.

natality (birth) rate The number of live births divided by the total population.

National Alliance on Mental Illness (NAMI) A national self-help group that supports the belief that major mental disorders are brain diseases that are of genetic origin and biological in nature and are diagnosable and treatable with medications.

National Ambient Air Quality Standards (NAAQSs) Standards created by the EPA for allowable concentration levels of outdoor air pollutants.

National Electronic Telecommunications System (NETS) The electronic reporting system used by state health departments and the Centers for Disease Control and Prevention.

National Institute for Occupational Safety and Health (NIOSH) A research body within the Centers for Disease Control and Prevention, U.S. Department of Health and Human Services, that is responsible for developing and recommending occupational safety and health standards.

National Institute of Mental Health (NIMH) The nation's leading mental health research agency, housed in the National Institutes of Health.

National Institute on Drug Abuse (NIDA) The federal government's lead agency for drug abuse research; part of the National Institutes of Health.

National Institutes of Health (NIH) The research division of the U.S. Department of Health and Human Services. It is part of the U.S. Public Health Service.

National Mental Health Association (NMHA) A national voluntary health association that advocates for mental health and for those with mental illnesses; it has 600 affiliates in 43 states.

natural disaster A natural hazard that results in substantial loss of life or property.

natural experiment Naturally occurring circumstances in which subsets of the population have different levels of exposure to a supposed causal factor, in a situation resembling an actual experiment where human subjects would be randomly allocated to groups.

natural hazard A naturally occurring phenomenon or event that produces or releases energy in amounts that exceed human endurance, causing injury, disease, or death (such as radiation, earthquakes, tsunamis, volcanic eruptions, hurricanes, tornados, and floods).

NEDSS Base System (NBS) Information system created by the CDC to record and report notable disease information to the CDC.

needs assessment   "The process of identifying, analyzing, and prioritizing the needs of a priority population." (McKenzie, J. F., Neiger, B. L., and Thackeray, R. (2017). Planning, implementing, and evaluating health promotion programs: A primer (7th ed.). Pearson Education.)

neonatal death (neonatal mortality)   Death occurring during the first 28 days after birth.

neonatologist   A medical doctor who specializes in the care of newborns from birth to t months of age.

network model HMO   A type of HMO that contracts with more than one medical group practice.

neurodiversity   The idea that unique differences in brain function and behavior are not necessarily pathological and can represent strengths, and are perceived negatively primarily because of social factors like ignorance or stigma.

neuroleptic drug   Drug that reduces nervous activity; another term for antipsychotic drug.

nonallopathic provider   Independent provider who provides nontraditional forms of health care.

noncommunicable (noninfectious) disease   A disease that cannot be transmitted from infected host to susceptible host.

nonpoint source pollution   All pollution that occurs through the runoff, seepage, or falling of pollutants into the water where the source is difficult or impossible to identify.

nontarget organisms   All other susceptible organisms in the environment, for which a pesticide was not intended.

notifiable diseases   Diseases for which health officials request or require reporting for public health reasons.

observational study   An analytic, epidemiologic study in which an investigator observes the natural course of events, noting exposed and unexposed subjects and disease development.

occupational disease   An abnormal condition or disorder, other than one resulting from an occupational injury, caused by an exposure to environmental factors associated with employment.

occupational health nurse (OHN)   A registered nurse (RN) whose primary responsibilities include prevention of illness and promotion of health in the workplace.

occupational illness   An abnormal condition or disorder, other than an occupational injury, caused by an exposure to environmental factors associated with employment.

occupational injury   An injury that results from exposure to a single incident in the work environment.

occupational medical practitioner (OMP)   A practitioner (physician) whose primary concern is preventive medicine in the workplace.

Occupational Safety and Health Act of 1970 (OSH Act)   Comprehensive federal legislation aimed at assuring safe and healthful working conditions for working men and women.

Occupational Safety and Health Administration (OSHA)   The federal agency located within the U.S. Department of Labor and created by the OSH Act, which is charged with the responsibility of administering the provisions of the OSH Act.

Office of National Drug Control Policy (ONDCP)   The headquarters of the United States' drug control effort, located in the executive branch of the federal government, and headed by a director appointed by the president.

official health agency   See *governmental health agency*.

old   Those 65 years of age and older.

old-age dependency ratio   The dependency ratio that includes only the old.

Older Americans Act of 1965 (OAA)   Federal legislation to improve the lives of older adults.

old old   Those 85 years of age and older.

open-panel HMO   An organization in which private practice physicians are contracted by a health maintenance organization to deliver care in their own offices.

operationalize   To define a concept so that it can be measured.

osteopathic provider   Independent healthcare provider whose remedies emphasize the inter-relationships of the body's systems in prevention, diagnosis, and treatment.

outbreak   An event similar to an epidemic except that it is used for a limited geographic area.

outcome evaluation   The evaluation that focuses on the end result of the program.

outpatient care facilities   Any facility in which the patient receives care and does not stay overnight.

outpatient commitment   Laws mandating involuntary psychiatric treatment for individuals who do not understand their illness to protect the individual from harm and safeguard the public.

over-the-counter (OTC) drug   Drug (except tobacco and alcohol) that can be legally purchased without a physician's prescription.

ownership   A feeling that one has a stake in or "owns" the object of interest.

ozone (O_3)   An inorganic molecule considered to be a pollutant in the atmosphere because it harms human tissue, but considered beneficial in the stratosphere because it screens out UV radiation.

packaged pricing   Several related health services are included in one price.

pandemic   An outbreak of disease over a wide geographic area, such as a continent or multiple continents.

parity   The concept of equality in healthcare coverage for people with mental illness and those with other medical illnesses or injuries.

participation and relevance   "Community organizing should 'start where the people are' and engage community members as equals." (Minkler, M., & Wallerstein, N. (2012). Improving health through community organization and community building: Perspectives from health education and social work. In M. Minkler (Ed.), *Community organizing and community building for health and welfare* (3rd ed., pp. 37–58). Rutgers University Press.)

passive immunity Occurs when a person receives antibodies against a disease rather than their immune system producing them.

passive smoking The inhalation of environmental tobacco smoke by nonsmokers.

patient-centered medical home "A care delivery model whereby patient treatment is coordinated through their primary care physician to ensure they receive the necessary care when and where they need it, in a manner they can understand" (applies to patients of all ages.) (American College of Physicians. (2016). *What is the patient-centered medical home?* Available from https://www.acponline.org /running_practice /delivery_and_payment_models/pcmh /understanding /what.htm)

Patient Protection and Affordable Care Act (ACA) Federal legislation that expands eligibility for Medicaid and increases access to private insurance for low-income Americans not covered by employer-provided health insurance.

pathogenicity The capability of a communicable disease agent to cause disease in a susceptible host.

pay-for-performance (P4P) purchasing A payment system that offers financial rewards to providers and facilities for meeting, improving, or exceeding quality measures or other performance goals.

peer counseling program School-based program in which students discuss alcohol and other drug-related problems with peers.

peer support Support from other people who themselves are coping with mental illness; it reduces people's social isolation, improves their access to services, and provides useful advice for managing the disorder.

pest Any organism—multicelled animal, plant, or microbe—that has an adverse effect on human interests.

pesticide Synthetic chemical developed and manufactured for the purpose of killing pests.

pharmaceuticals and personal care products (PPCPs) Synthetic chemicals found in everyday consumer healthcare products and cosmetics.

phasing in Implementation of an intervention with small groups instead of the entire population.

philanthropic foundation An endowed institution that donates money for the good of humankind.

photochemical smog Haze or fog formed when air pollutants interact with sunlight, also known as brown smog.

physical dependence A physiologic state in which discontinued drug use results in clinical illness.

physician assistant (PA) Healthcare professionals who practice medicine with physician supervision. (Woolsey, C. V. (n.d.). *What is a physician assistant? A patient's guide to the physician assistant.* Available from http://www.pg?pa .org/index.html

pilot test A trial run of an intervention.

placebo Treatment of no therapeutic effect, usually given to a group within an experimental study to serve as comparison to another group receiving the intervention of interest.

pneumoconiosis Fibrotic lung disease caused by the inhalation of dusts, especially mineral dusts.

point-of-service (POS) option An option of a health maintenance organization plan that allows enrollees to be at least partially reimbursed for selecting a healthcare provider outside of the plan.

point source epidemic A type of epidemic where all cases were exposed at the same point in time.

point source pollution Pollution that can be traced to a single identifiable source.

polydrug use Concurrent use of multiple drugs.

population at risk Those in the population who are susceptible to a particular disease or condition.

population-based public health practice Incorporates interventions aimed at disease prevention and health promotion, specific protection, and case findings.

population health "The health outcomes of a group of individuals, including the distribution of such outcomes within the group." (Kindig, D., & Stoddart, G. (2003). What is population health? *American Journal of Public Health, 93*(3), 380–383.)

postneonatal death (postneonatal mortality) Death that occurs between 28 days and 365 days after birth.

preconception health care Medical care provided to a women of reproductive age to promote health prior to conception.

pre-existing condition A medical condition that had been diagnosed or treated, usually within 6 months before the date a health insurance policy goes into effect.

preferred provider organization (PPO) An organization that buys fixed-rate health services from providers and sells them to consumers.

premature infant One born following a gestation period of 38 weeks or less, or one born at a low birth weight.

premium A regular periodic payment for an insurance policy.

prenatal health care Medical care provided to a pregnant woman from the time of conception until the birth process occurs.

prepaid health care A method of paying for covered healthcare services on a per-person premium basis for a specific period of time prior to service being rendered. Also referred to as *capitation*.

preplacement examination A physical examination of a newly hired or transferred worker to determine medical suitability for placement in a specific position.

prevalence rate The number of new and old cases of a disease in a population in a given period of time, divided by the total number of that population.

prevention The planning for and taking of action to forestall the onset of a disease or other health problem.

preventive care Care given to healthy people to keep them healthy.

primary care Clinical preventive services, first-contact treatment services, and ongoing care for commonly encountered medical conditions.

primary data Original data collected by planners.

primary pollutants Air pollutants emanating directly from transportation, power and industrial plants, and refineries.

primary prevention Preventive measures that forestall the onset of illness or injury during the prepathogenesis period.

priority population (audience) Those whom a program is intended to serve.

private (proprietary or investor-owned) hospital A for-profit hospital.

problem drinker One for whom alcohol consumption results in a medical, social, or other type of problem.

pro-choice A medical/ethical position that holds that women have a right to reproductive freedom.

program planning A process by which an intervention is planned to help meet the needs of a priority population.

pro-life A medical/ethical position that holds that performing an abortion is an act of murder.

propagated epidemic curve An epidemic curve depicting a distribution of cases traceable to multiple sources of exposure.

prospective reimbursement "Uses pre-established criteria to determine in advance the amount of reimbursement." (Shi, L., & Singh, D. A. (2017). *Essentials of the U.S. health care system* (4th ed.). Jones & Bartlett Learning.)

prospective study An epidemiologic study that begins in the present and continues into the future for the purpose of observing the development of disease (e.g., cohort study).

protective factor Factors that increase an individual's ability to avoid risks or hazards, and promote social and emotional competence to thrive in all aspects of life.

provider Healthcare facility or health professional that provides healthcare services.

psychiatric rehabilitation Intensive, individualized services encompassing treatment, rehabilitation, and support delivered by a team of providers over an indefinite period to individuals with severe mental disorder to help them maintain stable lives in the community.

psychoactive drug Drug that alters sensory perceptions, mood, thought processes, or behavior.

psychological dependence A psychological state characterized by an overwhelming desire to continue use of a drug.

psychological power An individual sense of potency demonstrated in self-confident behavior.

psychopharmacologic therapy Treatment for mental illness that involves medications.

psychotherapy A treatment that involves verbal communication between the patient and a trained clinician.

public health Actions that society takes collectively to ensure that the conditions in which people can be healthy can occur.

public health practice Incorporates "the development and application of preventive strategies and interventions to promote and protect the health of populations." (Turnock, B. J. (2016). *Public health: what it is and how it works* (6th ed.). Jones & Bartlett Learning.)

public health preparedness The capability of the public health and healthcare systems, community, and individuals to prevent, protect against, quickly respond to, and recover from health emergencies, particularly those in which scale, timing, or unpredictability threatens to overwhelm routine capabilities.

public health professional A healthcare worker who works in a public health organization.

Public Health Service (PHS) An agency in the U.S. Department of Health and Human Services (HHS) that comprises eight of the 11 operating divisions of HHS.

public health system The organizational mechanism of those activities undertaken within the formal structure of government and the associated efforts of private and voluntary organizations and individuals.

public hospital A hospital that is supported and managed by governmental jurisdictions.

public policy The guiding principles and courses of action pursued by governments to solve practical problems affecting society.

quality management and utilization review The analysis of provided health care for its appropriateness by someone other than the patient and provider.

quarantine Limitation of freedom of movement of those who have been exposed to a disease and may be incubating it.

quasi-governmental health organizations Organizations that have some responsibilities assigned by the government but operate more like voluntary agencies.

race The categorization of parts of a population based on physical appearance due to particular historic social and political forces.

radiation A process in which energy is emitted as particles or waves.

radon A naturally occurring, colorless, tasteless, odorless, radioactive gas formed during the radioactive decay of uranium-238.

rate The number of events that occur in a given population in a given period of time.

recovery Outcome sought by most people with mental illness; includes increased independence, effective coping, supportive relationships, community participation, and sometimes gainful employment.

recycling The collecting, sorting, and processing of materials that would otherwise be considered waste into raw materials for manufacturing new products, and the subsequent use of those new products.

reform phase of public health The years 1900 to 1920, characterized by social movements to improve health conditions in cities and in the workplace.

refugee Someone who has been forced to flee their country because of persecution, war, or violence.

registered environmental health specialist (REHS; sanitarian) Environmental worker responsible for the inspection of restaurants, retail food outlets, public housing, and other sites to ensure compliance with public health codes.

registered nurse (RN)   One who has successfully completed an accredited academic program and a state licensing examination.

regulation   The enactment and enforcement of laws to control conduct.

rehabilitation center   A facility in which restorative care is provided following injury, disease, or surgery.

reimbursement   The monetary value that healthcare providers and facilities receive for providing services to patients.

reportable diseases   Conditions whose reporting is mandatory when encountered by health providers, hospitals, or laboratories.

resident   A physician who is training in a specialty.

resource-based relative value scale (RBRVS)   Reimbursement to physicians according to the relative value of the service provided.

Resource Conservation and Recovery Act of 1976 (RCRA)   The federal law that sets forth guidelines for the proper handling and disposal of hazardous wastes.

respite care   Planned short-term care, usually for the purpose of relieving a full-time informal caregiver.

restorative care   That which is provided after successful treatment or when the progress of an incurable disease has been arrested.

retirement communities   Residential communities that have been specifically developed for individuals in their retirement years or of a certain age.

retrospective study   An epidemiologic study that looks into the past for clues to explain the present distribution of disease.

risk factor   Factor that increases the probability of disease, injury, or death.

Roe v. Wade   1973 Supreme Court decision that made it unconstitutional for state laws to prohibit abortions in the first trimester for any reason and placed restrictions on the conditions under which states could regulate them in the second and third trimesters.

Rohypnol (flunitrazepam)   A powerful depressant in the benzodiazepine group that has achieved notoriety as a date-rape drug because its amnestic and sedative effects when combined with alcohol can last up to eight hours.

rollover protective structure (ROPS)   Factory-installed or retrofitted reinforced framework on a cab to protect the operator of a tractor in case of a rollover.

runoff   Water that flows over land surfaces (including paved surfaces), typically from precipitation.

Safe Drinking Water Act (SDWA)   The federal law that regulates the safety of public drinking water.

safety engineer   Safety professionals employed by a company for the purpose of reducing unintentional injuries in the workplace.

safety programs   Those parts of the workplace health and safety program aimed at reducing unintentional injuries on the job.

salad bowl   Concept of integrated American society that refers to its global leadership, rich heritage, and a cultural profile that has evolved from centuries worth of both indigenous peoples and immigrants and their traditions, language, culinary preferences, and myriad other customs.

sanitary landfill   Waste disposal site on land suited for this purpose and on which waste is spread in thin layers, compacted, and covered with a fresh layer of clay or plastic foam each day.

sanitation   The practice of establishing and maintaining healthy or hygienic conditions in the environment.

school health advisory council   An advisory group composed of school, health, and community representatives who act collectively to advise the school district or school on aspects of coordinated school health, also known as school wellness council.

school health coordinator   A trained professional at the state, district, or school level who is responsible for managing, coordinating, planning, implementing, and evaluating school health policies, programs, and resources.

school health education   The development, delivery, and evaluation of a planned curriculum, kindergarten through grade 12.

school health policies   Written statements that describe the nature and procedures of a school health program.

school health services   Health services provided by school health workers to appraise, protect, and promote the health of students.

scope   Part of the curriculum that outlines what will be taught.

secondary data   Information that has been collected by someone else and is available for use by the planners.

secondary medical care   "Specialized attention and ongoing management for common and less-frequently encountered medical conditions, including support services for people with special challenges due to chronic or long-term conditions." (Turnock, B. J. (2016). *Public health: What it is and how it works* (6th ed.). Jones & Bartlett Learning.)

secondary pollutants   Air pollutants formed when primary air pollutants react with sunlight and other atmospheric components to form new harmful compounds.

secondary prevention   Preventive measures that lead to early diagnosis and prompt treatment of a disease or injury to limit disability and prevent more severe pathogenesis.

secondhand smoke   See *environmental tobacco smoke*.

Secretary's Task Force Report on Black and Minority Health   Published in 1985, a landmark report that first documented the health status disparities of minority groups in the United States.

self-funded insurance program   One that pays the healthcare costs of its employees with the premiums collected from the employees and the contributions made by the employer.

self-help group   Group of concerned members of the community who are united by a shared interest, concern, or deficit not shared by other members of the community (e.g., Alcoholics Anonymous).

senior center   Facility where elders can congregate for fellowship, meals, education, and recreation.

septic tank   A watertight concrete or fiberglass tank that holds sewage; one of two main parts of a septic system.

sequence   Part of the curriculum that states in what order the content will be taught.

sexual orientation   A person's emotional, romantic, or sexual feelings toward other people or no people.

sick building syndrome   A term to describe a situation in which the air quality in a building produces generalized signs and symptoms of ill health in the building's occupants.

sidestream tobacco smoke   The smoke that comes off the end of burning tobacco products.

silicosis   Acute or chronic lung disease caused by the inhalation of free crystalline silica.

sliding scale   The scale used to determine the fee for services based on ability to pay.

sludge   A semiliquid mixture of solid waste that includes bacteria, viruses, organic matter, toxic metals, synthetic organic chemicals, and solid chemicals.

SMART objectives   Those that are specific, measurable, achievable, realistic, and time-phased.

smokeless tobacco   Includes oral snuff, loose leaf chewing tobacco, plug chewing tobacco, and nasal snuff.

social capital   "Social capital refers to the social norms and networks that build trust and enable individuals to pursue shared objectives; it can vary considerably between communities and across time." Cronin, C. E., Franz, B., & Garlington, S. (2021). *Population health partnerships and social capital: Facilitating hospital-community partnerships*. SSM - Population Health, 13, 100739. https://doi.org/10.1016/j.ssmph.2021.100739

social determinants of health (SODH)   The nonmedical factors that influence health outcomes. They are the conditions in which people are born, grow, work, live, and age, and the wider set of forces and systems shaping the conditions of daily life.

Social Security Administration (SSA)   An independent federal agency that administers programs that provide financial support to special groups of Americans.

socio-ecological approach (ecological perspective)   Individuals influence and are influenced by their families, social networks, the organizations in which they participate (workplaces, schools, religious organizations), the communities of which they are a part, and the society in which they live.

socioeconomic status   Relating to a combination of social and economic factors.

solid waste   Solid refuse from households, agriculture, mining, and businesses.

solid waste management (integrated waste management)   The collection, transportation, and disposal of solid waste.

sound-level meter   Instrument used to measure sound.

source reduction   A waste management approach involving the reduction or elimination of use of materials that produce an accumulation of solid waste.

specialty hospital   A stand-alone, single-specialty (e.g., women's health, surgery, cardiac, or orthopedic) facility not within the walls of a full-service hospital.

spectrum of healthcare delivery   The array of types of care—from preventive to continuing, or long-term, care. It comprises four levels of care.

spiritual era of public health   A time during the Middle Ages when the causation of communicable disease was linked to spiritual forces.

staff model HMO   A health maintenance organization that hires its own staff of healthcare providers.

standard of acceptability   A comparative mandate, value, norm, or group.

stimulant   A drug that increases the activity of the central nervous system.

stir fry   See *salad bowl.*

structural racism   The totality of ways in which societies foster racial discrimination through mutually reinforcing systems of housing, education, employment, earnings, benefits, credit, media, health care, and criminal justice. These patterns and practices in turn reinforce discriminatory beliefs, values, and distribution of resources.

student assistance program (SAP)   School-based drug education program to assist students who have alcohol or other drug problems.

Substance Abuse and Mental Health Services Administration (SAMHSA)   The agency within the U.S. Department of Health and Human Services that provides leadership in drug abuse prevention and treatment. It houses the Center for Substance Abuse Prevention and the Center for Substance Abuse Treatment.

Substance use disorder (SUD)   is the disorder defined by the American Psychiatric Association's Diagnostic and Statistical Manual of Mental Disorders, fifth edition (DSM-5-TR; 2022), and combines substance abuse, and substance dependence into a single condition called substance use disorder.

sudden infant death syndrome (SIDS)   Sudden unanticipated death of an infant in whom, after examination, there is no recognized cause of death.

summative evaluation   The evaluation that determines the effect of a program on the priority population.

Supplemental Security   Program of the Social Security Administration that provides cash benefits to elderly, blind, and disabled Americans with minimal resources.

surface water   Precipitation that does not infiltrate the ground or return to the atmosphere by evaporation; the water in streams, rivers, and lakes.

Sustainable Development Goals (SDGs)   A set of goals adopted by the United Nations Member States focused on ending poverty and inequality, protecting the planet, and ensuring health for all adopted by all.

Synar Amendment   A federal law that requires states to set the minimum legal age for purchasing tobacco products at 18 years and that requires states to enforce this law.

synesthesia   Impairment of mind (by hallucinogens) characterized by a sensation that senses are mixed (e.g., seeing sounds and hearing images).

tardive dyskinesia   Irreversible condition of involuntary and abnormal movements of the tongue, mouth, arms, and legs, which can result from long-term use of certain antipsychotic drugs (such as chlorpromazine).

target organism (target pest)   The organism (or pest) for which a pesticide is applied.

task force   A temporary group that is brought together for dealing with a specific problem.

terrorism   Calculated use of violence (or threat of violence) against civilians to attain goals that are political or religious in nature.

tertiary medical care   Specialized and technologically sophisticated medical and surgical care for those with unusual or complex conditions.

tertiary prevention   Measures aimed at rehabilitation following significant pathogenesis.

The Joint Commission   The predominant organization responsible for accrediting healthcare facilities.

thermal inversion   A condition that occurs when warm air traps cooler air at the surface of the Earth.

third-party payment system   A health insurance term indicating that bills from a healthcare provider for services rendered to a patient are paid by the insurer.

Thorazine   See *chlorpromazine*.

Title X   A portion of the Public Health Service Act of 1970 that provides funds for family planning services for low-income people.

tolerance   Physiological and enzymatic adjustments that occur in response to the chronic presence of drugs, which are reflected in the need for ever-increasing doses.

top-down funding   A method of funding in which funds are transmitted from the federal or state government to the local level.

total dependency ratio   The dependency ratio that includes both youth and old.

Total Worker Health   "Policies, programs, and practices that integrate protection from work-related safety and health hazards with promotion of injury and illness prevention efforts to advance worker well-being." (Centers for Disease Control and Prevention, National Institute for Occupational Safety and Health. (2016). *Total Worker Health*®. Available from http://www.cdc.gov/niosh/twh)

Transinstitutionalization   Transferring patients from one type of public institution to another, usually as a result of policy change rather than improved treatment effectiveness.

treatment   (for drug abuse and dependence) Care that removes the physical, emotional, and environmental conditions that have contributed to drug abuse and/or dependence.

21st Century Cures Act   Legislation that funds comprehensive programs for addressing challenges to recovery, including the criminalization of mental illness, gaps in community-based services, and inadequate numbers of service providers.

ultraviolet (UV) radiation   Radiation energy with wavelengths of 10 to 400 nanometers.

unauthorized immigrant   An individual who entered this country without permission.

unconscious (implicit) bias   When someone holds a bias, but is not aware of its existence.

unintentional injury   An injury that occurred without anyone intending that harm be done.

unmodifiable risk factor   Factor contributing to the development of a noncommunicable disease that cannot be altered by modifying one's behavior or environment.

unsafe act   Any behavior that would increase the probability of an injury occurring.

unsafe condition   Any environmental factor or set of factors (physical or social) that would increase the probability of an injury occurring.

U.S. Census   The enumeration of the population of the United States that is conducted every 10 years.

vector   A living organism, usually an insect or other arthropod (e.g., mosquitoes, ticks, lice, fleas), that can transmit a communicable disease agent to a susceptible host.

vectorborne disease   A communicable disease transmitted by insects or other arthropods; for example, St. Louis encephalitis.

vectorborne disease outbreak (VBDO)   An occurrence of an unexpectedly large number of cases of disease caused by an agent transmitted by insects or other arthropods.

vehicle   An inanimate material or object that can serve as a source of infection.

vehicleborne disease   A communicable disease transmitted by nonliving objects; for example, typhoid fever can be transmitted by water.

visitor services   One individual taking time to visit with another who is unable to leave his or her residence.

vital statistics   Statistical summaries of vital records of major life events, such as births, deaths, marriages, divorces, and infant deaths.

volatile organic compounds (VOCs)   Compounds that exist as vapors over the normal range of air pressures and temperatures.

voluntary health agency   A nonprofit organization created by concerned citizens to deal with health needs not met by governmental health agencies.

voluntary hospital   A nonprofit hospital administered by a not-for-profit corporation or other charitable community organization.

wastewater   The aqueous mixture that remains after water has been used or contaminated by humans.

wastewater treatment   The process of improving the quality of wastewater (sewage) to the point that it can be released into a body of water without seriously disrupting the aquatic environment, causing health problems in humans, or causing nuisance conditions.

waterborne disease   A disease that is transmitted through contamination of water.

waterborne disease outbreak (WBDO)   A disease in which at least two persons experience a similar illness after the ingestion of drinking water or after exposure to water used for recreational purposes and epidemiological evidence implicates water as the probable source of the illness.

water pollution   Any physical or chemical change in water that can harm living organisms or make the water unfit for other uses.

watershed   The area of land from which all of the water that is under it or drains from it goes into the same place and drains in one point; for example, the Mississippi River watershed drains and collects all the water from the land extending from east of the Rocky Mountains to the Appalachian Mountains and from the upper Midwest all the way south to the Gulf of Mexico.

weathering   Concept in which the age of a person's body is significantly older than its years due to sociological disadvantage.

Whole School, Whole Community, Whole Child (WSCC) model   A model that focuses on addressing the educational and health needs of children within the context of the school setting, which is a critical component of the local community.

Women, Infants, and Children (WIC)   A special supplemental food program for women, infants, and children, sponsored by the U.S. Department of Agriculture.

workers' compensation laws   A set of federal laws designed to compensate those workers and their families who suffer injuries, disease, or death from workplace exposure.

worksite health and wellness promotion (WHWP) programs   Workplace-based programs aimed at improving the health and wellness of employees by identifying and acting on existing health conditions and by encouraging employees to optimize their health by improving health behavior and lifestyle choices.

World Health Assembly   A body of delegates of the member nations of the World Health Organization.

World Health Organization (WHO)   The most widely recognized international governmental health organization.

years of potential life lost (YPLL)   The number of years lost when death occurs before the age of 65 or 75.

young old   Those 65 to 74 years of age.

youth dependency ratio   The dependency ratio that includes only youth.

youth gang   An association of peers, bound by mutual interests and identifiable lines of authority, whose acts generally include illegal activity and control over a territory or an enterprise.

zoonosis   A communicable disease transmissible under natural conditions from vertebrate animals to humans.

INDEX